Neurology of the Infant

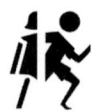

Fondazione Pierfranco e Luisa Mariani
Viale Bianca Maria 28
20129 Milan, Italy

Telephone: +39 02 795458
Fax: +39 02 76009582
Publications coordinator: Valeria Basilico
e-mail: publications@fondazione-mariani.org

www.fondazione-mariani.org

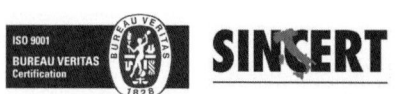

Neurology of the Infant

Edited by
Francesco Guzzetta

This special publication is produced in cooperation between
John Libbey Eurotext and the Mariani Foundation in Milan,
on the occasion of the 25th anniversary of the Mariani Foundation,
which has dedicated it efforts to child neurology since 1984

Mariani Foundation Paediatric Neurology Series: 21
Series Editor: Maria Majno

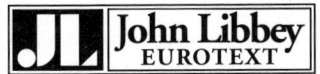

ISBN: 978-2-7420-0731-8

Cover illustration: Detail from *Prospettiva di rovine con figure*, by Marco and Sebastiano Ricci (Palazzo Chiericati, Vicenza).

Design elaboration by Costanza Magnocavallo.

Technical and language editor: Oliver Brooke

Published by

Éditions John Libbey Eurotext
127, avenue de la République, 92120 Montrouge, France
Tél. : +33 (0)1 46 73 06 60
Fax : +33 (0)1 40 84 09 99
e-mail : contact@jle.com
www.jle.com

© 2009 John Libbey Eurotext. All rights reserved.

Unauthorized duplication contravenes applicable laws.

It is prohibited to reproduce this work or any part of without authorisation of the publisher or of the Centre Français d'Exploitation du Droit de Copie (CFC), 20, rue des Grands Augustins, 75006 Paris, France.

Contents

Preface		VII
Chapter 1	Developmental assessment: neurological examination *Eugenio Mercuri, Giovanni Baranello and Daniela Ricci*	1
Chapter 2	Developmental assessment: functional techniques *Andrea Guzzetta*	13
Chapter 3	Psychomotor development: the beginning of cognition *Francesco Guzzetta*	37
Chapter 4	Malformations of cortical development *Francesco Guzzetta, Cesare Colosimo and Tommaso Tartaglione*	55
Chapter 5	Early brain injuries: infantile cerebral palsy *Francesco Guzzetta*	91
Chapter 6	Congenital defects: a clinical approach *Giuseppe Zampino*	117
Chapter 7	Early intervention *Giovanni Cioni, Giulia D'Acunto and Paola Bruna Paolicelli*	137
Chapter 8	Metabolic disorders *Enrico Bertini and Carlo Dionisi-Vici*	159
Chapter 9	Brain tumours *Luca Massimi, Gianpiero Tamburrini and Concezio Di Rocco*	191
Chapter 10	Epilepsy in infancy *Francesco Guzzetta and Domenica Battaglia*	243

Chapter 11	Paroxysmal non-epileptic disorders *Federico Vigevano, Raffaella Cusmai and Nicola Specchio*	291
Chapter 12	The infant with neuromuscular disorders *Eugenio Mercuri, Paolo Alfieri and Marika Pane*	305
Chapter 13	Peripheral neuropathies *Francesco Guzzetta*	317

Preface

The extraordinary progress made in the field of neuroscience in the last twenty years has allowed huge advancement in understanding the complex mechanisms underlying human early development. As is well known, this period of life is characterized by formidable and rapid changes related to this first development of the innate biological program. Correspondingly, the effects of pathological events may be particularly severe, and include extensive disorders of function.

Clinical semeiology in infants is thus highly distinctive in that the normal functional patterns to which clinicians must attend are continuously changing with age. Consequently, possible abnormalities are not easily to interpret and treatment strategies often difficult to decide. This complexity makes the neurology of the infant almost a specific discipline – one that requires awareness of an ever-increasing amount of information deriving from studies of the physiology, semeiology, and pathology in newly developing human beings.

In preparing the book, I have had the good fortune of enjoying the collaboration of some outstanding investigators into the field of neurology. Addressed to a broad audience of physicians specializing in paediatrics or paediatric neurology, this work represents an attempt to bring together the most current information available about the main advances in infant neurology.

The first part is concerned with the *normal* neurologic development of infants and the assessment techniques used in paediatric neurology. The bulk of the volume, however, concentrates on the CNS disorders that can occur when normal development is compromised: cerebral palsy, congenital defects, epilepsy, metabolic and neuromuscular diseases, and brain tumors, to cite a few examples.

I apologize for any oversimplification that may have resulted from our wish to synthesize this knowledge, but nevertheless trust that this collection will be useful to the reader and, ultimately, of even more help to the small patients that paediatricians encounter in their daily practice.

Francesco Guzzetta

Chapter 1

Developmental assessment: neurological examination

Eugenio Mercuri, Giovanni Baranello and Daniela Ricci

Child Neuropsychiatry Unit, Policlinico Gemelli, Catholic University, Largo Agostino Gemelli 8, 00168 Rome, Italy
eumercuri@gmail.com

Various structured neurological examinations have been developed over the years in order to provide a standardized assessment of the neurological and neurobehavioural status of the infant after the neonatal period (Andre-Thomas *et al.*, 1960; Milani-Comparetti & Gidoni, 1967; Touwen, 1976; Saint-Anne Dargassies, 1977; Baird & Gordon, 1983; Ellison *et al.*, 1983; Palmer *et al.*, 1984; Campbell & Wilheim, 1985; Gorga *et al.*, 1985; Amiel-Tison & Grenier, 1986; Nickel *et al.*, 1989; Amiel-Tison & Stewart, 1989; Hempel, 1993; Kuenzle *et al.*, 1994). The assessment of neurological signs in the first year, however, requires not only good skills in performing the examination but also sound knowledge of motor milestones and the maturation of neurological signs, so as to be able to define what can be considered normal or abnormal at a given age.

Most of the available assessments combine neurological findings with behavioural characteristics and motor milestones and provide diagrams or instructions to help the clinician to interpret the neurological findings. The various examinations described are not all suitable for both clinical and research settings. Some are ideal for research studies but are time-consuming and cannot easily be undertaken in routine clinical settings; others are easier to perform but do not always provide structured validation of their data or reference data that could also be used in a research setting (Vohr, 1999).

In the past few years much work has been done to validate the Hammersmith Infant Neurological Examination (HINE) and to provide both reference data for clinicians and an optimality scoring system to be used in a research setting. The examination is based on the criteria employed in Dubowitz and Dubowitz's original neurological assessment of the newborn (Dubowitz & Dubowitz, 1981), using a proforma with instructions for carrying out the tests and diagrams to aid recording.

In this chapter we review our experience in using the HINE, its validation in low-risk preterm, near term and full term infants, and its application in infants with lesions.

Hammersmith Infant Neurological Examination

The infant examination has undergone several modifications over the years. The principle was that the assessment should be easy to perform and to score, and be relatively short so that it can be easily used in routine clinical work but also contain items reflecting different aspects of neurological function in relation to age. The latest version (Haataja et al., 1999) consists of 37 items divided into three sections. The first section includes items assessing tone and posture; the second includes eight items assessing the development of motor function; and the third evaluates behaviour, with items assessing the state of behaviour adapted from the Bayley scales (Bayley, 1993). A final section was added to assess the development of gross and fine motor function. The ability to acquire motor milestones is an important part of the neurological development of infants, and their absence is an important sign of abnormal neurological maturation.

A full description of the examination and its procedures is beyond the scope of this chapter and has been fully reported previously (Haataja et al, 1999 and 2001). Figure 1a–1c shows the various parts of the proforma and the various panels in Fig. 2 illustrate some of the tests being applied.

Timing and sequence of the recording

The examination should be carried out while the infant is awake and vigilant. The child should wear only a nappy. The posture and tone items should optimally be tested with the infant lying on a mat. The examiner can use toys to try to engage the child's confidence and cooperation.

Scoring the examination

The response to any item is indicated by circling one of the options. If a response does not fall clearly into one of the options offered but falls between two options then a mark is made across the vertical line that divides the options. In case of asymmetry, the observation is marked separately for the left and right side (in many boxes **L** [left] and **R** [right] are readily marked). Some items provide two drawings in the same box. In this case the one closest to what is observed is marked. In case of deviation from given responses the deviation is drawn on the figures.

Interpretation of the results

The examination was initially designed for infants over 6 months of age, and the proforma was structured in a way that could identify deviant neurological signs or at least signs requiring further assessment.

The frequency distribution of the findings in each item was calculated by analysing the results obtained in a cohort of 135 low-risk term infants at 12 and 18 months who had been recruited at birth and had no known perinatal or neonatal risk factors (Dubowitz et al., 1998; Mercuri et al., 1998; Dubowitz et al., 1999; Haataja et al., 1999).

Column 1 in the proforma represents the findings most frequently seen in the normal population (75 per cent or more), while those in column 2 are seen less frequently (in 25 per cent or less but in more than 10 per cent), and those in columns 3 are those seen in 10 per cent or less. An isolated finding outside column 1 or 2 does not always indicate a neurological abnormality, but rather that the finding observed is not one commonly found in a low-risk population and therefore should be reassessed. The risk of neurological abnormalities, however, increases in parallel with the increasing number of findings in columns 3 (Haataja et al., 1999).

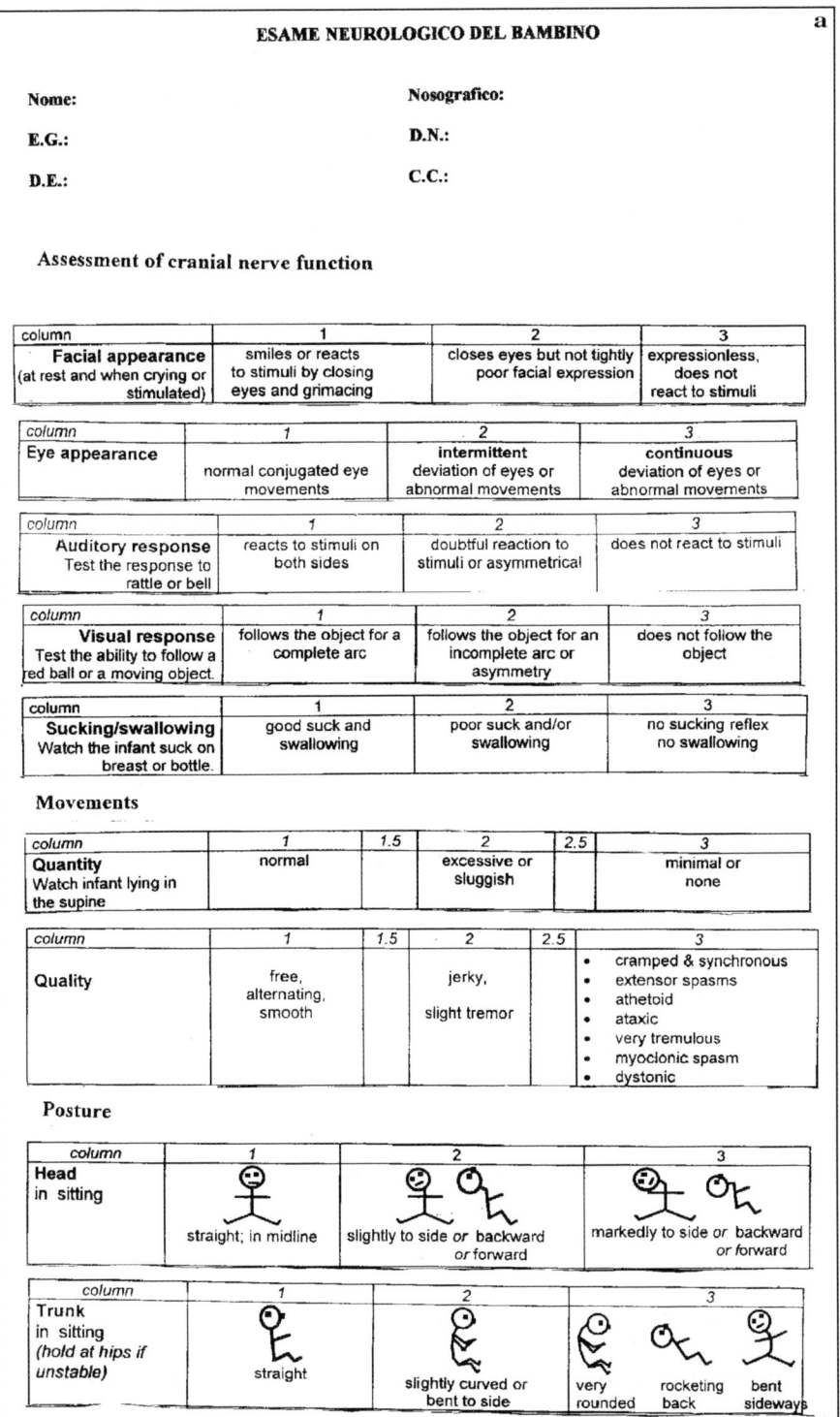

Fig. 1a–1c. Various parts of the proforma.

column	1	2	3
Arms *(at rest)*	in neutral position central straight *or* slightly bent	slight internal rotation *or* external rotation	marked internal rotation *or* external rotation *or* dystonic posture hemiplegic posture

column	1	2	3
Hands	hands open	intermittent adducted thumb *or* fisting	persistent adducted thumb *or* fisting

column	1	1.5	2	2.5	3
Legs in sitting	able to sit with straight back and legs straight or slightly bent (long sitting)		sit with straight back but knees bent at 15-20°		unable to sit straight unless knees markedly bent (no long sitting)
in supine and in standing	legs in a central position straight *or* slightly bent		slight internal rotation or external rotation at hips		marked internal rotation; external rotation *or* fixed extension or flexion or contractures at hips and knees

column	1	2	3
Feet in supine and in standing	central in neutral position	slight internal rotation *or* external rotation at the ankle	marked internal rotation *or* external rotation at the ankle
	toes straight midway between flexion and extension	intermittent tendency to stand on tiptoes or toes up or curling under	persistent tendency to stand on tiptoes or toes up or curling under

Tone

column	1	2	3
Scarf sign Take the infant's hand and pull the arm across the chest until there is resistence. Note the position of the elbow.	Range: R L R L	R L	R L or R L

column	1	1.5	2	3
Passive shoulder elevation Lift arm next to the infant's head. Note resistance at shoulder and elbow.	resistance but overcomed R L		no resistance R L	resistance not overcomed R L

Pronation/supination Steady upper arm while pronating and supinating forearm, note resistance	full pronation and supination, no resistance	full pronation and supination but resistance to be overcomed	full pronation and supination not possible, marked resistance

column	1	2	3
Adductors With the infant's legs extended, open them as far as possible. The angle formed by the legs is noted.	170-80° R L to R L	>170° R L	<80° R L

Chapter 1 Developmental assessment: neurological examination

Popliteal angle Legs are flexed at the hip simultaneously on to the side of the abdomen, then extended at the knee until there is resistance. Note angle between lower and upper leg.	Range: 170°-110° R L R L	~90° or > 170° R L R L	<80° R L

column	1	2	3
Ankle dorsiflexion With knee extended, dorsiflex ankle. Note the angle between foot and leg.	Range: 20°-85° R L R L	<20° or 90° R L R L	> 90° R L

column	1	2	3
Pulled to sit Pull infant to sit by wrists.			

column	1	2	3
Ventral suspension			

Reflexes and reactions

column	1	1.5	2	2.5	3
Tendon Reflexes	easily elicitable biceps knee ankle		brisk biceps knee ankle		clonus or absent biceps knee ankle

column	1	1.5	2	2.5	3
Arm protection Pull the infant by one arm from the supine position and note the reaction of the opposite side.	arm & hand extend R L		arm semi-flexed R L		arm fully flexed R L

column	1	2	3
Vertical suspension Hold infant under axilla, make sure legs do not touch any surface.	kicks symmetrically	kicks one leg more or poor kicking	no kicking even if stimulated or scissoring

column	1	1.5	2	2.5	3
Lateral tilting (describe side up). Infant held vertically, tilt quickly to horizontal. Note spine, limbs and head.	R L		R L		R L

column	1	2
Forward parachute Infant held vertically and suddenly tilted forwards. Note reaction of the arms.	(after 6 months)	(after 6 months)

c

Optimality scores

When we validated the examination in a cohort of low-risk full term infants tested at 12 and 18 months we also devised an optimality score, mainly for research purposes. The optimality score is based on the distribution frequency of the findings observed in full term infants examined at 12 and 18 months. The scoring system was devised so that for each item a score of 3 is given to the finding in column 1, a score of 2 to column 2, a score of 1 to column 3. If the finding falls between two columns, it is given the appropriate half score between the columns (for example, an item falling between score 1 and 2 is scored 1.5). In the case of asymmetries, the left and right sides are scored separately, and the mean of the separate scores taken as the score of this particular item. The examination is constructed to give subscores of all the tested subsections (cranial nerves, posture, movements, tone, reflexes, and reactions), and the global optimality score is achieved by adding up all the scores from individual items. Thus the global score can vary from a minimum of 0 to a maximum of 78. Based on the calculated frequency distribution of the global scores at 12 and 18 months, the optimality was set at or above the 10th centile, and suboptimality below the 10th centile. Accordingly, a global score equal to or above 73 was regarded as optimal at 12 months and equal to or above 74 optimal at 18 months (Haataja et al., 1999).

We have subsequently examined 74 infants between 3 and 8 months in order to establish whether the optimality scoring system could be applied to younger infants. Our results suggest that the optimality scoring system developed for infants at 12 and 18 months should not be applied in infants younger than 6 months, as many items show age-dependent changes; the system should also be used with caution between 6 and 9 months as a few items will still have a wider variability (Haataja et al., 2003).

Further validation in younger infants

The examination has subsequently been validated in infants younger than 10 months (Haataja et al., 2003) and it was found that while infants assessed between 6 and 11 months showed similar findings to those assessed between 12 and 19 months, those examined before 6 months had differences that were mainly related to immature axial tone and incomplete development of saving reactions (Haataja et al., 2003).

Applications

Preterm infants

At the time when we published the optimality score, we were frequently asked whether the score could also be used for infants born prematurely. We therefore carried out the HINE in a cohort of preterm infants whose gestational age ranged between 24 and 30.5 weeks. The infants were examined at between 9 and 18 months of chronological age (6 to 15 months of corrected age) and were scored with the optimality score system previously standardized in a cohort of low-risk term infants. The aim of the study was to establish the frequency distribution of the optimality scores in a low-risk cohort. The results showed no significant association with the degree of prematurity or the age of assessment in the low-risk preterm cohort. All infants with either normal scans or mild ventricular dilatation had either optimal scores or suboptimal scores which were never below 64. There were only a few items that appeared to be slightly different in preterm and full term infants. These were mainly those related to reflexes and reactions, such as lateral tilting, forward parachute or arm protection, or some of the items assessing tone, such as passive shoulder elevation or popliteal angle (Frisone *et al.*, 2002).

In order to establish a possible prognostic value of the HINE, it was also undertaken in a smaller cohort of preterm infants born within a similar range of gestational ages but with brain lesions on cranial ultrasound. Our results showed that the HINE, even when carried out in preterm infants as early as 9 months of chronological age, was able to predict motor outcome at 2 years.

Low-risk near term infants

The HINE has recently also been applied to a low-risk near-term population, followed longitudinally at 6, 9, and 12 months of corrected age. The inclusion criteria were normal or nearly normal neonatal ultrasound, a neurodevelopmental quotient above or equal to 80, and the absence of cerebral palsy or motor disability. The results showed no significant differences between infants born at 35 and 36 weeks but surprisingly, although the cohort was born only a few weeks before term age, when the optimality score developed for term infants at 12 months was applied to the near term cohort at 12 months corrected age, only 55 per cent of the near term infants showed optimal scores. The differences mainly reflected lower scores in the subsections of tone and reflexes. In contrast the scores for cranial nerves, movements, and posture were similar to those of term infants. These findings were rather more similar to the HINE scores reported in preterm infants with gestational age < 31 weeks, who also had similar differences in tone, posture, and reflexes compared with term infants (Romeo *et al.*, 2007).

Infants with neonatal lesions

The HINE has been used for over 20 years as a clinical tool in the follow-up of newborn infants at risk of neurological sequelae, for example preterm infants (Frisone *et al.*, 2002) and full term infants with neonatal encephalopathy (Mercuri *et al.*, 1999a; Haataja *et al.*, 2001) or with other congenital or acquired brain lesions (Dubowitz *et al.*, 1998). The use of an integrated approach – in combination with brain imaging and neurophysiological techniques – has enabled the identification of specific clinical patterns in infants with different types of brain lesions (Mercuri *et al.*, 1999a; Haataja *et al.*, 2001; Frisone *et al.*, 2002) and documentation of their onset and evolution over time (Bouza *et al.*, 1994).

Preterm infants with brain lesions

In preterm infants with severe brain lesions the range of optimality scores reflects the variability in motor outcome better than cranial ultrasound findings. Our experience in children with cystic periventricular leukomalacia (PVL) has highlighted the prognostic role of the examination. We have recently applied the HINE optimality score to a cohort of 24 infants with cystic PVL detected in the neonatal period who were examined at between 6 and 9 months of corrected age, and we found that the scores were related to the severity of motor sequelae at 2 years (Ricci *et al.*, 2006a). Scores below 40 were always associated with inability to sit independently at 2 years, scores between 41 and 60 were associated with independent sitting but not with walking, and those above 60 with the ability to walk independently at 2 years. These results confirmed that the optimality score obtained as early as 6 months of corrected age can be used to predict the severity of motor impairment in these infants.

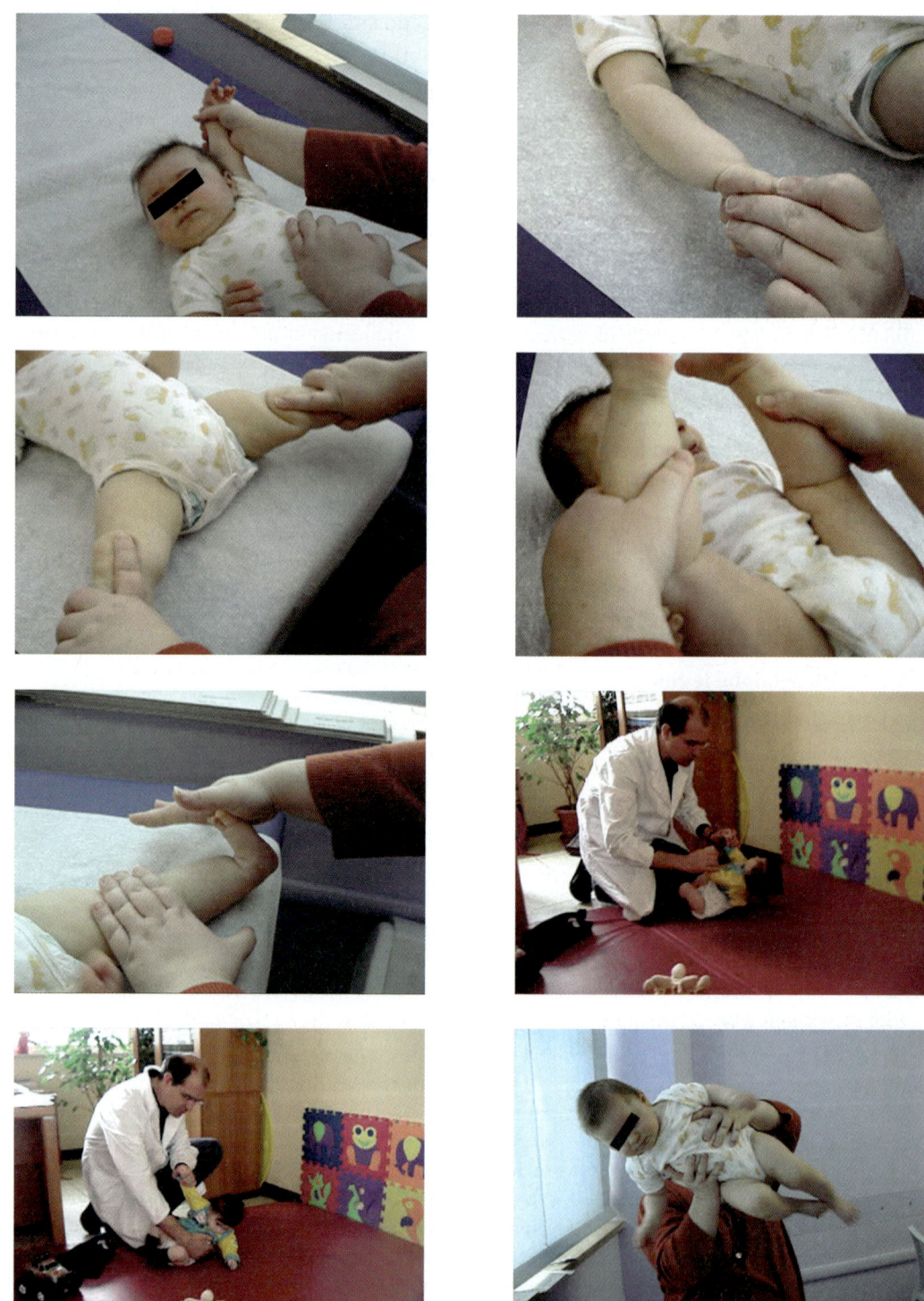

Fig. 2. Some of the tests being applied.

We were also able to demonstrate that reliable prognostic information can be achieved by examining individual clinical signs or patterns and not just by calculating the optimality score.

More specifically, we were also interested in establishing whether specific clinical patterns of neurological abnormalities could be related to the degree of impairment of motor outcome. We found that in our cohort some patterns – such as abnormal distribution of tone, with increased neck and trunk extensor tone and a posture of flexed arms and extended legs – were always associated with severe cerebral palsy and an inability to sit unsupported at 2 years. We also found in our cohort that arm protection, forward parachute, and vertical suspension were generally normal in the infants who achieved independent ambulation and abnormal in the infants who developed cerebral palsy and did not achieve independent sitting at 2 years, but the results were more variable in the group of infants who were able to sit but not to walk.

Full term infants with brain lesions

The HINE has also been used in infants with neonatal encephalopathy and focal infarction, which are major causes of morbidity in full term infants.

We applied the HINE and calculated the optimality score in 53 infants with hypoxic-ischaemic encephalopathy assessed at between 9 and 14 months of age. The range of scores reflected the motor outcome at 2 years (Haataja et al., 2001). Total scores of between 67 and 78 were always found in infants who achieved independent ambulation by 2 years, while scores between 40 and 67 predicted restricted mobility. Scores under 40 were found in infants who were not able to sit independently at 2 or 4 years. The distribution of scores was also related to the pattern of lesions on neonatal magnetic resonance imaging (MRI). Optimal scores were always found in infants with normal or minor basal ganglia and white matter abnormalities on the neonatal MRI. The scores decreased with increasing severity of basal ganglia involvement, with intermediate scores in infants with diffuse white matter lesions but normal basal ganglia. The lowest scores were found in infants with the most severe basal ganglia and white matter lesions.

Assessing the infants longitudinally from the neonatal period up to 12 to 24 months of age, we were also able to determine a different neurological pattern according to the severity of the brain lesions. Infants with normal brain MRI or mild white matter changes may present with minor neurological abnormalities in the first 2 weeks after birth but they show normal neurological development when assessed after the third week and throughout the first 2 years (Dubowitz et al., 1998; Mercuri et al., 1999a). In contrast, infants with severe basal ganglia lesions – with or without associated white matter lesions – have abnormal axial and limb tone, reduced visual alertness and poor sucking from the time of the initial assessment in the first weeks after birth and these abnormalities persist at 5–7 weeks, 6 months, and 12 months (Dubowitz et al., 1998; Ricci et al., 2006b).

A different profile of neurological development was found in the group of infants with less severe basal ganglia lesions or diffuse white matter changes. Assessments carried out in the first weeks after birth showed reduced axial and limb tone, reduced visual alertness and often poor sucking, but when the examination was repeated at 5–7 weeks of age there was a dramatic improvement in all aspects assessed, with results falling within the normal range for age. This improvement proved to be consistent for sucking and vision abilities but was only transient for axial and limb tone and movements, highlighting the timing of tone changes from hypotonia to hypertonia and supporting the importance of performing sequential neurological examinations in order to follow the evolution of clinical signs.

Infants with cerebral infarction

Neonatal cerebral infarction in full term infants is now considered to be more common than previously estimated (Mercuri et al., 1999b). The incidence of motor problems is quite variable, ranging from 8 to 100 per cent of the cases in different studies, probably reflecting the population studied. In our experience hemiplegia occurs in 20 to 30 per cent of cases with neonatal presentation.

The timing of the appearance of the first clinical signs of hemiplegia is variable and reflects to some extent the severity of motor impairment, with early clinical signs generally related to more severe motor sequelae. In the neonatal period, the neurological examinations in infants with cerebral infarction can be quite variable, ranging from normal to the presence of marked asymmetry in tone and movement (Mercuri et al., 1999b). An early sign is usually generalized hypotonia but, as most of these infants present with convulsions in the first 72 hours after birth and they are often on anticonvulsant drugs, the significance of this finding is uncertain. The first signs of limb tone asymmetry can be detected after a few weeks, but it generally consists of a relative hypotonia more than hypertonia of the affected side, and it can easily be missed or misjudged. This underlies the importance of looking carefully for subtle tone signs in infants with focal lesions, particularly the popliteal angle, the adductors angle, shoulder elevation, and lateral tilting for active trunk tone. The assessment of spontaneous movements can also show early asymmetries between 9 and 16 weeks, mainly in kicking and reaching, even when no clear tonal asymmetries are detected (Guzzetta et al., 2003). Reflexes and reactions can also show early asymmetries after 12 weeks, mainly asymmetry of kicking in vertical suspension (Bouza et al., 1994) with a relative paucity of kicking on the affected side, and asymmetry of the arm protective reaction, seen when a child is pulled up from supine by one arm (Bouza et al., 1994).

After 9 months of age asymmetries can also be detected in other limb tone items such as pronation/supination of the forearm and ankle dorsiflexion, and functional asymmetry can become more evident, with the development of a strong hand preference in all children with hemiplegia by 12 months. These infants usually tend to reach over and to manipulate toys using the non-affected hand. In infants with severe hemiplegia dystonic posture of the hand and hand fisting are typical findings after 5–6 months of age. The involvement of the lower limb is generally less severe. These infants develop an asymmetrical gait with hyperextension of the knee and a tendency to tiptoe when they achieve the standing position.

At variance with the other groups of patient we have described, the HINE score in patients with infarction does not always reflect the severity of hemiplegia. In many cases neurological abnormalities may be present but these are mainly asymmetries of tone and posture that are scored as the average of the individual scores for each side. This will only slightly reduce the total score, which is often still close to optimal, either because the normal scores from the non-hemiplegic side compensate for the abnormal side or because both sides, while different, may be within the optimal range. It is of interest, however, that relatively good scores may be found in children who, even if though going on to develop hemiplegia, are nevertheless able to walk independently by 2 years of age.

Other applications

In the past few years the protocol has been used in different environments including developing countries, where a clinical examination is often the only diagnostic and prognostic tool available. A short version of the examination – the Shoklo Neurological Test – has been developed for rural settings aimed at screening and following up the short and long term adverse effects of serious infections, drugs and toxins in children aged from 9 to 36 months of age (Haataja et al., 2002). The examination includes some items assessing hand coordination and others assessing tone and behaviour from the HINE. We selected only such items as could be reliably performed even by less experienced health workers, for example paramedics. The test was validated in a cohort of British low-risk term infants and shown to correlate favourably with the Griffiths Developmental Scales. In order to evaluate the usefulness of The Shoklo Neurological Test under less optimal conditions, it was applied to a cohort of 128 infants from a Karen refugee camp. After appropriate training, the paramedical staff performed well in quality control situations, showing an inter-tester agreement of 95 per cent. These results are very encouraging and suggest that the test may be used in resource-poor settings for clinical and research purposes (Haataja et al., 2002).

References

Amiel-Tison, C. & Grenier, A. (1986): *Neurological assessment during the first years of life*. New York: Oxford University Press.

Amiel-Tison, C. & Stewart, A. (1989): Follow up studies during the first five years of life: a pervasive assessment of neurological function. *Arch. Dis. Child.* **64**, 496–502.

Andre-Thomas, A., Chesni, Y. & Saint-Anne Dargassies, S. (1960): *The neurological examination of the infant*. Clinics in Developmental Medicine 1. London: Heineman.

Baird, H.W. & Gordon, E.C. (1983): *Neurological evaluation of infants and children*. Clinics in Developmental Medicine, vol. 84/85. London: Heinemann.

Bayley, N. (1993): *Bayley scales of infant development*, 2nd edition. San Antonio: The Psychological Corporation (BSID-II).

Bouza, H., Rutherford, M., Acolet, D., Pennock, J.M. & Dubowitz, L.M. (1994): Evolution of early hemiplegic signs in full-term infants with unilateral brain lesions in the neonatal period: a prospective study. *Neuropediatrics* **25**, 201–207.

Campbell, S.K. & Wilheim, I.J. (1985): Development from birth to 3 years of age of 15 children at high risk for central nervous system dysfunction. *Phys. Ther.* **65**, 463–469.

Dubowitz, L. & Dubowitz, V. (1981): *The neurological assessment of the preterm and full term infant*. Clinics in Developmental Medicine, vol. 79. London: Heinemann.

Dubowitz, L., Mercuri, E. & Dubowitz, V. (1998): An optimality score for the neurologic examination of the term newborn. *J. Pediatr.* **133**, 406–416.

Dubowitz, L., Dubowitz, V. & Mercuri, E. (1999): *The neurological assessment of the preterm and full term newborn infant*, 2nd edition. Clinics in Developmental Medicine, vol. 148. London: MacKeith Press.

Ellison, P.H., Browning, C.A., Larson, B. & Denny, J. (1983): Development of a scoring system for the Milani-Comparetti and Gidoni method of assessing neurologic abnormality in infancy. *Phys. Ther.* **63**, 1414–1423.

Frisone, M.F., Mercuri, E., Laroche, S., Foglia, C., Maalouf, E.F., Haataja, L., Cowan, F. & Dubowitz, L. (2002): Prognostic value of the neurologic optimality score at 9 and 18 months in preterm infants born before 31 weeks' gestation. *J. Pediatr.* **140**, 57–60.

Gorga, D., Stern, F.M. & Ross, G. (1985): Trends in neuromotor behavior of preterm and fullterm infants in the first year of life: a preliminary report. *Dev. Med. Child Neurol.* **27**, 756–766.

Guzzetta, A., Mercuri, E., Rapisardi, G., Ferrari, F., Roversi, M.F., Cowan, F., Rutherford, M., Paolicelli, P.B., Einspieler, C., Boldrini, A., Dubowitz, L., Prechtl, H.F. & Cioni, G. (2003): General movements detect early signs of hemiplegia in term infants with neonatal cerebral infarction. *Neuropediatrics* **34**, 61–66.

Haataja, L., Mercuri, E., Regev, R., Cowan, F., Rutherford, M., Dubowitz, V. & Dubowitz, L. (1999): Optimality score for the neurologic examination of the infant at 12 and 18 months of age. *J. Pediatr.* **135**, 153–161.

Haataja, L., Mercuri, E., Guzzetta, A., Rutherford, M., Counsell, S., Flavia Frisone, M., Cioni, G., Cowan, F. & Dubowitz, L. (2001): Neurologic examination in infants with hypoxic-ischemic encephalopathy at age 9 to 14 months: use of optimality scores and correlation with magnetic resonance imaging findings. *J. Pediatr.* **138**, 332–337.

Haataja, L., McGready, R., Arunjerdja, R., Simpson, J.A., Mercuri, E., Nosten, F. & Dubowitz, L. (2002): A new approach for neurological evaluation of infants in resource-poor settings. *Ann. Trop. Paediatr.* **22,** 355–368.

Haataja, L., Cowan, F., Mercuri, E., Bassi, L., Guzzetta, A. & Dubowitz, L. (2003): Application of a scorable neurologic examination in healthy term infants aged 3 to 8 months [letter]. *J. Pediatr.* **143,** 546.

Hempel, M.S. (1993): *The neurological examination for toddler-age*. Thesis, University of Groningen, Netherlands.

Kuenzle, C., Baenziger, O., Martin, E., Thun-Hohenstein, L., Steinlin, M., Good, M., Fanconi, S., Boltshauser, E. & Largo, R.H. (1994): Prognostic value of early MR imaging in term infants with severe perinatal asphyxia. *Neuropediatrics* **4,** 191–200.

Mercuri, E., Dubowitz, L., Paterson-Brown, S. & Cowan, F. (1998): Incidence of cranial ultrasound abnormalities in apparently well neonates on a postnatal ward: correlation with antenatal and perinatal factors and neurological status. *Arch. Dis. Child. Fetal Neonatal Ed.* **79,** F185–189.

Mercuri, E., Guzzetta, A., Haataja, L., Cowan, F., Rutherford, M., Counsell, S., Papadimitriou, M., Cioni, G. & Dubowitz, L. (1999a): Neonatal neurological examination in infants with hypoxic ischaemic encephalopathy: correlation with MRI findings. *Neuropediatrics* **30,** 83–89.

Mercuri, E., Rutherford, M., Cowan, F., Pennock, J., Counsell, S., Papadimitriou, M., Azzopardi, D., Bydder, G. & Dubowitz, L. (1999b): Early prognostic indicators of outcome in infants with neonatal cerebral infarction: a clinical, electroencephalogram, and magnetic resonance imaging study. *Pediatrics* **103,** 39–46.

Milani-Comparetti, A. & Gidoni, E.A. (1967): Routine developmental examination in normal and retarded children. *Dev. Med. Child Neurol.* **9,** 31–638.

Nickel, R.E., Renken, C.A. & Gallenstein, J.S. (1989): The infant motor screen. *Dev. Med. Child Neurol.* **31,** 35–42.

Palmer, F.B., Shapiro, B.K., Wachtel, R.C., Ross, A. & Accardo, P.J. (1984): Primitive reflex profile: a quantitation of primitive reflexes in infancy. *Dev. Med. Child Neurol.* **24,** 375–383.

Ricci, D., Cowan, F., Pane, M., Gallini, F., Haataja, L., Luciano, R., Cesarini, L., Leone, D., Donvito, V., Baranello, G., Rutherford, M., Romagnoli, C., Dubowitz, L. & Mercuri, E. (2006a): Neurological examination at 6 to 9 months in infants with cystic periventricular leukomalacia. *Neuropediatrics* **37,** 247–252.

Ricci, D., Guzzetta, A., Cowan, F., Haataja, L., Rutherford, M., Dubowitz, L. & Mercuri, E. (2006b): Sequential neurological examinations in infants with neonatal encephalopathy and low apgar scores: relationship with brain MRI. *Neuropediatrics* **37,** 148–153.

Romeo, D.M., Cioni, M., Guzzetta, A., Scoto, M., Conversano, M., Palermo, F., Romeo, M.G. & Mercuri, E. (2007): Application of a scorable neurological examination to near-term infants: longitudinal data. *Neuropediatrics* **38,** 233–238.

Saint-Anne Dargassies, S. (1977): Neurological development in the full-term and premature neonate. Amsterdam: Elsevier.

Touwen, B. (1976): *Neurological development in infancy*. Clinics in Developmental Medicine, vol. 58. London: Heinemann.

Vohr, B.R. (1999): The quest for the ideal neurologic assessment for infants and young children. *J. Pediatr.* **135,** 140–142.

Chapter 2

Developmental assessment: functional techniques

Andrea Guzzetta

Department of Developmental Neurosciences, IRCCS Stella Maris,
via dei Giacinti 2, 56128 Calambrone Pisa, Italy
aguzzetta@inpe.unipi.it

Functional techniques that are currently used to measure *in vivo* electromagnetic, metabolic, or haemodynamic changes in the brain include electroencephalography (EEG), magneto-encephalography (MEG), proton magnetic resonance spectroscopy (1H-MRS), functional magnetic resonance imaging (fMRI), positron emission tomography (PET), and single-photon emission computed tomography (SPECT). These techniques share the capacity to explore brain functional processes and to map them both spatially and temporally, but show huge differences in terms of their neurophysiological principles, technical aspects, reliability and level of invasiveness.

During infancy, the most widely used functional techniques are without doubt those based on EEG, both in the clinical and the research domain. This is mainly because EEG recordings are minimally invasive and require little collaboration from the patient, aspects especially necessary at this age. Moreover, with the great technological advances of the last decades – and particularly with digitization of the signal – it has become possible to acquire EEG signals in neonates and infants at high sampling rates, very high densities, and with effective artefact reduction. Most of the other functional techniques are not routinely used in clinical practice in the infant, their application being limited to research studies carried out by dedicated laboratories.

In this chapter we will focus mainly on EEG-based techniques, evoked potentials, and the cerebral function monitor (CFM). With the exception of fMRI – a method that is attracting increasing attention in infant studies and promises to make an important contribution to our understanding of brain development under normal and pathological conditions – we will not cover the other less widely used techniques, as this would go beyond the scope of the chapter.

Electrophysiological techniques

Electrophysiological techniques provide useful information on brain function in all neonatal and infantile diseases of the central nervous system (CNS). They are not invasive and can be used directly at the infant's bedside. The EEG consists on the direct recording of cerebral electrical activity followed, when needed, by off-line processing of the raw signal. This is necessary, for example, for the evoked potentials, which correspond to the changes of cerebral electrical activity evoked by an external stimulus, or for the amplitude-integrated EEG, also known as cerebral function monitoring (CFM), a highly compressed and filtered trace suitable for prolonged recordings.

In this early stage of CNS development, electrical activities undergo rapid age-related changes; hence it is crucial to evaluate the maturational features of EEG activity correctly, in order to relate the findings to what is expected for the patient's age.

The EEG

Technical aspects

Despite remarkable technological progress, EEG recording in the infant or neonate is much more challenging than at other stages of life. These patients are obviously not able to cooperate and, particularly in neonates, the recording is frequently carried out in an intensive care unit, where the presence of other electrical instruments can generate persisting artefacts. The new computer-aided electroencephalographs, equipped with battery-operated amplifiers and A/D converters, have significantly improved EEG quality under these extreme conditions. In neonates and infants, electrodes are usually applied to the scalp using ring-shaped double adhesive plasters or directly with a conductive-adhesive paste. In infants the EEG is recorded using the same technique as in adults (collodion-applied electrodes, latex cups, and so on), but it is important to make sure that the infant is allowed to rest and sleep safely and comfortably. More recently, a new easy-to-use type of web-like high density structure, requiring no abrasion, has been developed for infant use (Geodesic Sensor Net).

The number of electrodes varies according to age. In neonates no more than eight or 10 active electrodes are generally applied (Fp1-2, C3-4, O1-2, T3-4 + Cz and Pz or Fz of the International 10–20 System). After the neonatal period, a complete montage is usually possible. Polygraphic channels are also used in both neonates and infants (Fig. 1). They generally include electro-

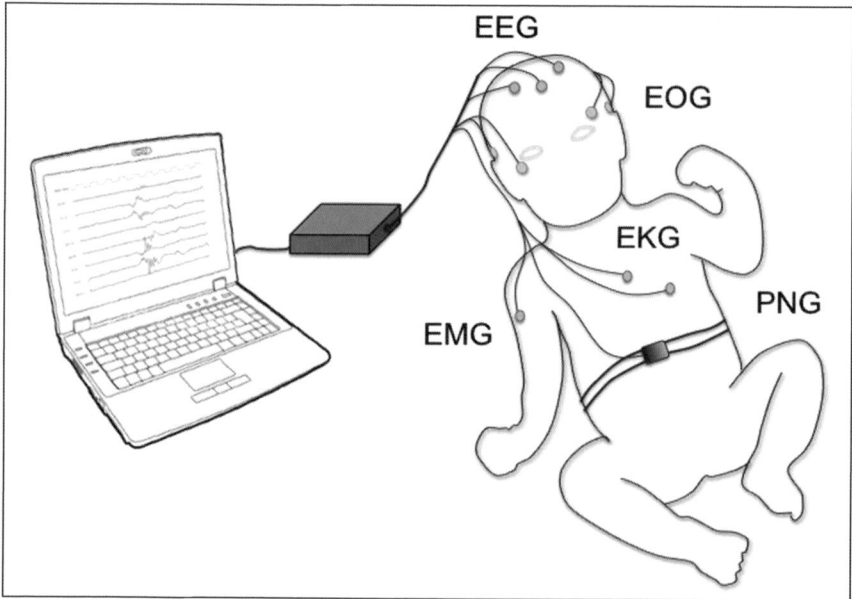

Fig. 1. Graphic representation of an infant polygraphic EEG digital system. EEG, electroencephalogram; EKG, electrocardiogram; EMG, electromyogram; EOG, electro-oculogram; PNG, pneumogram.

myography (EMG) of different muscles (deltoid, chin, other muscles of legs and arms, and so on), pneumography (PNG – recorded by means of a nasal thermistor or a strain gauge transducer applied to the chest or the abdomen), electrocardiogram (EKG), and electro-oculogram (EOG – recorded by means of a piezoelectric accelerometer applied to the eyelid, or electrodes applied at the outer canthi). Recordings must include an entire sleep-wake cycle in neonates and should therefore last at least 45 to 90 minutes. In infants it is also generally necessary to record some phases of both wakefulness and sleep, to demonstrate the maturational features or detect possible paroxysmal abnormalities of drowsiness, sleep and arousal.

Normal neonatal EEG

Cerebral electrical activity undergoes rapid modifications in the early phases of life. In the neonate these changes are particularly fast and do not depend on the interval since birth, but rather on the postmenstrual age (PMA) at the time of recording. Hence, EEG features of all healthy neonates at a specific PMA are similar, irrespective of the postnatal age (Anders *et al.*, 1971; Dreyfus-Brisac, 1972; Nolte & Haas, 1978; Anderson *et al.*, 1985; Lombroso, 1985; Ferrari *et al.*, 1992; Stockard-Pope & Werner, 1992; Biagioni *et al.*, 1994). This finding strongly indicates that the maturation of cerebral electrical activity in preterm infants – as well as other aspects of CNS functioning – is related to the infant's corrected age (CA), within a developmental continuum from conception to childhood. In this section normal features of neonatal EEG activity will be illustrated for each stage of PMA, from early preterm birth to the end of the first month post-term.

In recent years significant improvements in neonatal care allowed many young preterm infants to survive, despite their low birth weight and their very low gestational age. This gives us the opportunity to explore brain electrical activity in a very early phase of development, when cortical foldings are still poorly developed and glial cells are still migrating from the germinal matrix to the cortex (Battin *et al.*, 1998; Kostovic & Jovanov-Milosevic, 2005).

At around 23 to 25 weeks PMA, the EEG activity is constantly discontinuous: bursts of activity are interposed with long periods of flattening (up to 40 to 50 seconds) (Biagioni *et al.*, 2000; Vecchierini *et al.*, 2003; Lamblin *et al.*, 2004). This pattern is detectable in healthy neonates up to the end of the neonatal period, although it is progressively replaced by continuous activity. At this age, bursts consist of high amplitude (up to 450 μV), very slow (up to 0.5 Hz) waves, often asynchronous between the two hemispheres. These delta waves are sometimes superimposed on low amplitude (generally less than 60–70 μV) 8–22 Hz rhythms and, much more clearly, on trains of high amplitude (up to 200 μV) 3.5–7 Hz activities, characterized by an almost sinusoidal appearance and by a larger representation in the occipital regions. This often asynchronous theta rhythm constitutes the first rhythmic activity detectable in humans and is generally called the 'occipital saw-tooth' pattern (Fig. 2) (Hughes *et al.*, 1990; Biagioni *et al.*, 2000).

Around 26 to 28 weeks PMA, the temporal organization of brain electrical activity is still constantly discontinuous. Fast 8–22 Hz rhythms are now higher in amplitude and superimposed on slow waves, giving rise to a waveform called 'delta brush' (Stockard-Pope & Werner, 1992; Biagioni *et al.*, 1994). The occipital saw-tooth pattern gradually migrates to the temporal regions, and thus takes the name of 'temporal saw-tooth' (Fig. 3) (Anderson *et al.*, 1985; Stockard-Pope & Werner, 1992).

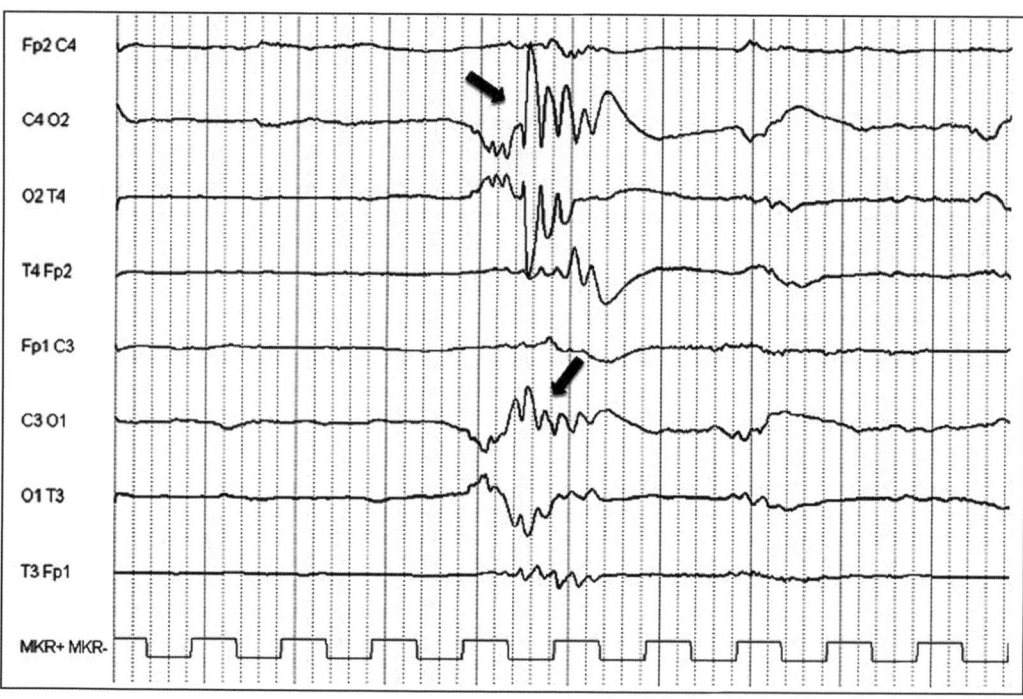

Fig. 2. Tracing recorded at 26 weeks' PMA in an infant with normal outcome. Occipital saw-tooth (arrow) is represented on posterior regions.

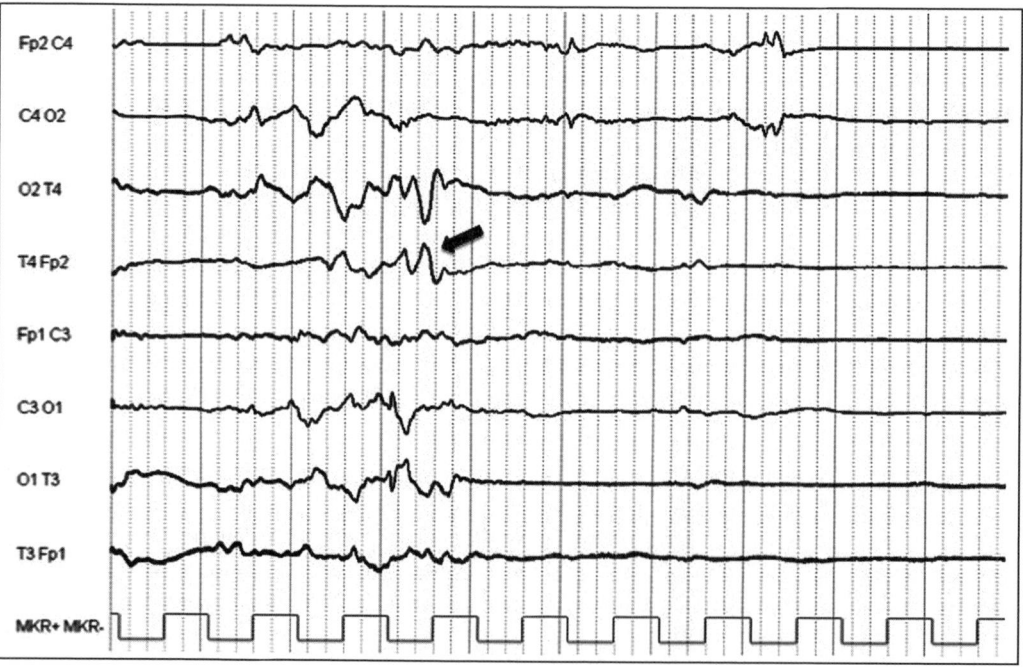

Fig. 3. Tracings recorded at 29 weeks' PMA in an infant with normal outcome. Note the presence of temporal saw-tooth (arrow), better expressed on the right temporal lobe.

From 29 to 32 weeks PMA, in periods generally corresponding to behaviourally active phases, bursts of slow waves are much longer and intervals are much shorter, so that a beginning of continuous activity becomes observable (Nolte & Haas, 1978). Delta brushes gradually increase their amplitude and their representation, whereas temporal saw-tooth activity is less predominant. When the infant is quiet, the tracing is constantly discontinuous: within bursts, both slow waves and fast activity are higher than in younger neonates and the temporal saw-tooth activity is still observable. At this age, it is possible to detect for the first time a certain organization of behavioural states, with a more reliable concordance among different physiological variables (such as body movements, eye movements, regularity of respiration, and EEG activity) (Curzi-Dascalova & Mirmiram, 1996).

At 33 to 36 weeks of PMA, a bursting tendency is no longer observable in continuous patterns during phases of wakefulness and active sleep. During quiet sleep the detectable discontinuous EEG is characterized by shorter intervals (generally less than 20 seconds) and longer bursts than in the earlier stages; delta brushes are now very obvious (their amplitude reaches 200 μV), whereas temporal saw-tooth activity definitively disappears (Biagioni *et al.*, 1994). From around 35 weeks a differentiation of a new continuous pattern can be observed, characterized by a relatively lower amplitude (less than 50–60 μV) and by irregular theta and delta band activity with superimposed very low amplitude 8–22 Hz rhythms (Fig. 4). This last pattern generally relates to phases of wakefulness and to those phases of active sleep following quiet sleep. During the phases of active sleep which precede quiet sleep, we observe a continuous pattern with a larger representation of the delta band (up to 100 μV high) and 8–22 Hz activities (Nolte & Haas, 1978; Stockard-Pope & Werner, 1992). Some polyphasic high amplitude sharp waves appear in the frontal regions, often synchronous between the two hemispheres: these waveforms are known as 'frontal sharp transients' or 'encoches frontales' (Stockard-Pope & Werner, 1992).

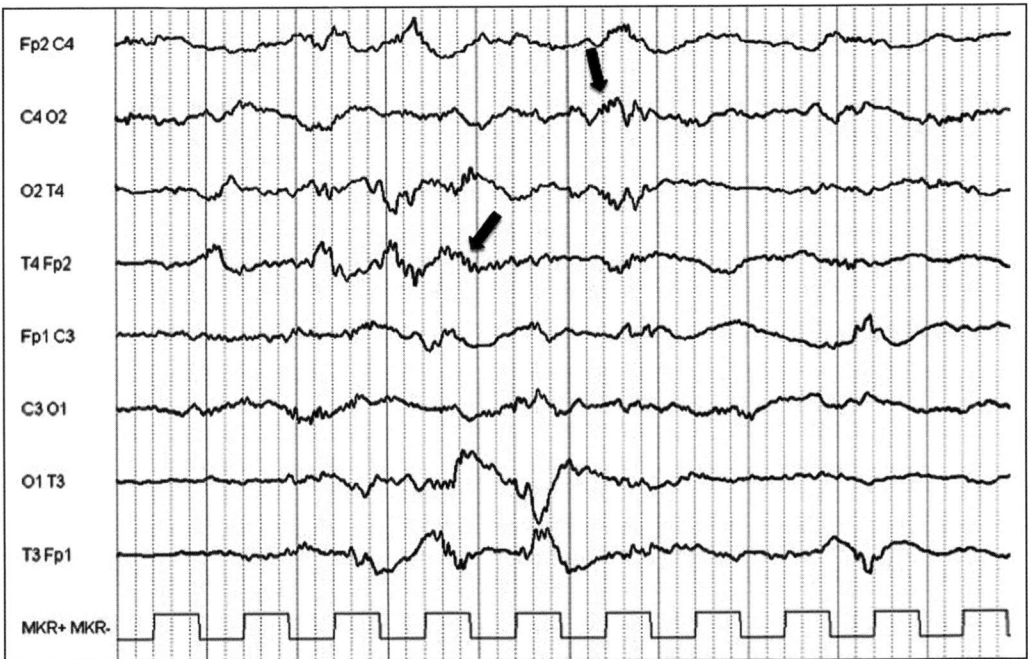

Fig. 4. Tracings recorded at 33 weeks' PMA in an infant with normal outcome. Note the presence of delta brush (arrows), and the absence of temporal saw-tooth.

Approaching term age, the neonatal EEG includes five different classical patterns (Dreyfus-Brisac, 1972; Nolte & Haas, 1978; Ferrari et al., 1992; Stockard-Pope & Werner, 1992). During wakefulness a continuous low amplitude (less than 50–60 µV) pattern is observable, characterized by irregular theta and delta frequencies (*activité moyenne*); 8–22 Hz rhythms are no longer observable during wakefulness after 37 to 38 weeks of PMA. In the active sleep periods that precede quiet sleep, a medium amplitude (up to 90–100 µV) mixed theta-delta continuous pattern is detectable (mixed); in this pattern it is possible to see superimposed 8–22 Hz activities until 38 to 39 weeks. Conversely, phases of active sleep following quiet sleep are characterized by a low voltage (less than 50–60 µV) predominant theta continuous pattern, with short trains of regular 4–5 Hz activities (low voltage irregular); no fast rhythm is detectable in this pattern. Quiet sleep still predominantly relates to a discontinuous pattern (*tracé alternant*): at term age bursts are characterized by up to 200 µV-high delta waves superimposed on low amplitude 8–22 Hz activities; intervals are short (generally less than 10 seconds) and relatively rich in activity. At the same time, a new continuous pattern appears in quiet sleep phases, characterized by high amplitude (up to 200 µV) delta activity (high voltage slow). During the first month of post-term age, the progressive disappearance of 8–22 Hz activities (delta brushes) in quiet sleep can also be observed. A high voltage slow pattern becomes predominant in this behavioural state, although it is possible to recognize a bursting tendency in quiet sleep until 44 weeks PMA (Nolte & Haas, 1978). Moreover, the mixed pattern tends to disappear as the infants more frequently fall asleep in quiet sleep (and therefore phases of active sleep preceding quiet sleep are no longer observable).

Normal EEG from 1 to 24 months of corrected age

After the fast and dramatic changes of the neonatal period, EEG activity gradually acquires features of more mature ages. In the first 2 years of life, wakefulness patterns are characterized by predominant low voltage theta activities (up to 50–60 µV). EEG reactivity to eye closure generally appears at around 4 months CA (Kellaway, 1987). Rhythmic activities in posterior regions are much slower than in adults and are included in the lower theta band (4–4.5 Hz). The frequency of the posterior rhythm is around 6.5–7 Hz at 1 year CA (Biagioni et al., 2002), and often reaches the limits of the alpha band at the age of 2 years (Kellaway, 1987). Rhythmic activity in the rolandic regions during quiet wakefulness also appears and develops in this same period, with similar frequencies. Phases of drowsiness (both before and after sleep) are characterized from the third month CA by high amplitude (up to 200 µV), regular 3.5–5.5 Hz diffuse activities, the so-called hypnagogic hypersynchrony (Kellaway, 1987).

Sleep EEG features at 1–24 months CA are much more similar to those detected in adults than those observable in neonates. Discontinuous patterns are no longer detectable after 1 month CA. The 'low voltage, irregular' pattern described above, typical of active sleep, generally disappears within the second month CA. At around 44 weeks of PMA, the first 11–16 Hz low voltage activities, represented more in central regions, are already detectable during sleep: they constitute the 'pre-spindles' – precursors of the more mature waveforms observed at older ages (Nolte & Haas, 1978). In infancy and up to the second year of life, spindles are sometimes asynchronous in the two hemispheres, and are represented (more often than in childhood) even in deep phases of sleep (Fig. 5). Vertex sharp waves and K-complexes also appear within the first 2 to 3 months CA. It is important to stress that K-complexes are usually constituted only by a high amplitude diffuse polyphasic sharp wave at this age (that is, they are rarely followed by a spindle as in older patients). Moreover, vertex sharp waves, typical of the first sleep phases, usually show a very sharp appearance, so that sometimes it is not easy to distinguish

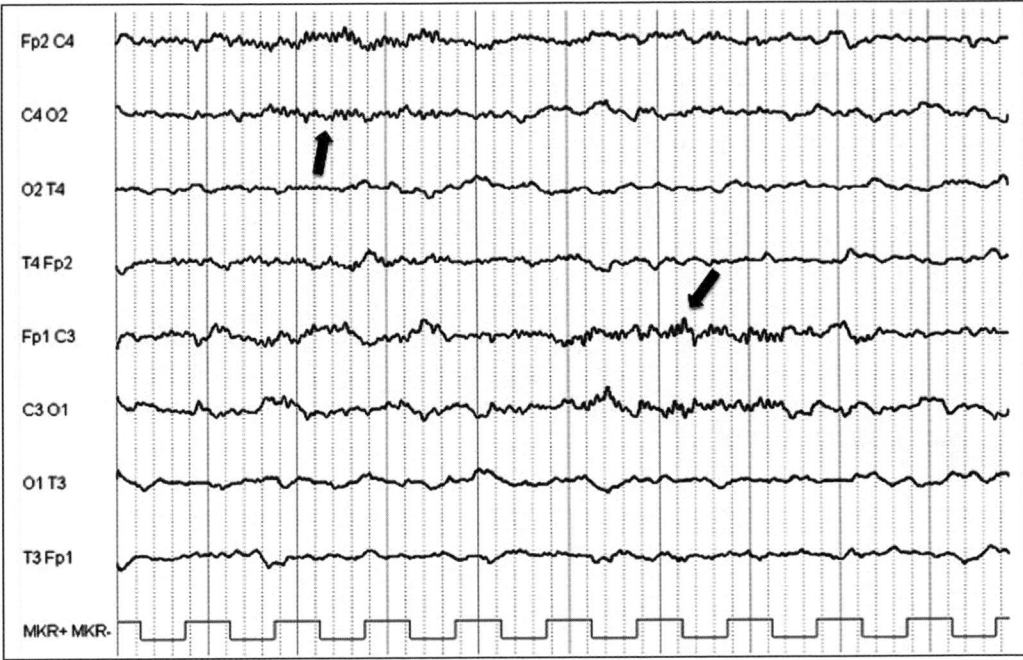

Fig. 5. EEG recorded in a 5-month-old healthy infant during sleep. The tracing shows a normal activity with symmetrical and asynchronous spindles, more represented on fronto-central regions (arrows).

them from epileptiform abnormalities. As far as sleep organization is concerned, the differentiation of classical sleep states according to EEG criteria (I, II, III, IV, and REM) is much less clear than at older ages.

Abnormal neonatal EEG

Background abnormalities: Background EEG abnormalities have been shown to have the highest significance for both diagnosis and prognosis in all CNS diseases of neonates (Monod et al., 1972; Pezzani et al., 1986; Holmes & Lombroso, 1993; Biagioni et al., 1996a; Hayakawa et al., 1997; Biagioni et al., 1999; Lamblin et al., 2004). An accurate examination of amplitude, temporal organization and morphology of EEG activities is therefore mandatory for a precise assessment of brain function. Some background EEG abnormalities observed in newborns are very similar to those in older patients, while others are specific for this age.

A constant low voltage represents a very severe abnormality. This definition includes tracings characterized by persistent low voltage activity, without any state-related pattern differentiation. According to some investigators (Monod et al., 1972; Lombroso, 1985), it is possible to distinguish between inactive EEG (amplitude $< 2\ \mu V$) and low voltage (< 5–$10\ \mu V$). It is important to bear in mind that, when EEG amplitude is very reduced, it is often hard to distinguish between residual cerebral activity and artefacts. Moreover, EEG amplitude can also depend on interelectrode distances and filtering. This very pathological pattern can be detected in both preterm and full term infants in association with a severe hypoxic-ischaemic brain insult. Of course, as in the early preterm period, inactive intervals can be very prolonged even in normal individuals (see above); in these infants an EEG can be classified as low voltage only when this feature is persistent. It is also important to consider that in some cases a constant low voltage is only observable within the first hours of life (for example, after a severe insult) and is subsequently replaced by other pathological EEG patterns (Biagioni *et al.*, 2001), such as constantly discontinuous tracings (see below).

Constantly discontinuous tracings, also known as burst suppression patterns, are characterized by medium to high voltage bursts separated by low activity intervals. As discontinuous patterns are normal not only in preterm but also in full term neonates, it is important to define this entity precisely in order to distinguish between normal and abnormal findings. Two main rules should be followed. First, no tracing can be classified as constantly discontinuous (or burst suppression) before 37 weeks' PMA. Second, a term age EEG can be considered as constantly discontinuous only when a discontinuous pattern is present in all phases of sleep and even during wakefulness, unless the infant is so seriously sick that no behavioural state is observable (for example, comatose patients). In all cases the tracing must be long enough to ensure that the discontinuous pattern is not related to a particular sleep phase (such as a normal *tracé alternant*, typical of quiet sleep).

A constantly discontinuous EEG is a frequent finding in hypoxic-ischaemic encephalopathy in full term neonates. This finding carries a severe prognosis (only constant low voltage is probably worse), especially when it persists after the first few days of life (Biagioni *et al.*, 1999; Menache *et al.*, 2002). Some quantitative characteristics of constantly discontinuous patterns in neonates are believed to be particularly significant from a prognostic point of view. Very low amplitude patterns (< 10 µV or even < 5 µV) predict a severe outcome, so that some authorities define a constantly discontinuous pattern as 'burst suppression' only when interval activity is very depressed. According to some recent data, interval length is the most reliable parameter to predict subsequent evolution (intervals lasting more than 20 to 30 seconds always relate to a bad outcome) (Biagioni *et al.*, 1999; Menache *et al.*, 2002). Timing of recording is also significant. Full term infants with perinatal asphyxia should have an EEG as soon as possible after birth: if this first tracing is constantly discontinuous (or low voltage), it should be repeated during the following days. Rapid EEG normalization (that is, the appearance of continuous activity and state-related EEG patterns) can also lead to a normal outcome. Conversely, when constantly discontinuous patterns persist until the eighth or ninth day of life, the evolution is always unfavourable (Biagioni *et al.*, 1999). Besides perinatal asphyxia, constantly discontinuous patterns can also be observed in other disorders of the CNS, such as early infantile epileptic encephalopathies (Ohtahara & Yamatogi, 2003). In these severe neonatal syndromes the constantly discontinuous pattern acquires a specific paroxysmal significance *(tracé paroxystique)* and is always accompanied by prolonged EEG discharges. Finally, a discontinuous pattern is also sometimes detectable in other metabolic, genetic and degenerative disorders of the neonate, or may be related to the effect of high doses of anticonvulsant drugs (Ferrari *et al.*, 2001).

Interhemispheric asymmetry also constitutes a background abnormality carrying a serious prognosis (Fig. 6). Nevertheless, before formulating unfavourable prognostic hypotheses, it is important to exclude technical reasons that could account for such an EEG finding. First, malfunctioning of electrodes on one side can give rise to flattening of traces on some leads. Second, some frequent neonatal conditions can increase the electrical resistance on one side and therefore reduce the amplitude of the EEG signal (for example, scalp oedema or cephalhaematoma). Third, it is well known that a slight asymmetry is normal in neonates, especially at low PMAs (Anderson *et al.*, 1985). However, when the asymmetry is significant (that is, > 50 per cent) and technical problems are excluded, this EEG pattern is generally an expression of an underlying pathology (such as cerebral infarction or haemorrhage). In the case of underlying

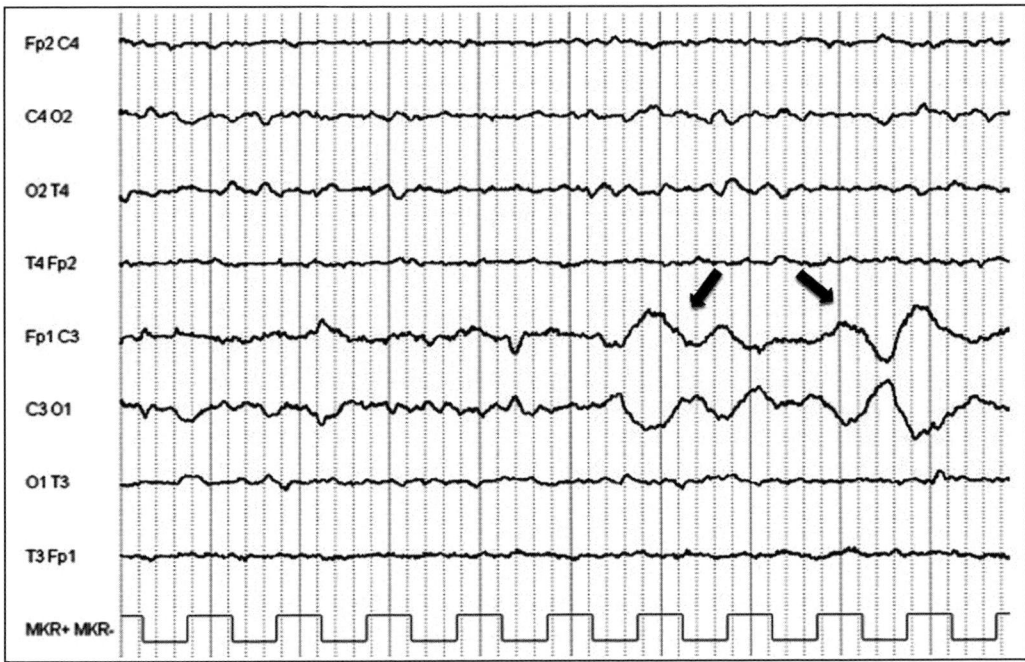

Fig. 6. EEG recorded at term in an infant with an arterial stroke in the territory of the left middle cerebral artery. Note the slow activity in the left central regions (arrows).

pathology we observe a reduced amplitude in the affected hemisphere (Ferrari et al., 2001). In other conditions, such as cortical dysplasia and in particular hemimegalencephaly, EEG activity in the affected hemisphere is higher and slower, with interposed frequent paroxysmal EEG discharges (Wertheim et al., 1994).

EEG dysmaturity constitutes a specific neonatal background abnormality. The definition includes EEG tracings showing maturational features that are not appropriate for the PMA at recording. The rapid changes in the maturational characteristics of brain electrical activity during the neonatal age were described earlier. At a certain PMA, EEG recordings are considered to be dysmature when age-specific criteria are not met (Lombroso, 1985; Biagioni et al., 1996a). For example, the EEG of a 28-week-old preterm infant with scarce representation of temporal saw-tooth activity and that of a 34-week-old neonate with marked persistence of the same waveform are both dysmature. It is important to stress that dysmaturity does not mean having characteristics overlapping those of normal tracings recorded at a previous age but, rather, a general alteration of maturational features. EEG dysmaturity is not frequent in full term neonates and in these infants it generally constitutes a minor anomaly. In contrast, it is a frequent finding in preterm infants with brain damage (Ferrari et al., 1992; Biagioni et al., 1996a; Hayakawa et al., 1997). The prognostic significance of EEG dysmaturity is generally high: in a study of ours, almost all preterm infants who had normal EEG maturational features also had a normal outcome, whereas some neonates with mildly dysmature EEG, and most of those with a severely dysmature EEG, had an unfavourable evolution (Biagioni et al., 1996a). Some investigators distinguish between an acute phase of disorganization of maturational aspects (that is, increased discontinuity, modifications of amplitude, and so on) and chronic stage maturational abnormalities (such as the representation and shape of age-specific waveforms) (Hayakawa *et al.*, 1997; Watanabe *et al.*, 1999; Kato *et al.*, 2004). The timing of the recording is crucial: when the EEG is done during the very first days of life, it often appears abnormal even in relatively healthy preterm infants, probably because of the neonate's unstable condition (Eaton *et al.*, 1994). In contrast, at a postnatal age of over 2 weeks it is possible to find reorganization of brain electrical activity (and from a maturational point of view) in infants with severe brain damage (for example, periventricular leukomalacia). Therefore, for optimal prediction of the neurological outcome, we suggest recording the EEG between the fourth and the 13th day of life (Biagioni *et al.*, 1996a).

Abnormal EEG transients: In neonates, as in other stages of life, it is possible to detect some abnormal transient EEG features. These abnormalities (spikes and sharp waves, delta and theta sharp rhythmic activities, alpha discharges) must be distinguished from the physiological waveforms described above, which constitute typical maturational findings at different PMAs (that is, occipital and temporal saw-tooth pattern, delta brushes, *encoches frontales*, and so on). Abnormal transient neonatal EEG features can be observed as interictal abnormalities or can give rise to more or less diffuse EEG discharges corresponding to epileptic phenomena (neonatal seizures). In the latter case, as well as at other stages of life, we can detect a sequence of differing transient epileptiform activity (for example, an alpha discharge first, followed by prolonged theta/delta sharp rhythmic activities, and finally by a degrading train of sharp waves). A detailed description of electroclinical findings in neonatal seizures is beyond the scope of this chapter.

Spikes and sharp waves are frequently observable as interictal abnormalities in neonates (Biagioni *et al.*, 1996b) and have been considered as quasi-normal features (Monod *et al.*, 1972), especially when they are infrequent and represented more in the context of discontinuous patterns. Spikes are obviously shorter in duration (< 80–100 ms) and are less frequent than sharp waves in neonates. A particular kind of sharp wave is the so-called positive rolandic sharp wave, characterized by predominant positive polarity, large amplitude and specific localization in central regions (Dreyfus-Brisac, 1972; Marret *et al.*, 1992; Aso *et al.*, 1993; Baud *et al.*, 1998; Vermeulen *et al.*, 2003). These transient features have been associated with different brain lesions in preterm infants, such as intraventricular haemorrhages, hydrocephalus and white matter lesions. In our experience these abnormalities are more frequently detectable in cases of severe periventricular leukomalacia and occur some weeks after the hypoxic-ischaemic insult (that is, at around the time cysts are observable on an ultrasound scan). Positive temporal sharp waves also relate to brain lesions in preterm infants, although their prognostic significance is still debated (Castro Conde *et al.*, 2004).

Delta and theta sharp rhythmic activities certainly have an epileptic significance (both ictal and interictal) (Fig. 7). It is important to distinguish these activities from other physiological maturational transient patterns such as the preterm infant's temporal or occipital theta (temporal and occipital saw-tooth). First, the preterm infant's theta is characteristic of specific PMAs (whereas theta sharp rhythmic activities are more frequent at around full term). Second, occipital-temporal saw-tooth activity shows a very regular (almost sinusoidal) appearance, whereas these epileptiform abnormalities are generally sharp, sometimes with interposed spikes, giving rise to something similar to spike-wave complexes (Biagioni *et al.*, 1996b). Finally, alpha discharges are generally characterized by low amplitude activity within the alpha band. Distinguishing between this waveform and the 8–22 Hz activity that constitutes the rapid component of 'delta brush' is often not easy. A lack of underlying slow waves, a regular appearance (the delta brush is usually sharp), and the associated representation of other epileptiform abnormalities (for example, sharp waves) in the same location can help the diagnosis (Biagioni *et al.*, 1996b).

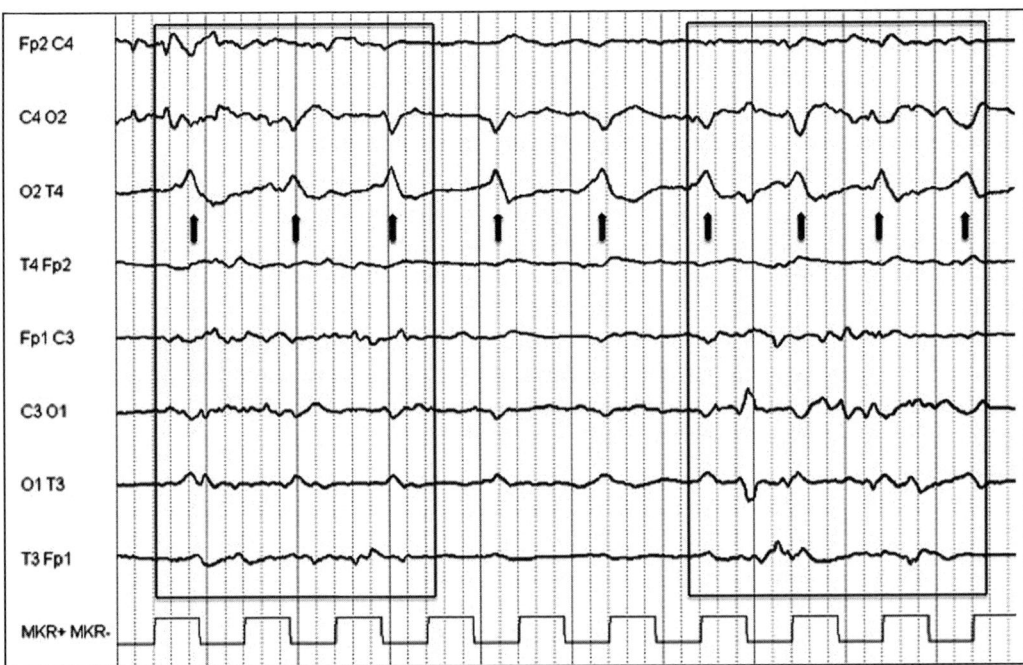

Fig. 7. EEG recorded on day 2 in an infant born at 40 weeks postmenstrual age with birth asphyxia. The tracing is constantly discontinuous (bursts are shown in the squares), with paroxysmal abnormalities consisting in delta sharp waves on the right occipital region (arrows), diffusing to the left occipital region.

Abnormal EEG from 1 to 24 months of corrected age

As stressed above, there is a significant change in the normal organization of cerebral electrical activity after the end of the first month CA. This same change is also observable in infants with pathology. Obviously, in this age range it is also possible to distinguish between background EEG abnormalities on the one hand and ictal-interictal (or epileptiform or, even better, paroxysmal) abnormalities on the other. Nevertheless, in infancy, changes in background activity and paroxysmal waveforms are often so strictly linked to each other (particularly in infantile epileptic encephalopathies) that it is hard to define a precise border between them. Major background EEG abnormalities – such as constant low voltage, interhemispheric asymmetry, and a constantly discontinuous pattern – can also be identified after the neonatal period in the case of acute hypoxic-ischaemic insults or in other severe CNS diseases (such as trauma, intoxication, encephalitis, metabolic disorders, tumours, and so on).

The characteristics and also the prognostic significance of these EEG abnormalities are similar to those described above for the neonate (Limperopoulos *et al.*, 2001). Maturational abnormalities, in contrast, are generally not detectable at this age. In particular, although in some conditions it is possible to register the absence or abnormal shape of some specific physiological EEG features (for example, rhythmic activities in posterior regions corresponding with eye closure, sleep spindles, and so on), in no child is it possible to observe in the same recording activities that are typical of two different age periods (as in the dysmature pattern of the newborn). For example, posterior rhythms are sometimes absent in infants with damage to the visual cortex or pathways but, when present, these activities have a normal frequency for the age (Biagioni *et al.*, 2002).

The most frequent background EEG abnormality in infants with previous perinatal hypoxic-ischaemic haemorrhagic encephalopathy is probably the excess of slow waves. This finding is characterized by high voltage (up to 300 µV) 0.5–3.5 Hz activities, diffuse or localized in some regions of one or both hemispheres, observable during both wakefulness and sleep. Slow waves can be constantly detectable or intermittent (that is, organized in bursts), and paroxysmal abnormalities (sharp waves, spikes) are always interposed (see above). When the excess of slow waves is marked, diffuse and constant, with several interposed spikes and poly-spikes, we are faced with a severe disorganization of cerebral electrical activity giving rise to the so-called hypsarrhythmic pattern (Rando et al., 2004). This last finding is characteristic of the most severe infantile epileptic encephalopathies, such as West syndrome. A full description of ictal and interictal EEG patterns in infantile spasms or in other epileptic syndromes of infancy is obviously beyond the scope of this chapter. Nevertheless, it is important to stress that serial EEG recordings constitute a mandatory prognostic tool in the follow-up of at-risk newborns, not only for psychomotor development but also for early diagnosis of severe epileptic syndromes.

In infants with symptomatic infantile spasms there is a long preclinical phase preceding the hypsarrhythmic pattern. During this period (generally beginning in the second month post-term) bursts of abnormal slow waves and interposed spikes gradually appear in some cerebral regions (Suzuki et al., 2003). Afterwards, these abnormalities increase their amplitude, spread to other locations and become more frequent. Moreover, besides spikes and poly-spikes, it is possible to detect briefs runs of rapid (10–22 Hz) rhythms, particularly corresponding with awakening and drowsiness (Vigevano et al., 2001). When these rhythms become synchronous in the two hemispheres and are accompanied by a short suppression, clinical spasms appear, although generally in a 'subtle' way, such as slight head flexion, slight shoulder movement, eye deviation, staring, arousal, and so on. At this stage, the EEG is not yet properly hypsarrhythmic and the psychomotor impairment typical of West syndrome is not yet observed (Rando et al., 2004).

To summarize, serial EEGs in at-risk newborns permit an early diagnosis (and early pharmacological treatment with possibly better results) in symptomatic infantile spasms. As far as the correlation between neonatal EEG abnormalities and the subsequent occurrence of infantile spasms is concerned, it is probably true that early background EEG abnormalities (for example, dysmature EEG in preterm infants, and constantly discontinuous pattern in full term infants) are more predictive than transient abnormal neonatal EEG features (Okumura & Watanabe, 2001). Finally, in our experience, there is almost always a 'free' interval between the disappearance of neonatal background EEG abnormalities and the appearance of the excess of slow waves leading to a pre-hypsarrhythmic pattern. Therefore, the prognostic value of EEGs recorded at the end of the first month post-term is generally low.

Cerebral function monitoring

Technical aspects

Cerebral function monitoring (CFM), also known as amplitude-integrated EEG, is a method of neurophysiological assessment suitable for prolonged recordings and is very common in neonatal intensive care units. It consists of an amplitude-integrated electroencephalogram, characterized by a single-lead trace (generally P3-P4 of the International 10–20 System). Signal processing consists of amplification, frequency filtration, and amplitude compression and rectification (Thornberg & Thiringer, 1990). Frequencies below 2 Hz and above 20 Hz are eliminated and, within this same range, higher frequencies are enhanced. The final result of this process is a very compressed trace; the lower edge of the tracing reflects a possibly stable measurement of non-rhythmic activities, the so-called 'minimum level of cerebral activity', whereas the upper edge reflects both rhythmic and non-rhythmic activities (the so-called 'maximum level of cerebral activity'). The width of the trace indicates the variability of the signal. Amplitudes are reported on a semilogarithmic scale and range between 0 and 100 µV.

Normal CFM patterns

The normal neonatal CFM tracing usually shows periods characterized by different amplitudes. This finding is also observable in preterm infants but it is more evident at term, when it is easy to distinguish between phases of broad bandwidth, corresponding to periods of quiet sleep, and phases of narrow bandwidth, corresponding to active sleep or wakefulness (Thornberg & Thiringer, 1990). Similar variations are observable from the 31st or 32nd week of PMA and again probably reflect modifications of the sleep-wake condition. By comparing CFM traces of full term and preterm infants, it can be seen that at low PMAs the bandwidth is generally broader and the minimum level of cerebral activity is located at a lower level (1.9 ± 0.5 µV in the low PMA preterm infant). Approaching term, the CFM trace becomes narrower – largely because of a raising of the lower edge – and well defined, state-related amplitude variations are detectable (Thornberg & Thiringer, 1990). Obviously, it is not possible to recognize in the CFM tracing the maturational patterns that characterize the EEG in preterm infants, such as temporal saw-tooth or delta brush patterns. This technique of recording rather reflects the development of the general organization of brain electrical activities, such as the differentiation of state-related patterns, the increase in minimum level of cerebral activity (which probably relates to increased amplitudes within inter-burst intervals of discontinuous EEG patterns), and a progressive reduction in maximum voltages.

Abnormal CFM patterns

CFM is now widely employed in neonatal intensive care units, as it is easy to use and allows on-line monitoring of cerebral activity (de Vries & Hellstrom-Westas, 2005). Its interpretation is also easy, even without specific knowledge of clinical neurophysiology, and therefore it is suitable for paediatricians and neonatologists. Despite the oversimplification of this recording technique, research results indicate a high diagnostic and prognostic value of CFM in neonates, in particular in full term infants with hypoxic-ischaemic encephalopathy (Eken *et al.*, 1995; Hellstrom-Westas *et al.*, 1995; al Naqeeb *et al.*, 1999; Toet *et al.*, 1999). Specific abnormalities of full term CFM have been described by various investigators. The classification used by Toet and colleagues (Toet *et al.*, 1999) is as follows:

(a) Isoelectric tracing (flat tracing): very low voltage, mainly inactive, with activity below 5 µV;
(b) Continuous extremely low voltage: continuous pattern of very low voltage (around or below 5 µV);
(c) Burst suppression: discontinuous pattern; periods of very low voltage are intermixed with bursts of higher amplitude;
(d) Discontinuous normal voltage: discontinuous trace where the voltage is predominantly above 5 µV.

Isoelectric tracings and continuous low voltage patterns consistently relate to a very poor outcome, whereas burst suppression is also compatible with a normal evolution (Hellstrom-Westas *et al.*, 1995), especially when non-persistent in subsequent recordings (Toet *et al.*, 1999). Other investigators have applied a quantitative classification, based on the voltage of the upper and lower edges of the trace (al Naqeeb et al., 1999). Moderately abnormal amplitudes (upper margin > 10 µV, lower margin < 5 µV) are associated with a negative outcome in most cases, whereas suppressed amplitudes (upper margin < 10 µV, lower margin < 5 µV) never result in a normal evolution.

Fewer reports are available on CFM background abnormalities in preterm infants. Indeed, while the most frequent anomalies of the full term infant's background electrical activity (that is, what is observable on the EEG as a constant low voltage or a burst suppression) are recognizable by means of CFM, the specific alterations of maturational features that characterize the EEG of pathological preterm infants do not seem able to modify CFM, nor can specific abnormal transient activity, such as positive sharp waves, be distinguished on such a compressed trace. Nevertheless, there is some evidence that the occurrence of continuous CFM activity and the appearance of differentiated state-related patterns indicate a positive prognosis in low PMA preterm infants, whereas low voltage traces indicate a poor prognosis (Hellstrom-Westas et al., 1991; Hellstrom-Westas, 1992).

As far as the recognition of neonatal epileptic phenomena is concerned, some descriptions of specific CFM patterns are available in published reports. Al Naqeeb and colleagues (al Naqeeb et al., 1999) reported that seizures are characterized by a sudden increase in voltage, accompanied by a narrowing of the bandwidth and followed by a period of suppression. Hellstrom-Vestas (1992) described repeated periods of increased voltage activity on the CFM, consisting of the so-called saw-tooth pattern and corresponding to low voltage discharges on the EEG. Another common CFM correlate of prolonged EEG discharges is prolonged plateaus of high voltage in both the lower and the upper edges. Nevertheless, it is also widely reported that brief or focal seizure activity can be missed by this technique (Hellstrom-Westas, 1992; Toet et al., 2002; Rennie et al., 2004), necessitating its use in association with standard EEG methods.

Evoked potentials

Essential information on the integrity of the nervous system, and in particular of the central and peripheral sensory pathways, is provided by the study of evoked potentials, consisting of the electrical responses to repeated visual, auditory, or somatosensory stimulation. By averaging a large number of responses it is possible to increase the signal to noise ratio, so detecting low amplitude electrical potentials generated by the stimulation. Evoked potentials have been shown to be of great value in assessing the maturation of the nervous system from birth onwards, and in the prediction of neurodevelopmental outcome after early insult. All three main types of evoked potentials – that is, visual evoked potentials (VEPs), brain stem auditory evoked potentials (BAEPs), and somatosensory evoked potentials (SEPs) – can be assessed from birth, even in preterm newborns, although in the latter there are greater technical restrictions and the technique is therefore less often used in clinical practice. Various adjustments from the adult settings are required in order to apply this technique to neonates and older infants, including hardware features, the number and frequency of the stimuli, filtering and post-processing. The positive and negative deflections following the stimulus are analysed in terms of general wave morphology, amplitude and latency of the single peaks, and interpeak intervals. All these aspects have different maturational and clinical meanings which have to be carefully assessed in relation to developmental changes, and normative data specific to the laboratory and the setting used. In the following section, the three main types of evoked potentials used in clinical practice during infancy will be considered. In particular, for each technique we provide information on the main methodological issues, the maturation profile of the responses, and the current clinical value and application.

Visual evoked potentials

VEPs are generated by the activation of neuronal populations in the occipital cortex and represent the summation of dendritic synaptic potentials of these neurons (Freeman & Thibos, 1975). The exact locations of the generator sources of the VEP are not well defined in humans; however, increasing data seem to support the hypothesis of different circumscribed neuronal generators in the mesial and lateral occipital cortex, with different latencies of activation and timing of maturation (Arroyo et al., 1997). There are two major classes of VEP stimulation: luminance and pattern. The first is usually delivered as a uniform flash of light, the flash VEP (FVEP); while the second may be presented in either a reversal or an onset-offset fashion, the pattern VEP (PVEP). PVEPs are considered more stable and reliable and are therefore the criterion standard in collaborative adult patients; however, their use is limited during infancy as they can only be elicited in individuals who are capable of prolonged fixations on the stimulus.

Flash VEPs: FVEPs are commonly used from birth in infants at risk of neurodevelopmental disabilities. The analysis time is usually set at 1000 ms, as the major components of the response emerge between 200 and 500 ms. The stimulus frequency should be low enough (< 1 Hz) to allow the visual system to return to its resting state. The behavioural state of the infant should be consistent over recordings, as this can affect both amplitude and latency. The first deflection elicited during development is visible in preterm neonates at around 24 weeks' gestational age (GA), and consists of a large negative wave occurring at approximately 300 ms (N300) (Fig. 8). The N300 shortens in latency as the infant matures, at a rate of 4.6–5.5 ms per week (Tsuneishi et al., 1995). The second visible component emerges at around 34 weeks GA, consisting of a positive peak occurring at about 200 ms (P200). At term the response consists of a negative-positive-negative complex which will gradually achieve adult characteristics during the first 6 months of life, with a progressive decrease of the three main peak latencies.

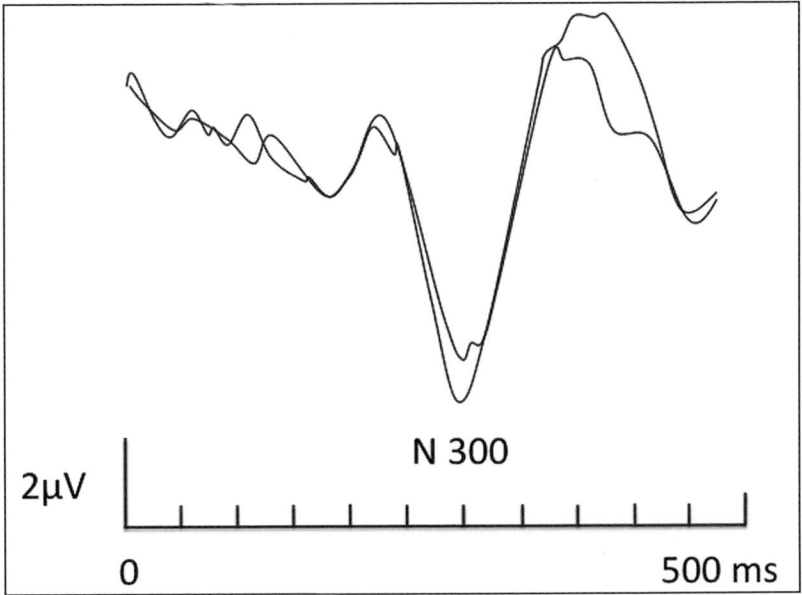

Fig. 8. Flash visual evoked potentials (FVEP) in a preterm infant born at 32 weeks' gestational age with birth asphyxia, who on ultrasound had a periventricular flare persisting for 14 days. FVEP were recorded at 3 weeks and showed normal wave morphology and latency. The outcome at 1 year was normal.

The main clinical application of FVEP in infancy is without doubt related to the early prediction of both visual impairment and neurological outcome in neonates with different types of prenatal and perinatal disorders. This technique has been shown to be a very good predictor of visual impairment of central origin (CVI), both in term infants with perinatal asphyxia (McCulloch & Skarf, 1991; McCulloch & Taylot, 1992) and in preterm infants with cystic leukomalacia (de Vries *et al.*, 1987; Eken *et al.*, 1996). Good correlation between FVEP responses and behavioural assessment of visual acuity (for example, acuity cards) has been shown in these infants, with an overall increase in predictive power with the combined use of the two approaches.

The clinical value of FVEP in the prediction of neurodevelopment has been shown to be different in preterm and full term infants. Several studies have failed to show a clear-cut correlation between abnormal FVEP and outcome in preterm infants (Beverley *et al.*, 1990; Shepherd *et al.*, 1999). Nevertheless, two main features of the response have been shown to be often associated with adverse outcome: a delayed N300 before term, and an absent P200 at term. Conversely, a very strong correlation with neurodevelopmental outcome has been shown consistently in studies in the term infant with birth asphyxia (Whyte *et al.*, 1986; McCulloch & Skarf, 1991; Muttitt *et al.*, 1991; Taylor *et al.*, 1992). A persistent abnormality of the FVEP during the first week of life has been shown to be the best predictor of an abnormal outcome, while a normal response by the end of the first week is usually associated with normal development. This type of profile is similar to what has been shown in comparable populations with EEG background activity, and probably shares the same pathophysiological basis. Other types of evoked potentials have been used in this type of patient and an even stronger predictive value has been shown, in particular by the somatosensory evoked potentials (see below).

Pattern VEPs: Different types of PVEP can be used during infancy. The pattern reversal VEP, based on black and white checkerboards, has been the most widely studied both in both children and adults, showing a relatively low intra- and intersubject variability of waveform and peak latency. However, its use early in infancy has been limited by poor cooperation at this age, particularly in infants with neurological problems. This technique has been used in preterm infants with inconsistent results, as the morphology of the waveform becomes more stable only as the infant approaches term. For this reason its application during the neonatal period for prognostic purposes in at-risk newborns has been limited. During the first months of life a rapid decrease in the latency of all peaks occurs. The adult-like latency of the P100 peak is reached by about 1 year of age with large checkerboards, and later with smaller ones. The variability in the maturational profile is, however, extremely high. This gradual decrease in latency might have a potential application as an index of neuronal development, but full evidence is not yet available (Porciatti *et al.*, 2002). Another type of PVEP which has recently been applied in early infancy is the orientation-reversal steady state VEP. This is based on high rate stimulations (4 or 8 Hz), generating a sinusoidal waveform which can eventually undergo statistical post-processing analysis of temporal coherence. This technique has been used in particular in the assessment of cortical visual maturation during the first year of life, and has shown high power in predicting cerebral visual impairment and neurodevelopment in newborns at risk (Mercuri *et al.*, 1995; Mercuri *et al.*, 1998).

Brain stem auditory evoked potentials

BAEPs are generated by the activation of neuronal populations within the auditory brain stem pathway in response to an acoustic stimulus. They consist of a relatively stable response composed of seven sequential positive waves arising during impulse transmission between the auditory nerve, pons and midbrain. The most important components of the potential during infancy are waves I, III and V (Fig. 9) (Stockard-Pope & Werner, 1992). Wave I is produced in the eighth nerve by the transformation into impulses of tone-specific responses in the hair cells; wave III is formed at the level of the cochlear nucleus of the brain stem, while wave V is produced at the level of the rostral part of the pons and the caudal part of the midbrain. The I–V interpeak latency has been shown to be unaffected by click intensity after a certain threshold and independent of peripheral auditory function; it has therefore been considered a reliable measure of central auditory conduction time (Eggermont & Don, 1980).

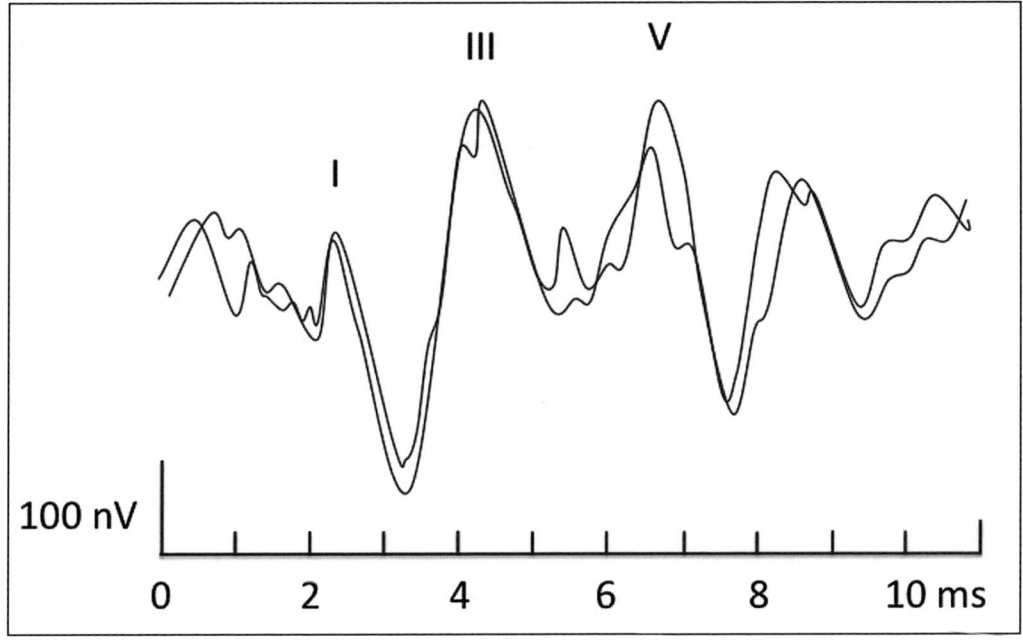

Fig. 9. Brain stem auditory evoked potentials (BAEP) at 35 weeks postmenstrual age in an infant born at 34 weeks' gestational age. Age-adequate latencies and amplitudes are found.

BAEPs are commonly used from birth in infants at risk of sensorial or neurodevelopmental disabilities. The analysis time is usually set between 15 and 20 ms, as the waves normally arise in the first 10 ms after the stimulus. A repetition rate of 10 per second can safely be used. The stimulus is presented monoaurally and its intensity has to be calibrated above the hearing threshold in order to get a full response. A contralateral masking is advisable to avoid trans-bone conduction to the opposite ear. The three major waves of the potential can be recognized from 25 weeks GA onwards. All peak latencies decrease gradually with age, with the V wave decreasing faster. This results in an overall reduction of the I–V interpeak interval with time. The effect of preterm exposure to auditory stimulation on the maturation of the auditory system has been investigated, with equivocal results, in part because of the different inclusion criteria used and therefore the risk level of the population studied. At term the morphology of the potential can easily be compared with adult responses, but the latencies are significantly higher. Adult-like responses are reached at about 2 years of age. It has to be noted that a high interindividual variability has been consistently reported in cross-sectional studies; however, the intra-individual maturation rate is fairly regular. As a general rule, a prolonged latency of wave I associated with a normal I–V peak interval is suggestive of a peripheral abnormality, while a normal latency of wave I associated with a prolonged I–V interpeak interval indicates a disorder of central conduction time. In both cases an early diagnosis of a hearing defect is mandatory, especially with regard to language development, as it has been shown to be more easily preserved when treatment is started within the first 6 months of life (Murray *et al.*, 1985). For this reason, when abnormal results are detected, repeated assessment once every 2 months should be carried out.

The use of BAEPs as a predictor of neurological outcome in infants with brain insults has also been extensively investigated. The features that are most commonly associated with abnormal development include absence or low amplitude of later peaks and prolonged I–V conduction intervals (Murray *et al.*, 1985). The majority of studies investigating the predictive value of this technique, however, stress the presence of a large number of false negatives with respect to neurological outcome. This is mainly caused by the frequent sparing of the deep structures explored by BAEPs in many infants with brain lesions and an abnormal outcome. This finding – together with the high prognostic value of other neurophysiological techniques such as EEG, VEPs, and SEPs – has limited the application of this type of potential as a predictor of neurological outcome.

Somatosensory evoked potentials

SEPs are generated by the activation of neuronal populations within the somatosensory pathway in response to a sensory stimulation – that is, the peripheral nerve, posterior column of the spinal cord and, following decussation, the medial lemniscus, thalamus and parietal cortex. In neonates and infants, the peripheral stimulation most commonly used is electrical stimulation of the median or tibial nerve (Laureau & Marlot, 1990; George & Taylot, 1991; Boor & Goebel, 2000). The peripheral somatosensory pathways can be assessed reliably over Erb's point (that is, the site at the lateral root of the brachial plexus 2–3 cm above the clavicle) (Laureau *et al.*, 1988) and over the spinal cord (Laureau & Marlot, 1990). These subcortical responses are more constantly recordable and stable than the cortical responses during the first 6 months of life, as the early maturation of peripheral nerve and posterior column fibres is significantly faster than that of the more central structures (Laureau *et al.*, 1988; Boor & Goebel, 2000).

The cortical responses are assessed by means of contralateral rolandic scalp electrodes. The first cortical response to median nerve stimulation, termed N19 in adults, is called N1 in newborns and young infants. The early N1 deflection is measurable in most normal preterm infants from at least the seventh gestational month, and presents a latency markedly longer than in term infants and adults (Taylor & Wynn-Williams, 1986). From birth and up to about 3 years of age, there is a developmental trend of shortening of the peak latencies, increase in the amplitudes, and decrease in the duration of the waveform (Laureau *et al.*, 1988). This increased conduction velocity is secondary to the myelination and maturation of the pathways; while after the age of 3 years an opposing mechanism is more dominant – that is, elongation of the pathway resulting from physical growth causes the latencies to start to lengthen. A similar general pattern of maturation can also be shown after tibial nerve stimulation.

One of the major clinical applications of SEPs during infancy concerns the prediction of neurodevelopmental outcome of preterm and term infants at neurological risk. The prognostic power of SEPs in preterm newborns with brain lesions has been widely studied, with unclear results. When the median nerve was assessed, either a low sensitivity or a low specificity was reported in the various studies, possibly reflecting differences in methodology and an overall limited prognostic value of the technique. In this population a greater prognostic value has been shown by studies assessing the tibial nerve, probably as a consequence of the frequency of lower limb involvement following preterm lesions. Another important field of application of infant SEPs is the asphyxiated term infant. General agreement has been reached by different investigators on the high value of this technique in predicting an abnormal outcome in newborns with hypoxic-ischaemic encephalopathy. The technique is particularly sensitive during the first 72 hours after delivery, when it appears more powerful than ultrasound or other types of evoked potential (Eken *et al.*, 1995).

Functional magnetic resonance imaging in newborns and infants

fMRI is a non-invasive technique based on the principle that brain functional activity is associated to regional changes in MR signal. In particular, fMRI takes advantage of the paramagnetic properties of deoxygenated haemoglobin, the concentrations of which change locally during neuronal activity, generating an endogenous contrast known as BOLD effect (blood-oxygenation-level-dependent) (Ogawa *et al.*, 1998) (Fig. 10). In the past 10 years, fMRI has been applied more consistently to newborns and infants; nevertheless, several important methodological issues still make it a technique suitable only for a few highly specialized centres. A detailed description of the specific aspects that distinguish adult and infant fMRI is beyond the scope of this chapter. It is important to emphasize, however, that one of the major issues in infant fMRI is the model of haemodynamic response (HRF) which best fits the temporal profile of HRF at this early stage – an aspect on which the scientific debate seems to be still open (Poldrack *et al.*, 2002; Seghier *et al.*, 2006). This is further complicated by the fact that infant studies are usually carried out during sleep following mild sedation (in most studies with chloral hydrate), a factor that could affect the sign (negative/positive) and site of the activations (Born *et al.*, 2002).

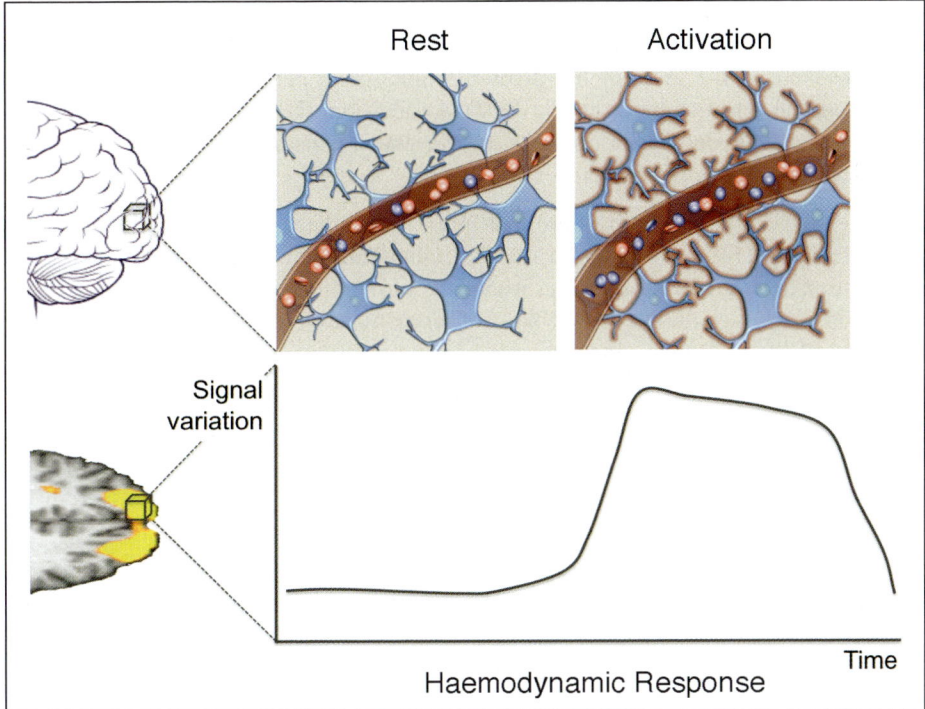

Fig. 10. Graphic representation of the haemodynamic response associated with brain function, on which the functional magnetic resonance imaging blood-oxygen-level-dependent (BOLD) contrast is based. During neuronal firing, the blood flow is increased and the brain extracts greater quantities of oxygen, transforming oxyhaemoglobin in deoxyhaemoglobin.

Most of the fMRI studies in infants and neonates have explored the visual system, usually with the aim of localizing primary visual areas and exploring structure-function correlations during development in both normal and pathological conditions (Born et al., 1996; Yamada et al., 1997; Born et al., 1998; Martin et al., 1999; Born et al., 2000; Liu et al., 2000; Morita et al., 2000; Yamada et al., 2000; Konishi et al., 2002; Muramoto et al., 2002; Seghier et al., 2005). The importance of these studies lies on their having identified significant differences relative to older subjects, which shed some light on early visual development and plasticity of the visual system, particularly in infants with congenital brain damage (Born et al., 2000; Seghier et al., 2004; Seghier et al., 2005). The two main differences compared with older children and adults concerned the site of visual activation and the sign of the BOLD responses. Activations following visual stimulations are generally located in regions of the occipital cortex that are more anterior than at older ages, for reasons that are still poorly understood (Born et al., 1998; Martin et al., 1999; Morita et al., 2000). Also, at variance with older subjects, BOLD responses are mostly negative during early infancy – that is, visual regions are apparently more active during rest condition than during stimulation. This phenomenon might be related to the age-dependent rate of oxygen consumption, which is maximum at an earlier age, in the phase of active synaptogenesis (Muramoto et al., 2002).

Another area in which infant fMRI has found important applications is represented by the auditory and language systems, as a result in particular of pioneering work by Dehaene-Lambertz's and coworkers (Dehaene-Lambertz et al., 2002; Dehaene-Lambertz et al., 2006). In a series of papers on early development of speech perception, not limited to the use of fMRI, these investigators have shown how the complex brain network involved in speech perception includes the superior temporal sulcus bilaterally, with a significant functional asymmetry toward the left hemisphere at the level of the planum temporale, a network anatomically similar to that of adults (Dehaene-Lambertz et al., 2002). In addition, these same regions are activated by speech with a well defined temporal structure and a capacity for memorizing sentences (Dehaene-Lambertz et al., 2006).

On the whole, these studies demonstrate that infant fMRI, despite its methodological pitfalls, is a suitable technique for early exploration of brain function. This can be of particular relevance in infants with congenital brain damage, where the possibility to perform longitudinal assessments of brain function from the early phases of reorganization could open the way to a deeper understanding of the underlying mechanisms of neuroplasticity.

References

al Naqeeb, N., Edwards, A.D., Cowan, F.M. & Azzopardi, D. (1999): Assessment of neonatal encephalopathy by amplitude-integrated electroencephalography. *Pediatrics* **103,** 1263–1271.

Anders, T., Emde, R. & Parmelee, A. (1971): *A manual of standardized terminology, techniques and criteria for scoring of the states of sleep and wakefulness in newborn infants.* Los Angeles: UCLA Brain Information Service/BRI Publications Office.

Anderson, C.M., Torres, F. & Faoro, A. (1985): The EEG of the early premature. *Electroencephalogr. Clin. Neurophysiol.* **60,** 95–105.

Arroyo, S., Lesser, R.P., Poon, W.T., Webber, W.R. & Gordon, B. (1997): Neuronal generators of visual evoked potentials in humans: visual processing in the human cortex. *Epilepsia* **38,** 600–610.

Aso, K., Abdab-Barmada, M. & Scher, M.S. (1993): EEG and the neuropathology in premature neonates with intraventricular hemorrhage. *J. Clin. Neurophysiol.* **10,** 304–313.

Battin, M.R., Maalouf, E.F., Counsell, S.J., Herlihy, A.H., Rutherford, M.A., Azzopardi, D. & Edwards, A.D. (1998): Magnetic resonance imaging of the brain in very preterm infants: visualization of the germinal matrix, early myelination, and cortical folding. *Pediatrics* **101**, 957–962.

Baud, O., d'Allest, A.M., Lacaze-Masmonteil, T., Zupan, V., Nedelcoux, H., Boithias, C., Delaveaucoupet, J. & Dehan, M. (1998): The early diagnosis of periventricular leukomalacia in premature infants with positive rolandic sharp waves on serial electroencephalography. *J. Pediatr.* **132**, 813–817.

Beverley, D.W., Smith, I.S., Beesley, P., Jones, J. & Rhodes, N. (1990): Relationship of cranial ultrasonography, visual and auditory evoked responses with neurodevelopmental outcome. *Dev. Med. Child Neurol.* **32**, 210–222.

Biagioni, E., Bartalena, L., Boldrini, A., Cioni, G., Giancola, S. & Ipata, A.E. (1994): Background EEG activity in preterm infants: correlation of outcome with selected maturational features. *Electroencephalogr. Clin. Neurophysiol.* **91**, 154–162.

Biagioni, E., Bartalena, L., Biver, P., Pieri, R. & Cioni, G. (1996a): Electroencephalographic dysmaturity in preterm infants: a prognostic tool in the early postnatal period. *Neuropediatrics* **27**, 311–316.

Biagioni, E., Boldrini, A., Bottone, U., Pieri, R. & Cioni, G. (1996b): Prognostic value of abnormal EEG transients in preterm and full-term neonates. *Electroencephalogr. Clin. Neurophysiol.* **99**, 1–9.

Biagioni, E., Bartalena, L., Boldrini, A., Pieri, R. & Cioni, G. (1999): Constantly discontinuous EEG patterns in full-term neonates with hypoxic-ischaemic encephalopathy. *Clin. Neurophysiol.* **110**, 1510–1515.

Biagioni, E., Frisone, M.F., Laroche, S., Rutherford, M., Counsell, S., Cioni, G., Azzopardi, D., Mercuri, E. & Cowan, F. (2000): Occipital sawtooth: a physiological EEG pattern in very premature infants. *Clin. Neurophysiol.* **111**, 2145–2149.

Biagioni, E., Mercuri, E., Rutherford, M., Cowan, F., Azzopardi, D., Frisone, M.F., Cioni, G. & Dubowitz, L. (2001): Combined use of electroencephalogram and magnetic resonance imaging in full-term neonates with acute encephalopathy. *Pediatrics* **107**, 461–468.

Biagioni, E., Cioni, G., Cowan, F., Rutherford, M., Anker, S., Atkinson, J., Braddick, O.J., Canapicchi, R., Guzzetta, A. & Mercuri, E. (2002): Visual function and EEG reactivity in infants with perinatal brain lesions at 1 year. *Dev. Med. Child Neurol.* **44**, 171–176.

Boor, R. & Goebel, B. (2000): Maturation of near-field and far-field somatosensory evoked potentials after median nerve stimulation in children under 4 years of age. *Clin. Neurophysiol.* **111**, 1070–1081.

Born, A.P., Rostrup, E., Leth, H., Peitersen, B. & Lou, H.C. (1996): Change of visually induced cortical activation patterns during development. *Lancet* **347**, 543.

Born, A.P., Leth, H., Miranda, M.J., Rostrup, E., Stensgaard, A., Peitersen, B., Larsson, H.B. & Lou, H.C. (1998): Visual activation in infants and young children studied by functional magnetic resonance imaging. *Pediatr. Res.* **44**, 578–583.

Born, A.P., Miranda, M.J., Rostrup, E., Toft, P.B., Peitersen, B., Larsson, H.B. & Lou, H.C. (2000): Functional magnetic resonance imaging of the normal and abnormal visual system in early life. *Neuropediatrics* **31**, 24–32.

Born, A.P., Law, I., Lund, T.E., Rostrup, E., Hanson, L.G., Wildschiødtz, G., Lou, H.C. & Paulson, O.B. (2002): Cortical deactivation induced by visual stimulation in human slow-wave sleep. *Neuroimage* **17**, 1325–1335.

Castro Conde, J.R., Martínez, E.D., Campo, C.G., Pérez, A.M. & McLean, M.L. (2004): Positive temporal sharp waves in preterm infants with and without brain ultrasound lesions. *Clin. Neurophysiol.* **115**, 2479–2488.

Curzi-Dascalova, L. & Mirmiran, M. (1996): *Manuel des techniques d'enregistrement et d'analyse des stades de sommeil et de veille chez le prématuré et le nouveau-né à term-e.* Paris: Inserm.

Dehaene-Lambertz, G., Dehaene, S. & Hertz-Pannier, L. (2002): Functional neuroimaging of speech perception in infants. *Science* **298**, 2013–2015.

Dehaene-Lambertz, G., Hertz-Pannier, L., Dubois, J., Mériaux, S., Roche, A., Sigman, M. & Dehaene, S. (2006): Functional organization of perisylvian activation during presentation of sentences in preverbal infants. *Proc. Natl. Acad. Sci. USA* **103**, 14240–14245.

de Vries, L.S., Connell, J.A., Dubowitz, L.M., Oozeer, R.C., Dubowitz, V. & Pennock, J.M. (1987): Neurological, electrophysiological and MRI abnormalities in infants with extensive cystic leukomalacia. *Neuropediatrics* **18**, 61–66.

de Vries, L.S. & Hellstrom-Westas, L. (2005): Role of cerebral function monitoring in the newborn. *Arch. Dis. Child. Fetal Neonatal Ed.* **90**, F201–F207.

Dreyfus-Brisac, C. (1972): *The electroencephalogram of fullterm newborns and premature infants. Handbook of electroencephalography and clinical neurophysiology*, pp. 6–23. Amsterdam: Elsevier.

Eaton, D.G., Wertheim, D., Oozeer, R., Dubowitz, L.M. & Dubowitz, V. (1994): Reversible changes in cerebral activity associated with acidosis in preterm neonates. *Acta Paediatr.* **83**, 486–492.

Eggermont, J.J. & Don, M. (1980): Analysis of the click-evoked brainstem potentials in humans using high-pass noise masking. II. Effect of click intensity. *J. Acoust Soc. Am.* **68**, 1671–1675.

Eken, P., Toet, M.C., Groenendaal, F. & de Vries, L.S. (1995): Predictive value of early neuroimaging, pulsed Doppler and neurophysiology in full term infants with hypoxic-ischaemic encephalopathy. *Arch. Dis. Child. Fetal Neonatal Ed.* **73**, F75–F80.

Eken, P., de Vries, L.S., van Nieuwenhuizen, O., Schalij-Delfos, N.E., Reits, D. & Spekreijse, H. (1996): Early predictors of cerebral visual impairment in infants with cystic leukomalacia. *Neuropediatrics* **27**, 16–25.

Ferrari, F., Torricelli, A., Giustardi, A., Benatti, A., Bolzani, R., Ori, L. & Frigieri, G. (1992): Bioelectric brain maturation in fullterm infants and in healthy and pathological preterm infants at term post-menstrual age. *Early Hum. Dev.* **28**, 37–63.

Ferrari, F., Biagioni, E., Boldrini, A., Roversi, M.F. & Cioni, G. (2001): *Neonatal electroencephalography.* In: *Fetal and neonatal neurology and neurosurgery,* ed. M.I. Levene & M. Whittle. London: Churchill Livingstone.

Freeman, R.D. & Thibos, L.N. (1975): Visual evoked responses in humans with abnormal visual experience. *J. Physiol. (Lond.)* **247**, 711–724.

George, S.R. & Taylor, M.J. (1991): Somatosensory evoked potentials in neonates and infants: developmental and normative data. *Electroencephalogr. Clin. Neurophysiol.* **80**, 94–102.

Hayakawa, F., Okumura, A., Kato, T., Kuno, K. & Watanabe, K. (1997): Disorganized patterns: chronic-stage EEG abnormality of the late neonatal period following severely depressed EEG activities in early preterm infants. *Neuropediatrics* **28**, 272–275.

Hellstrom-Westas, L. (1992): Comparison between tape-recorded and amplitude-integrated EEG monitoring in sick newborn infants. *Acta Paediatr.* **81**, 812–819.

Hellstrom-Westas, L., Rosen, I. & Svenningsen, N.W. (1991): Cerebral function monitoring during the first week of life in extremely small low birthweight (ESLBW) infants. *Neuropediatrics* **22**, 27–32.

Hellstrom-Westas, L., Rosen, I. & Svenningsen, N.W. (1995): Predictive value of early continuous amplitude integrated EEG recordings on outcome after severe birth asphyxia in full term infants. *Arch. Dis. Child. Fetal Neonatal Ed.* **72**, F34–F38.

Holmes, G.L. & Lombroso, C.T. (1993): Prognostic value of background patterns in the neonatal EEG. *J. Clin. Neurophysiol.* **10**, 323–352.

Hughes, J.R., Miller, J.K., Fino, J.J. & Hughes, C.A. (1990): The sharp theta rhythm on the occipital areas of prematures (STOP): a newly described waveform. *Clin. Electroencephalogr.* **21**, 77–87.

Kato, T., Okumura, A., Hayakawa, F., Kuno, K. & Watanabe, K. (2004): Electroencephalographic aspects of periventricular hemorrhagic infarction in preterm infants. *Neuropediatrics* **35**, 161–166.

Kellaway, P. (1987): Intensive monitoring in infants and children. *Adv. Neurol.* **46**, 127–137.

Konishi, Y., Taga, G., Yamada, H. & Hirasawa, K. (2002): Functional brain imaging using fMRI and optical topography in infancy. *Sleep Med.* **3** (suppl. 2), S41–S43.

Kostovic, I. & Jovanov-Milosevic, N. (2005): The development of cerebral connections during the first 20–45 weeks' gestation. *Semin. Fetal Neonatal Med.* **11**, 415–422.

Lamblin, M.D., André, M., Auzoux, M., Bednarek, N., Bour, F., Charollais, A., Cheliout-Heraut, F., D'Allest, A.M., De Bellecize, J., Delanoe, C., Furby, A., Frenkel, A.L., Keo-Kosal, P., Mony, L., Moutard, M.L., Navelet, Y., Nedelcoux, H., Nguyen, T.T., Nogues, B., Plouin, P., Salefranque, F., Soufflet, C., Touzery de Villepin, A., Vecchierini, M.F., Wallois, F. & Esquivel-Walls, E. (2004): Indications d'EEG dans le nouveau-né. *Arch. Pediatr.* **11**, 829–833.

Laureau, E. & Marlot, D. (1990): Somatosensory evoked potentials after median and tibial nerve stimulation in healthy newborns. *Electroencephalogr. Clin. Neurophysiol.* **76**, 453–458.

Laureau, E., Majnemer, A., Rosenblatt, B. & Riley, P. (1988): A longitudinal study of short latency somatosensory evoked responses in healthy newborns and infants. *Electroencephalogr. Clin. Neurophysiol.* **71**, 100–108.

Limperopoulos, C., Majnemer, A., Rosenblatt, B., Shevell, M.I., Rohlicek, C., Tchervenkov, C. & Gottesman, R. (2001): Association between electroencephalographic findings and neurologic status in infants with congenital heart defects. *J. Child Neurol.* **16**, 471–476.

Liu, G.T., Hunter, J., Miki, A., Fletcher, D.W., Brown, L. & Haselgrove, J.C. (2000): Functional MRI in children with congenital structural abnormalities of the occipital cortex. *Neuropediatrics* **31**, 13–15.

Lombroso, C.T. (1985): Neonatal polygraphy in full-term and premature infants: a review of normal and abnormal findings. *J. Clin. Neurophysiol.* **2**, 105–155.

Marret, S., Parain, D., Jeannot, E., Eurin, D. & Fessard, C. (1992): Positive rolandic sharp waves in the EEG of the premature newborn: a five year prospective study. *Arch. Dis. Child.* **67**, 948–951.

Martin, E., Joeri, P., Loenneker, T., Ekatodramis, D., Vitacco, D., Hennig, J. & Marcar, V.L. (1999): Visual processing in infants and children studied using functional MRI. *Pediatr. Res.* **46**, 135–140.

McCulloch, D.L. & Skarf, B. (1991): Development of the human visual system: monocular and binocular pattern VEP latency. *Invest. Ophthalmol. Vis. Sci.* **32,** 2372–2381.

McCulloch, D.L. & Taylor, M.J. (1992): Cortical blindness in children: utility of flash VEPs. *Pediatr. Neurol.* **8,** 156.

Menache, C.C., Bourgeois, B.F. & Volpe, J.J. (2002): Prognostic value of neonatal discontinuous EEG. *Pediatr. Neurol.* **27,** 93–101.

Mercuri, E., von Siebenthal, K., Tutuncuoglu, S., Guzzetta, F. & Casaer, P. (1995): The effect of behavioural states on visual evoked responses in preterm and full-term newborns. *Neuropediatrics* **26,** 211–213.

Mercuri, E., Braddick, O., Atkinson, J., Cowan, F., Anker, S., Andrew, R., Wattam-Bell, J., Rutherford, M., Counsell, S. & Dubowitz, L. (1998): Orientation-reversal and phase-reversal visual evoked potentials in full-term infants with brain lesions: a longitudinal study. *Neuropediatrics* **29,** 169–174.

Monod, N., Pajot, N. & Guidasci, S. (1972): The neonatal EEG: statistical studies and prognostic value in full-term and pre-term babies. *Electroencephalogr. Clin. Neurophysiol.* **32,** 529–544.

Morita, T., Kochiyama, T. & Yamada, H. (2000): Difference in the metabolic response to photic stimulation of the lateral geniculate nucleus and the primary visual cortex of infants: a fMRI study. *Neurosci. Res.* **38,** 63–70.

Muramoto, S., Yamada, H. & Sadato, N. (2002): Age-dependent change in metabolic response to photic stimulation of the primary visual cortex in infants: functional magnetic resonance imaging study. *J. Comput. Assist. Tomogr.* **26,** 894–901.

Murray, A.D., Javel, E. & Watson, C.S. (1985): Prognostic validity of auditory brainstem evoked response screening in newborn infants. *Am. J. Otolaryngol.* **6,** 120–131.

Muttitt, S.C., Taylor, M.J., Kobayashi, J.S., MacMillan, L. & Whyte, H.E. (1991): Serial visual evoked potentials and outcome in term birth asphyxia. *Pediatr. Neurol.* **7,** 86–90.

Nolte, R. & Haas, G. (1978): A polygraphic study of bioelectrical brain maturation in preterm infants. *Dev. Med. Child Neurol.* **20,** 167–182.

Ogawa, S., Menon, R.S., Kim, S.G. & Ugurbil, K. (1998): On the characteristics of functional magnetic resonance imaging of the brain. *Annu. Rev. Biophys. Biomol. Struct.* **27,** 447–474.

Ohtahara, S. & Yamatogi, Y. (2003): Epileptic encephalopathies in early infancy with suppression-burst. *J. Clin. Neurophysiol.* **20,** 398–407.

Okumura, A. & Watanabe, K. (2001): Clinico-electrical evolution in pre-hypsarrhythmic stage: towards prediction and prevention of West syndrome. *Brain Dev.* **23,** 482–487.

Pezzani, C., Radvanyi-Bouvet, M.F., Relier, J.P. & Monod, N. (1986): Neonatal electroencephalography during the first twenty-four hours of life in full-term newborn infants. *Neuropediatrics* **17,** 11–18.

Poldrack, R.A., Pare-Blagoev, E.J. & Grant, P.E. (2002): Pediatric functional magnetic resonance imaging: progress and challenges. *Top. Magn. Reson. Imaging* **13,** 61–70.

Porciatti, V., Pizzorusso, T. & Maffei, L. (2002): Electrophysiology of the postreceptoral visual pathway in mice. *Doc. Ophthalmol.* **104,** 69–82.

Rando, T., Bancale, A. & Baranello, G. (2004): Visual function in infants with West syndrome: correlation with EEG patterns. *Epilepsia* **45,** 781–786.

Rennie, J.M., Chorley, G., Boylan, G.B., Pressler, R., Nguyen, Y. & Hooper, R. (2004): Non-expert use of the cerebral function monitor for neonatal seizure detection. *Arch. Dis. Child. Fetal Neonatal Ed.* **89,** F37–F40.

Seghier, M.L., Lazeyras, F., Zimine, S., Maier, S.E., Hanquinet, S., Delavelle, J., Volpe, J.J. & Huppi, P.S. (2004): Combination of event-related fMRI and diffusion tensor imaging in an infant with perinatal stroke. *Neuroimage* **21,** 463–472.

Seghier, M.L., Lazeyras, F., Zimine, S., Saudan-Frei, S., Safran, A.B. & Huppi, P.S. (2005): Visual recovery after perinatal stroke evidenced by functional and diffusion MRI: case report. *BMC Neurol.* **5,** 17.

Seghier, M.L., Lazeyras, F. & Huppi, P.S. (2006): Functional MRI of the newborn. *Semin. Fetal Neonatal Med.* **11,** 479–488.

Shepherd, A.J., Saunders, K.J., McCulloch, D.L. & Dutton, G.N. (1999): Prognostic value of flash visual evoked potentials in preterm infants. *Dev. Med. Child Neurol.* **41,** 9–15.

Stockard-Pope, J. & Werner, S. (1992): *Atlas of neonatal electroenchephalography.* New York, Raven Press.

Suzuki, M., Okumura, A., Watanabe, K., Negoro, T., Hayakawa, F., Kato, T., Itomi, K., Kubota, T. & Maruyama, K. (2003): The predictive value of electroencephalogram during early infancy for later development of West syndrome in infants with cystic periventricular leukomalacia. *Epilepsia* **44,** 443–446.

Taylor, P.K. & Wynn-Williams, G.M. (1986): A modified mirror projection visual evoked potential stimulator for presenting patterns in different orientations. *Electroencephalogr. Clin. Neurophysiol.* **64,** 81–83.

Taylor, M.J., Murphy, W.J. & Whyte, H.E. (1992): Prognostic reliability of somatosensory and visual evoked potentials of asphyxiated term infants. *Dev. Med. Child Neurol.* **34,** 507–515.

Thornberg, E. & Thiringer, K. (1990): Normal pattern of the cerebral function monitor trace in term and preterm neonates. *Acta Paediatr. Scand.* **79,** 20–25.

Toet, M.C., Hellström-Westas, L., Groenendaal, F., Eken, P. & de Vries, L.S. (1999): Amplitude integrated EEG 3 and 6 hours after birth in full term neonates with hypoxic-ischaemic encephalopathy. *Arch. Dis. Child. Fetal Neonatal Ed.* **81,** F19–F23.

Toet, M.C., van der Meij, W., de Vries, L.S., Uiterwaal, C.S. & van Huffelen, K.C. (2002): Comparison between simultaneously recorded amplitude integrated electroencephalogram (cerebral function monitor) and standard electroencephalogram in neonates. *Pediatrics* **109,** 772–779.

Tsuneishi, S., Casaer, P., Fock, J.M. & Hirano, S. (1995): Establishment of normal values for flash visual evoked potentials (VEPs) in preterm infants: a longitudinal study with special reference to two components of the N1 wave. *Electroencephalogr. Clin. Neurophysiol.* **96,** 291–299.

Vecchierini, M.F., d'Allest, A.M. & Verpillat, P. (2003): EEG patterns in 10 extreme premature neonates with normal neurological outcome: qualitative and quantitative data. *Brain Dev.* **25,** 330–337.

Vermeulen, R.J., Sie, L.T. & Jonkman, E.J. (2003): Predictive value of EEG in neonates with periventricular leukomalacia. *Dev. Med. Child Neurol.* **45,** 586–590.

Vigevano, F., Fusco, L. & Pachatz, C. (2001): Neurophysiology of spasms. *Brain Dev.* **23,** 467–472.

Watanabe, K., Hayakawa, F. & Okumura, A. (1999): Neonatal EEG: a powerful tool in the assessment of brain damage in preterm infants. *Brain Dev.* **21,** 361–372.

Wertheim, D., Mercuri, E., Faundez, J.C., Rutherford, M., Acolet, D. & Dubowitz, L. (1994): Prognostic value of continuous electroencephalographic recording in full term infants with hypoxic ischaemic encephalopathy. *Arch. Dis. Child. Fetal Neonatal Ed.* **71,** F97–F102.

Whyte, H.E., Taylor, M.J., Menzies, R., Chin, K.C. & MacMillan, L.J. (1986): Prognostic utility of visual evoked potentials in term asphyxiated neonates. *Pediatr. Neurol.* **2,** 220–223.

Yamada, H., Sadato, N. & Konishi, Y. (1997): A rapid brain metabolic change in infants detected by fMRI. *Neuroreport* **8,** 3775–3778.

Yamada, H., Sadato, N. & Konishi, Y. (2000): A milestone for normal development of the infantile brain detected by functional MRI. *Neurology* **55,** 218–223.

Chapter 3

Psychomotor development: the beginning of cognition

Francesco Guzzetta

Catholic University, Largo Agostino Gemelli 8, 00168 Rome, Italy
fguzzetta@rm.unicatt.it

The development of cognition starts at birth or even earlier. Over the last century, our knowledge of neonatal competence was progressively modified, moving from a view of the newborn as a passive object of external stimulation, unstructured and without any organization, to that of an individual capable of complex, highly differentiated abilities in an interactive relationship with the environment. In this chapter we will try to follow the development and emergence of mature cognitive competence in infancy, starting with the initial neonatal skills, the so-called pre-cognitive abilities.

My starting point is the management of the neonatal state, and in particular alertness, motor and sensory competence, and highly complex functioning, including a rudimentary form of learning.

State management: the emergence of alertness

The notion of behavioural states in newborn infants and during early infancy refers to patterns of behaviour expressing distinct brain activities during the sleep-wake cycle. First introduced in assessment techniques by Prechtl and Beintema (Prechtl & Beintema, 1964), they emphasize the infant's ability to organize behavioural sleep-wake states including waking active, quiet alert, fuss or cry, drowse or transition, active sleep, and quiet sleep states (Table 1).

Table 1. Behavioural states in early infancy

Sleep states
State 1: Sleep with regular breathing, eyes closed, no spontaneous activity except startles or jerky movements at quite regular intervals; no eye movements.
State 2: Sleep with eyes closed; rapid eye movements may often be observed under closed lids; low activity level with random movements, smoother than in state 1; irregular respiration.

Awake states
State 3: Drowsy or semi-dozing; minimal activity level with smooth movements; minimal reactivity. This state is considered to be 'transitional'.
State 4: Alert, eyes open with bright look and appropriate changes in facial expression as stimulation occurs.
State 5: Eyes likely to be open; considerable motor activity with thrusting movements of the extremities; reactive to external stimulation. Some infants may pass from lower states (1, 2, or 3) directly to state 5.
State 6: Crying, characterized by intense, loud, rhythmic, and sustained cry vocalizations, difficult to be stopped. It is important to distinguish between crying as a state and the fuss/cry vocalizations that can occur in state 5 and even in state 3.

The emergence of sleep states is a relevant aspect of development. Increasingly in the last months of gestation and during the neonatal period the infant shows distinct cyclic patterns of *active sleep*, corresponding to a definite behavioural (rapid eye movements, REM) and electrophysiological pattern; and *quiet sleep*, with a different electrophysiological and neurobehavioural pattern, characterized by the absence of rapid eye movements (non-REM) (Peirano et al., 2003). Distinct patterns of the basic sleep-wake states begin in the foetus at around 30 weeks of gestation. The development of sleep-wake patterns follows a programmed path during infancy, with sleep time globally lasting 16 to 17 hours per day during the first year of life, initially taken in cycles throughout the 24 hours and then shifting to the night-time (Parmelee et al., 1961; Anders & Keener, 1985). In preterm infants an indeterminate sleep pattern is mainly present. The proportion of sleep states changes with age, with a decrease in active sleep compared with quiet sleep (Anders & Keener, 1985). Active sleep is characterized by intense endogenous neuronal firing in most areas of the brain. It acts as an inducer of CNS development, which accounts for its prevalence at younger ages (Roffwarg et al., 1966).

Awake patterns include two states of alertness (Wolff, 1965; Wolff, 1966). Alertness as a state of readiness to receive inputs is the foundation of attention. In early infancy alertness is considered to be the ability to attain (rather than maintain) the alert state. It begins in the neonatal period, and during the first 2 to 3 months of life is modulated mainly by exogenous events, with a dramatic increase in the time spent in alertness over this period (Berg & Berg, 1979). This early attention (in the first 3 months of life) is determined by low-order subcortical structures linked to arousal (Karmel et al., 1991), mainly the brain stem with its reticular activating system (Moruzzi & Magoun, 1949). Four ascending pathways to neocortical areas have been identified that are associated with attention and cognitive function (Doty, 1995). Among these, the noradrenergic system, with the locus ceruleus and the cholinergic pathway, seems to be particularly implicated in cognitive function, namely behavioural alertness (Usher et al., 1999) and sustained attention (Robbins et al., 1989). Sensory stimulation such as vestibular inputs – as occurs in caregiving activities (picking up and manipulating the infant) – elicits alertness in young infants (Becker et al., 1993), possibly producing changes in norepinephrine in cortical areas (Colombo, 2001).

Neonatal 'pre-cognitive' competence

Motor activity

Though cortical organization is largely incomplete, neonates already have various functional abilities. As the subcortical component appears to prevail, performance is still immature (Mercuri et al., 2007). An evident manifestation of this immaturity occurs in motor *function* (see chapter 1) with its *primitive reflexes* (Table 2) and its uncontrolled and uncoordinated motility, the organization of which is nevertheless guided by some specific agency. In foetal and early infant life (the first 6 months), there is in fact a 'spontaneous' movement repertoire in some way regulated by the CNS and defined as *general movements* (GM). GM were studied by the Prechtl school (Einspieler & Prechtl, 2005) and are complex movements involving the whole body in an apparently irregular and scattered way, waxing and waning, with a gradual beginning and termination. They progress with age, becoming increasingly fluent and elegant, with patterns that are more and more complex and variable. When there is CNS impairment, they deteriorate, becoming monotonous and limited, so that it is possible to identify two specific abnormal GM patterns

Table 2. Primitive reflexes in the newborn

Primitive reflex description	Time of disappearance
Sucking: touching the roof of the baby's mouth will induce sucking	2 months
Stepping: on holding the baby under the arms and allowing the dorsal surfaces of the feet to touch a flat surface, a step will occur	2–3 months
Supporting: holding the baby under the arms and allowing the soles of the feet touch a flat surface, extension of the legs for a few seconds will occur	2–4 months
Rooting reflex: stroking the corner of the mouth causes head turning and mouth opening in the direction of the stroking	3 months
Palmar grasping: placing an object in the open palm will cause hand grasping	3–4 months
Galant: stroking the mid-paravertebral areas when the infant is lying prone will cause the back to curve towards the stroked side	3–6 months
Asymmetrical tonic neck reflex: turning the head on one side while the infant is lying supine will cause extension of the homolateral arm and leg and the flexion of contralateral limbs	4 months
Moro: when support is withdrawn from the neck and head, the baby will spread the arms and legs out widely, extend the neck and cry	6 months
Walking: when the baby is supported bending forward and the soles of the feet touch a flat surface, 'walking' will occur with the placing of one foot in front of the other	8 months
Babinsky reflex: stroking the sole of the foot firmly causes the big toe to bend dorsally and the other toes to fan out	12 months

that are reliably predictive of later cerebral palsy: the cramped-synchronized GMs (rigid and stereotyped), and the absence of GMs of fidgety character (fluent and variable) (Cioni, 2003; Einspieler & Prechtl, 2005; Cioni *et al.*, 2007).

Orienting

Responsiveness – that is, the ability to respond to exogenous stimulation – is already present at birth. It can be studied in the two main sensory fields as the ability to orient towards salient stimulations, visual or auditory.

Orienting is expressed through behavioural and physiological changes associated with the detection of a novel stimulus – at birth as a simple reflex (Sokolov, 1963). During the first 6 to 8 weeks, ocular saccades towards a novel target are driven exogenously (reflexive saccades) and seem to be controlled by the superior colliculus. At this time, there is a lack of fixation control – an 'obligatory looking' or sticky fixation (Hood, 1995) – so that disengagement from the attended target is particularly difficult (see below, *Development of visual attention*). Similarly, salient auditory stimuli provoke the phenomenon of acoustic orienting in young infants. The characteristics of a stimulus to be regarded as novel vary with time (see below, *Habituation*) or with the experience of the subject.

Orienting in infants is generally measured through ocular/head turning; alternatively, especially in auditory orienting, as heart rate deceleration or motor quieting (Morrongiello & Clifton, 1984), in both infants and foetuses (Lecanuet *et al.*, 1992). The behavioural procedure for assessing grating acuity (the spatial threshold for resolving dark and white stripes) is based on an innate trend from the first weeks of life to orient visual attention towards a patterned target rather than a homogeneous target *(preferential looking)*. Characteristics of the auditory stimuli reflecting some innate selectivity in orienting and in the recovery of the orienting response (see below) are reported in specific reviews (Gomes *et al.*, 2000).

Habituation

Generally defined as decreased responsiveness over repeated stimulation, habituation in early infancy is usually measured by changes in motor response, heart rate, and galvanic skin resistance to sensory stimuli such as light or the sound of a rattle or bell. In older infants more complex measures are used such as looking time or manipulation. If a novel stimulus is presented after habituation to an earlier stimulus, there will be a renewed response (recovery of the response or dishabituation). Habituation should not be considered as the mere effect of fatigue of receptors (sensory) or effectors (reactive movements), but as a true learning process (Zelazo, 1991; Slater, 1995a; Rose & Rankin, 2001), even in the simple case of renewed responsiveness following a change in an acoustic tone to which the infant has been habituated. Habituation appears to derive from an internal representation that is constantly compared with the actual stimulus. When the stimulus is mismatched to the representation (forming a novel stimulus), attention to the external stimulus increases, with recovery of the response. This represents a primary form of cognitive processing (pre-cognitive ability) with respect to attention and memory paradigms. If we consider habituation as a form of information processing, it may be used to predict cognitive development at an older age (Bornstein, 1998).

Techniques of assessment in the first 2 months

Considering the newborn as an active individual capable of self-regulation and interaction with the environment, making adaptation and a relationship with the carer possible, scales were constructed to measure the complex degrees of competence of neonates and young infants. The first tool widely used was the Neonatal Behavior Assessment Scale (NBAS) devised by Brazelton, subsequently revised in 1984 and 1995 (Brazelton, 1984; Brazelton & Nugent, 1995). The NBAS is a neurobehavioural assessment scale that includes various aspects of newborn reactivity and the ability to self-regulate that contribute to the emerging parent-child relationship. Neurobehaviour is a term used to indicate at this very early age a condition that includes neurological and behavioural aspects. Psychosocial features, expressing in some way high cortical function, and biological features, consisting of neurological competence, are intrinsically and reciprocally connected in every activity, even in the newborn, so that neurophysiology at the onset of infancy directly mediates 'psychological' processes. In the seven-cluster scoring method developed by Lester and Brazelton to show changes of patterns over time (Lester & Brazelton, 1982), several variables are examined. Besides motor performance (tone, reflexes, quality of movements), which is usually included in a neurological examination, the method considers behavioural features such as habituation, orientation, range and regulation of states, and autonomic stability (Table 3).

Table 3. Neonatal Behavior Assessment Scale (NBAS): cluster of items (Lester & Brazelton, 1982)

(1) Habituation (ability to inhibit repeated discrete stimuli while asleep)
(2) Orientation (ability to attend to visual and auditory stimuli)
(3) Range of states (measures of behavioural states)
(4) Regulation of state (infant's ability to regulate state when exposed to increasing levels of stimulation)
(5) Autonomic stability (homeostatic adjustments in the central nervous system)

The NBAS is a reliable tool for assessing the competence of both healthy neonates (Lundquist & Sabel, 2000) and abnormal neonates (newborns at developmental risk) (Jiron *et al.*, 1998). The negative influence of prenatal and neonatal factors has also been studied in order to prevent anomalies (Emory *et al.*, 1999). The ability to predict development has been demonstrated both in short term and long term follow-up studies (Lundqvist-Persson, 2001; Wolf *et al.*, 2002; Canals *et al.*, 2003; Canals *et al.*, 2006). However, the scale has been most successfully used to increase parental awareness and for the prevention of disorders (Grimanis *et al.*, 1998; Nugent & Brazelton, 2000), especially when infants are at high risk (Beeghly *et al.*, 1995; Cardone & Gilkerson,1995; Gomes-Pedro *et al.*, 1995; Cantavella & Leonhardt, 1996).

Scales deriving from the classical NBAS are those aimed at assessing preterm infants' behavior (APIB) (Als *et al.*, 1982) and more recently the Neonatal Intensive Care Unit Network Neurobehavioral Scale (NNNS) (Lester & Tronick, 2004).

The NNNS is a more complete and standardized assessment technique, encompassing neurobehavioural responses and regulatory capacities of normal and impaired infants at different gestational ages. The NNNS assessment can be carried out from 30 weeks' gestational age to an upper limit of 46 to 48 weeks conceptional age – that is, weeks of gestational age at birth plus weeks since birth, corresponding to 2 months' corrected age, when standardized infant assessments can be administered reliably (Table 4).

Table 4. The Neonatal Intensive Care Unit Network Neurobehavioral Scale Procedures (NNNS) (Lester & Tronick, 2004)

Domains	Items	Domains	Items
Pre-examination observation	Initial state observation (infant asleep and covered)	Upright responses Placing	Stepping Ventral suspension Incurvation
Habituation	Response decrement to light Response decrement to rattle Response decrement to bell	Infant prone Crawling Pick up	Stimulation needed Head raise in prone Infant cuddle in arm Cuddle on shoulder
Unwrap and supine posture	Skin colour Skin texture Movement Response decrement to tactile stimulation of the foot	Infant supine on examiner's lap	Orientation (order not predetermined): Animate visual and auditory Animate visual
Lower extremity reflexes	Plantar grasp Babinski Ankle clonus Leg resistance Leg recoi Power of active leg movements Popliteal angle	Infant spin	Animate auditory Inanimate visual and auditory Inanimate visual Inanimate auditory Tonic deviation of head and eyes Nystagmus
Upper extremities and facial reflexes	Scarf sign Forearm resistance Forearm recoil Power of active arm movements Rooting Sucking Hand grasp Truncal tone Pull-to-sit	Infant supine in crib Post-examination observation	Defensive response Asymmetrical tonic neck reflex Moro reflex State observation

First developed to assess the effects of prenatal drug exposure on child outcome, NNNS includes a neurological examination and a separate stress/abstinence scale in addition to behavioural items examined by Brazelton. It is applicable to newborns – normal healthy, preterm, or at risk – as an unstructured examination, bearing in mind that each item should be administered when the infant is in a predefined state, for example habituation should be examined in state 1 or 2, and no item should be administered in state 6.

Summary scores are calculated for 13 main fields (habituation, attention, handing, quality of movement, regulation, non-optimal reflexes, asymmetrical reflexes, stress/abstinence, arousal, hypertonicity, hypotonicity, excitability, and lethargy) (Lester & Tronick, 2004). This makes it possible to draw up a profile of abnormalities in young infants which can be used in different studies, particularly those concerning drug exposure in pregnancy (Napiorkowski et al., 1996; Law et al., 2003; de Moraes Barros et al., 2006; Salisbury et al., 2007).

Development up to 4 months

Development in the first 3 to 4 months of life results in the infant reaching some important milestones in cortical maturation, corresponding to the acquisition of distinct sensory-motor functions. In this context, visual function seems to play a major role.

Smooth reflexive pursuit can already be elicited in neonates (Shea & Aslin, 1990). To do this, targets should be presented at a moderate and constant speed. A rapid increase in the velocity and accuracy of pursuit occurs at 3 to 4 months of age, for intervention at that time of a factor of cortical maturation (Richards & Hunter, 1998).

Following the seminal work of Zeki (Zeki, 1974; Zeki, 1978), cortical areas specific for motion information (V5 or MT, in the temporal region) and for recognition of object features (V3 and V4, in the parietal region) have been defined (Milner & Goodale, 1995). Two functional streams, ventral and dorsal, serve these areas (Ungerleider & Mishkin, 1982), respectively accounting for 'where' objects are located and 'what' their features are (colour, form, face recognition). These streams are linked to the anatomical magnocellular and parvocellular streams, morphologically distinct from the levels of ganglion cells and the lateral geniculate nucleus up to V1, V4, and MT cortical areas (Van Essen & Maunsell, 1983) (Fig. 1).

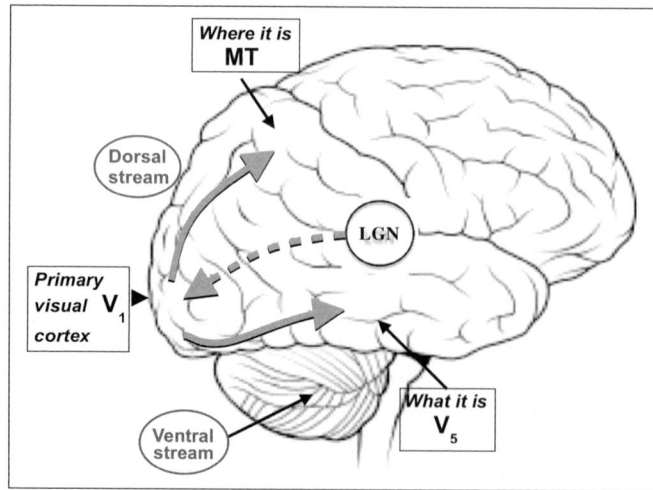

Fig. 1. Functional visual streams. LGN, lateral geniculate nucleus.

Nevertheless, it seems that the distinction between 'where' and 'what' categories (rather than the location of the different properties) needs to be considered as two ways of visual coding with distinct functions: one linked to perception (regardless of whether static or moving) and the other interconnected with motor areas for controlling action (Milner & Goodale, 1995). That is why, rather than referring to two separated streams, it would be better to refer to different modules that subserve complex functions based on larger anatomo-functional areas including attention, memory, and motor areas: "The relatively fast, dorsal, 'action' stream has a very short memory and is for automatic 'unconscious' immediate response, whereas the ventral stream controls 'conscious' awareness and interactions with more long lasting elaborate memory stores" (Atkinson, 2007).

Functional maturation of cortical modules for colour, orientation, ocular disparity, and motion occurs between birth and 3 to 4 months. Within the first month colour discrimination is weak or absent. Red-green discrimination appears in the second month, while the whole colour discrimination finally emerges beyond 3 months of age. Similarly, the selectivity of cortical neurons to differences in orientation is present even in the very early weeks of life and increases progressively, rapid development occurring over the first 3 months. Maturation is measured by electrophysiological techniques such as orientation-reversal visual evoked potentials (OR-VERP), capable of detecting a VEP response time-locked to a change in orientation of the pattern of stripes.

Binocular correlation or disparity depends on cortical mechanisms, and there is evidence that sensitivity to binocular disparity begins in infants at about 3 to 4 months (Atkinson, 2000). Simple reflexive ocular saccades present at birth are controlled by subcortical mechanisms, but intentional eye movements need the intervention of the quoted cortical networks within parietal, temporal, and frontal lobes. Maturation of voluntary eye movements occurs by 3 to 4 months of age and may be measured when two targets presented in competition in the visual field elicit a gaze shift from one to the other. This allows the eyes to be disengaged from the central to the peripheral visual field in order to focus on an interesting object, and marks the acquisition of free scanning. The test of fixation shift proposed by Atkinson and Braddick (Atkinson & Braddick, 1985) (Fig. 2) has been the one mainly used to examine visual maturation in preterm infants (Atkinson, 1991; Foreman *et al.*, 1991) or brain-injured infants (Hood & Atkinson, 1990; Guzzetta *et al.*, 2002).

In parallel, maturation of auditory function in the first months of life is critical. Infants become active listeners, able to discriminate both tones and speech sounds. Discrimination of sound contrasts may be assessed by mismatch negativity (MMN) an event related early potential corresponding to responses to changes in stimulus parameters. MMN, marked by the achievement of brain stem myelination and the marginal layer of the cortex maturation occurs exactly in the perinatal age when a clear separation develops between the primary auditory cortex of the transverse temporal gyrus and the secondary auditory cortex of the superior temporal gyrus (Moore & Linthicum Jr, 2007). This early cortical stage of sound discrimination has been proposed (Hickoka & Poppe, 2004) as a processing system founded on two processing streams like that of visual function: a ventral stream that subserves sound features up to word meaning and anatomically projects toward posterior middle temporal gyrus, and a dorsal stream involved in articulatory representations and projecting toward the posterior Sylvian fissure and eventually the frontal areas. Soon before this dissociation into two streams there is a first processing of auditory inputs located at the left superior temporal gyrus and coding not only the sub-lexical aspects of the perception of speech but also of the production. In this framework there will be all the steps of the language development.

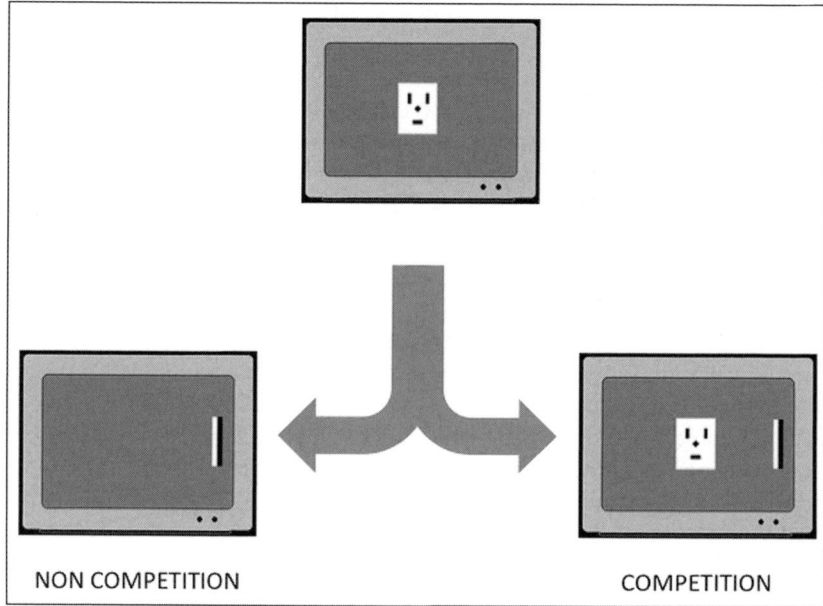

Fig. 2. Fixation shift assessment in orienting towards an interesting visual object in a non-competition setting (when a peripheral target is presented in absence of the central target) or in a competition setting (when the two targets are presented contemporarily in the visual field and the infant gaze shifts from one to another target); the latter shift ability is reached at about 3 months.

This 3 to 4 month period comprises the first stage of the maturation of exploratory 'free' eye movements, preceding that of the action module controlling exploratory reaching and grasping. Its achievement coincides with the time when motor maturation achieves the first praxia – that is, the first finalized movements that mark the start of true cognitive operations (primary circular reactions) according to Piaget's model (Fig. 3). It is noteworthy that, like the acquisition of disengagement in visual skill, mature grasping becomes possible when the infant develops the capacity for voluntary hand relaxation. The ideal line that can to drawn at this time between perceptive and cognitive competences – corresponding, respectively, to cortical areas for decoding sensory inputs and for categorizing and storing information – cannot be demonstrated at older ages.

'True' cognitive development

Motor abilities in infancy develop following anatomical maturation (mainly cortical organization and myelination), initially by overcoming the subcortical movement organization characteristic of the newborn (see above). The progressive achievement of gross motor milestones, recently assessed in the world population (de Onis et al, 2004), shows some variability owing to physiological variations, but primarily it follows a predefined functional hierarchy according to a cranio-caudal maturation process. This gross motor maturation, aimed initially at locomotion, develops successively with rolling-over ability, creeping, crawling, shuffling, and walking. In parallel, fine motor development achieved by increasingly mature coordination enables infants to reach for and grasp objects, manipulate them, and operate with them.

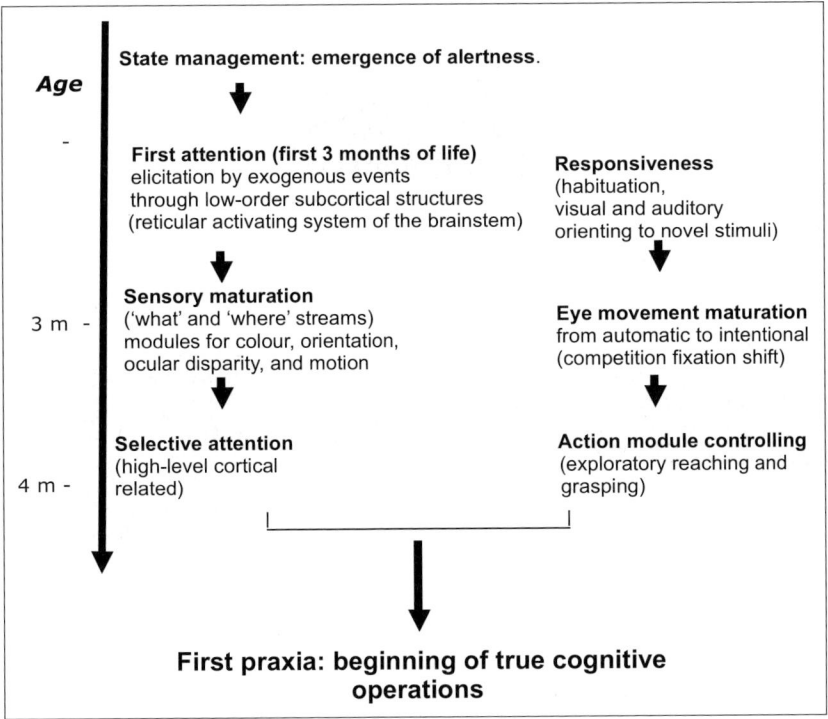

Fig. 3. Evolution of the elaboration ability of inputs (left column) and outputs (right column).

All these motor actions include a cognitive aspect and their development also reflects cognitive development. Similarly, sensory maturation, primarily visual, makes cognitive experiences possible. Thus motor and sensory achievements are both sources of cognitive performance and are barely separable in infancy.

The two main models on which cognitive development is based are the Piaget theory of genetic epistemology and the information processing theory. Piaget was not a psychologist but rather a developmental biologist who studied the biological influences on how learning occurs and how an organism adapts to its environment with increasingly complex adaptive behaviours produced by the stepwise organization of mental abilities. According to Piaget's theory, there are two processes which constitute this adaptation: *assimilation*, consisting of the ability to transform the environment so as to assimilate it into pre-existing cognitive structures (schemata); and *accommodation*, the process of changing internal mental structures so as to learn from the environment. Adaptations occur when existing schemata must be modified to account for a new experience. As the environment is assimilated, structures are accommodated. So throughout early life the child adapts to the environment in an increasingly complex way.

Among the four successive stages conceived in Piaget's model of cognitive development, the first concerns infancy. This is called the sensorimotor stage and includes six substages (Table 5), proceeding from the reflex stage of the newborn (that is, organized pattern of sensorimotor functioning associated with the reflex development), to the beginning of symbolic representation in the last months of the infancy. This occurs when the notion of object permanence (that is, objects continue to 'exist' even when they cannot be directly perceived) is achieved. Furthermore, to the acquisition of symbolic representation is linked the maturation of language (the system of symbols used to

Table 5. Sensorimotor stage according to Piaget

Developmental substages and approximate age of occurrence	Behaviour
Reflex schema (0–1 m)	Development of reflexes such as grasping or sucking
Primary circular reaction phase (1–4 m)	Development and consolidation of habits: reflexive behaviours (responses to a stimulus) occurring in stereotyped repetition such as sucking the thumb
Secondary circular reactions phase (4–8 m)	Development of coordination between vision and prehension: repetition of change actions to reproduce interesting consequences such as kicking one's feet to move a mobile suspended over the crib; getting a response from another person
Coordination of secondary circular reactions (8–12 m)	Beginning of object permanence; responses become coordinated into more complex sequences, actions take on an 'intentional' character; learning of procedures that make interesting things last
Tertiary circular reactions (12–18 m)	Discovery of new ways to obtain the same goal (active experimentation)
Internalization of schemes; the beginning of symbolic representation (18–24 m)	Development of mental representation; emergence of an internal representational system; mental combinations to solve simple problems; deferred imitation

communicate). A receptive vocabulary is first acquired at the end of the first year of life, whereas expressive ability begins in the second year (with the utterance of the first words at 12 to 14 months), as holophrastic words (a single word implying the meaning of a complete sentence).

Specific aspects of Piaget's theory have been criticized in the sense that it does not consider the importance of the infant's sensory and perceptual abilities in a thorough enough way. Furthermore, imitation and object permanence may occur earlier. Finally, there is a physiological variability in development caused by various endogenous and exogenous factors. Many neo-Piagetian theorists have emerged in recent years, but Piaget's framework for understanding the clinical development of the infant remains valid.

The information processing (IP) perspective shows that thinking is analogous to the working of a computer. The information (Fig. 4) is collected by sensory receptors and is processed in its travels through the brain structures. IP is based on three main processes: *encoding*, the way of recording information in a form usable to memory; *storage* of information in the memory; and *retrieval* of information from the memory to be used. From infancy onwards, the IP structures remain relatively constant. The processes are innate, relatively automatic, dependent on CNS integrity, and are present throughout life (for example, habituation in early infancy implies some memory). Thus, IP measurements are likely to be related to cognitive development and its disorders.

Assessment scales in infancy

Various standardized psychometric tests in infancy are available. These consist of reliable tools to measure the infant's skill in different specific fields against the 'normal' population. Standardization allows comparisons to be made between the patient's data and the normative data. It enables the test to be scored objectively and provides possible cut-off points to identify abnormal populations. The standardization of a test does not ensure its psychometric validity, which needs further assessment evaluating various different psychometric properties such as

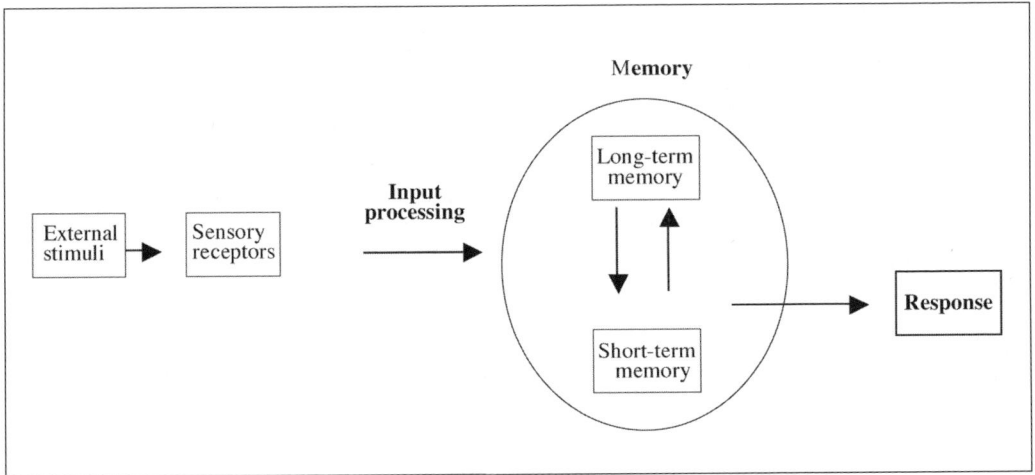

Fig. 4. Information processing model, from external stimuli to responses.

internal consistency, test-retest and inter-rater reliability, and predictive validity (Johnson & Marlow, 2007). In fact, the aim of the test is not only to give information about the development of the infant but also to help predict the outcome.

Traditional scales are generally poorly predictive because of the discontinuity of cognitive development. Discontinuity, as evidenced by a poor correlation between early assessment results and outcome (McCall, 1979; Largo et al., 1990; Slater, 1995b), is mainly explained by the measures used in infancy which are only able to detect specific age-related abilities, and by the discontinuous character of development as it passes from sensory-motor to mature cognition.

The assessment of infant development is specially aimed at identifying individuals with developmental delay. In infancy, there are techniques for screening that are easy to administer but give poor results, being capable only of identifying children who are needing detailed analysis (Frankenberg et al., 1992; Aylward, 1995). A characteristic of all scales relating to infancy is that the features to be measured include different domains (sensory, motor, cognitive), and it is difficult to integrate these; for example, motor disability may be an obstacle to assessing cognitive performance. Thus the choice of the scale paradigm has been guided by the need for a defined measurement objective and satisfactory validity.

Multi-domain developmental assessments

As already said, the interpretation of performance in infancy is not easy because the different abilities are strictly interdependent. Generally, development examinations involve all the domains of infant skills: sensory, motor, and cognitive. Moreover, cognition – especially in the early months – is barely distinguishable from sensory-motor abilities.

Among the various tools of developmental assessment (Table 6), we will consider two of the currently most frequently used scales in Western countries: the Bayley Scales of Infant Development and the Griffiths Mental Development Scales.

Table 6. Main multidomain assessment tools in infancy

Assessment	Age range
Bayley Scales of Infant Development III (BSID III) (Bayley, 2006)	1 m to 42 m
Brunet-Lézine (Brunet-Lézine, 1997)	Birth to 3 y
Early Learning Accomplishment Profile (Glover et al., 1995)	Birth to 3 y
Griffiths Mental Development Scales (Luiz et al., 2004)	Birth to 8 y
Merrill-Palmer Scales of Development (Roid & Sampers, 2004)	Birth to 6.5 y
Mullen Scales of Early Learning (Mullen, 1995)	Birth to 68 m
Provence Profile (Provence et al., 1995)	Birth to 3 y

Bayley Scales of Infant Development

The Bayley Scales of Infant Development (BSID) (standard revision in 1993: BSID-II) measure mental and motor development and test the behaviour of infants aged 15 days to 42 months, in order to assist in the diagnosis and treatment of infants with developmental delay or disabilities (Bayley, 1993). Their standardization is among the best, with adequate psychometric properties in all fields except for the behavioural scales, which are evidently weaker. However, their predictive validity – as in other scales – generally appears poor (Hack et al., 2005). There are three domains (motor, cognitive, and behavioural) scored along 14 different age groups. Cognitive abilities such as memory, learning, problem-solving ability, and verbal communication are tested by mental scales. The motor scales evaluate the child's ability to control the axial muscles and to move (sitting, standing, and walking), to coordinate large muscle movements (gross motor skills), and to perform fine manipulations with the fingers and hands (fine motor skills). Finally, the Infant Behavior Record (IBR) assesses the child's social and emotional development using a standardized description.

Periodic revision and standardization of the test has prevented it from suffering from the Flynn effect (Flynn, 1999), yielding higher normative mean scores in the more recent editions than in the previous one.

The last revision of the test (BSID III) (Bayley, 2006) increased the number of scales included. Three scales now refer to motor, cognitive, and language skills, while two involve other parent-reported scales concerning social-emotional development and adaptive behaviour. Moreover, the floor and ceiling scores have been extended so that they are more adequate at assessing low functioning and impaired development.

Griffiths Mental Development Scales

The Griffiths Mental Development Scales include an infant section (from birth to 23 months) and an extended edition for children from 2 to 8 years. The Griffiths Scales administration needs a 5-day training course with an appropriate examiner certification. The infant scales, developed in 1954 (Griffiths, 1954) and revised in 1996 (Griffiths, 1996) and 2004 (Luiz et al., 2004), assess infant skills in five domains: locomotor, personal-social, hearing and language, eye and hand coordination, and performance. For each domain, it is possible to obtain developmental subquotients the sum of which provides the general quotient (GQ). As in other scales, and particularly infant scales, there are many limitations, particularly poor test-retest reliability and weaker utility for infants with disabilities. As far as predictive ability is concerned, Ivens and Martin (Ivens & Martin, 2000) corrected the raw scores of each scale and the GQ into score equivalents for ICD10 ranges of mental retardation, allowing some continuity between early scores and outcome. However, the Griffiths scales are mainly used in the follow-up of at-risk populations and show good predictive ability in specific cases (Barnett *et al.*, 2004; Guzzetta *et al.*, 2008).

Assessment of the cognitive development

Tests specifically designed to assess cognitive competence are not numerous. An old test with only historical value is the Cattell Infant Intelligence Scale (Cattell, 1940). On the other hand, the Uzgiris-Hunt Scales (Uzgiris & Hunt, 1975) are still in use in some countries (for example, Italy and Spain).

The Uzgiris-Hunt Scales are an ordinal test constructed according to a piagetian model of development. They cover six different areas of sensorimotor development: object permanence, means-end relations, gestural and vocal imitation, operational causality, spatial cognition, and object schemes. As they do not provide developmental quotients, the results refer to the sequential organization of development, to some extent disentangling development from the age variable. This makes it possible to use the scales in older children with developmental delay. Results may also be compared with the approximate age at which normal children reach the ceiling on each scale, as reported in several studies (Bates *et al.*, 1979; Uzgiris & Hunt, 1987; Guzzetta *et al.*, 1993; Dall'Oglio *et al.*, 1994). Being derived from Piaget's hypothesis of six sensorimotor stages and the sequential organization of development, the test allows the structural and hierarchical aspects of development to be discerned in normal and abnormal infants.

Information processing

Information processing has several advantages (Guzzetta *et al.*, 2007):

1) It is easy to link the results with the molecular processes of cognition (for example, visual function).
2) It can improve the anatomo-functional investigation of children with impaired abilities.
3) Most importantly, it enables the continuity of the cognitive development to be assessed, allowing the results to have a better prognostic value.

The continuity of cognitive development has its basis in the fundamental cognitive processes for acquiring information (encoding, storage and retrieval). Numerous tools based on information processing have been proposed for measuring the mental abilities of infants (McCall & Carriger, 1993). They generally measure the ability to discriminate a new stimulus from the one previously encoded, taking advantage of the infant's preference for novelty. A test of selective attention to visual novelty has been extensively used to measure encoding and retention of information during infancy, and there is now enough evidence that recognition memory and novelty preference in infancy are predictive of later cognitive competence (Guzzetta *et al.*, 2006).

In the Fagan Test of Infant Intelligence (FTII) (Fagan & Sheperd, 1989), a familiarization phase with a particular stimulus precedes the presentation of the novel stimulus on a screen for a variable time (depending on age). The familiar and novel stimuli are then simultaneously presented for two successive trials (in left-right and right-left positions) and the time spent by the infant looking at the stimuli is recorded. The novelty score (time spent looking at the novel stimulus divided by the total time looking at both familiar and novel stimuli), calculated over 10 trials, is finally compared with standard values.

The main fields of application of the information processing model in infancy are the examination of visual attention, processing speed, and visual recognition memory. The measurement of developmental changes in *visual attention* in infancy may provide a key to its maturation. Fixation, pursuit, looking duration, quality of saccades, and shift rates express visual maturation with the progressive acquisition of visual attention; this seems to be associated with increasingly good visual recognition memory (Colombo, 1993). Measures of looking duration and shift rate in infancy discriminate well between groups of normal and variously disturbed infants, and can predict IQ scores at later ages to some degree (Rose et al., 1989; Rose et al., 1991; Rose et al., 1992; Sigman et al., 1997).

A deficit in *processing speed* may limit several cognitive abilities, lowering the general intelligence competence (Vernon, 1987). Available tests for measuring processing speed in infancy are based on the assessment of reaction time in initiating saccades in a visual expectation paradigm (Haith et al., 1988), or on the measurement of the time needed to encode information with a 'continuous familiarization' task (time of familiarization) (Rose et al., 2002). Processing speed measurement also seems to have predictive value for later cognitive development (Dougherty & Haith, 1997).

Visual recognition memory (VRM), based on the novelty preference in infancy for looking at a new stimulus in comparison with an old one, generally uses the paired comparison paradigm (Fantz, 1964; Fagan, 1970). As described above, VRM is expressed as a novelty score. There is evidence that this increases significantly across the first year of life (Ross-Sheehy et al., 2003).

The one test of VRM so far published (Fagan & Sheperd, 1989) was not standardized, but data are available concerning the stability and validity (discriminating and predictive) of the test (Rose et al., 2003). The discriminating value of VRM has been proven in various different risk groups, including preterm infants, infants with neonatal respiratory distress syndrome and infants exposed *in utero* to negative factors such as alcohol, cocaine, nutritional deficiency, and so on. VRM seems to have a high predictive value in relation to both general mental competence and the molecular aspects of information processing ability, such as memory or speed of processing. The median predictive correlation of infant VRM with later cognition is definitely higher than that of any other test used, at around 0.45 (McCall & Carriger, 1993). Some cut-off points have been proposed as being predictive of mental retardation: for example, a cut-off of 54 per cent novelty preference at 7 months allowed the identification of children who later presented with definite mental delay, with good sensitivity and specificity (Rose et al., 1988; Fagan & Haiken-Vasen, 1997).

References

Als, H., Lester, B.M., Tronick, E.C. & Brazelton, T.B. (1982): Towards a research instrument for the assessment of preterm infants' behavior (A. P. I. B.). In: *Theory and Research in Behavioral Pediatrics*, eds. H.E. Fitzgeral, B.M. Lester & M.W. Yogman, Vol. 1, pp. 85–132. New York, NY: Plenum.

Anders, T.F. & Keener, M. (1985): Developmental course of night time sleep-wake patterns in full-term and premature infants during the first year of life. *Sleep* **8,** 173–192.

Atkinson, J. (1991): Review of human visual development: crowding and dyslexia. In: *Vision and visual dyslexia*, vol. 13, ed. J.F. Stein, pp. 44–57. London: Macmillan.

Atkinson, J. (2000): *The developing visual brain*. Oxford: Oxford University Press.

Atkinson, J. (2007): New paediatric behavioural and electrophysiological tests of brain function for vision and attention to predict cognitive and neurological outcomes. In: *Progress in epileptic spasms and West syndrome*, eds. F. Guzzetta, B. Dalla Bernardina & R. Guerrini, pp. 83-114. London: John Libbey.

Atkinson, J. & Braddick, O.J. (1985): Early development of the control of visual attention. *Perception* **14,** A25.

Aylward, G.P. (1995): *The Bayley Infant Neurodevelopmental Screener.* San Antonio, Texas: The Psychological Corporation.

Barnett, A.L., Guzzetta, A., Mercuri, E., Henderson, S.E., Haataja, L., Cowan, F. & Dubowitz, L. (2004): Can the Griffiths scales predict neuro-motor and perceptual-motor impairment in term infants with neonatal encephalopathy? *Arch. Dis. Child.* **89,** 637–643.

Bates, E., Benigni, L., Bretherton, I., Camaioni, L. & Volterra, V. (1979): *The emergence of symbols: cognition and communication in infancy.* New York: Academic Press.

Bayley, N. (1993): *Bayley scales of infant development,* 2nd edition. San Antonio, Texas: The Psychological Corporation.

Bayley, N. (2006): *Bayley scales of infant and toddler development,* 3rd edition. San Antonio, Texas: Harcourt Assessment Inc.

Becker, P.T., Grunwald, P.C., Moorman, J. & Strur, S. (1993): Effects of developmental care on behavioural organization in very-low-birth-weight infants. *Nurs. Res.* **42,** 214–220.

Beeghly, M., Brazelton, T.B., Flannery, K., Nugent, J.K., Barrett, D.E. & Tronick, E.Z. (1995): Specificity of pediatric intervention effects in early infancy. *J. Dev. Behav. Pediatr.* **16,** 158–166.

Berg, W.K. & Berg, K.M. (1979): Psychophysiological development in infancy: state, sensory function, and attention. In: *Handbook of infant development,* ed. J.D. Osofsky, pp. 203–243. New York: John Wiley.

Bornstein, M.H. (1998): Stability in mental development from early life: methods, measures, models, meanings and myths. In: *The development of sensory, motor and cognitive capacities in early infancy: from perception to cognition,* ed. F. Simion, pp. 301–332. London: Taylor & Francis.

Brazelton, T.B. (1984): *Neonatal behavioral assessment scale,* 2nd ed. London: Spastics International Medical Publications.

Brazelton, T.B. & Nugent, J.K. (1995): *Neonatal behavioral assessment scale,* 3rd ed. London: Mac Keith Press.

Brunet-Lézine, J. (1997): *Echelle de développement psychomoteur de la première enfance.* (Forme révisée). Paris: EAP.

Canals, J., Fernández-Ballart, J. & Esparò, G. (2003): Evolution of neonatal behavior assessment scale scores in the first month of life. *Infant Behav. Dev.* **26,** 227–237.

Canals, J., Esparò G. & Fernandez-Ballart, J.D. (2006): Neonatal behaviour characteristics and psychological problems at 6 years. *Acta Paediatr.* **95,** 1412–1417.

Cantavella, F. & Leonhardt, M. (1996): Behavioral assessment of the blind neonate: an early intervention. *Ab Initio, The Brazelton Center Newsletter,* 3 (3).

Cardone, I.A. & Gilkerson, L.V. (1995): Family administered neonatal activities (FANA). In: *Neonatal behavioral assessment scale,* 3rd edition, ed. T.B. Brazelton & J.K. Nugent, pp. 111–116. London: Mac Keith Press.

Cattell, P. (1940): *Cattell infant intelligence scale.* San Antonio, Texas: Psychological Corporation.

Bates, E., Benigni, L., Bretherton, I., Camaioni, L. & Volterra, V. (1979): *The emergence of symbols: cognition and communication in infancy.* New York: Academic Press.

Cioni, G. (2003): Observación de los Movimientos Generales en recién nacidos y lactantes: Valor pronóstico y diagnóstico. *Rev. Neurol.* **37,** 30–35.

Cioni, G., Einspieler, C. & Paolicelli, A. (2007): Other approaches to neurological assessment. In: *Neurological assessment in the first two years of life,* eds. G. Cioni & E. Mercuri, pp. 49–68. London: Mac Keith Press.

Colombo, J. (1993): *Infant cognition: predicting later intellectual functioning.* Newbury Park: Sage.

Colombo, J. (2001): The development of visual attention in infancy. *Annu. Rev. Psychol.* **52,** 337–367.

Dall'Oglio, A.M., Bates, E., Volterra, V., Di Capua, M. & Pezzini, G. (1994): Early cognition, communication and language in children with focal brain injury. *Dev. Med. Child Neurol.* **36,** 1076–1098.

de Moraes Barros, M.C., Guinsburg, R., de Araújo Peres, C., Mitsuhiro, S., Chalem, E. & Laranjeira, R.R. (2006): Exposure to marijuana during pregnancy alters neurobehavior in the early neonatal period. *J. Pediatr.* **149,** 781–787.

de Onis, M., Garza, C., Victora, C.G., Bhan, M.K. & Norum, K.R. (2004): The WHO Multicentre Growth Reference Study (MGRS): Rationale, planning, and implementation. *Food and Nutrition Bulletin* **25** (Suppl. 1), S3-S84.

Doty, R.W. (1995): Brainstem influences on forebrain processes, including memory. In: *Neurobehavioral plasticity: learning, development, and the response to brain insults,* eds. N.E. Spear, L.P. Spear & M.L. Woodruff. Hillsdale, New Jersey: Erlbaum.

Dougherty, T.M. & Haith, M.M. (1997): Infant expectations and reaction time as predictors of childhood speed of processing and IQ. *Dev. Psychol.* **33,** 146–155.

Einspieler, C. & Prechtl, H.F. (2005): Prechtl's assessment of general movements: a diagnostic tool for the functional assessment of the young nervous system. *Ment. Retard. Dev. Disabil. Res. Rev.* **11,** 61–67.

Emory, E., Pattillo, R., Archibold, E., Bayorh, M. & Sung, F. (1999): Neurobehavioral effects of low-level lead exposure in human neonates. *Am. J. Obstet. Gynecol.* **181,** S2–S11.

Fagan, J.F. (1970): Memory of the infant. *J. Exp. Child Psychol.* **9,** 217–226.

Fagan, J.F. & Sheperd, P. (1989): *The Fagan test of infant intelligence.* Cleveland: Infantest Corporation.

Fagan, J.F. & Haiken-Vasen, J.H. (1997): Selective attention to novelty as measure of information processing. In: *Attention, development, and psychopathology*, eds. J.A. Burack & J.T. Enns. New York: Guildford.

Fantz, R.L. (1964): Visual experience in infants: decreased attention to familiar patterns relative to novel ones. *Science* **146,** 668–670.

Foreman, N., Fielder, A., Price, D. & Bowler, V. (1991): Tonic and phasic orientation in full-term and preterm infants. *J. Exp. Child Psychol.* **51,** 407–422.

Flynn, J.R. (1999): Searching for justice. The discovery of IQ gains over time. *Am. Psychol.* **54,** 5–20.

Frankenberg, W.K., Dodds, J.B., Archer, P. & Bresnick, B. (1992): The Denver II: a major revision and re-standardisation of the Denver Developmental Screening Test. *Pediatrics* **89,** 91–97.

Glover, E.M., Preminger, J.L. & Sanford, A.R. (1995): *Early learning accomplishment profile*, revised edition (E-LAP). Lewisville, North Carolina: Kapitan Press.

Gomes, H., Molholm, S., Christodoulou, C., Ritter, W. & Cowan, N. (2000): The development of auditory attention in children. *Bioscience* **5,** 108–120.

Gomes-Pedro, J., Patricio, M., Carvalho, A., Goldschmidt, T., Torgal-Garcta, F. & Monteiro, M.B. (1995): Early intervention with Portuguese mothers: a two years follow-up. *Dev. Behav. Pediatr.* **16,** 21–28.

Griffiths, R. (1954): *The abilities of babies.* London: University of London Press.

Griffiths, R. (1996): *The Griffiths mental development scales from birth to 2 years. Manual. The 1996 revision.* Henley: Association for Research in Infant and Child Development Test Agency.

Grimanis, M., Nugent, K.J., Vo, D., Beck, D. & Brazelton, T.B. (1998): The Brazelton scale boosts maternal awareness and cognitive growth: implications for early intervention. *Ab Initio, The Brazelton Center Newsletter.*

Guzzetta, A., Mazzotti, S., Tinelli, F., Bancale, A., Ferreti, G., Battini, R., Bartalena, L., Boldrini, A. & Cioni, G. (2006): Early assessment of visual information processing and neurological outcome in preterm infants. *Neuropediatrics* **37,** 278–285.

Guzzetta, F. (2007): West syndrome: epilepsy-induced neurosensory disorders and cognitive development. In: *Progress in epileptic spasms and West syndrome*, ed. F. Guzzetta, B. Dalla Bernardina & R. Guerrini, pp. 131–142. London: John Libbey.

Guzzetta, F., Crisafulli, A. & Isaya Crinó, M. (1993): Cognitive assessment of infants with West syndrome: how useful is it for diagnosis and prognosis? *Dev. Med. Child Neurol.* **35,** 379–387.

Guzzetta, F., Frisone, M.F., Ricci, D., Randò, T. & Guzzetta, A. (2002): Development of visual attention in West syndrome. *Epilepsia* **43,** 757–763.

Guzzetta, F., Veredice, C. & Guzzetta, A. (2007): Cognitive development in the first two years of life. In: *Neurological assessment in the first two years of life*, eds. G. Cioni & E. Mercuri, pp. 158–168. London: Mac Keith Press.

Guzzetta, F., Cioni, G., Mercuri, E., Fazzi, E., Biagioni, E., Veggiotti, P., Bancale, A., Baranello, G., Epifanio, R., Frisone, M.F., Guzzetta, A., La Torre, G., Mannocci, A., Randò, T., Ricci, D., Signorini, S. & Tinelli, F. (2008): Neurodevelopmental evolution of West syndrome: a 2-year prospective study. *Eur. J. Paediatr. Neurol.* **12,** 387–397.

Hack, M., Taylor, H.G., Drotar, D., Schluchter, M., Cartar, L., Wilson-Costello, D., Klein, N., Friedman, H., Mercuri-Minich, N. & Morrow, M. (2005): Poor predictive validity of the Bayley scales of infant development for cognitive function of extremely low birth weight children at school age. *Pediatrics* **116,** 333–341.

Haith, M.M., Hazan, C. & Goodman, G.S. (1988): Expectation and anticipation of dynamic visual events by 3.5-month-old babies. *Child Dev.* **59,** 467–479.

Hickoka, G. & Poppe, D. (2004): Dorsal and ventral streams: a framework for understanding aspects of the functional anatomy of language. *Cognition* **92,** 67–99.

Hood, B.M. (1995): Shifts of visual attention in the infant: a neuroscientific approach. In: *Advances in infancy research*, eds. C. Rovee-Collier & L. Lippsitt, pp. 163–216. Norwood, New Jersey: Ablex.

Hood, B. & Atkinson, J. (1990): Sensory visual loss and cognitive deficits in the selective attentional system of normal infants and neurologically impaired children. *Dev. Med. Child Neurol.* **32,** 1067–1077.

Ivens, J. & Martin, N. (2000): A common metric for the Griffith scales. *Arch. Dis. Child.* **87,** 109–110.

Jiron, P., Costas, C., Botet, F. & De Cáceres, M. (1998): The effects of acute fetal distress on neonatal behaviour measured by the Brazelton scale. *An. Esp. Pediatr.* **48,** 163–166.

Johnson, S. & Marlow, N. (2007): Assessment of the development of high risk infants in the first two years.. In: *Neurological assessment in the first two years of life*, eds. G. Cioni & E. Mercuri, pp. 120–157. London: Mac Keith Press.

Karmel, B.Z., Gardner, J.M. & Magnano, C.L. (1991): Attention and arousal in early infancy. In: *Newborn attention: biological constraints and the influence of experience*, eds. M.J.S. Weiss & P.R. Zelazo, pp. 339–376. Norwon, New Jersey: Ablex.

Largo, R.H., Graf, S., Kundu, S., Hunziker, U. & Molinari, L. (1990): Predicting developmental outcome at school age from infant tests of normal, at-risk and retarded infants. *Dev. Med. Child Neurol.* **32,** 30–45.

Law, K.L., Stroud, L.R., LaGasse, L.L., Niaura, R., Liu, J. & Lester, B.M. (2003): Smoking during pregnancy and newborn neurobehavior. *Pediatrics* **111,** 1318–1323.

Lecanuet, J.C., Granier-Deferre, C. & Jacquet, A. (1992): Decelerative cardiac responsiveness to acoustic stimulation in the near term fetus. *Q. J. Exp. Psychol.* **44B,** 279–303.

Lester, B.M. & Tronick, E.Z. (2004): The Neonatal Intensive Care Unit Network neurobehavioral scale procedures. *Pediatrics* **113,** 641–667.

Lester, B.M. & Brazelton, T.B. (1982): Cross-cultural assessment of neonatal behavior. In: *Cultural perspectives on child development*, eds. D.A. Waquer & H.W. Stepherson, pp. 20–53. San Francisco: W.H. Freeman.

Luiz, D., Barnard, A., Knoesen, N. & Kotras, N. (2004): *Griffiths mental development scales – extended revised (GMDS-ER)*. Amersham: Association for Research in Infant and Child Development.

Lundqvist-Persson, C. (2001): Correlation between level of self-regulation in the newborn infant and developmental status at two years of age. *Acta Paediatr.* **90,** 345–350.

Lundquist, C. & Sabel, K. (2000): Brief report: The Brazelton Neonatal Behavioral Assessment Scale detects differences among newborn infants of optimal health. *J. Pediatr. Psychol.* **25,** 577–582.

McCall, R.B. (1979): The development of intellectual functioning in infancy and the prediction of later IQ. In: *Handbook of infant development*, ed. J.D. Osofsky, pp. 707–740. New York: John Wiley.

McCall, R.B. & Carriger, M.S. (1993): A meta-analysis of infant habituation and recognition memory performance as predictors of later IQ. *Child Dev.* **64,** 57–79.

Mercuri, E., Haataja, L. & Dubowitz, L. (2007): Neurological assessment in normal young infants. In: *Neurological assessment in the first two years of life*, eds. G. Cioni & E. Mercuri, pp. 24–37. London: Mac Keith Press.

Milner, A.D. & Goodale, M.A. (1995): *The visual brain action*. Oxford: Oxford University Press.

Moore, J.K. & Linthicum Jr, F.H. (2007): The human auditory system: a timeline of development. *Intern. J Audiology* **46**, 460-478.

Morrongiello, B.A. & Clifton, R.K. (1984): Effects of sound frequency on behavioral and cardiac orienting in newborn and five-month-old infants. *J. Exp. Child Psychol.* **38,** 429–446.

Moruzzi, G. & Magoun, H.H. (1949): Brain stem reticular formation and activation of the EEG. *Electroencephalogr. Clin. Neurophysiol.* **1,** 455–473.

Mullen, E.M. (1995): *Mullen scales of early learning*. Los Angeles: Western Psychological Services.

Napiorkowski, B., Lester, B.M., Freier, M.C., Brunner, S., Dietz, L., Nadra, A. & Oh, W. (1996): Effects of in utero substance exposure on infant neurobehavior. *Pediatrics* **98,** 71–75.

Nugent, J.K. & Brazelton, T.B. (2000): Preventive infant mental health: uses of the Brazelton Scale. In: *WAIMH handbook of infant mental health*, eds. J.O. Osofsky & H.E. Fitzgerald, pp. 159–202. New York: John Wiley.

Parmelee, A.H., Shulz, H.R. & Disbrow, M.A. (1961): Sleep patterns of the newborn. *Pediatrics* **58,** 241–250.

Peirano, P., Algarín, C. & Uauy, R. (2003): Sleep-wake states and their regulatory mechanisms throughout early human development. *J. Pediatr.* **143** (4 Suppl.), S70–S79.

Prechtl, H. & Beintema, D. (1964): The neurological examination of the full-term newborn infants. In: *Clinics in Developmental Medicine, N° 12*. London: Heinemann.

Provence, S., Erikson, J., Vater, S. & Palmeri, S. (1995): Infant-toddler developmental assessment (IDA). Chicago: Riverside Publishing.

Richards, J.E. & Hunter, S.K. (1998): Attention and eye movements in young infants: neural control and development. In: *Cognitive neuroscience of attention: a developmental perspective*, ed. J.E. Richards, pp. 131–162. Mahwah, New Jersey: Erlbaum.

Robbins, T.W., Everitt, B.J., Marston, H.M., Wilkinson, J., Jones, G.H. & Page, K.J. (1989): Comparative effects of ibotenic acid- and quisqualic acid-induced lesions of the substantia nigra nominate on attentional function in the rat: further implications for the role of the cholinergic neurons of the nucleus basalis in cognitive processes. *Behav. Brain Res.* **35,** 221–240.

Roffwarg, H.F., Muzio, J. & Dement, W.C. (1966): Ontogenetic development of the human sleep-wakefulness cycle. *Science* **152,** 604–619.

Roid, G.H. & Sampers, J.L. (2004): *Merrill-Palmer-R scales of development manual.* Wood Dale, Illinois: Stoelting Company.

Rose, J.K. & Rankin, C.H. (2001): Analyses of habituation in Caenorhabditis elegans. *Learn. Mem.* **8,** 63–69.

Rose, S.A., Feldman, J.F. & Wallace, J.F. (1988): Individual differences in infants' information processing: reliability, stability, and prediction. *Child Dev.* **59,** 1177–1197.

Rose, S.A., Feldman, J.F., Wallace, I.F. & McCarton, C. (1989): Infant visual attention: relation to birth status and developmental outcome during the first five years. *Dev. Psychol.* **25,** 560–576.

Rose, S.A., Feldman, J.F., Wallace, I.F. & McCarton, C. (1991): Information processing at 1 year: relation to birth status and developmental outcome during the first five years. *Dev. Psychol.* **27,** 723–737.

Rose, S.A., Feldman, J.F. & Wallace, I.F. (1992): Infant information processing in relation to six-year cognitive outcome. *Child Dev.* **63,** 1126–1141.

Rose, S.A., Jankowski, J.J. & Feldman, J.F. (2002): Speed of processing and face recognition at 7 and 12 months. *Infancy* **3,** 435–455.

Rose, S.A., Feldman, J.F. & Jankowski, J.J. (2003): The building blocks of cognition. *J. Pediatr.* **143,** S54–S61.

Ross-Sheehy, S., Oakes, L.M. & Luck, S.J. (2003): The development of visual short-term memory capacity in infants. *Child Dev.* **74,** 1807–1822.

Salisbury, A.L., Lester, B.M., Seifer, R., Lagasse, L., Bauer, C.R., Shankaran, S., Bada, H., Wright, L., Liu, J. & Poole, K. (2007): Prenatal cocaine use and maternal depression: effects on infant neurobehavior. *Neurotoxicol. Teratol.* **29,** 331–340.

Shea, A.L. & Aslin, R.N. (1990): Oculomotor responses to step-ramp targets by young human infants. *Vis. Res.* **30,** 1077–1092.

Sigman, M.D., Cohen, S.E. & Bechwith, L. (1997): Why does infant attention predict adolescent intelligence? *Infant Behav. Dev.* **20,** 133–140.

Slater, A. (1995a): Visual perception and memory at birth. In: *Advances in infancy research*, vol. 9, ed. C. Rovee-Collier & L.P. Lipsitt, pp. 107–162. Norwood, New Jersey: Ablex.

Slater, A. (1995b): Individual differences in infancy and later IQ. *J. Child Psychol. Psychiatry* **36,** 69–112.

Sokolov, E.N. (1963): Higher nervous functions. The orienting reflex. *Annu. Rev. Physiol.* **25,** 545–580.

Ungerleider, L.G. & Mishkin, M. (1982): Two cortical visual systems. In: *Analysis of visual behaviour*, eds. D.J. Ingle, M.A. Goodale & R.J. Mansfield, pp. 549–586. Cambridge, Massachusetts: MIT Press.

Usher, M., Cohen, J.D., Servan-Schreiber, D., Rajkowski, J. & Aston-Jones, G. (1999): The role of locus coeruleus in the regulation of cognitive performance. *Science* **283,** 549–554.

Uzgiris, I.C. & Hunt, J. (1975): *Assessment in infancy: ordinal scales of psychological development.* Urbana: University of Illinois Press.

Uzgiris, I.C. & Hunt, J. (1987): *Research with scales of infant development.* Hillsdale, New Jersey: Erlbaum.

Van Essen, D.C. & Maunsell, J.H. (1983): Hierarchical organization and functional streams in visual cortex. *Trends Neurosci.* **6,** 370–375.

Vernon, P.A. (1987): *Speed of processing and intelligence.* Norwood, New Jersey: Ablex.

Wolf, M.J., Koldewijn, K., Beelen, A., Smit, B., Hedlund, R., & de Groot, I.J.M. (2002): Neurobehavioral and developmental profile of very low birthweight preterm infants in early infancy. *Acta Paediatr.* **91,** 930–938.

Wolff, P.H. (1965): The development of attention in young infants. *Ann. N. Y. Acad. Sci.* **118,** 815–830.

Wolff, P.H. (1966): The causes, controls, and organization of behavior in the neonate. *Psychol. Issues* **5,** 7–11.

Zeki, S. (1974): Functional organization of a visual area in the posterior bank of the superior temporal sulcus of the rhesus monkey. *J. Physiol. (Lond.)* **236,** 549–573.

Zeki, S. (1978): Functional specialization in the visual cortex of the rhesus monkey. *Nature* **274,** 423–428.

Zelazo, P.R. (1991): Habituation and recovery of neonatal orienting to auditory stimuli. In: *Newborn attention: biological constraints and the influence of experience*, eds. M.J. Weiss & P.R. Zelazo, pp. 120–141. Brazelton Center Newsletter, 5.

Chapter 4

Malformations of cortical development

Francesco Guzzetta, Cesare Colosimo and Tommaso Tartaglione

Catholic University, Largo Agostino Gemelli 8, 00168 Rome, Italy
fguzzetta@rm.unicatt.it

Since the second half of the 19th century, when neuropathologists began to find a relationship between brain malformations and clinical features and in particular epilepsy, scientific knowledge in this field has increased progressively. However, developments in three fields in particular resulted in the enormous advances in our knowledge of brain cortical malformations and their clinical effects. These were the development of magnetic resonance imaging (MRI) in the 1980s, with its ability to reveal the appearance of human brain *in vivo*; the formidable evolution of genetics, with identification of genes involved in cerebral cortical development; and the increasing surgical treatment of epilepsy which has provided samples of malformed cortex for new neuropathological studies.

Cortical malformations may arise from a disruption of normal developmental events, including three distinct stages. The earliest consists of stem cell proliferation and differentiation in the germinal ventricular (VZ) and subventricular zones (SVZ) of the dorsal telencephalon, and in the ganglionic eminences. Second, after the end of mitotic divisions, the cells migrate radially from the VZ and SVZ and tangentially from the ganglionic eminences towards the meningeal surface; successive migration waves reach the final site in a chronological inside-outside fashion. The third stage concerns the organization of the six layers of the cortical mantle where the intercellular connections are defined, involving synaptogenesis and programmed cellular death. The process is finally completed with myelination.

The range of the timing of these often overlapping events is between 2 months of gestation and adult life. A synoptic presentation of these stages with their timing and consequent abnormalities is shown in Table 1. We refer readers to the seminal works on this subject for detailed information (Rakic, 1985; Rakic, 1995; Caviness & Takahashi, 1995; Volpe, 2008).

Table 1. Developmental events of cortical formation

Timing	Main normal events	Cortical malformations
2–4 months	Proliferation in ventricular and subventricular zones and differentiation (symmetrical and asymmetrical divisions)	Microcephalies, macrencephalies, exceeding proliferation
3–5 months	Radial and tangential migration	Lissencephaly, agyria-pachygyria, heterotopias, etc.
5 months → postnatal	Organization (subplates, lamination, neurite outgrowth, synaptogenesis, apoptosis, glial proliferation, and differentiation)	Cortical dysplasias, polymicrogyria, schizencephaly

Neuroimaging

The diagnosis of cortical malformations has made formidable progress following the introduction of new neuroimaging techniques and particularly magnetic resonance imaging (MRI). The multiplanar capability and high resolution of MRI remains unmatched by any other current imaging technique in the detection of brain lesions and particularly of cortical brain malformations. Techniques such as the volumetric acquisition of thin contiguous slices, three dimensional (3D) linear and curvilinear reformatting, and surface rendering have enhanced the ability of MRI to display normal or altered brain anatomy with precision.

Functional MRI using the blood oxygenation level dependent technique (BOLD) has the ability to provide physiological information about brain regions activated during various tasks, and allows pre-surgical evaluation of the relations between lesions and the eloquent brain areas. MR-tractography (based upon diffusion anisotropy of the white matter) can also provide information about white matter tracts involved by lesions. In addition, metabolic imaging using MR spectroscopy has now emerged as a supplementary tool to investigate the neurochemical status of the central nervous system, with widespread applications in diseased brains.

All these MR-based imaging modes are now routinely available on high-field commercial imaging systems and continue to evolve rapidly, improving the way we study the central nervous system, its functions, and its common disorders.

The MRI protocol should be tailored to the age of the child. The white matter signal changes on T1w images are related to the normal evolution of the cerebral myelination and become complete within the first 10–12 months; therefore up to this age high resolution 3D T1w images are suboptimal because of their reduced intrinsic contrast. Similarly, cerebral myelination on T2w images appears generally completed within the second year of life, and an adult-like appearance is found on fluid-attenuated inversion recovery (FLAIR) T2-weighted images only at 3–4 years of age.

Thus in the first year of life the MR protocol is generally based upon two-dimensional (2D) SE T1-w and highly T2-w turbo spin echo (TSE/FSE) sequences, using axial and coronal planes (≤ 3 mm thickness). Diffusion-weighted images (DWI) are added to exclude acute brain damage in suspected neonatal respiratory distress; moreover, we strongly suggest the use of diffusion tensor images (DTI) to determine the integrity of the white matter tracts.

Beyond 10 months of age, a typical basic MRI protocol to study patients with cortical malformations comprises turbo-spin-echo T2-weighted acquisitions along axial and coronal planes, obtained with contiguous slices (covering the entire brain with 3 mm thick slices). This is followed by volume T1-weighted acquisition, obtained with the 3D gradient-echo technique

(< 1 mm thickness); 3D images may be reformatted in any orientation and used for volumetric measurements. FLAIR images should not be employed before the third year of life.

Contrast medium injection is confined to a few specific clinical radiological scenarios, particularly when a differential diagnosis from cortical tumours is needed.

Classification

Recent advances in genetics have had revolutionary consequences for the classification of cortical malformations. The classical concepts, mainly founded on a morphologic basis (Barkovich *et al.*, 2001), became confusing as knowledge about gene mutations and their consequences increased (Table 2). Considering the aetiological aspects, a critical point was the overlapping function of genetic and environmental factors in inducing cortical malformations.

A classification according to phenotypic criteria alone risks being inconsistent, and new proposals suggest classifying malformations under the different mutated genes (Sarnat, 2000). On the other hand, no unequivocal correlation between phenotype and genotype exists (the same phenotype can result from mutations of multiple genes, and the same gene mutation may produce different phenotypes), so updated classifications generally consider both genetic and morphological axes (Sarnat & Flores-Sarnat, 2002; Barkovich *et al.*, 2005). We will refer predominantly to the Barkovich classification (2005), though other classifications that focus on genetic expression present additional analytic criteria. This is the case with the Sarnat & Flores-Sarnat classification (2002) which, for example, considers neuroblast migration according to the time of disruption (initial, middle, or late), along with the respective known underlying genetic mutations. An up-to-date presentation of the influence on cortical development of the principal genes with detected mutations is shown in Fig. 1.

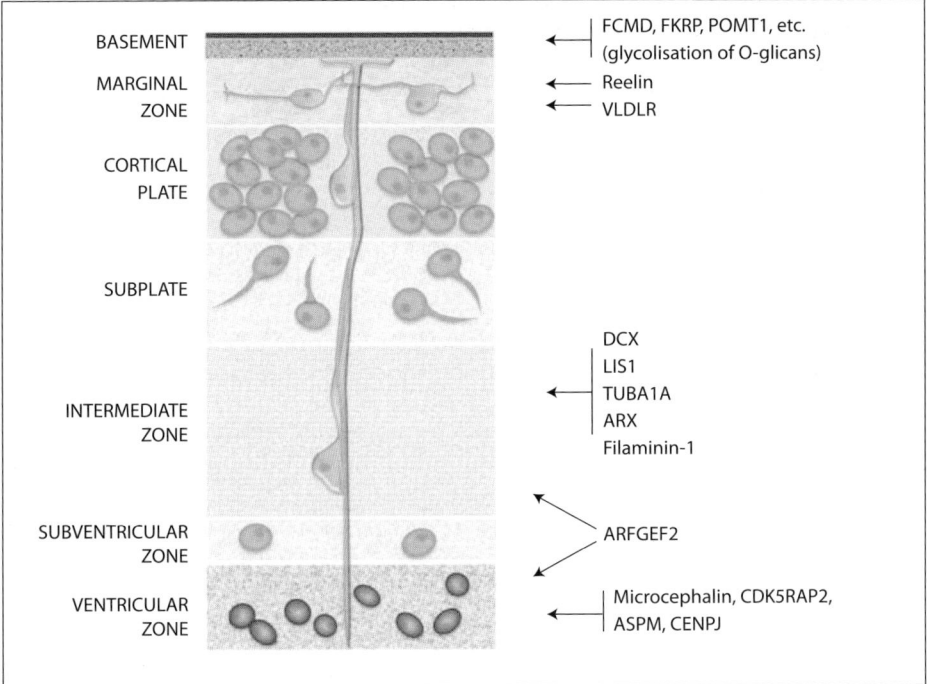

Fig. 1. Influence on cortical development of main genes whose mutations have been so far detected. For the meaning of acronyms see table 2.

Table 2. The most frequent gene mutations associated with cortical development disorders

Class and name	Inheritance	Mutated gene	Chromosome	Function of gene product	Brain malformation
Proliferation/apoptosis disorders					
Primary microcephaly	Autosomal recessive	Micro-cephalin	8p23	Inhibition CDK1 phosphorylation, which prevents mitosis	Microcephalia vera
		MCPH2	19q13.1-q13.2		
		CDK5RAP2	9q31.2–q34.1	Involved in centrosomal function	
		MCPH4	15q15-q21		
		ASPM	1q31	Essential for normal mitotic spindle function in embryonic neuroblasts	
		CENPJ	13q12.2	Centrosomal protein that may have a role in microtubule nucleation	
Tuberous sclerosis	Autosomal dominant	TSC1	9q34.13	(Hamartin) activation of MTOR and downstream signalling elements, resulting in tumour development and neurological disorders	Cortical tubers and subependymal nodules
		TSC2	16p13.3	(Tuberin)	
Agyria-pachygyria-band spectrum					
ILS or SBH	Autosomal dominant	LIS1	17p13.3	(PAF-AH) regulation of microtubule organization and function, critical for neuronal migration	Classical lissencephaly or band heterotopia
		TUBA1A	12q13.12	(α-tubulin)	
Miller-Dieker syndrome		LIS1 + YWHAE	17p13.3	Co-deletion of YWHAE with LIS1, acting as a modifier locus	Severe lissencephaly
	X-linked	DCX	Xq22.3-q24	(Doublecortin)	Subcortical band heteropia or lissencephaly
Lissencephaly with cerebellar hypoplasia	Autosomal recessive	RELN	7q22	(Reelin) disruption of Dab1 pathway that leads at the end stages of radial migration (accumulation of neurons beneath the preplate)	Pachygyria with simple moderate thickened gyri and cerebellar hypoplasia
		VLDLR	9q24	Defect in very low density lipoprotein receptor binding with the protein Reelin	

Agyria-pachygyria-band spectrum					
XLAG	X-linked	ARX	Xp22.1-p21.3	Interacts via its homeodomain with IPO13, a mediator of direct nucleocytoplasmic transport	Lissencephaly with moderate increase in thickness of cortex and with a posterior-to-anterior gradient
Infantile spasms with severe dyskinetic quadriparesis			Xp22.1-p21.3	Inhibition of tangential migration of GABAergic inhibitory interneurons	Foci of abnormal cavitation on T1 and increased signal intensity on T2 in putamina
Cobblestone complex					
MEB or WWS	Autosomal recessive	POMT1	9q34.1	Glia limitans integrity perturbed by defective glycosylation of O-glycans (deficit of *O*-mannosyltransferase 1)	Cobblestone lissencephaly
MEB or WWS		POMT2	14q24.3	(deficit of *O*-mannosyltransferase 2)	
MEB disease		POMGnT1	1p32-34	(deficit of mannosyl-glucosamintransferase)	
MEB disease		LARGE	22q12.3-q13.1	Molecular recognition of dystroglycan by LARGE is a key determinant in the biosynthetic pathway to produce mature and functional dystroglycan	
FCMD mutation		FCMD	9q31	(Fukutin) glycosylation of α-dystroglycan	
MEB or WWS		FKRP	19q13.3	(Fukutin-related protein)	
Heterotopia					
FLNA mutation	X-linked dominant	FLNA	Xq28	(Filaminin A) links proteins at the plasma membrane and the cytoskeleton (adhesion, motility and signal transduction)	Periventricular nodular heterotopia (PNH)
ARFGEF2 mutation	Autosomal recessive	ARFGEF2	20q13.13	Favours transport to the cell surface of molecules such as E-cadherin and β-catenin, enhancing proliferation and migration	Microcephaly and PNH

Abnormal cortical organization					
BFPP	Autosomal recessive	GPR56	16q12.2–21	(G-protein-coupled receptor), expressed in neuronal progenitor cells of the ventricular and subventricular germinal zones	BFPP, myelination defects, cerebellar cortical dysplasia
Polymicrogyria	Autosomal dominant	PAX6	11p13	Expressed by radial glia in developing neocortex, produces many cortical projection neurons for deep cortical layers (large cortical neurons)	Polymicrogyria
Rolandic seizures, oromotor dyspraxia	X-linked	SRPX2	Xq22	Role in the development and/or function of the perisylvian region critical for language and cognitive development	Perisylvian polymicrogyria
CCA, microcephaly and PMG	Autosomal dominant	TBR2	3p21	Expressed by intermediate progenitor cells in developing neocortex	Polymicrogyria, microcephaly and CCA

ILS, isolated lissencephaly; SBH, subcortical band heterotopia; XLAG, X-linked lissencephaly with corpus callosum agenesis and ambiguous genitalia; MEB, muscle-eye-brain syndrome; WWS, Walker-Warburg syndrome; FLNA, filaminin; ARGEF2, ADP-ribosylation factor guanine nucleotide exchange factor-2; BFPP, bilateral frontoparietal polymicrogyria; CCA, corpus callosum agenesis; PMG, polymicrogyria: MTOR, mammalian target of rapamycin; PAF.AH, platelet-activating factor acetylhydrolase.

Proliferation and differentiation

Normal cortical development involves in the early phase of proliferation (2–4 months of gestation), neuronal proliferation, and the generation of radial glia inside the ventricular zone of the germinal matrix, and for some regions of the forebrain in the subventricular zone. Later on, from 5 months of gestation up to approximately 1 year, glial proliferation predominates.

Developmental disorders of the proliferation stage are believed to come both from disturbed intrinsic cell proliferation mechanisms, which control neuron number, and from abnormal programmed cell death (Price, 2004; Rakic, 2005). The study on abnormal proliferation/apoptosis (according the classification by Barkovitch et al., 2001) provides a new insight into the mechanisms whereby neuron numbers and the formation of correct lamination and cortical convolutions are controlled (Francis et al., 2006).

Malformations related to the proliferation phase, according to the most recent classification of Barkovich et al. (2005), consist of two groups. The first group includes all the disorders of abnormal proliferation or apoptosis, both excessive or defective, often with multifactorial causes (McConnell, 1995; Desai & McConnell, 2000; Marin-Padilla et al., 2002; Marin-Padilla et al., 2003). The second group includes abnormal cell types. Along with these two genetic categories, a third category involving the acquired (destructive) forms may also be included (Table 3).

Table 3. Malformations due to abnormal encephalic growth

A. Acquired (secondary) microcephaly, due to intrauterine or postnatal destructive brain injuries

B. Congenital malformations
1. Due to abnormal neuronal and glial proliferation or apoptosis
   a. Microcephaly with normal to thin cortex
   b. Microlissencephaly (extreme microcephaly with thick cortex)
   c. Microcephaly with extensive polymicrogyria
   d. Megalencephalies
2. Due to abnormal proliferation (abnormal cell types)
   a. Non-neoplastic
      i. Cortical hamartomas of tuberous sclerosis
      ii. Cortical dysplasia with balloon cells
      iii. Hemimegalencephaly
   b. Neoplastic (associated with disordered cortex): dysembryoplastic neuroepithelial tumour, ganglioglioma, gangliocytoma

Decreased proliferation/increased apoptosis or increased proliferation/decreased apoptosis: abnormalities of brain size

The abnormalities of brain size include microcephalies and megalencephalies. In microcephalies the size of the head is significantly smaller than normal: according to the classification of Barkovich et al. (2001), the cranial circumference should be more than 2 SD below the mean, though others place the cut-off at −3 SD (Goodman & Gorlin, 1983). Apart from acquired (secondary) microcephalies (Abuelo, 2007), caused by accidents occurring during intrauterine life or postnatally (intrauterine or postnatal destructive diseases), congenital microcephalies are characterized by an error in the programmed development of the proliferation phase.

On the basis of clinical, morphological and genetic data, congenital microcephalies are classified into at least four main categories: primary microcephaly or *microcephalia vera*, extreme microcephaly with simplified gyral pattern (MSGP), microlissencephaly, and microcephaly with polymicrogyria or other cortical dysplasias often associated with corpus callosum agenesis (Table 3) (Barkovich et al., 2005; Francis et al., 2006).

Microcephaly

Microcephalia vera is difficult to confirm because it overlaps with other unidentified forms. Conventionally, the cranial circumference should be between −2 and −3 SD (Barkovich et al., 2001) or the brain should weigh less than 500 g in adults with no other associated malformations (Mochida & Walsh, 2001). A correct description, however, should be confined to the autosomal recessive cases (Evrard et al., 1989).

Primary microcephaly is characterized by size preponderance of the face over the calvarium, a markedly small brain with a normal or later a thin cortex, surrounded by enlarged extracerebral CSF spaces (Fig. 2). Morphological features of the brain (from pathological and MRI studies) include a simplified but grossly conserved gyral pattern.

Studies by Rakic (2003) suggested that early proliferation provides the cell precursors of the radial columns of cortical cells, so producing their tangential expansion. In microcephalia vera this proliferation is relatively preserved (with near normal gyration), while later cell division is impaired, determining the decrease in the number of vertically arranged cells and producing a thinner cortex (Francis et al., 2006).

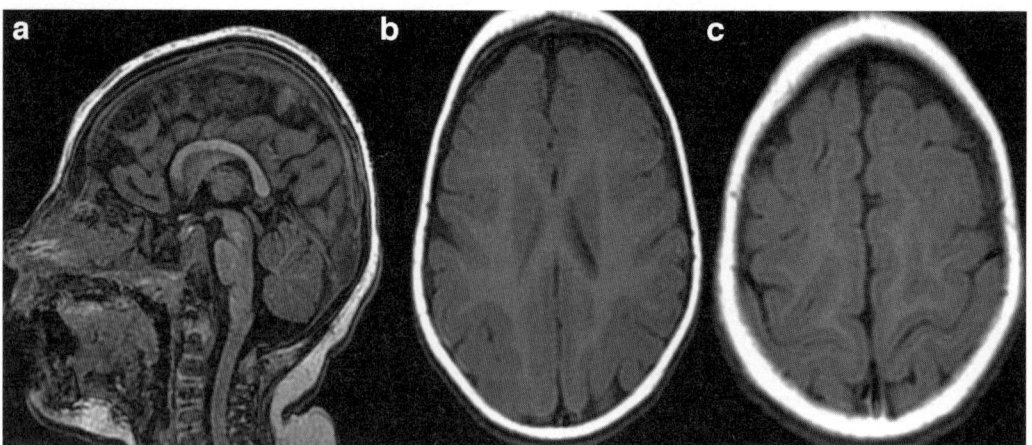

Fig. 2. Microcephaly with normal cortex. Sagittal (a) and axial (b,c) T1w images. Brain and skull are smaller than normal. No apparent change of brain cortex.

Genetic mapping has revealed six genetic loci, named MCPH1–MCPH6 (Francis *et al.*, 2006), and four genes have been already cloned (*ASPM* at MCPH5 locus on chromosome 1q31, *MCPH1* (microcephalin) at MCPH1 locus on chromosome 8p23, *CDK5RAP2* at MCPH3 locus on chromosome 9q31.2–q34.1, and *CENPJ* at MCPH6 locus on chromosome 13q12.2) (Bond *et al.*, 2002; Jackson *et al.*, 2002, Bond *et al.*, 2005). *ASPM* (abnormal spindle-like microcephaly associated) codes for a protein apparently essential for mitotic spindle function in embryonic neuroblasts. The expression of *ASPM* in mouse is restricted to the proliferative zones of the cortex, thus showing its relevance to neurogenesis. *Microcephalin*, on the other hand, codes for a protein that regulates chromosome condensation before its segregation in mitosis; mutations in *microcephalin* thus produce an impairment of the cell cycle during neurogenesis. Finally, cyclin-dependent kinase 5 regulatory subunit-associated protein 2 *(CDK5RAP2)* and centromere protein J *(CENPJ)*, expressed in neuroepithelial tissue, are involved in centrosomal function. All these genes are thus implicated in controlling neuron proliferation and consequently affect the neuron destiny (cell fate choice) in human brain.

The clinical presentation is characterized by the relative preservation of development with no severe mental retardation. Motor deficit and seizures are rarely observed. Some severe clinical forms are associated with very rare genetic mutations (Barkovich *et al.*, 2005).

Extreme microcephaly with a simplified gyral pattern

Extreme microcephaly with a simplified gyral pattern (MSGP; Mochida & Walsh, 2001) is the second main form of microcephaly. The brain architecture in this case is strongly affected because of a definitely simplified gyral pattern with an extremely thin cortex. Brain volume is much reduced (cranial circumference more than 3 SD below the mean according to Barkovich *et al.*, 2001) with a normally laminated but immature cortex.

These morphological characteristics are revealed by MRI which can show reduced brain volume, with thin, smooth cortex, and a simplified gyral pattern (oligogyria), surrounded by extremely enlarged CSF spaces.

Neuropathological features include a reduced germinal zone with cysts and abnormal neuronal loss (Fallet-Bianco, 2000). Both precursor cell proliferation and late cell divisions seem to be impaired (Francis *et al.*, 2006). Genetic heterogeneity with a continuum towards microcephalia vera is presumed because of the lack of identification of specific genetic loci. Infants with this form of microcephaly have diffuse motor disabilities and resistant seizures. They usually die in the neonatal period or in early infancy.

Microlissencephaly

In microlissencephaly (MLIS) (Dobyns & Truwit, 1995), in contrast to MSGP, there is a thickened and disorganized cortex. Isolated or associated with other syndromes (Pena-Shokeir syndrome, lethal multiple pterigium syndrome, type III lissencephaly) (Francis *et al.*, 2006), it is characterized by an extremely small agyric brain with incomplete lamination and evidence of neuronal degeneration.

Widening of cortex thickness is the key factor differentiating microlissencephaly from microcephalia vera. Neuroimaging shows a markedly small brain with a simplified gyral pattern, and shallow sulci or even complete agyria. The corpus callosum may be absent and the cortex shows variable thickening. MLIS may be associated with cerebellar hypoplasia in the group of *lissencephalies with cerebellar hypoplasia* (LCH), in which, according to Barkovich's definition, six different types of LCH are recognized, with possible cerebellar or brain stem hypoplasia, or both.

So far no gene locus has been found. Based on studies in the mouse, it seems that microlissencephaly may be the result of a disequilibrium between cell proliferation and cell death of either neuronal progenitors or postmitotic neurons (Francis *et al.*, 2006). Affected infants generally die early in the neonatal period.

Megalencephaly

An excessive proliferative disorder may be the cause of megalencephaly accompanied by an enlargement of the skull (macrocephaly). Macrocephalies (Table 4) consist of a group of heterogeneous conditions including a physiological variant of brain size. Macrocephalies without megalencephaly may be due to hydrocephalus, subdural haematoma, enlargement of the subarachnoid spaces, or a thickened calvarium. Megalencephaly is generally divided into developmental and metabolic types. Metabolic megalencephaly comprises storage or neurodegenerative diseases (for example, Alexander's disease, Canavan disease), whereas developmental megalencephalies are caused by proliferative disorders, identified in the brain by excessive cellular proliferation occurring in various syndromes, including neurocutaneous syndrome and vanishing white matter disease. When unilateral, it is named hemimegalencephaly. We deal with this in the next section.

Table 4. Macrocephalies

Classification of macrocephalies
(1) Without megalencephaly (hydrocephalus, subdural haematoma, etc.)
(2) With megalencephaly
(a) metabolic (Alexander's disease, Canavan disease, Tay-Sachs disease, etc.)
(b) developmental, isolated or syndromic (Sotos syndrome, Gorlin syndrome, etc.) (Olney, 2007)

Non-neoplastic forms of abnormal proliferation (abnormal cell types)

Cortical malformations caused by abnormal proliferation with abnormal cell types are classified by Barkovich *et al.* (2005), in particular non-neoplastic forms including cortical hamartomas of tuberous sclerosis, cortical dysplasia with balloon cells, and hemimegalencephaly (Table 3).

All these forms are characterized by the presence of abnormal cells – 'balloon cells' (huge size, pale eosinophilic cytoplasm staining with neuronal or glial markers, or both, and one or more eccentric nuclei) – resulting from a disorder of differentiation at an early (stem cell) stage (Robain, 1996).

There is evidence that in these disorders (focal cortical dysplasia (FCD), hemimegalencephaly, and tuberous sclerosis) there is an enhanced activation of the mTOR cascade. The mTOR pathway is supposed to regulate cell growth and thus may provide an explanation for the malformations associated with aberrant cell size. Using new genetic methodologies (single nucleotide polymorphism (SNP) array and gene sequencing, gene and protein expression profile techniques) to determine how mTOR activation leads to cortical maldevelopment, a common pathogenesis for these disorders may be identified (Crino, 2007).

Cortical hamartomas of tuberous sclerosis

Tuberous sclerosis is a neurocutaneous syndrome inherited as an autosomal dominant disease with high penetrance, characterized by the presence of hamartomata in multiple organ systems including the brain (cortical tubers) (Crino *et al.*, 2006).

Cortical tubers are characterized by focal disruption of the cortical architecture, with prominent dysmorphic neurons, balloon and giant cells, and increased numbers of astrocytes (Scheithauer & Reagan, 1999; Crino, 2004). As well as cortical tubers, subependymal nodules may be found in the walls of the lateral ventricles. These are composed of abnormal glial cells and multi-nucleated cells of indeterminate origin, progression of which may produce subependymal giant cell tumours typically located in the region of the foramen of Monroe and associated with the risk of developing obstructive hydrocephalus.

Mutations of either of two tumour suppressor genes – *TSC1* (mapped on the chromosome 9q34) or *TSC2* (mapped on the chromosome 16p13) – are the cause of tuberous sclerosis complex (TSC) (Kwiatkowski & Manning, 2005). They code, respectively, for two proteins (hamartin and tuberin) which play an important role in a signalling pathway that regulates cell proliferation and differentiation (Kwiatkowski & Manning, 2005; Sarbassov *et al.*, 2005). Biallelic mutation of either *TSC1* or *TSC2* has been observed in most hamartomas from TSC patients (Cheadle *et al.*, 2000; Chan *et al.*, 2004). TSC hamartomas show a loss of the tumour-suppressor genes *TSC1* and *TSC2* and thus of hamartin-tuberin complex; this – through its GAP (GTPase-activating protein) – induces a critical negative regulation of mTORC1 (mammalian target of rapamycin complex 1) with its downstream effector, resulting in the development of tumours and neurological disorders. Similarly, in subependymal giant cell astrocytomas there are markers of mTORC1 activation (Chan *et al.*, 2004). Studies on genotype/phenotype correlation showed that mutations in *TSC2* produce more severe symptoms (Au *et al.*, 2007).

In about 20 per cent of patients there is no evidence of mutation (Kwiatkowski, 2003). As well as brain, the disease may involve skin, kidneys, heart, eyes, teeth, and other organs where tumours may develop. The severity of TSC, the manifestations of which may occur later in life, ranges from mild skin abnormalities to severe neurological and renal signs. Neurological symptoms include epilepsy with early severe seizures, predominantly infantile spasms, developmental delay, and behavioural disorders. Studies report the presence of pervasive developmental disorders in a large proportion of cases.

Medically intractable seizures caused by balloon cell lesions may be managed surgically. This can be especially effective in selected patients (Maldhavan *et al.*, 2007). Studies identifying candidates for surgery may use new diagnostic tools to identify more epileptogenic tubers (Iida et al., 2005).

In almost all individual with TSC, dermatological signs are present: hypomelanic macules ('ash leaf spots'), usually the only visible sign of TSC at birth; facial angiofibromas in a butterfly distribution; ungual or subungual fibromas, very rare in childhood; and shagreen patches, wrinkled like orange peel, usually found in the axillae. In a variable proportion of cases other benign tumours of the heart (rhabdomyoma, mostly present at birth) or of the kidneys (angiomyolipomas) as well as of the eyes (retinal astrocytic hamartomas, revealed by ophthalmic examination as greyish or yellowish-white lesions) may be observed.

Cortical tubers are identical – by histology, neuroimaging, and clinical manifestations – to focal cortical dysplasia with balloon cells. They are most common in the cerebral hemispheres but may occur in the cerebellum as well.

Computed tomography (CT) shows cortical tubers in children as foci of low attenuation, typically expanding a gyrus. Calcifications are sometimes found in the tubers. In unmyelinated brain, MRI shows lesions on T1-weighted images as hyperintense in both grey and white matter; on T2-weighted images they appear as hypointense in white matter (Fig. 3). MRI can also show a funnel-like extension of the lesion towards the ventricular surface. As the white matter myelinates, the appearance of the lesions changes: when myelination is complete, they appear either as hyperintense when compared with surrounding white matter on T2-weighted images, or isointense as well as slightly hypointense when compared with surrounding normal white matter on T1-weighted images.

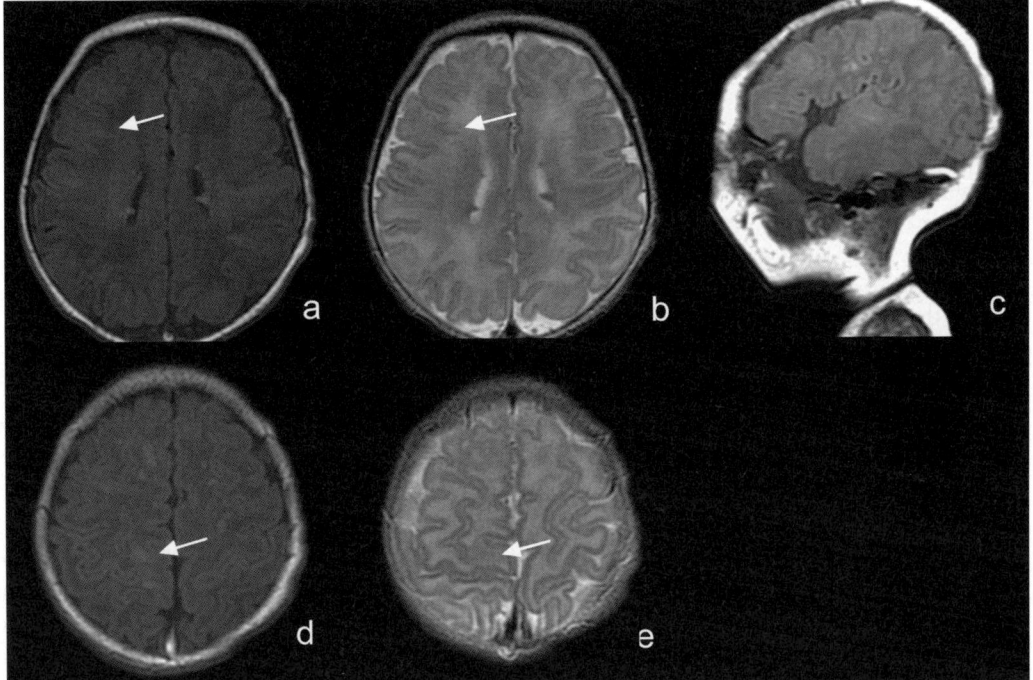

Fig. 3. Tuberous sclerosis. Axial T1w (a,c) and T2w (b,d) images; c) Sagittal T1w image. Infant with unmyelinated brain: cortical tubers appear as slightly hyperintense on T1w and slightly hypointense on T2-w images in both gray and white matter; typical subependimal hamartomas are also evident.

Calcified cortical tubers sometimes appear bright on Tl-weighted images, while tubers with degenerative changes may show mild enhancement which should not be misinterpreted as malignant degeneration.

Hemimegalencephaly

Hemimegalencephaly (HME) is a rare sporadic congenital brain malformation consisting of hypertrophy of all or part of a cerebral hemisphere (Flores-Sarnat, 2002). Exceptionally, there is also hypertrophy of the ipsilateral cerebellum (Fitz et al., 1978; Sener, 1997; Di Rocco & Iannelli, 2000).

Enlargement of a large part of an entire hemisphere or part of a hemisphere (generally, the posterior quadrant), with thickened cortex and ipsilateral ventricular dilatation, as well as white matter and basal ganglia changes, are typical features of hemimegalencephaly (Kalifa et al., 1987; Barkovich & Chuang, 1990). Histologically, there is a disruption of cortical lamination with diffuse dysmorphic and balloon cells spreading into the white matter; neuronal heterotopia, polymicrogyria, and marked gliosis are other abnormalities found (Bosman et al., 1996).

Neuroimaging (Fig. 4) shows gross asymmetry with enlargement of all parts of one hemisphere and, possibly, of the ipsilateral half of the brain stem and cerebellar hemisphere. The cerebral cortex is irregularly thickened and includes a variable spectrum of disorders including lissencephaly, pachygyria and polymicrogyria. The gyri are broad and flat, and the sulci are shallow. Typically the affected hemisphere contains a dilated ventricle. In neonates, white matter changes are characterized by hyperintensity on T1wi and hypointensity on T2wi; in older children the affected white matter is hyperintense compared with normal on T2wi, and the white matter volume is increased. Calcifications, better demonstrated on CT, can involve white matter and grey matter. Polymicrogyric hemispheres are larger than lissencephalic ones.

Patients with hemimegalencephaly present with an asymmetrically enlarged skull, contralateral hemiparesis with hemianopia, developmental delay, and epilepsy. These features may be isolated in many cases (Sasaki et al., 2000; Tinkle et al., 2005) or occur in the context of a syndrome. The onset of seizures is very early, even in the neonatal period, and they are often resistant to drug treatment, so that infants are often candidates for surgical management. Early surgical treatment involves either anatomical hemispherectomy (Di Rocco & Iannelli, 2000) or, to avoid additional complications, a functional anatomical approach – that is, the disconnection (without ablation) of the affected hemisphere (Schramm et al., 2001). If the surgery is carried out within the first year, a favourable outcome is possible, especially in relation to seizure evolution (Battaglia et al., 1999; Devlin et al., 2003; Lettori et al., 2007).

Syndromic hemimegalencephaly comprises at least one third of the cases, mainly the neurocutaneous syndromes (Tinkle et al., 2005). The epidermal nevus syndrome and other neurocutaneous syndromes (proteus syndrome, encephalocraniocutaneous lipomatosis, hypomelanosis of Ito, Klippel-Trenaunay syndrome, and tuberous sclerosis) are the most commonly reported. Some of these (for example, epidermal nevus or hypomelanosis of Ito) may not be present in infancy and only develop later, so that an early diagnosis may not be possible. Intriguingly, the association between hemimegalencephaly and tuberous sclerosis (because of the histopathological similarities of the two diseases) suggests a common genetic origin, although so far no known genetic mutation has been reported in hemimegalencephaly.

We will deal with focal cortical dysplasia in the section on abnormal organization (see below).

Chapter 4   Malformations of cortical development

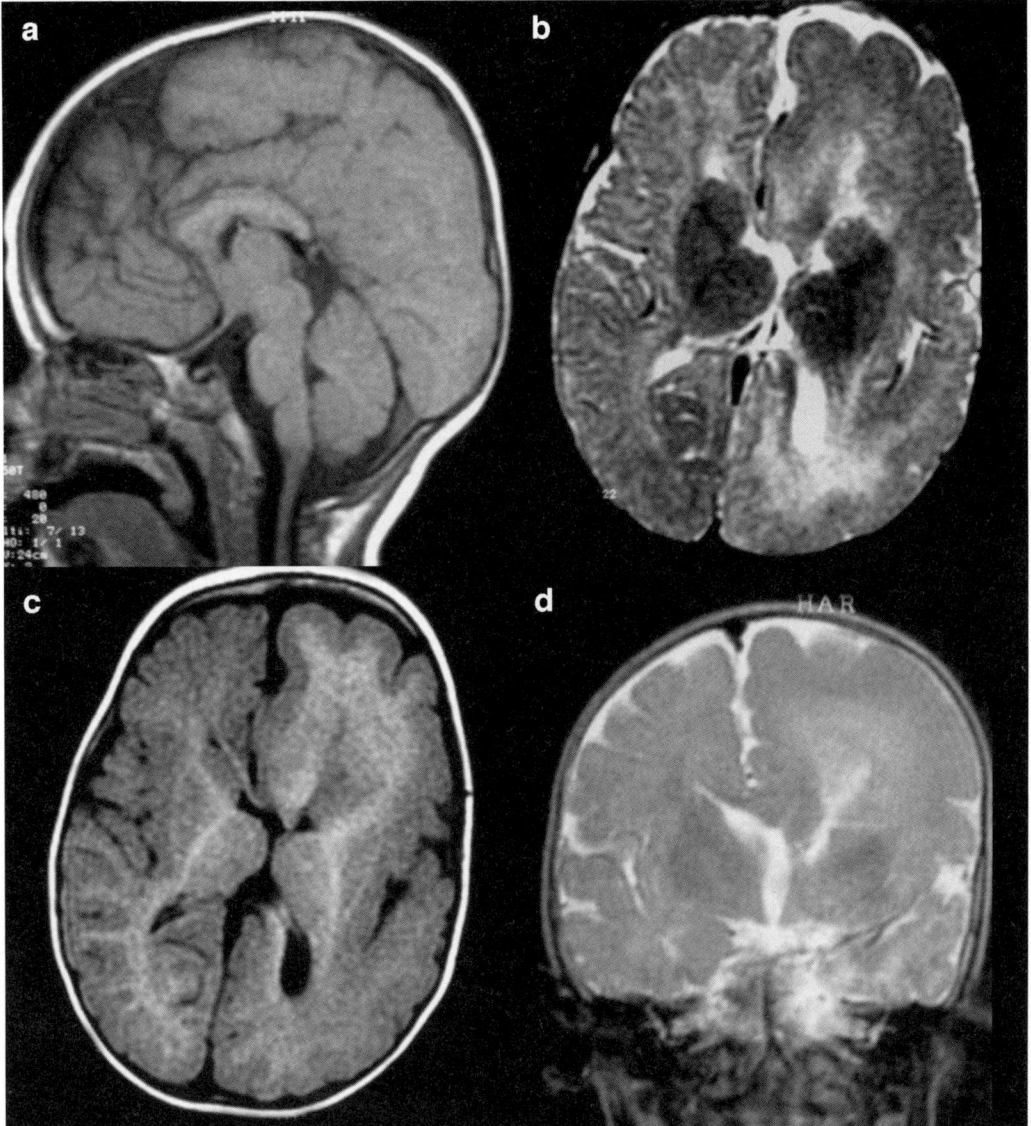

Fig. 4. Hemimegalencephaly
a) Sagittal T1w image; b, c) axial T2w and T1w images; d) coronal T2w image.
MR images show enlargement of left cerebral hemisphere; cerebral cortex is irregularly thickened, gyri are broad and flat with shallow peripheral sulci.
MR T2w images show also a diffuse hyperintensity of the inner WM of the left hemisphere that is increased in volume.

Migration

Migration consists of movement of postmitotic nerve cells from the sites of origin to the definitive location (the cortex and the deep nuclei), generally guided by radial glial cells that make up the columnar pattern of brain architecture. Recently, a tangential migration not derived from the germinal zones of the dorsal telencephalon has also been recognized, especially for the GABAergic cortical interneurons. This seems to be at least partially generated in the lateral, medial, and caudal ganglionic eminences (LGE, MGE, and CGE) and migrates tangentially into the cerebral cortex, though its route remains controversial (Kriegstein & Noctor, 2004). The function of radial glia as a mere guide for radial migration is also controversial, but its role as the progenitor cell of neurons and glia has now been recognized (Rakic, 2003).

The period of migration in the human is predominantly from the third to the fifth month of gestation. The first migration aims at the formation of the preplate, which is subsequently split by the arrival of cortical plate neurons into a marginal zone and a subplate (Marin-Padilla, 1978). Lamination of cortical plate is formed by an inside-outside process, so that the deepest layer is formed first and the successive waves migrate through the predecessors up to the marginal zone (Caviness & Takahashi, 1995). Particularly relevant in humans is the subplate, a kind of transient neuronal population that develops predominantly in the third trimester of gestation in parallel with the cortical plate (Kostovic & Rakic, 1990; Meyer et al., 2000). Subplate neurons have an important function in the developing brain. They are established at sites where thalamocortical and corticocortical afferents form synaptic contacts enabling them subsequently to reach cortical targets that contribute to an adequate cortical organization. Moreover, they form guides for the projections from the cerebral cortex towards subcortical targets (Ghosh & Shatz, 1992; Ghosh & Shatz, 1993; Volpe, 2008).

Malformations resulting from abnormal migration are divided in Barkovich's classification (Barkovich et al., 2005) into different groups, including the lissencephaly spectrum and the heterotopias. Another category should, however, be considered, consisting of non-genetic malformations secondary to acquired lesions occurring early in development. These include white matter ischaemic or haemorrhagic infarction interrupting the radial glial fibres that guide migratory neuroblasts (Sarnat & Flores-Sarnat, 2004) (Table 5).

Table 5. Malformations due to abnormal neuronal migration

(A) Genetic malformations (caused by gene mutations)
1. Lissencephalies/subcortical band heterotopia spectrum
    a. *LIS1* mutations
    b. *TUBA1A* mutations
    c. *DCX* mutations
    d. *ARX* mutations
    e/f. *RELN* and *VLDLR* mutations: pachygyria with extreme cerebellar hypoplasia
    g. Other lissencephaly/pachygyria syndromes

2. Cobblestone complex (congenital muscular dystrophy syndromes)
    a. *POMT1* and *POMT* mutations (WWS or MEB disease)
    b. *POMGnT1* mutation: MEB disease
    c. *LARGE* mutation: MEB disease
    d. *FCMD* mutation
    e. *FKRP* mutation: MEB disease or WWS

(B) Heterotopias Subependymal heterotopia (periventricular nodular heterotopia, PNH) Subcortical heterotopia (other than band heterotopia): subcortical heterotopic nodules, columnar (transmantle) heterotopia, ribbon heterotopia, etc. Leptomeningeal heterotopia
(C) Acquired malformations Migration disorders due to ischaemic, haemorrhagic, or toxic early lesions of white matter

MEB, muscle-eye-brain disease; WWS, Walker-Warburg syndrome.

Agyria-pachygyria-band spectrum

Classical lissencephaly

Classical lissencephaly (smooth brain) is caused by a defect of early migration, both tangential and radial, and is characterized by an abnormally thick cortex. Tangential migration is especially involved in the X-linked type of lissencephaly in which expression of *DCX* (the causative gene) is predominantly in non-radially oriented cells of the SVZ (Meyer *et al.*, 2002). The name 'lissencephaly' derives from the appearance of the brain surface, with absent (agyria) or decreased (pachygyria) convolutions and shallow sulci (Barkovich *et al.*, 2005). The defective migration prevents neurons from reaching their final destination. A disrupted lamination shows only four layers consisting of a superficial pyramidal layer, normally located more deeply, under the marginal layer and above a cell-sparse and a dense inner cell layer, possibly reflecting incomplete migration of neurons (Jellinger & Rett, 1976).

Subcortical band heteropia (SBH) results from a partial migration defect. In this there is a bilateral band of heterotopic neurons within the white matter which parallels an apparently normal cortex. SBH, though in some ways differing pathologically from lissencephaly (heterotopia rather than cortical dysplasia), will be dealt here for genetic reasons: the causative gene mutations and the mechanism of the migration defect are in fact common in these two conditions, forming the so-called agyria-pachygyria-band spectrum.

Neuroimaging shows a continuous spectrum of findings, ranging from *complete lissencephaly* (Fig. 5) to localized forms of subcortical band of heterotopia (SBH) (Fig. 6). Dobyns *et al.* (1999a) proposed a six tiered grading system for lissencephaly and SBH (see Table 6), as follows:

- Lissencephaly (Agyria, Dobyns' grade 1) is rare, the brain is small with a smooth surface, complete lack of sulci, and vertically oriented sylvian fissures; cortical thickness is around 10 mm.
- Diffuse agyria (Agyria-pachygyria, Dobyns' grade 2–4) presents with a few shallow sulci subdividing the cortical mantle in broad coarse gyri. In the less severe cases portions not completely agyric can be found.
- Subcortical band heterotopia (Dobyns' grade 5–6) is due to a partial migration defect and is characterized by a bilateral band of heterotopic neurons within the white matter deep to the cortical mantle, paralleling an apparently normal cortex. The gyral pattern can be normal with normal thickness and shallow sulci, or can be pachygyric.

Table 6. Grading system for classical lissencephaly and subcortical band heterotopia (Dobyns *et al.*, 1999b)

1) Diffuse agyria
2) Diffuse agyria with a few shallow sulci
3) Mixed agyria and pachygyria
4) Diffuse or partial pachygyria only
5) Mixed pachygyria and subcortical band of heterotopia
6) Subcortical band of heterotopia only

There are three genes with germline or more rarely mosaicism mutations related to this spectrum. Cases of classical lissencephaly in acquired intrauterine diseases such as fetal cytomegalovirus infection are described as well (Dobyns *et al.*, 1992). The genes involved are: *LIS1* on chromosome 17p13.3 (Reiner *et al.*, 1993); *DCX* on chromosome Xq22.3-q24, mostly mutated in SBH (des Portes *et al.*, 1998; Gleeson *et al.*, 1998); and rarely *TUBA1A* on chromosome 12q13.12 (Poirier *et al.*, 2007), transmitted as an autosomal recessive disease. This mutation is mostly observed in classical lissencephaly.

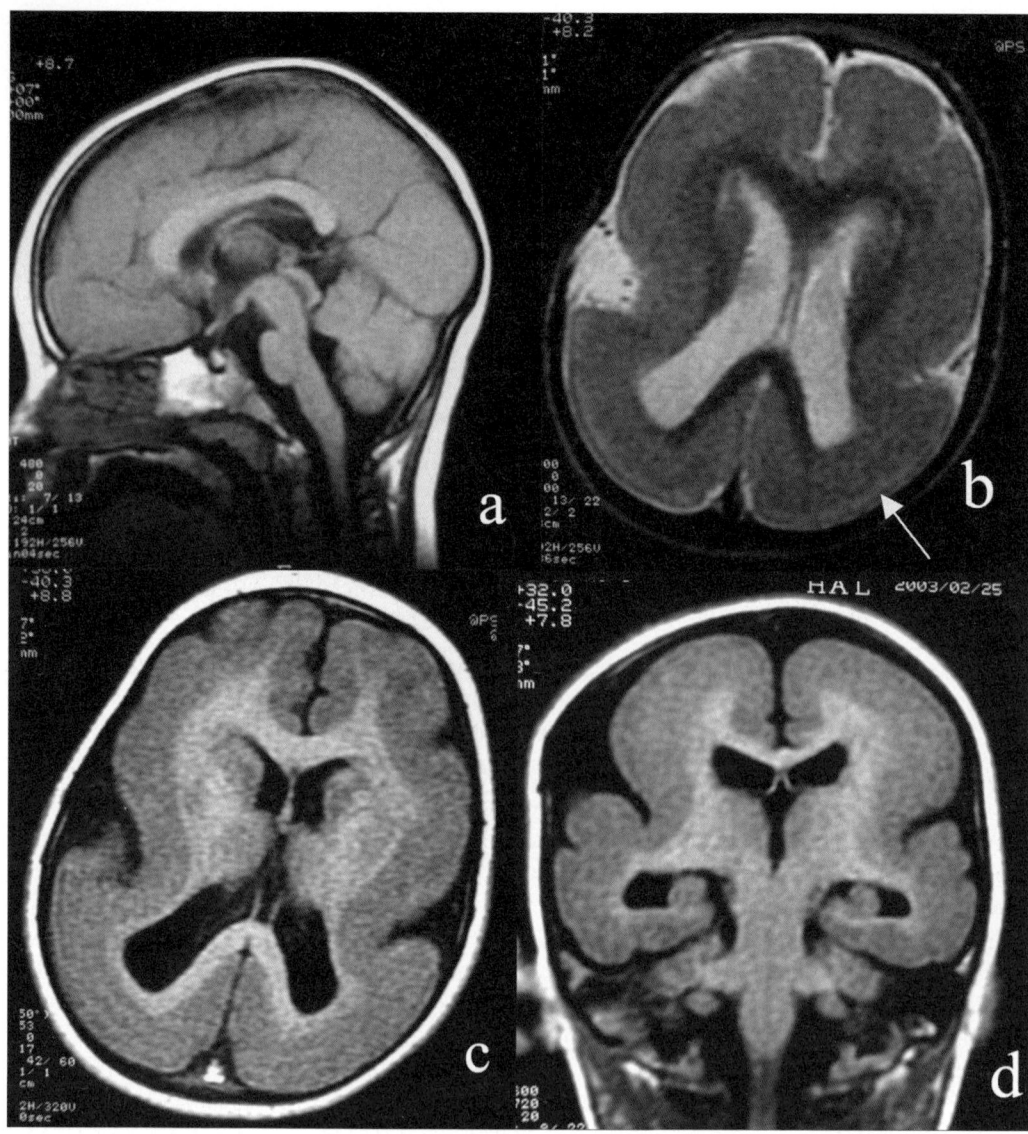

Fig. 5. Lissencephaly type 1.
a) Sagittal T1w image; b, c) Axial FSE T2w and T1w images; d) Coronal FSE T1w image.
MRI show a small brain, with smooth surface, quite complete lack of sulci, vertically oriented Sylvian fissures, with characteristic 'eight' pattern; cortical thickness is > 10 mm; the bright subcortical band on T2w image (arrow) is related to cells-sparse layer. Corpus callosum is dismorphic.

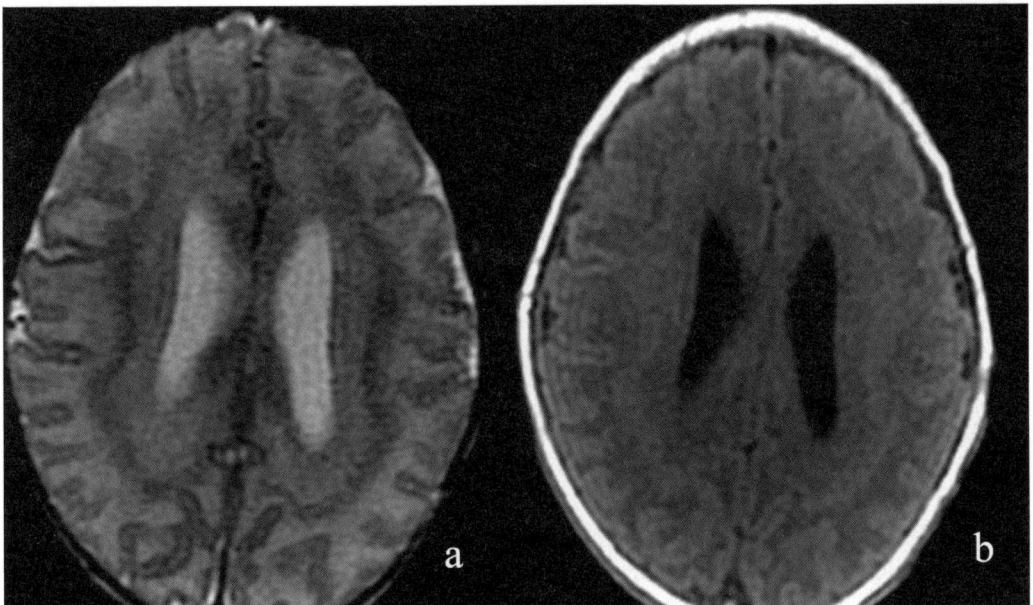

Fig. 6. Subcortical band of heterotopia in neonate ('double cortex').
a, b: Axial T2w and T1w FSE images.
In a neonate with moderate microcephaly MRI show a band of gray matter in both fronto-parietal corona radiata. The overlying cortex is thin, with shallow sulci. The heterotopic band is hypointense on T2w images and hyperintense on T2w and hyperintense on T1w images with respect to the normal unmyelinated with matter.

LIS1, *TUBA1A*, and *DCX* encode, respectively, for proteins PAF-AH (platelet activating factor acetylhydrolase, an enzyme that degrades the bioactive factor), α-tubulin, and doublecortin, which play a role in the regulation of nuclear microtubule organization and function, critical for neuronal migration; they block microtubule-directed nuclear movement in ventricular zone neuroblasts converting postmitotic neurons to bipolar migratory cells (Francis *et al.*, 2006).

Phenotypic expression of *LIS1* mutation, generally with posterior predominance (Piltz *et al.*, 1998; Gleeson *et al.*, 2000), varies according to the type of mutation – that is, deletion including the entire gene or intragenic mutations, among which truncating mutations are associated with more severe malformations, while missense mutations show milder malformations (pachygyria) and lesser clinical impairment (Cardoso *et al.*, 2000). Fluorescence in situ hybridization (FISH) analysis of the 17p13.3 region and *LIS1* sequencing does not show any abnormality in about 40 per cent of patients with phenotypic pattern of *LYS1* mutation. Using the multiplex ligation-dependent probe amplification assay (MLPA), small genomic deletions/duplications have been found in 76 per cent of the apparently normal *LYS1* loci, the proportion of patients in whom a molecular diagnosis is possible being at present 87 per cent. Posterior predominance is also observed in the rare forms of *TUBA1A* mutations. In Miller-Dieker syndrome, where the 17p deletion involves the *LIS1* gene together with other contiguous loci (among which is *YWHAE* gene, acting as a modifier locus) (Cardoso, 2003), a severe lissencephaly is observed with typical facial dysmorphisms (Kato & Dobyns, 2003).

Mutations of the *DCX* gene generally express a phenotype in which the involvement of the anterior part of the brain is predominant (Pilz *et al.*, 1998; Gleeson *et al.*, 2000). They produce SBH in females and classical lissencephaly in hemizygous males; however, there are exceptional cases of boys with missense *DCX* mutations (Guerrini & Marini, 2006). Girls with missense mutations in DCX and normal MRI have been rarely observed (possibly cases of unbalanced X inactivation) (Guerrini *et al.*, 2003).

In lissencephalic infants with the *LIS1* mutation, analysis of mutations in parents should be carried out because of possible germinal mosaicism (giving a 1 per cent risk of recurrence).

Molecular analysis of *DCX* should also be done in mothers of boys with DCX lissencephaly even if the mother has normal MRI, and prenatal diagnosis should be requested in cases of maternal germinal mosaicism (Guerrini & Filippi, 2005).

Developmental delay and mental retardation, motor disabilities and epilepsy are the main clinical features of all these conditions. The severity of clinical signs may vary according to the grade of malformation; cases with mild phenotypes are rare (Gleeson *et al.*, 2000; Leventer *et al.*, 2001). Epilepsy is present in almost all cases (90 per cent); typically in lissencephaly there is early onset infantile spasms.

Other gene mutations in malformed cortex type lissencephaly

Pachygyria with simple thickened gyri and cerebellar hypoplasia (lissencephaly with cerebellar hypoplasia, LCH) is associated with mutations of two genes, *RELN* (Hong *et al.*, 2000) and *VLDR* (Boycott *et al.*, 2005), related to the Reelin-Dab1 signalling pathway that is relevant for neuronal migration and lamination (Tissir & Goffinet, 2003). *RELN* (mapped on chromosome 7q22) codes for the protein Reelin secreted by Cayal-Retzius cells in the marginal zone and binding to the very low density lipoprotein receptor (VLDLR) (coded by the *VLDLR* gene, mapped on chromosome 9q24). It is expressed by migrating cells and induces tyrosine phosphorylation of the cytoplasmic adapter Dab1. The disruption of this pathway at the end stage of radial migration would lead to cortical malformation ('type-Reelin' pachygyria), characterized by an accumulation of neurons beneath the preplate (Lambert de Rouvroit & Goffinet, 1998). The rare reports of these mutations suggest that it is an autosomal recessive disease. Typically, in humans pachygyria is associated with cerebellar hypoplasia as in the reeler mouse mutant (Lambert de Rouvroit & Goffinet, 1998; D'Arcangelo, 2006). Six subtypes of LCH (a to f) have been identified, based on the phenotype; in two of the six the causative gene mutation has been identified. Clinically, non-progressive ataxia with developmental delay is usually observed.

An X-linked lissencephaly with corpus callosum agenesis and ambiguous genitalia (XLAG) has also been reported (Dobyns *et al.*, 1999b; Bonneau *et al.*, 2002). This X-linked disease is associated with mutations of the *aristaless*-related homeobox gene *(ARX)* mapped on Xp22.1-p21.3 and coding for a protein important for cortical lamination and organization (Miura *et al.*, 1997). It affects only males; carrier females may show corpus callosum hypo- or agenesis and rarely epilepsy with normal development or mild developmental delay (Bonneau *et al.*, 2002; Kato *et al.*, 2004). *ARX* expression in the telencephalon involves the VZ and the ganglionic eminence (Ohira *et al.*, 2002), thus involving radial and tangential migration; mutations altering the latter, which includes GABAergic interneurons, may explain the severe forms of epileptic disorder (early infantile spasms) quite often seen in affected boys. The disruption of both radial and tangential migration is evident in brain neuropathology, with a severe cortical dislamination associated with sparse heterotopic neurons within the white matter, dysplastic basal ganglia, and corpus callosum agenesis (Bonneau *et al.*, 2002).

The clinical phenotype of XLAG comprises lissencephaly with a posterior-to-anterior gradient and only a moderate increase in cortical thickness, intractable epilepsy of neonatal onset, severe hypotonia, poor responsiveness, ambiguous genitalia with micropenis and cryptorchidism, and early death (Dobyns *et al.*, 1999b; Bonneau *et al.*, 2002).

MRI findings in XLAG consist of posterior agyria and frontal pachygyria associated with corpus callosum agenesis. Cortical thickness is increased, in the range of 6 to 7 mm. Basal ganglia regions are poorly delineated, ventricles are dilated, and periventricular white matter is abnormal, sometimes containing multiple heterotopic islands of grey matter.

Phenotypical expressivity of the mutations of the *ARX* gene, however, encompasses a wide range of variability, extending from different forms of malformation such as hydranencephaly and abnormal genitalia (HYD/AG) or Proud syndrome (mental retardation, agenesis of the corpus callosum and abnormal genitalia, ACC/AG) to conditions without malformations including infantile spasms, Partington syndrome, and other non-syndromic types of mental retardation (Stromme *et al.*, 2002). Recently, a phenotype of infantile spasms with severe dyskinetic quadriparesis and basal ganglia cystic lesions has been described in ARX mutations with pathological expansion of single alanine repeats (Guerrini *et al.*, 2007). Disruption of tangential migration of GABAergic inhibitory interneurons could explain brain excitability (infantile spasms) and other neurological defects, confirming the notion of 'interneuronopathy' (Kato, 2006).

Cobblestone complex

Type II or cobblestone lissencephaly

Cobblestone lissencephaly is characterized by a loss of convolutions and a non-homogeneous dimpled cortical surface (Dobyns *et al.*, 1985). The disorder of cortical organization is caused by disruption of the glia limitans, a special marginal structure of the extracellular matrix on which radial glial fibres terminate and which guides neuron migration and organization. Glia limitans integrity is perturbed by defective glycosylation of O-glycans, as in deficiency of *O*-mannosyltransferase 1 (coded by *POMT1* gene, mapped on chromosome 9q34.1) (Beltran-Valero de Bernabe *et al.*, 2002) and *O*-mannosyltransferase 2 (POMT2, mapped on 14q24.3) (van Reeuwijk *et al.*, 2005), or of mannosyl-glucosamintransferase (coded by *POMGnT1* gene mapped on chromosome 1p33-34) (Yoshida *et al.*, 2001), as well as by mutations of other genes involved in the glycosylation of α-dystroglycan (*FCMD*, fukutin, mapped on chromosome 9q31 and *FKRP*, fukutin-related protein, mapped on chromosome 19q13.3) (Kobayashi *et al.*, 1998; Brockington *et al.*, 2001). Phenotypes of these mutations comprise muscle dystrophy, ocular abnormalities and cortical malformations. Walker-Warburg syndrome, Fukuyama congenital muscular dystrophy, and muscle-eye-brain syndrome (Fukuyama congenital muscular dystrophy plus retinal abnormality) are the corresponding phenotypes, related more to the kind of mutation than to the mutated gene (Barkovich *et al.*, 2005). Walker-Warburg or HARD+/–E syndrome is a congenital condition characterized by hydrocephalus (H), agyria (A), retinal dysplasia (RD), with or without encephalocele (+/–E). The disorder, often associated with congenital muscular dystrophy, is usually lethal within the first few months of life. Fukuyama congenital muscular dystrophy shows generalized muscle weakness and hypotonia from early infancy, and mental retardation. In muscle-eye-brain syndrome there is a combination of congenital muscular dystrophy and involvement of the central nervous system and the eyes.

Another mutated gene, a member of the N-acetylglucosaminyltransferase gene family, designated *LARGE* and mapped on chromosome 22q12.3-q13.1, accounts for a muscle-eye-brain syndrome – a brain malformation consisting of pachygyria, abnormalities of the brain stem and pons, and increased signal intensity in the white matter at MRI (Brockington *et al.*, 2005). However, a large proportion of patients with lissencephaly type 2 or cobblestone lissencephaly do not have any mutation, while mutations of the relevant genes are often not associated with cobblestone lissencephaly.

Neuroimaging of the cobblestone complex is characterized by irregular cortical thickening with a mixture of agyria, pachygyria, and polymicrogyria, with reduced sulcation. The white matter is diffusely hyperintense on T2w images, owing to gliosis and oedema, and the ventricles are enlarged (colpocephalic ventriculomegaly or, possibly, hydrocephalus). The brain stem and vermis are hypoplastic or dysplastic, or both (Barkovich, 1996).

Heterotopias

Heterotopias are disorders occurring in the last phase of migration and consist of collections of nerve cells inside the white matter, appearing as an effect of their arrest during the radial migration. The arrest can occur either at the beginning of migration, in the subependymal region (periventricular heterotopia), or inside the white matter, focally or diffusely (subcortical heterotopia, a form of which is subcortical band heterotopia or double cortex), or even over the cortex in the leptomeningeal space (leptomeningeal heterotopia), typically found in the foetal-alcohol syndrome.

Clinically, these disorders are heterogeneous in their aetiology, localization, and extension. A common sign is the frequent association with an epileptic disorder. The cause may be a problem occurring during intrauterine life (ischaemia, toxic exposure, and so on). In various diseases of known genetic origin, the heterotopias can also be associated with metabolic disorders (for example, non-ketotic hyperglycinaemia, GM2-gangliosidosis, and Leigh disease), neurocutaneous syndromes, chromosomal syndromes (trisomy 13, 18, and 21), and multiple congenital anomaly syndromes. The clinical spectrum of the migration disorders encompasses a large group of phenotypes where the genetic aetiology has been identified in several cases, including different kinds of heterotopia with focal or diffuse cortical dysplasias, while environmental factors may play a causal role in other cases. The cortex corresponding to heterotopic neurons may be functionally disturbed, as shown by its epileptogenicity (Munari *et al.*, 1996).

Subcortical heterotopias present as irregular collections of grey matter nodules located inside the white matter, between the ventricles and a microgyric cortex. They are very heterogeneous in location and extension. There is no known genetic cause. The whole hemisphere including the basal ganglia is usually small. Neuropathologists distinguish heterotopia as either nodular or laminar (Friede, 1989); the ambiguous laminar definition has now been made more precise, being divided into a band heterotopia and a possible form of subcortical heterotopia (Norman *et al.*, 1995); the latter was later indicated by Barkovich (2000) to have a curvilinear profile in neuroimages in contrast to the apparently more common nodular aspect. Moreover, Barkovich (2000) observed blood vessels and fluid inside the heterotopic region, apparently communicating with the subarachnoid space. Clinical signs may include epilepsy and other neurological symptoms.

On neuroimaging (Fig. 7), focal subcortical heterotopias appear as large, somewhat heterogeneous masses that are isointense to cortical grey matter on all MRI sequences. They sometimes appear as multinodular grey matter masses and at other times are composed of swirling, curvilinear bands of grey matter. The portion of the hemisphere that is affected is almost always small, and the cortex overlying the heterotopia is thin, with shallow sulci – an appearance resembling polymicrogyria.

Chapter 4 Malformations of cortical development

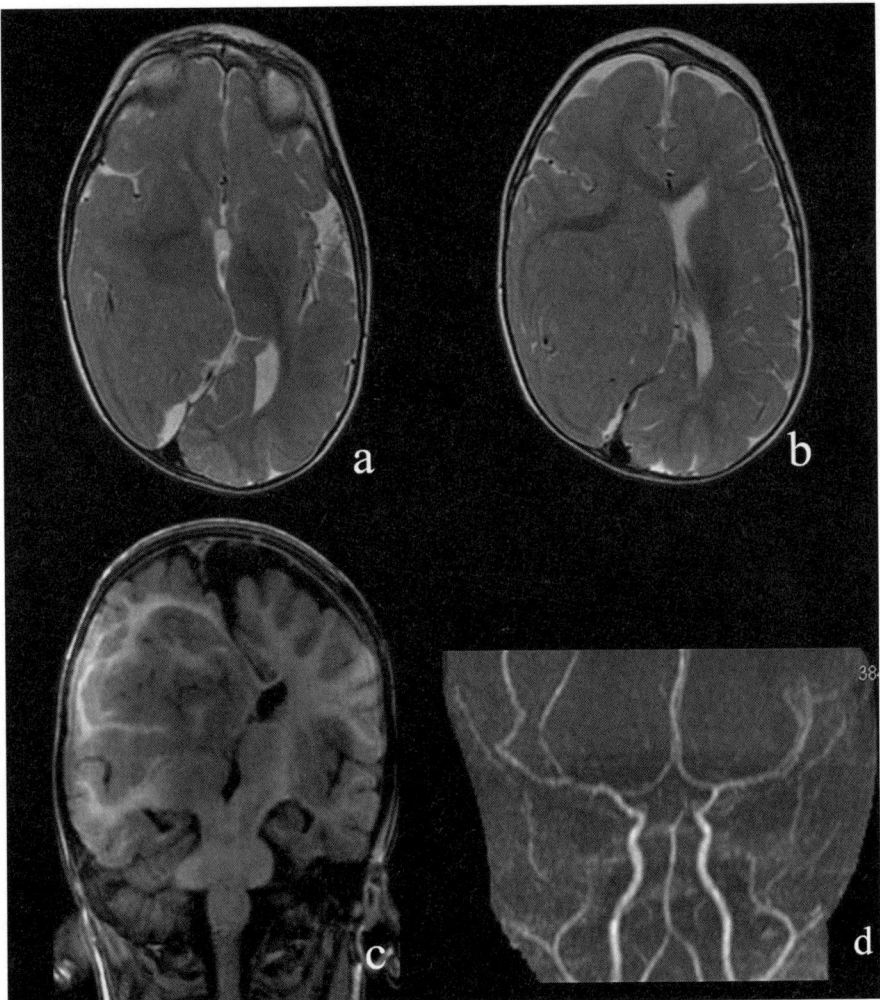

Fig. 7. Subcortical giant heterotopia.
a, b) Axial T2w mages; c) Coronal IR T1w-images; d) Angio-RM 3DTOF images.
A large right hemispheric pseudo-mass, isointense to gray matter emanates from the lateral aspect of the right thalamus and compress the right lateral ventricle, extends across the interhemispheric fissure and appears to mildly distort the left hemisphere. Some vessels originating from the right ACM, surrounded by CSF spaces, are visible inside the lesion. Angio-MR image shows more vertical orientation of right Sylvian vessels compared to the other side with two arterial branches approaching the heterotopia. Note that the right basal ganglia are small or dysplastic.
The involved right hemisphere is abnormally small, the right thalamus is rotated and caudally displaced. Also the right internal capsula and corona radiata are laterally and anteriorly displaced. The overlying cortex is thin, with shallow sulci.

Because the white matter in the affected portion of the cerebrum is reduced, the heterotopy may appear to exert a mass effect on the adjacent ventricle or on the interhemispheric fissure and may thus be mistaken for a tumour.

Periventricular nodular heterotopias (PNH) consist of nodular subependymal collections of heterotopic neurons including multiple neuron types and interneurons (Hannan *et al.*, 1999), caused by a complete defect of migration. Imaging studies (Fig. 8) reveal subependymal

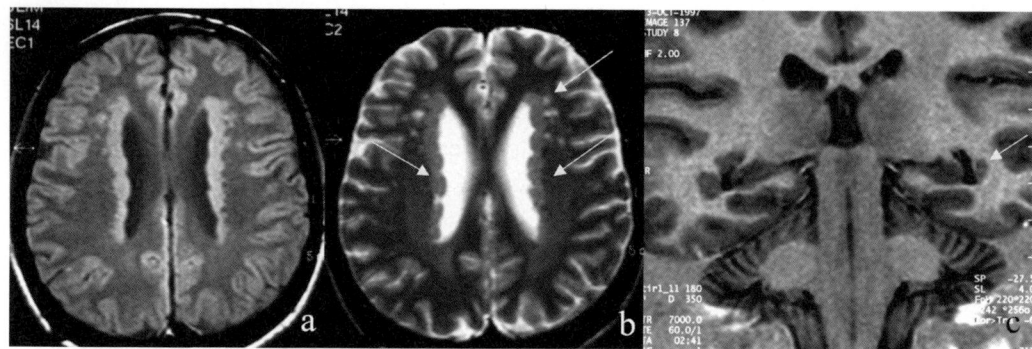

Fig. 8. Subependimal Heterotopy.
Fig. a, b: Axial FLAIR and T2w images; Fig. c: Coronal IR T1w image.
MRI shows multiple and confluent ectopic nodules of gray matter (arrows) located in the subependimal region of both lateral ventricles.

heterotopias as smooth, ovoid nodules that are isointense with grey matter on all imaging sequences. The long axis of the nodule is parallel to the adjacent ventricular wall. The heterotopia can be located in the wall of the ventricle and may be seen to protrude into the ventricular lumen. There are about 15 distinct PNH syndromes (Parrini et al., 2006), among which the most common is the bilateral PNH in females. About 50 per cent of familial cases and only a small proportion of sporadic cases are carriers of a mutation of the filaminin 1 gene (FLNA) (Fox et al., 1998); rare cases with unilateral PNH have been described (Sheen et al., 2001; Guerrini et al., 2004). Mapping on Xq28, this is an X-linked dominant disorder predominantly involving females, in whom random lyonization (X-inactivation) of mutated cells produces a somatic mosaicism; heterozygous females may have a normal or heterotopic cortex.

The phenotype is rarely found in heterozygous males as it is generally lethal in the embryonic period (Moro et al., 2002); rare living males with this genetic mutation have been described, possibly with only a partial loss of FLNA function in their cells (Guerrini et al., 2004).

The *FLNA* gene codes for the F-actin-binding cytoplasmic cross-linking phosphoprotein filamin A, which may link proteins at the plasma membrane and the cytoskeleton. Its central role in many cell functions, such as adhesion, motility and signal transduction, is well known. In the mouse *FLNA* expression is poor in the proliferating ventricular zone (Nagano et al., 2002), and it is highly expressed only in postmitotic migrating neurons, confirming its role in nerve cell migration out of the ventricular zone (Francis et al., 2006). Unfortunately, the hypothesis has not been confirmed in the mouse by the presence of known migration disorders sustained by *FLNA* mutation.

FLNA seems to provide the contact between postmitotic neurons and radial glial cells inducing the migration (Fox et al., 1998). Another function arises from the orthogonal branching of actin filaments, relevant for coagulation and vascular development; this could explain embryonic lethality in males (Guerrini & Marini, 2006), as shown by an affected male dying from a severe haemorrhage (Fox et al., 1998). A broad clinical spectrum including developmental delay and epilepsy is phenotypical of *FLNA* mutations, with a partial phenotypic correlation between the extent and location of the heterotopia and the severity of the clinical signs (Guerrini et al., 2004).

Bilateral PNH may be caused by mutation of other genes. It is rarely due to mutations of the ADP-ribosylation factor guanine nucleotide exchange factor-2 (*ARFGEF2*) – mapped on chromosome 20q13.13 (Sheen et al., 2004) – which encodes for a protein required for vesicle and membrane trafficking from the trans-Golgi network. The vesicle trafficking favours transport to the cell surface of molecules such as E-cadherin and β-catenin, enhancing proliferation and migration. The disruption of cortical development caused by *ARGEF2* mutation is observed as an autosomal recessive disease with microcephaly and bilateral PNH, clinically characterized by severe impairment of development and early onset epilepsy.

Recently, an association of PNH with chromosomal rearrangements such as 5p15.1 and 5p15.33 duplication (Sheen *et al.*, 2003) or 1p36 and 7q11.23 deletion (Ferland *et al.*, 2006; Neal *et al.*, 2006) has been observed. In addition, there are descriptions of sporadic syndromes with bilateral PNH (Parrini *et al.*, 2006).

Organization

In the phase of cortical organization, the architectural structure of the cortex is achieved between 5 months of gestation and a few years after birth, following processes summarized by Volpe (2008) in six stages: settlement of subplate neurons, attainment of orientation of neurons in their proper layer, dendritic arborization, synaptogenesis, cell and synaptic death, and finally glial proliferation and differentiation. Any error in the completion of this programme from genetic or acquired causes produces a cortical malformation (Table 7).

Table 7. Malformations caused by abnormal cortical organization

A. Polymicrogyria and schizencephaly
(1) Unilateral or bilateral polymicrogyria syndromes (perisylvian, parasagittal, frontoparietal, parieto-occipital, frontal, multilobar)
    a. Bilateral frontoparietal polymicrogyria (BFPP)
    b. Perisylvian polymicrogyria (PSP)
(2) Schizencephaly (polymicrogyria involving clefts, open or closed lips)
(3) Polymicrogyria or schizencephaly as part of multiple congenital anomaly/mental retardation syndromes (Adams-Oliver syndrome, Aicardi syndrome, etc.)

B. Focal cortical dysplasias
C. Acquired forms, due to *in utero* accidents such as ischaemia or infections

Polymicrogyria

Proliferation and pattern disorders are possibly classifiable as cortical malformations: they comprise a polymicrogyric cortex and schizencephaly, often observed together in the same patient.

The polymicrogyric brain surface is characterized macroscopically by an area with 'fewer and coarser gyri having an irregular, embossed surface with many smooth bulges' (Friede, 1989), mimicking pachygyria. Microscopical neuropathology shows an abnormally folded cortex, with numerous small packed microgyri, fused together at the level of the molecular layer.

On MRI (Fig. 9), polymicrogyria can show two main patterns of presentation. The first is seen in the neonate or young infant with unmyelinated white matter and is characterized by a thin cortex (< 3 mm) with irregular cortical margins; the second is seen after 3–4 years and is characterized by a thick cortex (6–8 mm) with irregular outer and inner surfaces, sometimes with a 'bumpy' or a 'smooth' aspect.

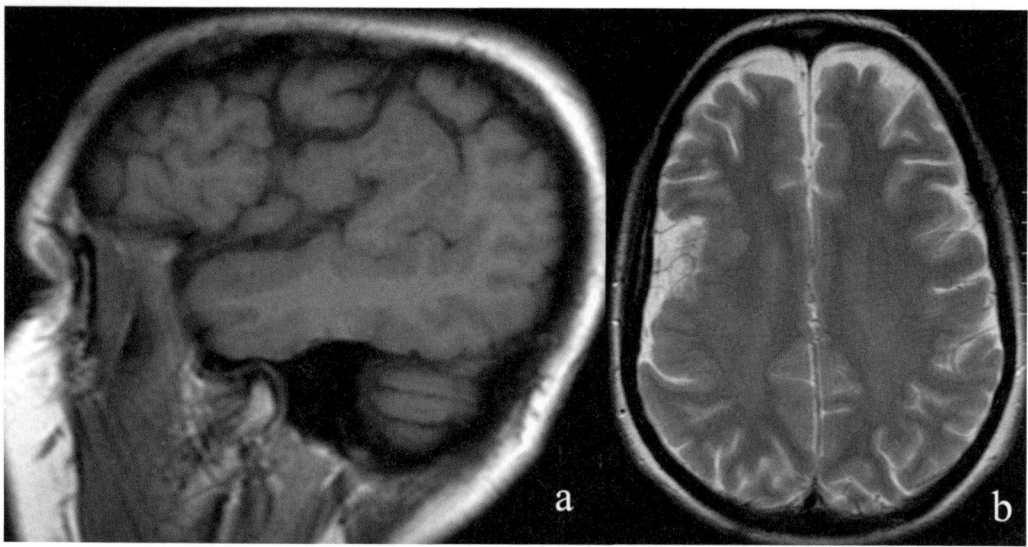

Fig. 9. Perisylvian polimicrogyria. a) sagittal FSE T1w image; b) axial FSE T2w image. The perisylvian cortex is irregularly thickened (6-8 mm) with ill-defined cortical-subcortical junction and in ward infolding. Note also the reduced size of the right cerebral hemisphere.

It is important to note that a polymicrogyric cortex can look normal if routine spin-echo thick image sections (5 mm or more) are acquired, or if the subcortical white matter is incompletely myelinated. High resolution thin (1–2 mm) T1w images are mandatory to demonstrate polymicrogyria.

Regarding the underlying white matter, a diffuse hyperintensity on T2w images underlying the dysplastic cortex (found in 20 to 27 per cent of patients) is commonly encountered, probably related to dilated perivascular spaces. Moreover, large cortical veins are frequently found adjacent to the dysplastic cortex (51 per cent), especially in regions where there is a large infolding of thickened cortex (Hayashi *et al.*, 2002). Proton MR spectroscopy seems to be normal in regions of polymicrogyria (Li *et al.*, 1998).

Two histological types of polymicrogyria are described. Both are characterized by cortical disruption with possibly different underlying mechanisms. Four-layered polymicrogyria is characterized by an intracortical laminar necrosis mainly involving the fifth layer and impairing later migration. It probably causes the packing of gyri (Ferrer *et al.*, 1986). No recognisable lamination is observed in unlayered polymicrogyria, the origin of which would thus seem to be an earlier disorder of cortical development. However, the two types of polymicrogyria may coexist in the same malformed brain (Harding & Copp, 1997), suggesting a continuum of the same malformation.

Polymicrogyria involves some cortical regions selectively (perisylvian, parasagittal, frontoparietal, parieto-occipital, frontal) or may sometimes extend diffusely (multilobar). Clinical features are very heterogeneous and range from normal to severe neurological involvement and refractory epilepsy, depending on the extent and location of the cortical abnormalities. Like schizencephaly, polymicrogyria may be caused by genetic (several possible genes) and environmental causes, namely *in utero* accidents such as ischaemia or infections. The paired-box transcription factor (*PAX6*), a gene frequently associated with polymicrogyria, codes for a transcription factor relevant in human brain development.

Among the localized forms, bilateral frontoparietal polymicrogyria (BFPP) and perisylvian polymicrogyria (PSP) have been well defined, and some genetic substrates recognized. One gene identified for the BFPP codes a G-protein-coupled receptor (GRP56), mapped to chromosome 16q12.2–21 (Piao *et al.*, 2002). GRP56 expression in the mouse preferentially involves the proliferating zones (VZ and SVZ). This suggests that the condition arises from a proliferation disorder regulating a graded cortical patterning (Piao *et al.*, 2004). Observed in several families with recessive pedigrees, BFPP has heterogeneous neurological features often associated with epilepsy (partial seizures and atypical absences). Recently, some neuropathological similarities (myelination defects, cerebellar cortical dysplasia with cysts, frequent involvement of the medial aspects of the cerebral hemispheres) and genetic similarities (N-glycosylation defects) with the so-called cobblestone complex have been emphasized, suggesting that BFPP should be classified as a cobblestone malformation (Guerrini *et al.*, 2008).

Different gene mutations have been identified in perisylvian polymicrogyria (PSP). An *SPRX2* gene mutation may be associated with PSP. Bilateral perisylvian polymicrogyria has been reported in a case of mutation in the methyl-CpG binding protein (*MECP2*) gene on X28 (Geerdink *et al.*, 2002) and in a patient carrying the *A3243G* mutation on mitochondrial transfer RNA for the leucine 1 (*MTTL1*) gene (Keng *et al.*, 2003). Moreover, several families have been observed with all the possible variation of pedigrees (Guerreiro *et al.*, 2000). Children with bilateral perisylvian polymicrogyria have been described, showing a deletion of chromosome 22q11.2, the critical region of Di George syndrome (Bingham *et al.*, 1998; Sztriha *et al.*, 2004). Other chromosomal abnormalities in children with all forms of polymicrogyria have, however, also been reported, so that karyotype studies are highly recommended (Jansen & Andermann, 2005).

Characteristically, PSP results in cerebral palsy with facio-pharyngo-glosso-masticatory diplegia (Kuzniecky *et al.*, 1993) and developmental language disorder, associated with epilepsy that is often resistant to antiepileptic drugs; in some children electrical status epilepticus during sleep can develop (Guerrini *et al.*, 1998).

Schizencephaly is a defect of the cortex consisting of a full thickness cleft involving one hemisphere or both hemispheres symmetrically, with a communication between the ventricle and the extra-axial subarachnoid spaces. The cortex of the cleft lips is polymicrogyric. The clefts, which are generally found in the perisylvian region, have widened or contiguous walls; when bilateral they may be substituted on one side by a zone of polymicrogyric cortex.

The pathogenesis of schizencephaly is controversial: a defect in proliferation/migration or focal ischaemia involving the radial glia has been evoked (Guerrini & Filippi, 2005).

MRI shows a unilateral or bilateral CSF-filled cleft, bordered by polymicrogyric grey matter, extending from the pial surface to the ventricular wall (Barkovich, 1993). The clefts can be of 'open' or 'closed' lip type. The open lip cleft (Fig. 10) is characterized by complete separation of the cleft walls, resulting in a complete communication of the extracerebral sulci with the homolateral ventricle. The closed lip cleft (Figs. 11 and 12) is characterized by apposition and fusion of the walls of the cleft, resulting in a narrow and variably obliterated furrow that extends from the pial surface to a dimple located along the lateral ventricular wall (Tortori-Donati, 2005). Polymicrogyria and subependymal heterotopia are frequently associated. Large drainage vessels are often encountered in the CSF spaces corresponding to the cortical malformation. Schizencephaly occurs sporadically, though some familial cases have been reported (Hosley *et al.*, 1992).

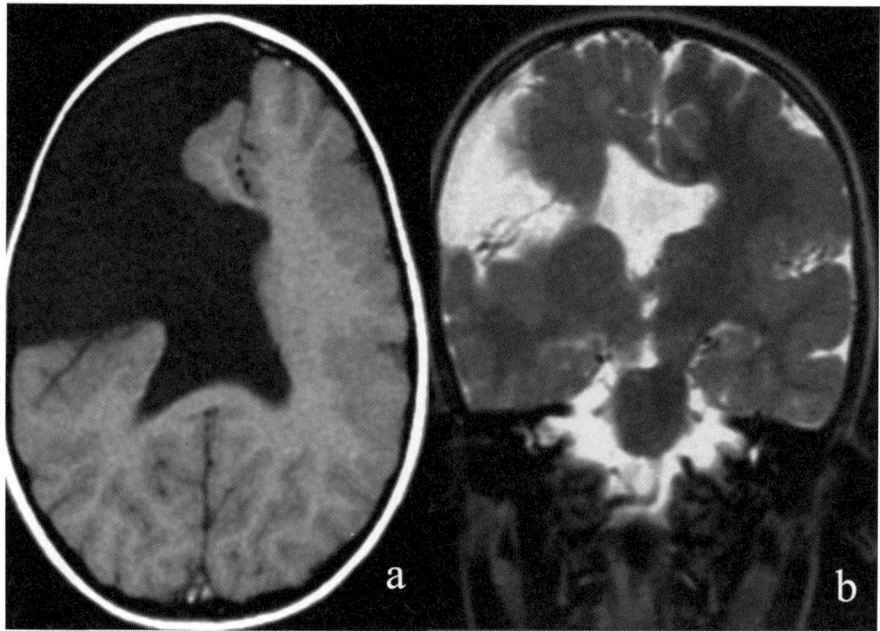

Fig. 10: Schizencephaly open lips. a) Axial T1w image; b) Coronal T2w image.
MR imaging shows a unilateral CSF filled cleft, bordered by polimycrogyric gray matter, extending from pial surface to ventricular wall. The cleft is characterized by the complete separation of the cleft walls resulting in a complete communication of extracerebral sulci with the homolateral ventricle.

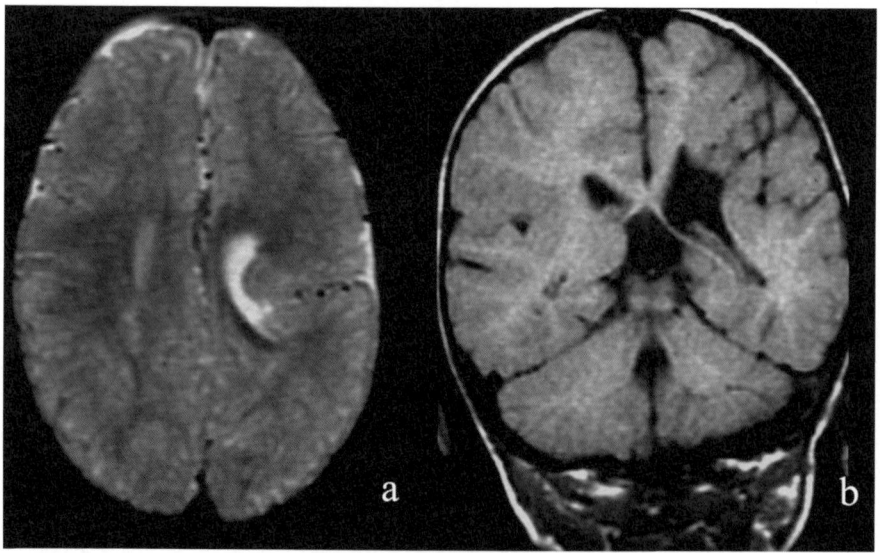

Fig. 11: Schizencephaly closed lips. a) Axial T2w image; b) Coronal T1w image.
MR imaging shows a unilateral CSF filled cleft, bordered by polimycrogyric gray matter, extending from pial surface to the ventricular wall. It is evident an apposition and fusion of the walls of cleft, resulting in a narrow obliterated furrow that extends from the pial surface to a dimple located site along the lateral ventricular wall. In the CSF spaces corresponding to the cortical malformation are evident multiple anomalous vessels.

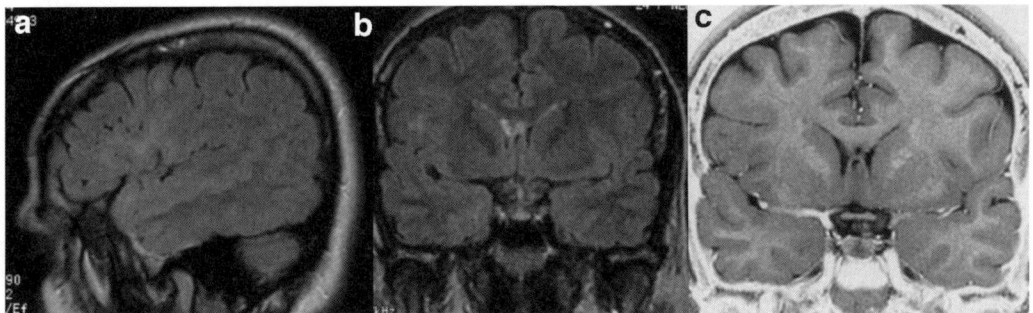

Fig. 12. Focal cortical dysplasia non Taylor type. a, b) Sagittal and coronal FLAIR images; c) Coronal T1w image.
MR FLAIR images show subcortical frontal ill-defined hyperintense alteration with normal adjacent cortex. The signal alteration spares the subependimal region.

A heterozygous mutation of the homeobox gene *EMX2* on the chromosome 10q26.1 has been described in some Italian families (Brunelli *et al.*, 1996; Faiella *et al.*,1997; Granata *et al.*, 1997), but not in other cohorts (Barkovich *et al.*, 2001). EMX2 is a homeodomain transcription factor expressed in progenitor cells and related to the 'empty spiracles' in the developing *Drosophila* head. Its mutation in the mouse produces defects in cortical areas but not schizencephaly. However, the role of *EMX2* mutation in human schizencephaly is not certain at present (Merello *et al.*, 2008). Clinical features include different degrees of mental retardation and cerebral palsy, unilateral in asymmetrical forms, related to the size and location of the clefts and to the presence of associated cerebral malformations. The severity of epilepsy is not related to the extent of the malformation (Granata *et al.*, 1997).

Focal cortical dysplasia

Among the different types of cortical dysplasia caused by developmental disorders of proliferation, migration or organization, localized cortical changes of unknown origin are frequent findings in cortical specimens from children operated on for refractory epilepsy. Their extension is generally focal but may encompass an entire lobe or more. The term 'focal cortical dysplasia' (FCD) was firstly used by Taylor *et al.* (1971); successively, histopathological studies have defined different types of pathology which seem to correspond to clinical and neuroimaging features.

In the absence of known genetic causes, the aetiology of FCD seems to be multifactorial, with gene mutations (abnormalities in the Wnt/Notch signalling pathway) (Aronica *et al.*, 2003) or acquired events, such as *in utero* ischaemic or infectious injuries, interfering with the normal differentiation and organization of neurons (Rakic, 1988; Rickert, 2006).

The similar features of the cytoarchitecture of some forms of FCD to those of the cortical tubers of tuberous sclerosis, as well as of hemimegalencephaly, may suggest a common developmental origin.

The classification of Palmini and Lüders (2002) (Table 8) describes four main forms of FCD, according to their cytological characteristics. FCD 1A comprises cases with disorganization of the cortical layering and in particular an increase in cell concentration (glia and neurons) in layer 1. In FCD 1B, several giant neurons are scattered throughout the cortical grey matter. The presence of abnormal cells is typical of FCD type 2: dysmorphic neurons in FCD 2A to which are added balloon cells (huge size, pale eosinophilic cytoplasm and one or more eccentric nuclei), mainly concentrated at the grey-white matter junction or dispersed in the white matter in FCD type 2B (Taylor-type cortical dysplasia).

Table 8. Histopathological classification of focal cortical dysplasia (according to Palmini & Lüders, 2002)

FCD 1A: Focal architectural abnormalities of the cortex
FCD 1B: Focal architectural abnormalities plus giant or immature neurons
FCD 2A: Focal architectural abnormalities plus dysmorphic neurons
FCD 2B: Focal architectural abnormalities with dysmorphic neurons and balloon cells.
Mild cortical dysplasia. Ectopic neurons within or adjacent to layer 1 or microneuronal heterotopia outside layer 1

Besides these identified dysplasias, a mild form with only ectopic neurons occurs. In addition, there is a controversial notion of 'microdysgenesia' as a subtle disorganization of cortical architecture (Meencke & Janz, 1985; Mischel et al., 1995).

Definition of the timing of these different kinds of cortical disruption is not easy. For all the types of architectural abnormalities, a postmigrating disorder of cortical organization may be evoked; in contrast, dysmorphic and balloon cells in the Taylor-type of cortical dysplasia are connected with earlier phases of proliferation/differentiation. That is why Barkovich et al. (2005) classified the latter among the malformations caused by abnormal neuronal and glial proliferation or apoptosis, in particular a condition of aberrant neuronal-glial differentiation, together with tuberous sclerosis and hemimegalencephaly with which histopathological affinities exist; the other forms are listed under the malformations caused by abnormal organization.

In parallel, from a clinical point of view – that is, the clinical features and severity, the neuroimaging characteristics, and the aetiological data – only two subtypes of FCD are generally recognized: FCD with dysplasia alone, and FCD with balloon cells or Taylor-type cortical dysplasia (Barkovich et al., 2001). The form with dysplasia alone is characterized by neuroimaging features (Fig. 12) of cortical bands of normal/increased or decreased thickness, a cortical-white matter junction that is not necessarily blurred, and generally no changes in the white matter; on the other hand in Taylor's form there is a definite diffuse increase in cortical thickness, blurring of the cortical-white matter junction due to excessive spillover of neurons and/or balloon cells into the white matter, and hyperintensity of the subcortical white matter on T2-weighted sequences (Fig. 13). This corresponds to histopathological abnormalities ranging from moderate myelin axonal damage to microcystic or mineralizing degeneration with excessive astrocytosis (Colombo et al., 2003; Lawson et al., 2005). It is not rare, especially in infancy, for there to be an absence of MRI changes, so it is mandatory to repeat the MRI after the second year of life. In contrast, cases with disappearance of imaging changes detected in infancy are also described (Eltze et al., 2005).

Clinically, FCD presents with early onset and often refractory epilepsy, severe developmental delay and focal neurological deficits; these features, along with a lesser effectiveness of epilepsy surgery, seem more severe in FCD type 1 (Lawson et al., 2005).

Chapter 4 Malformations of cortical development

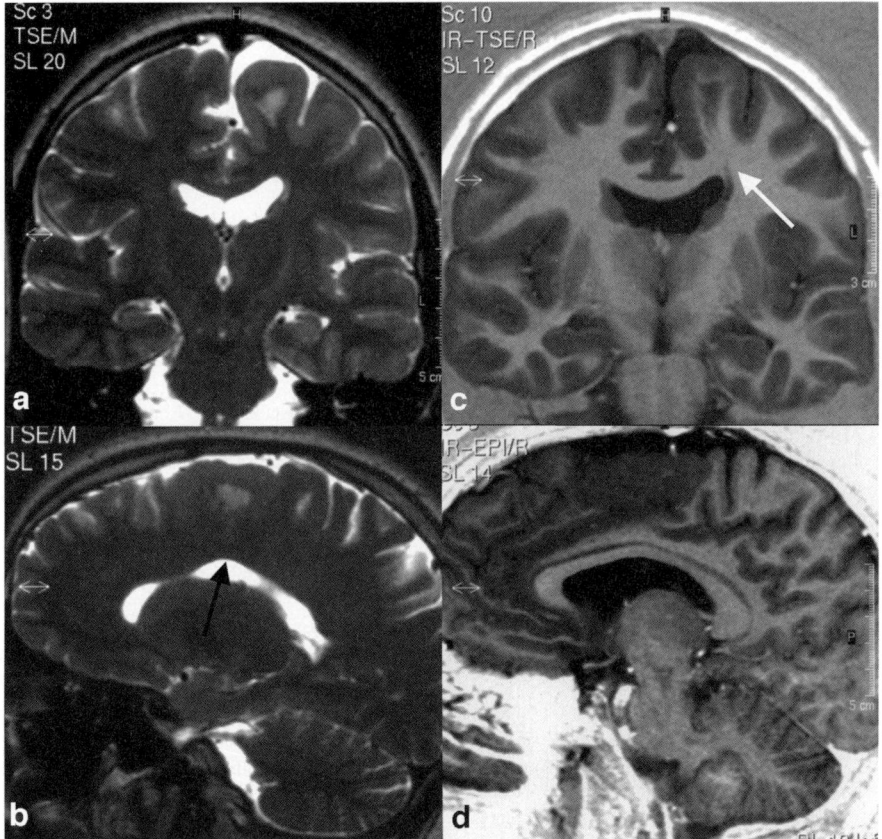

Fig. 13. Focal cortical dysplasia Taylor type II. a, b) Coronal T2w and T1w images; c, d) Sagittal T2w and T1w images.
MR images show focal cortical thickening of the left superior frontal gyrus; the subcortical WM is diffusely hyperintense on T2w and hypointense on T1w images. The parenchymal signal alteration extends from the cortex to the ependymal ventricular surface, that is focally attracted to the lesion.

References

Abuelo, D. (2007): Microcephaly syndromes. *Semin. Pediatr. Neurol.* **14,** 118–127.

Aronica, E., Gorter, J.A., Jansen, G.H., et al. (2003): Expression and cell distribution of group I and group II metabotropic glutamate receptor subtypes in taylor-type focal cortical dysplasia. *Epilepsia* **44**, 785–795.

Au KS, Williams AT, Roach ES, et al. (2007): Genotype/phenotype correlation in 325 individuals referred for a diagnosis of tuberous sclerosis complex in the United States. *Genet. Med.* **9,** 88–100.

Barkovich, A.J. (1993): Formation, maturation and disorders of brain neocortex. *Am. J. Neuroradiol.* **13,** 423–446.

Barkovich, A.J. (1996): Imaging of the cobblestone lissencephalies. *Am. J. Neuroradiol.* **17,** 615–618.

Barkovich, A.J. (2000): Morphologic characteristics of subcortical heterotopia: MR imaging study. *Am. J. Neuroradiol.* **21,** 290–295.

Barkovich, A.J. & Chuang, S.H. (1990): Unilateral megalencephaly: correlation of MR imaging and pathologic characteristics. *AJNR Am J Neuroradiol.* 11, 523–531.

Barkovich, A.J., Kuzniecky, R.I., Jackson, G.D., Guerrini, R. & Dobyns, W.B. (2001): Classification system for malformations of cortical development: update 2001. *Neurology* **57,** 2168–2178.

Barkovich, A.J., Kuzniecky, R.I., Jackson, G.D., Guerrini, R. & Dobyns, W.B. (2005): A developmental and genetic classification for malformations of cortical development *Neurology* **65,** 1873–1887.

Battaglia, D., Di Rocco, C., Iuvone, L., Acquafondata, C., Iannelli, A., Lettori, D., et al. (1999): Neuro-cognitive development and epilepsy outcome in children with surgically treated hemimegalencephaly. *Neuropediatrics* **30**, 307–313.

Beltrán-Valero de Bernabé, D., Currier, S., Steinbrecher, A., Celli, J., van Beusekom, E., et al. (2002): Mutations in the O-mannosyltransferase gene POMT1 give rise to the severe neuronal migration disorder Walker-Warburg syndrome. *Am. J. Hum. Genet.* **71**, 1033–1043.

Bingham, P.M., Lynch, D., McDonald-McGinn, D. & Zackai, E. (1998): Polymicrogyria in chromosome 22 deletion sindrome. *Neurology* **51**, 1500–1502.

Bond, J., Roberts, E., Mochida, G.H., Hampshire, D.J., Scott, S., Askham, J.M., Springell, K., Mahadevan, M., Crow, Y.J., Markham, A.F., Walsh, C.A. & Woods, C.G. (2002): ASPM is a major determinant of cerebral cortical size. *Nat. Genet.* **32**, 316–320.

Bond, J., Roberts, E., Springell, K., Lizarraga, S.B., Scott, S., Higgins, J., Hampshire, D.J., Morrison, E.E., Leal, G.F., Silva, E.O., Costa, S.M., Baralle, D., Raponi, M., Karbani, G., Rashid, Y., Jafri, H., Bennett, C., Corry, P., Walsh, C.A. & Woods, C.G. (2005): A centrosomal mechanism involving CDK5RAP2 and CENPJ controls brain size. *Nat. Genet.* **37**, 353–355.

Bonneau, D., Toutain, A., Laquerriere, A., Marret, S., Saugier-Veber, P., Barthez, M.A., Radi, S., Biran-Mucignat, V., Rodriguez, D. & Gélot, A. (2002): X-linked lissencephaly with absent corpus callosum and ambiguous genitalia (XLAG): clinical, magnetic resonance imaging, and neuropathological findings. *Ann. Neurol.* **51**, 340–349.

Bosman, C., Boldrini, R., Dimitri, L., Di Rocco, C. & Corsi, A. (1996): Hemimegalencephaly. Histological, immunohistochemical, ultrastructural and cytofluorimetric study of six patients. *Childs Nerv Syst.* 12, 765–775.

Boycott, K.M., Flavelle, S., Bureau, A., et al. (2005): Homozygous deletion of the very low density lipoprotein receptor gene causes autosomal recessive cerebellar hypoplasia with cerebral gyral simplification. *Am. J. Hum. Genet.* **77**, 477–483.

Brockington, M., Yuva, Y., Prandini, P., et al. (2001): Mutations in the fukutin-related protein gene (FKRP) identify limb girdle muscular dystrophy 2I as a milder allelic variant of congenital muscular dystrophy MDC1C. *Hum. Mol. Genet.* **10**, 2851–2859.

Brockington, M., Torelli, S., Prandini, P., et al. (2005): Localization and functional analysis of the LARGE family of glycosyltransferases: significance for muscular dystrophy. *Hum. Mol. Genet.* **14**, 657–665.

Brunelli, S., Faiella, A., Capra, V., Nigro, V., Simeone, A., Cama, A. & Boncinelli, E. (1996): Germline mutations in the homeobox gene EMX2 in patients with severe schizencephaly. *Nat. Genet.* **12**, 94–96.

Cardoso, C. (2003): Refinement of a 400-kb critical region allows genotypic differentiation between isolated lissencephaly, Miller-Dieker syndrome, and other phenotypes secondary to deletions of 17p13.3. *Am. J. Hum. Genet.* **72**, 918–930.

Cardoso, C., Leventer, R.J., Matsumoto, N., Kuc, J.A., Ramocki, M.B., Mewborn, S.K., Dudlicek, L.L., May, L.F., Mills, P.L., Das, S., Pilz, D.T., Dobyns, W.B. & Ledbetter, D.H. (2000): The location and type of mutation predict malformation severity in isolated lissencephaly caused by abnormalities within the LIS1 gene. *Hum. Mol. Genet.* **9**, 3019–3028.

Caviness, V.S. & Takahashi, T. (1995): Proliferative events in the cerebral ventricular zone. *Brain Dev.* **17**, 159–163.

Caviness, V.S., Takahashi, T. & Nowakowski, R.S. (1995): Numbers, time and neocortical neurogenesis: a general developmental and evolutionary model. *Trends Neurosci.* **18**, 379–383.

Chan, J.A., Zhang, H., Roberts, P.S., Jozwiak, S., Wieslawa, G., Lewin-Kowalik, J., Kotulska, K. & Kwiatkowski, D.J. (2004): Pathogenesis of tuberous sclerosis subependymal giant cell astrocytomas: biallelic inactivation of TSC1 or TSC2 leads to mTOR activation. *J. Neuropathol. Exp. Neurol.* **63**, 1236–1242.

Cheadle, J.P., Reeve, M.P., Sampson, J.R. & Kwiatkowski, D.J. (2000): Molecular genetic advances in tuberous sclerosis. *Hum. Genet.* **107**, 97–114.

Colombo, N., Tassi, L., Galli, C., Citterio, A., Lo Russo, G., Scialfa, G. & Spreafico, R. (2003): Focal cortical dysplasia: MR imaging, histopathologic, and clinical correlations in surgical treated patients with epilepsy. *Am. J. Neuroradiol.* **24**, 724–733.

Crino, P.B. (2004): Molecular pathogenesis of tuber formation in tuberous sclerosis complex. *J. Child Neurol.* **9**, 716–725.

Crino, P.B. (2007): Focal brain malformations: a spectrum of disorders along the mTOR cascade. *Novartis Found. Symp.* **288**, 260–272.

Crinò, P.B., Nathanson, K.L. & Henske, E.P. (2006): The tuberous sclerosis complex. *N. Engl. J. Med.* **355**, 1345–1356.

D'Arcangelo, G. (2006): Reelin mouse mutants as models of cortical development disorders. *Epilepsy Behav.* **8**, 81–90.

Desai, A.R. & McConnell, S.K. (2000): Progressive restriction in fate potential by neural progenitors during cerebral cortical development. *Development* **127**, 2863–2872.

des Portes, V., Pinard, J.M., Billuart, P., Vinet, M.C., Koulako, V.A., Carrie, A., Gelot, A., Dupuis, E., Motte, J., Berwald-Netter, Y., Catala, M., Kahn, A., Beldjord, C. & Chelly, J. (1998): A novel CNS gene required for neuronal migration and involved in X-linked subcortical laminar heterotopia and lissencephaly syndrome. *Cell* **92**, 51–61.

Devlin, A.M., Cross, J.H., Harkness, W., Chong, W.K., Harding, B., Vargha-Khadem, F. & Neville, B.G. (2003: Clinical outcomes of hemispherectomy for epilepsy in childhood and adolescence. *Brain* **126**, 556–566.

Di Rocco, C. & Iannelli, A. (2000): Hemimegalencephaly and intractable epilepsy: complications of hemispherectomy and their correlations with the surgical technique. A report on 15 cases. *Pediatr. Neurosurg.* **33**, 198–207.

Dobyns, W.B., Gilbert, E.F. & Opitz, J.M. (1985): Further comments on the lissencephaly syndromes. *Am. J. Med. Genet.* **22**, 197–211.

Dobyns, W.B., Elias, E.R., Newlin, A.C., Pagon, R.A. & Ledbetter, D.H. (1992): Causal heterogeneity in isolated lissencephaly. *Neurology* **42**, 1375–1388.

Dobyns, W.B. & Truwit, C.L. (1995): Lissencephaly and other malformations of cortical development: 1995 update. *Neuropediatrics* **26**, 132-147.

Dobyns, W.B., Truwit, C.L., Ross, M.E., Matsumoto, N., Pilz, D.T., Ledbetter, D.H., Gleeson, J.G., Walsh, C.A. & Barkovich, A.J. (1999a): Differences in the gyral pattern distinguish chromosome 17-linked and X-linked lissencephaly. *Neurology* **53**, 270–277.

Dobyns, W.B., Berry-Kravis, E., Havernick, N.J., Holden, K.R. & Viskochil, D. (1999b): X-linked lissencephaly with absent corpus callosum and ambiguous genitalia. *Am. J. Med. Genet.* **86**, 331–337.

Eltze, C.M., Chong, W.K., Bhate, S., Harding, B., Neville, B.G. & Cross, J.H. (2006): Taylor-type focal cortical dysplasia in infants: some MRI lesions almost disappear with maturation of myelination. *Epilepsia* **46**, 1988–1992.

Evrard, P., de Saint-Georges, P., Kadhim, H.J. & Gadisseux, J.F. (1989): Pathology of prenatal encephalopathies. In: *Child neurology and developmental disabilities*, eds. J.H. French, S. Harel & P. Casaer. Baltimore: P.H. Brookes.

Fallet-Bianco, C. (2000): Microcephaly with simplified gyral pattern: neuropathological study. *Childs Nerv. Syst.* **16**, 47–71.

Faiella, A., Brunelli, S., Granata, T., D'Incerti, L., Cardini, R., Lenti, C., Battaglia, G. & Boncinelli, E. (1997): A number of schizencephaly patients including 2 brothers are heterozygous for germline mutations in the homeobox gene EMX2. *Eur. J. Hum. Genet.* **5**, 186–190.

Ferland, R.J., Gaitanis, J.N., Apse, K., Tantravahi, U., Walsh, C.A. & Sheen, V.L. (2006): Periventricular nodular heterotopia and Williams syndrome. *Am. J. Med. Genet. A* **140**, 1305–1311

Ferrer, I., Cusi, M.V., Liarte, A. & Campistol, J.A. (1986): Golgi study of the polymicrogyric cortex in Aicardi syndrome. *Brain Dev.* **8**, 518–525.

Fitz, C.R., Harwood-Nash, D.C. & Boldt, D.W. (1978): The radiographic features of unilateral megalencephaly. *Neuroradiology* **15**, 145–148.

Flores-Sarnat, L. (2002): Hemimegalencephaly: part 1. Genetic, clinical, and imaging aspects. *J. Child Neurol.* **17**, 373–384.

Fox, J.W., Lamperti, E.D., Ekşioğlu, Y.Z., Hong, S.E., Feng, Y., Graham, D.A., Scheffer, I.E., Dobyns, W.B., Hirsch, B.A., Radtke, R.A., Berkovic, S.F., Huttenlocher, P.R. & Walsh, C.A. (1998): Mutations in filamin 1 prevent migration of cerebral cortical neurons in human periventricular heterotopia. *Neuron* **21**, 1315–1325.

Francis, F., Meyer, G., Fallet-Bianco, C., Moreno, S., Kappeler, C., Socorro, A.C., Tuy, F.P., Beldjord, C. & Chelly, J. (2006): Human disorders of cortical development: from past to Present. *Eur. J. Neurosci.* **23**, 877–893.

Friede, R.L. (1989): *Developmental neuropathology*, 2nd edition. Berlin: Springer-Verlag.

Geerdink, N., Rotteveel, J.J., Lammens, M., Sistermans, E.A., Heikens, G.T., Gabreëls, F.J., Mullaart, R.A. & Hamel, B.C. (2002): MECP2 mutation in a boy with severe neonatal encephalopathy: clinical, neuropathological and molecular findings. *Neuropediatrics* **33**, 33–36.

Ghosh, A. & Shatz, C.J. (1992): Involvement of subplate neurons in the formation of ocular dominance columns. *Science* **255**, 1441–1443.

Ghosh, A. & Shatz, C.J. (1993): A role for subplate neurons in the patterning of connection from thalamus to neocortex. *Development* **117**, 1031–1047.

Gleeson, J.G., Allen, K.M., Fox, J.W., Lamperti, E.D., Berkovic, S., Schever, I., Cooper, E.C., Dobyns, W.B., Minnerath, S.R., Ross, M.E. & Walsh, C.A. (1998): Doublecortin, a brain-specific gene mutated in human X-linked lissencephaly and double cortex syndrome, encodes a putative signaling protein. *Cell* **92**, 63–72.

Gleeson, J.G., Luo, R.F., Grant, P.E., Guerrini, R., Huttenlocher, P.R., Berg, M.J., Ricci, S., Cusmai, R., Wheless, J.W., Berkovic, S., Scheffer, I., Dobyns, W.B. & Walsh, C.A. (2000): Genetic and neuroradiological heterogeneity of double cortex syndrome. *Ann. Neurol.* **47**, 265–269.

Goodman, R.M. & Gorlin, R.Y. (1983): *The malformed infant and child*. Oxford: Oxford University Press.

Granata, T., Farina, L., Faiella, A., et al. (1997): Familial schizencephaly associated with EMX2 mutation. *Neurology* **48**, 1403–1406.

Griffiths et al. (1994):

Guerreiro, M.M., Andermann, E., Guerrini, R., et al. (2000): Familial perisylvian polymicrogyria: a new familial syndrome of cortical maldevelopment. *Ann. Neurol.* **48**, 39–48.

Guerrini, R. & Filippi, T. (2005): Neuronal migration disorders, genetics, and epileptogenesis. *J. Child Neurol.* **20**, 287–299.

Guerrini, R. & Marini, C. (2006): Genetic malformations of cortical development. *Exp. Brain Res.* **173**, 322–333.

Guerrini, R., Genton, P., Bureau, M., Parmeggiani, A., Salas-Puig, X., Santucci, M., Bonanni, P., Ambrosetto, G. & Dravet, C. (1998): Multilobar polymicrogyria, intractable drop attack seizures, and sleep-related electrical status epilepticus. *Neurology* **51**, 504–512.

Guerrini, R., Moro, F., Andermann, E., et al. (2003): Nonsyndromic mental retardation and cryptogenic epilepsy in women with doublecortin gene mutations. *Ann. Neurol.* **54**, 30–37.

Guerrini, R., Mei, D., Sisodiya, S., et al. (2004): Germline and mosaic mutations of FLN1 in men with periventricular nodular heterotopia. *Neurology* **63**, 51–56.

Guerrini, R., Dobyns, W.B. & Barkovich, A.J. (2008): Abnormal development of the human cerebral cortex: genetics, functional consequences and treatment options. *Trends Neurosci.* **31**, 154–162.

Guerrini, R., Moro, F., Kato, M., et al. (2007): Expansion of the first PolyA tract of ARX causes infantile spasms and status dystonicus. *Neurology* **69**, 427–433.

Hannan, A.J., Servotte, S., Katsnelson, et al (1999): Characterization of nodular neuronal heterotopia in children. *Brain* **122**, 219–238.

Harding, B. & Copp, A. (1997): Malformations of the nervous system. In: *GreenWelds neuropathology*, eds. J. Graham & P.L. Lantos, pp. 521–538. London: Edward Arnold.

Hayashi, N., Tsutsumi, Y. & Barkovich, A.J. (2002): Polymicrogyria without porencephaly/schizencephaly. MRI analysis of the spectrum and the prevalence of macroscopic findings in the clinical population. *Neuroradiology* **44**, 647–655.

Hong, S.E., Shugart, Y.Y., Huang, D.T., Shahwan, S.A., Grant, P.E., Hourihane, J.O., Martin, N.D. & Walsh, C.A. (2000): Autosomal recessive lissencephaly with cerebellar hypoplasia (LCH) is associated with human reelin gene mutations. *Nat. Genet.* **26**, 93–96.

Hosley, M.A., Abroms, I.F. & Ragland, R.L. (1992): Schizencephaly: case report of familial incidence. *Pediatr. Neurol.* **8**, 148–150.

Iida, K., Otsubo, H., Mohamed, I.S., Okuda, C., Ochi, A., Weiss, S.K., Chuang, S.H. & Snead, O.C. (2005): Characterizing magnetoencephalographic spike sources in children with tuberous sclerosis complex. *Epilepsia* **46**, 1510–1517.

Jackson, A.P., Eastwood, H., Bell, S.M., Adu, J., Toomes, C., Carr, I.M., Roberts, E., Hampshire, D.J., Crow, Y.J., Mighell, A.J., Karbani, G., Jafri, H., Rashid, Y., Mueller, R.F., Markham, A.F. & Woods, C.G. (2002): Identification of microcephalin, a protein implicated in determining the size of the human brain. *Am. J. Hum. Genet.* **71**, 136–142.

Jansen, A. & Andermann, E. (2005): Genetics of the polymicrogyria syndromes. *J. Med. Genet.* **42**, 369–378.

Jellinger, K. & Rett, A. (1976): Agyria-pachygyria (lissencephaly syndrome). *Neuropadiatrie* **7**, 66–91.

Kalifa, G.L., Chiron, C., Sellier, N. et al. (1987) : Hemimegalencephaly: MR imaging in five children. *Radiology* **165**, 29–33.

Kato, M. (2006): A new paradigm for West syndrome based on molecular and cell biology. *Epilepsy Res.* **70** (Suppl. 1), S87–S95.

Kato, M. & Dobyns, W.B. (2003): Lissencephaly and the molecular basis of neuronal migration. *Hum. Mol. Genet.* **12**, 89–96.

Kato, M., Das, S., Petras, K., Kitamura, K., Morohashi, K., Abuelo, D.N., Barr, M., Bonneau, D., Brady, A.F., Carpenter, N.J., Cipero, K.L., Frisone, F., Fukuda, T., Guerrini, R., Iida, E., Itoh, M., Lewanda, A.F., Nanba, Y., Oka, A., Proud, V.K., Saugier-Veber, P., Schelley, S.L., Selicorni, A., Shaner, R., Silengo, M., Stewart, F., Sugiyama, N., Toyama, J., Toutain, A., Vargas, A.L., Yanazawa, M., Zackai, E.H. & Dobyns, W.B. (2004): Mutations of ARX are associated with striking pleiotropy and consistent phenotype-genotype correlation. *Hum. Mutat.* **23**, 147–159.

Keng, W.T., Pilz, D.T., Minns, B. & FitzPatrick, D.R. (2003): A3243G mitochondrial mutation associated with polymicrogyria. *Dev. Med. Child Neurol.* **45**, 704–708.

Kobayashi, K., Nakahori, Y., Miyake, M., Matsumura, K., Kondo-Iida, E., Nomura, Y., Segawa, M., Yoshioka, M., Saito, K., Osawa, M., Hamano, K., Sakakihara, Y., Nonaka, I., Nakagome, Y., Kanazawa, I., Nakamura, Y., Tokunaga, K. & Toda, T. (1998): An ancient retrotransposal insertion causes Fukuyama-type congenital muscular dystrophy. *Nature* **394**, 388–392.

Kostovic, I. & Rakic, P. (1990): Developmental history of the transient subplate zone in the visual and somatosensory cortex of the macaque monkey and human brain. *J. Comp. Neurol.* **297**, 441–470.

Kriegstein, A.R. & Noctor, S.C. (2004): Patterns of neuronal migration in the embryonic cortex. *Trends Neurosci.* **27**, 392–399.

Kuzniecky, R., Andermann, F., Guerrini, R. & Study, C.M.C. (1993): Congenital bilateral perisylvian syndrome: study of 31 patients. *Lancet* **341**, 608–612.

Kwiatkowski, D.J. (2003): Tuberous sclerosis: from tubers to mTOR. *Ann. Hum. Genet.* **67**, 87–96.

Kwiatkowski, D.J. & Manning, B.D. (2005): Tuberous sclerosis: a GAP at the crossroads of multiple signaling pathways. *Hum. Mol. Genet.* **14** suppl. 2, R251–R258.

Lambert de Rouvroit, C. & Goffinet, A.M. (1998): The reeler mouse as a model of brain development. *Adv. Anat. Embryol. Cell. Biol.* **150**, 1–106.

Lawson, J.A., Birchansky, S., Pacheco, E., Jayakar, P., Resnick, T.J., Dean, P. & Duchowny, M.S. (2005): Distinct clinicopathologic subtypes of cortical dysplasia of Taylor. *Neurology* **64**, 55–61.

Lettori, D., Battaglia, D., Sacco, A., Veredice, C., Chieffo, D., Massimi, L., Tartaglione, T., Chiricozzi, F., Staccioli, S., Mittica, A., Di Rocco, C. & Guzzetta, F. (2008): Early hemispherectomy in catastrophic epilepsy A neuro-cognitive and epileptic long-term follow-up. *Seizure* **17**, 49–63.

Leventer, R.J., Cardoso, C., Ledbetter, D.H. & Dobyns, W.B. (2001): LIS1 missense mutations cause milder lissencephaly phenotypes including a child with normal IQ. *Neurology* **57**, 416–422.

Li, L.M., Cendes, F., Bastos, A.C., Andermann, F., Dubeau, F. & Arnold, D.L. (1998): Neuronal metabolic dysfunction in patients with cortical developmental malformations. A proton magnetic resonance spectroscopic imaging study. *Neurology* **50**, 755–759.

Madhavan, D., Schaffer, S., Yankovsky, A., Arzimanoglou, A., Renaldo, F., Zaroff, C.M., LaJoie, J., Weiner, H.L., Andermann, E., Franz, D.N., Leonard, J., Connolly, M., Cascino, G.D. & Devinsky, O. (2007): Surgical outcome in tuberous sclerosis complex: a multicenter survey. *Epilepsia* **48**, 1625–1628.

Marin-Padilla, M. (1978): Dual origin of the mammalian neocortex and evolution of the cortical plate. *Anat. Embryol. (Berl.)* **52**, 109–126.

Marin-Padilla, M., Parisi, J.E., Armstrong, D.L., Sargent, S.K. & Kaplan, J.A. (2002): Shaken infant syndrome: developmental neuropathology, progressive cortical dysplasia, and epilepsy. *Acta Neuropathol. (Berl.)* **103**, 321–332.

Marin-Padilla, M., Tsai, R.J., King, M.A. & Roper, S.N. (2003): Altered corticogenesis and neuronal morphology in irradiation-induced cortical dysplasia: a Golgi-Cox study. *J. Neuropathol. Exp. Neurol.* **62**, 1129–1143.

McConnell, S.K. (1995): Constructing the cerebral cortex: neurogenesis and fate determination. *Neuron* **15**, 761–768.

Meencke, H.J. & Janz, D. (1985): The significance of microdysgenesia in primary generalized epilepsy: an answer to the considerations of Lyon and Gastaut. *Epilepsia* **26**, 368–371.

Merello, E., Swanson, E., De Marco, P., Akhter, M., Striano, P., Rossi, A., Cama, A., Leventer, R.J., Guerrini, R., Capra, V. & Dobyns, W.B. (2008): No major role for the EMX2 gene in schizencephaly. *Am. J. Med. Genet.* **146A**, 1142–1150.

Meyer, G., Schaaps, J.P., Moreau, L. & Goffinet, A.M. (2000): Embryonic and early fetal development of the human neocortex. *J. Neurosci.* **20**, 1858–1868.

Meyer, G., Perez-Garcia, C.G. & Gleeson, J.G. (2002): Selective expression of doublecortin and LIS1 in developing human cortex suggests unique modes of neuronal movement. *Cereb. Cortex* **12**, 1225–1236.

Mischel, P., Nguyen, L. & Vinters, H. (1995): Cerebral cortical dysplasiaassociated with pediatric epilepsy. Review of neuropathologia features and proposal for a grading system. *J. Neuropathol. Exp. Neurol.* **54**, 137–153.

Miura, H., Yanazawa, M., Kato, K. & Kitamura, K. (1997): Expression of a novel aristaless related homeobox gene 'Arx' in the vertebrate telencephalon, diencephalon and floor plate. *Mech. Dev.* **65**, 99–109.

Mochida, G.H. & Walsh, C.A. (2001): Molecular genetics of human microcephaly. *Curr. Opin. Neurol.* **14**, 151–156.

Moro, F., Carrozzo, R., Veggiotti, P., Tortorella, G., Toniolo, D., Volzone, A. & Guerrini, R. (2002): Familial periventricular heterotopia: missense and distal truncating mutations of the FLN1 gene. *Neurology* **58**, 916–921.

Munari, C., Francione, S. & Kahane, P. (1996): Usefulness of stereo EEG investigations in partial epilepsy associated with cortical dysplastic lesions and gray matter heterotopia. In: *Dysplasias of cerebral cortex and epilepsy*, eds. R. Guerrini, F. Andermann, R. Canapicchi, J. Roger, B. Zifkin & P. Pfanner P, pp. 383–394. Philadelphia: Lippincott-Raven.

Nagano, T., Yoneda, T., Hatanaka, Y., Kubota, C., Murakami, F. & Sato, M. (2002): Filamin A-interacting protein (FILIP) regulates cortical cell migration out of the ventricular zone. *Nat Cell Biol.* **4**, 495–501.

Neal, J., Raju, G.P., Bodell, A., Apse, K., Walsh, C.A. & Sheen, V.L. (2006): Periventricular heterotopia with complete agenesis of the corpus callosum: a case report. *J. Neurol.* **253**, 1358–1359.

Norman, M.G., McGillivray, B.C., Kalousek, D.K., Hill, A. & Poskitt, K.J. (1995): *Congenital malformations of the brain: pathologic, embryologic, clinical, radiologic and genetic aspects*, pp. 223–307. Oxford: Oxford University Press.

Ohira, R., Zhang, Y.H., Guo, W., Dipple, K., Shih, S.L., Doerr, J., Huang, B.L., Fu, L.J., Abu-Khalil, A., Geschwind, D. & McCabe, E.R. (2002): Human ARX gene: genomic characterization and expression. *Mol. Genet. Metab.* **77**, 179–188.

Olney, A.H. (2007): Macrocephaly syndromes. *Semin. Pediatr. Neurol.* **14**, 128–135.

Palmini, A. & Lüders, H.O. (2002): Classification issues in malformations caused by abnormalities of cortical development. *Neurosurg. Clin. N. Am.* **13**, 1–16.

Parrini, E., Ramazzotti, A., Dobyns, W.B., Koide, N., Yoshida, T. & Yokochi, T. (2006): Periventricular heterotopia: phenotypic heterogeneity and correlation with filamin A mutations. *Brain* **129**, 1892–1906.

Piao, X., Basel-Vanagaite, L., Straussberg, R., Grant, P.E., Pugh, E.W., Doheny, K., Doan, B., Hong, S.E., Shugart, Y.Y. & Walsh, C.A. (2002): An autosomal recessive form of bilateral frontoparietal polymicrogyria maps to chromosome 16q12.2–21. *Am. J. Hum. Genet.* **70**, 1028–1033.

Piao, X., Hill, R.S., Bodell, A., Chang, B.S., Basel-Vanagaite, L., Straussberg, R., Dobyns, W.B., Qasrawi, B., Winter, R.M., Innes, A.M., Voit, T., Ross, M.E., Michaud, J.L., Déscarie, J.C., Barkovich, A.J. & Walsh, C.A. (2004): G protein-coupled receptor-dependent development of human frontal cortex. *Science* **303**, 2033–2036.

Pilz, D.T., Matsumoto, N., Minnerath, S., Mills, P., Gleeson, J.G., Allen, K.M., Walsh, C.A., Barkovich, A.J., Dobyns, W.B., Ledbetter, D.H. & Ross, M.E. (1998): LIS1 and XLIS (DCX) mutations cause most classical lissencephaly, but different patterns of malformation. *Hum. Mol. Genet.* **7**, 2029–2037.

Poirier, K., Keays, D.A., Francis, F., Saillour, Y., Bahi, N., Manouvrier, S., Fallet-Bianco, C., Pasquier, L., Toutain, A., Tuy, F.P., Bienvenu, T., Joriot, S., Odent, S., Ville, D., Desguerre, I., Goldenberg, A., Moutard, M.L., Fryns, J.P., van Esch, H., Harvey, R.J., Siebold, C., Flint, J., Beldjord, C. & Chelly, J. (2007): Large spectrum of lissencephaly and pachygyria phenotypes resulting from de novo missense mutations in tubulin a 1A (TUBA1A). *Hum. Mutat.* **28**, 1055–1064.

Price, D.J. (2004): Lipids make smooth brains gyrate. *Trends Neurosci.* **27**, 362–364.

Rakic, P. (1985): Limits of nerogenesis in primate. *Science* **227**, 1054–1056.

Rakic, P. (1988): Defects of neuronal migration and the pathogenesis of cortical malformations. *Prog. Brain Res.* **73**, 15–37.

Rakic, P. (1995): A small step for the cell, a giant leap for mankind: a hypothesis of neocortical expansion during evolution. *Trends Neurosci.* **18**, 383–388.

Rakic, P. (2003): Developmental and evolutionary adaptations of cortical radial glia. *Cereb. Cortex* **13**, 541–549.

Rakic, P. (2005): Less is more: progenitor death and cortical size. *Nat. Neurosci.* **8**, 981–982.

Reiner, O., Carrozzo, R., Shen, Y., Wehnert, M., Faustinella, F., Dobyns, W.B., Caskey, C.T. & Ledbetter, D.H. (1993): Isolation of a Miller–Dieker lissencephaly gene containing G protein b-subunit-like repeats. *Nature* **364**, 717–721.

Rickert, C.H. (2006): Cortical dysplasia: neuropathological aspects. *Child Nerv. Syst.* **22**, 821–826.

Robain, O. (1996): Introduction to the pathology of cerebral cortical dysplasia. In: *Dysplasias of cerebral cortex and epilepsy*, eds. R. Guerrini, F. Andermann, R. Canapicchi, R.J. Zifkin & P. Pfanner, pp. 1–9. Philadelphia: Lippincott-Raven.

Sarbassov, D.D., Ali, S.M. & Sabatini, D.M. (2005): Growing roles for the mTOR pathway. *Curr. Opin. Cell Biol.* **17**, 596–603.

Sarnat, H.B. (2000): Molecular genetic classification of central nervous system malformations. *J. Child Neurol.* **15**, 675–687.

Sarnat, H.B. & Flores-Sarnat, L. (2002): Molecular genetic and morphologic integration in malformations of the nervous system for etiologic classification. *Semin. Pediatr. Neurol.* **9**, 335–344.

Sarnat, H.B. & Flores-Sarnat, L. (2004): Integrative classification of morphology and molecular genetics in central nervous system malformations. *Am. J. Med. Genet.* **126A**, 386–392.

Sasaki, M., Hashimoto, T., Shimada, M., Iinuma, K., Fushiki, S., Takano, T., Oka, E., Kondo, I. & Miike, T. (2000): Nation-wide survey on hemimegalencephaly in Japan. *No To Hattatsu* **32**, 255–260.

Scheithauer, B.W. & Reagan, T.J. (1999): Neuropathology. In: *Tuberous sclerosis complex*, ed. M.R. Gomez, pp. 101–144. New York: Oxford University Press.

Schramm, J., Kral, T. & Clusmann, H. (2001): Transsylvian keyhole functional hemispherectomy. *Neurosurgery* **49**, 891–900.

Sener, R.N. (1997): MR demonstration of cerebral hemimegalencephaly associated with cerebellar involvement (total hemimegalencephaly). *Comput. Med. Imaging Graph.* **21**, 201–204.

Sheen, V.L., Dixon, P.H., Fox *et al.* (2001): Mutations in the X-linked Wlamin 1 gene cause periventricular nodular heterotopia in males as well as in females. *Hum. Mol. Genet.* **10,** 1775–1783.

Sheen, V.L., Ganesh, V.S., Topcu, M., Sebire, G., Bodell, A., Hill, R.S., Grant, P.E., Shugart, Y.Y., Imitola, J., Khoury, S.J., Guerrini, R. & Walsh, C.A. (2004): Mutations in ARFGEF2 implicate vesicle trafficking in neural progenitor proliferation and migration in the human cerebral cortex. *Nat. Genet.* **36,** 69–76.

Sheen, V.L., Wheless, J.W., Bodell, A., Braverman, E., Cotter, P.D., Rauen, K.A., Glenn, O., Weisiger, K., Packman, S., Walsh, C.A. & Sherr, E.H. (2003): Periventricular heterotopia associated with chromosome 5p anomalies. *Neurology* **60,** 1033–1036.

Strømme, P., Mangelsdorf, M.E., Shaw, M.A., Lower, K.M., Lewis, S.M., Bruyere, H., Lütcherath, V., Gedeon, A.K., Wallace, R.H., Scheffer, I.E., Turner, G., Partington, M., Frints, S.G., Fryns, J.P., Sutherland, G.R., Mulley, J.C. & Gécz, J. (2002): Mutations in the human ortholog of Aristaless cause X-linked mental retardation and epilepsy. *Nat. Genet.* **30,** 441–445.

Sztriha, L., Guerrini, R., Harding, B., Stewart, F., Chelloug, N. & Johansen, J.G. (2004): Clinical, MRI, and pathological features of polymicrogyria in chromosome 22q11 deletion syndrome. *Am. J. Med. Genet.* **127A,** 313–317.

Taylor, D.C., Falconer, M.A., Bruton, C.J. & Corsellis, J.A. (1971): Focal dysplasia of the cerebral cortex in epilepsy. *J. Neurol. Neurosurg. Psychiatry* **34,** 369–373.

Tinkle, B.T., Schorry, E.K., Franz, D.N., Crone, K.R. & Saal, H.M. (2005): Epidemiology of hemimegalencephaly: a case series and review. *Am. J. Med. Genet.* **139,** 204–211.

Tissir, F. & Goffinet, A.M. (2003): Reelin and brain development. *Nat. Rev. Neurosci.* **4,** 496–505.

Tortori Donati, P. (2005): *Pediatric neuroradiology: brain malformations*, pp. 72–198. Berlin: Springer-Verlag.

van Reeuwijk, J., Janssen, M., van den Elzen, C., Beltran-Valero de Bernabé, D., Sabatelli, P., Merlini, L., Boon, M., Scheffer, H., Brockington, M., Muntoni, F., Huynen, M.A., Verrips, A., Walsh, C.A., Barth, P.G., Brunner, H.G. & van Bokhoven, H. (2005): POMT2 mutations cause alpha-dystroglycan hypoglycosylation and Walker Warburg syndrome. *J. Med. Genet.* **42,** 907–912.

Volpe, J.J. (2008): *Neurology of the newborn*. Philadelphia, Saunders.

Yoshida, A., Kobayashi, K., Manya, H., Taniguchi, K., Kano, H., Mizuno, M., Inazu, T., Mitsuhashi, H., Takahashi, S., Takeuchi, M., Herrmann, R., Straub, V., Talim, B., Voit, T., Topaloglu, H., Toda, T. & Endo, T. (2001): Muscular dystrophy and neuronal migration disorder caused by mutations in a glycosyltransferase, POMGnT1. *Dev. Cell* **1,** 717–724.

Chapter 5

Early brain injuries: infantile cerebral palsy

Francesco Guzzetta

Catholic University, Largo Agostino Gemelli 8, 00168 Rome, Italy
fguzzetta@rm.unicatt.it

Cerebral palsy, the most common physical disability in childhood, consists of a group of non-progressive disorders mainly and persistently affecting the motor system, but also involving other relevant functions (sensory, language, intelligence, behaviour). Epilepsy is a frequent complication. It is caused by 'a defect or lesion of the immature brain' (Bax, 1964), occurring before birth, at birth, or during infancy (during the first month according to some authors, for example Cans *et al.*, 2007). The notion of non-progressive disorders does not refer to clinical features – which may worsen during growth – but arises from biological considerations related to the static causal injury. Thus, as proposed by a recent definition (Rosenbaum *et al.*, 2007), 'cerebral palsy describes a group of permanent disorders of the development of movement and posture, causing activity limitation, *that are attributed to non-progressive disturbances that occurred in the developing foetal or infant brain*'. The motor involvement of the neurodevelopmental disorder seems to be an obligatory feature, though the same process needs to be considered in individuals with only disturbances of sensation, cognition, communication, perception or behaviour, or with a seizure disorder, caused by an early brain injury.

Functional disorders become manifest early in life, often after a clinically 'silent' period, the duration of which is becoming shorter and shorter as diagnostic tools improve, though sometimes the condition only emerges years after birth (MacLennan, 1999). On the other hand, very early diagnosis may be erroneous because of possible transient abnormalities, especially in preterm infants, so that 5 years is generally considered the optimal last age for confirming the diagnosis. Cumulative data on cerebral palsy are provided by information from numerous registries around the world (Cans *et al.*, 2004). According to several Western country studies (MacGillvray & Campbell, 1995; Stanley *et al.*, 2000; Hagberg *et al.*, 2001; Nelson, 2002; Winter *et al.*, 2002) the prevalence of cerebral palsy is between 1.0 and 2.5 per 1000 live births, and it is especially related to preterm birth. The number of patients with cerebral palsy appears to have increased since 1970, in keeping with an improved survival of preterm and very preterm infants at the cost of an increase in cerebral palsy risk (Hagberg *et al.*, 1993; Murphy *et al.*, 1993; MacGillivray & Campbell, 1995). The prevalence of cerebral palsy increases with decreasing gestational age (GA), and significantly for infants under 27 weeks of GA (Himpens *et al.*, 2008). Recent advances in obstetrics and neonatology have led to an improvement in preterm infant survival, especially in babies of <1500 g birth weight (Platt *et al.*, 2007; Robertson *et al.*, 2007), but generally there has been no decrease in neurological morbidity (Vohr *et al.*, 2000; D'Angio *et al.*, 2002; Wilson-Costello *et al.*, 2005; Vincer *et al.*, 2006; Tommiska *et al.*, 2007), though in some series a decline has recently been reported (Platt *et al.*, 2007; Robertson *et al.*, 2007).

There is evidence of a higher incidence of cerebral palsy in boys than in girls, which would seem to be linked to the greater vulnerability of the male brain to early insults (Johnston & Hagberg, 2007).

Causes

Genetics

A *genetic origin* of cerebral palsy is proven in a small proportion of cases (Hughes & Newton, 1992; McHale *et al.*, 1999), related to chromosomal anomalies, gene mutations, and contiguous gene syndromes (Menkes & Flores-Sarnat, 2006). However, reports of a high familial risk of cerebral palsy suggest that heritable factors may play a more general role (Bundey & Griffiths, 1977; Hemminki *et al.*, 2007). In some large series, a genetic origin has been presumed in about 40 per cent of cerebral palsy cases (Costeff, 2004), as a genetic causal co-factor is implicated in various aetiological subgroups of cerebral palsy (infections, vascular conditions, and so on) (Nelson & Chang, 2008).

Infection and inflammation

Maternal infections during the first months of gestation (rubella, cytomegalovirus, toxoplasmosis) are possible causes of cerebral palsy. Generally, intrauterine exposure to infection plays an important role in determining the development of cerebral palsy, as shown by studies on markers of infections such as chorioamnionitis, which is significantly associated with cerebral palsy as well as with cystic periventricular leukomalacia (Wu, 2002). In full term infants, markers of infection are associated with a ninefold increase in the risk of cerebral palsy (Grether & Nelson, 1997).

Infection and inflammation are supposed to act through several mediators, among which the cytokines seem to play an important role (Yoon *et al.*, 1997; Dammann & Leviton, 2000). There is evidence of an overexpression of tumour necrosis factor alpha (TNF-α), interleukin-1 beta (IL-1β) and interleukin-2 (IL-2) in injured brains. Receptors for these cytokines are observed on many inflammatory and neural cells in the white matter. Furthermore, antiphospholipid antibodies – indicators of autoimmune disease or previous infections – are associated with greater risk of cerebral palsy (Silver *et al.*, 1992).

Thrombophilia

Prenatal stroke is favoured by several inherited conditions – for example, factor V Leiden mutation (the most common genetic thrombophilia, present in about 6 per cent of European-derived populations) (High, 1998), prothrombin gene mutation, and defective homocysteine metabolism. Acquired fetal thrombophilia (for example, lupus anticoagulant) or maternal thrombophilia (physiological enhancement of coagulability in pregnancy) may also occur (Hagstrom *et al.*, 1998;

Harum *et al.*, 1999; Walker, 2000; Smith *et al.*, 2001; Hogeveen *et al.*, 2002). These disorders interact with other conditions linked to infections and cytokines (Smith *et al.*, 2001). The placenta and abnormalities of its vasculature have been found to be associated with antiphospholipid antibodies (Lochshin *et al.*, 1985; Salafia & Parke, 1997) and with factor V Leiden mutation (Dizon-Townson *et al.*, 1997). Thromboses in the placenta may give rise to emboli in the fetal circulation. These can pass through the patent foramen ovale to the fetal brain, causing strokes (Thorarensen *et al.*, 1997). Thus a complex mix of factors including infection, fetal or maternal thrombophilia and vascular factors may lead to ischaemic infarction (Gunther *et al.*, 2000).

Thyroxine deficiency

Low circulating thyroxine, usually present in very low birthweight infants, is associated with an increased risk of cerebral palsy (Reaus *et al.*, 1996), especially when there are other neonatal problems such as severe respiratory disease, low arterial blood pressure and so on (Reuss *et al.*, 1996; Leviton *et al.*, 1999).

Hypoxia-ischaemia

Asphyxia, with hypercarbia and acidosis, is one of the main aetiological factors in the pathogenesis of cerebral palsy. Generally, asphyxia is associated with ischaemia which worsens the brain damage. Though asphyxia apparently plays a central role in cerebral palsy, it has been difficult to prove this in the perinatal period (Nelson & Grether, 1998), because more than one risk factor is generally involved (for example, intrauterine exposure to infection or coagulation disorders) (Nelson & Grether, 1999).

Severe prenatal or perinatal hypoxaemia is mainly due to disorders of placental exchange, and postnatal hypoxaemia to respiratory insufficiency (respiratory distress) and severe right to left shunts. Ischaemia is particularly related to cardiac insufficiency resulting from severe hypoxaemia, as in intrauterine asphyxia, severe congenital heart disease or malformations, and patent ductus arteriosus (Volpe, 2008).

Brain injuries caused by asphyxia depend on the severity and the timing of the insult. Many other co-factors may contribute to produce the lesional effect on the brain (intrauterine growth retardation, prematurity, infections, metabolic disorders, and so on).

The lack of oxygen in brain tissue leads to neuronal cell death, immediate *(primary cell death)* or delayed *(secondary cell death)*, probably apoptotic in nature, with different neuropathological sequelae (gliosis, demyelination, cysts). The final effects are modulated by endogenous neuroprotective mechanisms (release of inhibitory neurotransmitters such as GABA, post-ischaemic change in cerebral blood flow, induction of anti-apoptotic neurotrophins, and so on).

Various types of injury may be present in the brain, often in a mixed form. The most common kind of lesion is selective neuronal necrosis, which may be diffuse or be located in the cerebral cortex or deep nuclei, or in the brain stem and ponto-subiculum (Volpe, 2008). Cerebral palsy, with a broad range of clinical expression (motor, sensory, cognitive, seizure), is a possible outcome, with specific clinical correlations relating to brain stem involvement – for example, oculomotor disturbances, ventilatory disorders, sucking and swallowing disorders. Injury to the supero-medial aspects of the cerebral convexities (parasagittal injuries) is another known neuropathological pattern in perinatal asphyxia. A defect in perfusion of the border zones between the end fields of the major cerebral arteries is the dominant ischaemic lesion in full term neonates. Tetraplegic cerebral palsy with greater involvement of upper limbs and mental retardation is the main clinical correlate.

The most frequent injury in hypoxic-ischaemic encephalopathies is periventricular leukomalacia (PVL), consisting of necrosis of the white matter in characteristic distributions. This involves the external angles of the lateral ventricles dorsally and laterally but it may extend more diffusely. Three grades of severity have been proposed (de Vries et al., 1992), according to the topography and evolution of PVL on ultrasound scanning: (i) periventricular hyperechogenicity lasting more than 7 days (PVL I); (ii) frontoparietal hyperechogenicity evolving towards small cysts (PVL II); and (iii) extensive formation of definite periventricular cysts (PVL III). However, the presence of cysts in PVL (cPVL) requires special attention, as these are especially predictive of a poor outcome. Though more prevalent in the most severe grade of PVL (PVL III), cPVL may also be found in the later stages of PVL II (particularly after 1 month), sometimes transiently (Pierrrat et al., 2001); in the latter case, ventricular dilatation may be the only indirect sign. That is why the use of early diffusion weighted magnetic resonance imaging (DWMRI) is of particular interest, as it is capable of detecting which area of increased echogenicity on ultrasound will evolve to become cystic (Inder et al., 1999). The main clinical correlate of PVL is spastic tetraplegia, with greater involvement of lower limbs than the upper (so called diplegia); more extensive lesions are also associated with mental retardation.

The most common type of PVL occurs in the third trimester of gestation. It can occur prenatally or in preterm neonates. The prenatal form, in particular, is a strong predictor of cerebral palsy, with more than 90 per cent of surviving infants affected (Hayakawa et al., 1999).

Focal and multifocal ischaemic brain necrosis with porencephalic cysts is another severe neuropathological pattern of hypoxic-ischaemic injury.

Haemorrhage

Haemorrhage into the cerebral ventricles – intraventricular haemorrhage (IVH), linked to the developmental anatomical characteristics at the end of the third trimester of gestation – is another major complication occurring in foetal/preterm life. Though the numbers of very premature infants and hence the IVH risk are increasing in developed countries, the prevalence of IVH has fallen significantly since the late 1980s because of success in prevention (Philip et al., 1989; Vohr et al., 2000).

The anatomical origin of IVH is usually the subependymal germinal matrix, from which blood erupts into the ventricular cavity. There are three grades of haemorrhagic severity (Volpe, 2008): (i) a form confined to the subependymal matrix (grade 1); (ii) a limited inpouring into the ventricle that does not cause distension (grade 2); (iii) extensive and expanding intraventricular bleeding (grade 3). In about 15 per cent of cases of IVH, periventricular haemorrhagic necrosis occurs because of venous infarction (Guzzetta et al., 1986; Volpe, 2008).

Progressive posthaemorrhagic ventricular dilatation (hydrocephalus) is a common acute or subacute sequel of IVH.

Grades 1 and 2 IVH, with no parenchymal lesions, are not associated with an increase in the incidence of cerebral palsy. Grade 3 is responsible for about one third of the cases with neurocognitive sequelae, the most impaired outcome occurring in patients with periventricular infarction, also called grade 4 IVH. With parenchymal lesions larger than 1 cm there is generally a high mortality and a poor neurocognitive outcome; normal development is rarely observed (Guzzetta et al., 1986). Among infants with localized forms of infarction, the outcome seems better (Volpe, 2008).

Hypoglycaemia

Glucose is presumably the most important energy substrate for neonatal and foetal brain (Vannucci & Vannucci, 2001). Symptomatic hypoglycaemia – that is, a condition in which a low blood glucose concentration, usually under 25 mg/dl (1.39 mmol/L), is associated with clinical symptoms (tremulousness, seizures, respiratory depression, irritability, hypotonia) – may be observed in preterm and high risk full-term infants, with an increase in chronic neurological sequelae. The mechanism of brain injury produced by severe hypoglycaemia is directly related to the lack of glucose availability, which enhances the vulnerability of the brain to hypoxic-ischaemic insults. The most frequent cause of hypoglycaemia in newborn infants is asphyxia with a consequent rapid anaerobic glucose consumption. The neuropathological pattern of hypoglycaemic damage is widespread neuronal injury with glial involvement (Anderson et al., 1967; Larroche, 1977), involving the posterior aspects of the brain in particular. The main sequelae are microcephaly with atrophic gyri and widened sulci, and diffuse demyelination.

Neuroimaging confirms these findings. Acute abnormalities (diffuse cortical and subcortical white matter damage) occur particularly in the parietal and occipital regions of the brain (Barkovich et al., 1998). When they are persistent, signal abnormalities consist of a reduction in white matter with diffuse demyelination, primarily located in the occipital lobes (Murakami et al., 1999).

Although, it is difficult to discriminate between the various different concurrent aetiological factors that may contribute to chronic disability, there is evidence that infants with severe, persistent, or recurrent symptomatic hypoglycaemia are at high risk of chronic neurodevelopmental sequelae (Lucas et al., 1988; Stenninger et al., 1998).

Hyperbilirubinaemia

Raised concentrations of unconjugated bilirubin may occur in neonates as a result of several disorders (haemolytic disease, mainly secondary to blood group incompatibility, polycythaemia, inherited defects of conjugation, and so on). It is well known that the neurotoxicity of hyperbilirubinaemia is dependent on various determinants including the concentration of serum unconjugated and free bilirubin, the bilirubin binding capacity of albumin, the transfer across the blood-brain barrier, and the degree of neuronal susceptibility. The neuropathological effects of hyperbilirubinaemia ('*kernicterus*', bilirubin staining of the basal nuclei, or *bilirubin encephalopathy*, a more inclusive term involving neuronal injury) are thus quite variable and a clear relationship is only found between the maximum serum bilirubin concentration and the percentage of encephalopathic infants (Avery et al., 1999). The worst outcome is in infants with serum bilirubin concentrations greater than 30 mg/dl (~ 500 μmol/L). Brain maturation is also a factor, in that premature infants may develop severe bilirubin encephalopathy in the absence of marked hyperbilirubinaemia.

Neuronal injury and bilirubin staining affect grey matter in several areas, mainly the basal ganglia but also the hippocampal cortex, various brain stem and cerebellar nuclei, and the anterior horn cells of the spinal cord. Neuroimaging confirms these particular locations (Penn et al., 1994; Yokochi, 1995). Patients with chronic bilirubin encephalopathy show typical clinical features (Volpe, 2008): there is an initial period of hypotonia with delayed motor milestones; this is followed after 1 year of age by the appearance of characteristic extrapyramidal movement abnormalities, often associated with gaze and auditory defects. Involvement of cognitive development is less common.

Aetiological pathways

Understanding the causes of a cerebral palsy is often difficult even though extensive epidemiological research is now available. It is increasingly evident that in most cases cerebral palsy does not have a single cause and that a series of concurrent aetiological factors interacts to produce causal pathways leading to the final outcome. The notion of an aetiopathogenic pathway (for example, ischaemic and inflammatory) as a complex route to the final result is now recognized (Stanley et al., 2000; Arpino et al., 2005). The presence of one type of insult (hypoxia-ischaemia) may make the foetus or infant more vulnerable to damage from another form of insult (such as infection). The predominant mechanisms of foetal brain damage are hypoxia-ischaemia caused by placental insufficiency from hypercoagulable states, abruption, or other causes, and inflammation from intrauterine infection (chorioamnionitis). We now know that the interacting roles of hypoxia-ischaemia and infective/inflammatory factors are crucial in the pathogenesis of PVL (Kadhim et al., 2005).

The synergistic mechanism of various factors in different combinations, among which the state of development appears central, produces the final outcome (Kendall & Peebles, 2005). Thus the notion of aetiopathogenic pathways instead of a single determinant has become dominant. Knowledge of these factors in individual cases is therefore crucial to the prevention of cerebral palsy and to the reduction of sequelae.

Prevention

A recent complete review considered all the tools used to prevent the casual agents or their effects (Nelson & Chang, 2008). Some of these (mild hypothermia in term infants, administration of magnesium sulphate to women in preterm labour) have been shown to be effective in preventing cerebral palsy. The best method of prevention, however, is likely to be a strategy aimed at tackling the individual aetiological factors – for example, birth asphyxia, prematurity, infection/inflammation, and multiple gestation.

Brain injury

As the chronic functional disorders of cerebral palsy are mediated by primary brain lesions occurring early in life, their aetiopathogenesis should be focused on brain injuries, their causes and how they translate into those functional disorders. The connection between the primary causes and the dysfunctional outcome is complex and the evidence of diagnostic tools is sometimes inconsistent (Table 1).

Table 1. Connection between causes and functional effects of primary brain damage

Primary causes: genetic or acquired (toxic, infectious, hypoxic-ischaemic, haemorrhagic, etc.)	→ **brain injury**	→ change in development of functions
(1)	(2)	(3)

(1) interacting mechanisms between genetic and acquired causes

(2) not shown by neuroimaging in a proportion of cases (10 per cent up to one third) (Bax et al., 2006; Wu et al., 2006a)

(3) not all brain-injured infants present significant changes in development; functional outcome is the result of the compensatory reorganization of functions (Vandermeeren et al., 2003; Guzzetta et al., 2007; Wilke et al., 2008)

Since the studies of Freud in 1897, there have been numerous reports about the neuropathological changes in cerebral palsy. In Table 2 we list the possible brain injuries found in association with cerebral palsy (Friede, 1989; Floyd, 2007). The pathological findings are dependent on the stage of maturation of the brain at the time of the insult and may involve the cortical neurogenesis of the first and second trimester of gestation, producing a disorder of development. If the insult occurs at a later stage, when the gross architecture of brain has been achieved and cortical organization is advanced, the result is a destructive lesion.

Table 2. Main neuropathological findings associated with cerebral palsy

Malformations	Acquired abnormalities of grey and white matter	Acquired abnormalities of white matter alone
Lissencephaly	Porencephaly	Hypoplastic white matter
Pachygyria-agyria	Multicystic encephalomalacia	Focal malacia
Micropolygyria	Embolic/thrombotic lesions in specific arterial distributions	Gliosis and demyelination
Nodular or laminar heterotopia		White matter astrocytosis
Cortical dysplasia	Border zone lesions	Delayed myelination
Hemimegalencephaly	Sclerotic microgyria (ulegyria)	
Microcephaly		

The neuropathology of cerebral palsy has been greatly assisted by recent advances in structural and functional neuroimaging, which have resulted in a great deal of progress in our understanding of the relations between causal injuries and the resulting types of dysfunction. Structural neuroimaging studies show the changes in brain structures that follow insults (Bekker & Vugt, 2001; Hoon, 2005; Glenn et al., 2007; Nagae et al., 2007) and provide useful information about whether the insult was of pre-, peri-, or postnatal origin. Moreover, neuroimaging allows us to study the development of lesions during the acute stage of the injury (Barkovich et al., 1995; Rutherford et al., 2006), while functional methods are being used to map regional sensory and cognitive processing (Cabeza & Nyberg, 2000; Gaillard, 2004; Berl et al., 2006), as well as to examine cortical reorganization (Johnston et al., 2001; Guzzetta et al., 2007; Stief O'Shaughnessy et al., 2008).

In more recent studies, there has been a focus on the lack of neuroimaging changes in a small proportion of cases (11 per cent when magnetic resonance imaging is employed) (Ashwal et al., 2004) with mild forms of cerebral palsy. These are predominantly ataxic patients, in most of whom there is a suspicion of a genetic origin (Bax et al., 2006).

Developmental focus

The stage of development is crucial in understanding the pathogenesis of early brain damage, not only the mechanism underlying the disorders of development in cerebral palsy, but also how different possible causes of cerebral palsy – such as hypoxia-ischaemia, infections, and oxidative stress – interact to cause the cortical damage and the consequent functional impairment (Volpe, 1996; Dammann et al., 2002; Kostovic & Judas, 2002; Kadhim et al., 2003).

Congenital malformations as well as destructive lesions are possible outcomes of such pathways, depending on the timing of the insult. Congenital malformations, including cortical dysplasias, are increasingly recognized as aetiological factors by modern neuroimaging techniques. Some of these have a genetic basis and are often associated with cerebral palsy (Nelson & Ellenberg, 1985; Nelson & Ellenberg, 1986; Blair & Stanley, 1993; Croen et al., 2001) as well as with other abnormalities, even outside the CNS (Coorssen et al., 1991).

In a recent meta-analysis of neuroimaging studies (Krägeloh-Mann & Horber, 2007), malformations accounted for about 10 per cent of cases of cerebral palsy. This finding was similar to that reported by Garne *et al.* (2008) in studies on the European Cerebral Palsy Database (SCPE). Bax *et al.* (2005) found that half the cases originated from infections acquired *in utero* such as cytomegalovirus, while the remainder were 'idiopathic' conditions (disorders of migration and cortical organization) possibly due to genetic causes.

An acquired aetiology may occur at any point in development and produces 'clastic' lesions consisting of destructive processes in formed tissues and the disruption of developmental pathways. The earlier this occurs, the more serious are the effects (Table 3).

Table 3. Effects of early damage on the development of the central nervous system

	Development disorders	Destructive effects
Cortex	• proliferation and migration disorders • cortical disorganization (unbalanced glutamatergic/GABAergic activity: GABA role in regulation of neuronal development)	• acquired late migration disorders (polymicrogyria, dysplasias) • cortical atrophy (neural necrosis/apoptosis)
Subcortical structures	Damage to: • 'Subplate neurons' • oligodendrocyte precursor* • GABAergic migrating neurons traversing axons from multiple neuronal systems	• axonal damage • oligodendrocyte damage (demyelination) • gliosis • cysts, porencephalies

• Oligodendrocyte precursor cells (OPCs) in the human telencephalon subplate arise from the ganglionic eminence, migrate to the subventricular zone, proliferate during mid-gestation, and disperse into the intermediate zone and cortex throughout the third trimester.

Post-injury reorganization

Mechanisms underlying reorganization after early brain lesions are relevant for our understanding of functional evolution and rehabilitation strategy. Functional recovery associated with brain damage early in life is better than with damage occurring later (Carr *et al.*, 1993; Ragazzoni *et al.*, 2002; Johnston, 2003).

Classifications

Cerebral palsy is usually classified according to topographic criteria or the type of motor disorder. In classical classifications, various physiological and topographic categories are considered, but matching the individual clinical pattern to a distinct category is difficult. The impairment of multiple functions makes each patient unique for prognosis and treatment. The category itself is hard to define – for example, the meaning of involvement of three limbs (triplegia) often remains ambiguous: is it an asymmetrical quadriplegia or a diplegia with superimposed hemiplegia? The same difficulty occurs with the mixture of functional effects (spasticity, rigidity, extrapyramidal signs) (Shapiro, 2004). The unreliability of these classifications was shown in a study in which trained clinicians were invited to classify several children with cerebral palsy topographically and physiologically, with diagnostic concordance in only about half the cases (Alberman, 1984).

Topographic classification

Topographic classification includes quadriplegia, the most severe form involving all four limbs; hemiplegia with a unilateral motor disorder; diplegia with the inferior limb involvement; and the less frequent mono- and triplegia.

Tetraplegic cerebral palsy

Tetraplegic cerebral palsy is the most severe form of cerebral palsy, involving all four limbs and the trunk. Spasticity is predominant with axial hypotonia; pseudobulbar signs (difficulty in swallowing with recurrent aspiration), central blindness, severe mental retardation, and seizures are other frequent features. Different subgroups of tetraplegic cerebral palsy have been proposed, such as a symmetrical four-limb type, a side asymmetrical type, and an upper-limb dominated type, with or without dystonic traits, all derived from injuries in different locations and of varying extent.

Generally, an extensive brain injury (porencephaly, diffuse encephalomalacia, sequelae of PVL III or type IV IVH, diffuse brain malformations) is revealed by neuroimaging.

Diplegic cerebral palsy

Originally called Little's disease, after the English surgeon William Little, diplegic cerebral palsy describes a bilateral spastic form of cerebral palsy with the lower limbs being more affected than the upper. The lower limbs are held in extension and adduction, resulting in the typical scissors gait with toe walking and frequent hip dislocation. In Ingram's classification of 1955, this condition was distinguished from quadriplegic cerebral palsy by a particular association with prematurity and a lesser incidence of mental retardation, pseudobulbar palsy, and seizures. However, the supposed association of diplegia with prematurity is controversial, and it is hard to distinguish between diplegia and conditions with three or four limb involvement in the individual case. The presence of mental retardation or seizures does not discriminate between the different subtypes of cerebral palsy. This is why the European Collaboration SCPE did not consider diplegia in its classification (Anon, 2000). To prove the inconsistency of any distinction between the two bilateral subtypes of cerebral palsy (tetraplegia and diplegia), Colver & Sethumadhavan (2003) analysed epidemiological studies and showed that difference in results found in various countries disappeared when the two forms of cerebral palsy were considered together.

Hemiplegic cerebral palsy

Hemiplegic cerebral palsy is a unilateral spastic paresis with the upper limbs more severely affected than the lower limbs. Intentional movements, especially hand functions, are impaired, principally pincer grasp of the thumb, extension of the wrist, and supination of the forearm. There is a hemiparetic posture with flexion of the elbow, wrist and knee, and an equinus posture of the foot. The affected leg may be shorter than the other and have contractures, but the age of walking may not be much later than in normal peers. Stereognosis and sensory functions of the affected limbs are often involved. Visual field defects, homonymous hemianopia and cranial nerve abnormalities are common. Epilepsy occurs in more than half the cases. Cognitive development may be preserved and generally there are no severe motor problems.

Pathology localized to one hemisphere is the cause of this form of cerebral palsy. Periventricular haemorrhagic infarction in a premature infant is a frequent cause. Stroke, predominantly occurring in the perinatal period, is the prevalent ischaemic cause. Other possible aetiological factors are cortical malformations and some other hypoxic-ischaemic causes (PVL, hypoxic-ischaemic encephalopathy) (Wu *et al.*, 2006b). According to Bax *et al* (2005), strokes are the cause of hemiplegia in 27 per cent of cases and asymmetrical PVL in 34 per cent.

Classification according to movement disorders

Motor disorders are of three main patterns: spasticity, dykinesia (dystonia and choreoathetosis), and ataxia (Surveillance of Cerebral Palsy in Europe, 2000). When isolated, hypotonia is generally not considered to be a form of cerebral palsy. Each child is classified according to the predominant type of motor disorder, with a mixed form in those cases when no one type dominates; however, the term 'mixed' should be combined with a detailed description of the components of the motor disorder (Rosenbaum *et al.*, 2007).

The establishment of nationwide registers is important. The Australian Cerebral Palsy Register (Love, 2007) recommends a descriptive report of clinical data following an agreed scoring system for motor disorders. In particular, it is proposed that the main motor abnormality in cerebral palsy, spasticity, should be classified according to the Australian Spasticity Assessment (Love, 2007) based on the muscle response to passive movements (Table 4).

Table 4. Scoring of the Australian Spasticity Assessment (Love, 2007)

0	No catch on rapid passive movement (RPM) (no spasticity).
1	Catch on RPM followed by release. There is no resistance to RPM throughout the rest of the range.
2	Catch occurs in second half of available range (after halfway point) during RPM and is followed by resistance throughout remaining range.
3	Catch occurs in the first half of range (up to and including half way point) during RPM and is followed by resistance throughout remaining range.
4	RPM is difficult; there is resistance to movement throughout the range.
5	RPM is not possible; body part appears fixed in flexion or extension during RPM but moves when passive movement is slow.

Spasticity, the most common finding in cerebral palsy, is characterized by muscle hypertonia in the affected areas, which enhances the stiffness and rigidity of movements. Its prevalence in the anti-gravity muscles produces contractures leading to permanent disabilities. Involuntary and uncontrolled movements are characteristic of dyskinetic cerebral palsy, including dystonic and choreoathetotic cerebral palsy. In the dystonic form, involuntary movements consist mainly of abnormal posture caused by sustained muscular contractions (trunk rotation, limb extension or flexion). Hyperkinesia (chorea or/and athetosis) and hypotonia are predominant in choreoathetotic cerebral palsy.

Children with the spastic and dyskinetic subtypes account for 94 per cent of all cases of cerebral palsy (Surveillance of Cerebral Palsy in Europe, 2000). Ataxic cerebral palsy is a less common form and presents later. It results in a loss of muscular coordination (gait, hand movements) associated with hypotonia and a slow intention tremor.

An objective functional scale – the Gross Motor Function Classification System (GMFCS) – was proposed by Palisano *et al.* (1997). This is based on five ordinal levels, ranging from the presence of all the abilities of their age-matched peers though with some impairment of speed and coordination (level 1) to the absence of postural control of the head and the trunk or of any voluntary control of movement (level 5). To cope with disabilities varying with age, four age bands were distinguished – less than 2 years, 2 to 4 years, 4 to 6 years, and 6 to 12 years – with detailed functional categories corresponding to the 5-level scale.

Although other systems for classifying the severity of movement disorders have been proposed, the GFMCS is the first to have its validity and reliability assessed (Wood & Rosenbaum 2000; Rosenbaum *et al.*, 2008).

The World Health Organisation International Classification of Functioning, Disability and Health (WHO, 2001) emphasizes the need to evaluate the functional consequences of motor disorders in cerebral palsy separately in the upper and lower limbs. Accordingly, functional classifications of specific abilities have been proposed in order to plan consequent interventions, such as the Manual Ability Classification System (MACS) aiming at classifying the ability to handle objects (Eliasson *et al.*, 2006), the Functional Mobility Scale (FMS) to measure changes in walking ability (Graham *et al.*, 2004), and the Bimanual Fine Motor Function (BFMF) assessment for upper limb function (Beckung & Hagberg, 2002). A similar test focusing on assessing the quality on upper limb abilities in children in a younger age range (18 months to 8 years) is the Quality of Upper Extremity Skills Test (QUEST) (DeMatteo *et al.*, 1992).

The construction of a scale based on the Communication Function Classification System (CSFC) analogous to the GFMCS and the MACS is now in progress (quoted by Rosenbaum *et al.*, 2008).

Enlarging the domains of classification

Although the traditional classification scheme generally concerns the distribution of affected limb patterns with the predominant type of tone or movement abnormality, a more accurate and comprehensive scheme should be considered for managing particular disorders in individual cases. The Definition and Classification of Cerebral Palsy, April 2006 (Rosenbaum *et al.*, 2007) proposes that more dimensions should be considered in the classification. As well as the traditional topographical and functional components, other important features should be considered in defining the disorder, as shown in Table 5.

Associated impairments

Various associated impairments can modulate the motor disorder. These are derived from the same pathophysiological processes and include sensory impairments, cognitive deficits, behavioural disorders, ongoing musculoskeletal problems, and seizures. The presence and severity of each abnormality should be reported in every case.

Sensory disorders are frequent in cerebral palsy, both visual, auditory and somatosensory. Visual function in particular is often impaired because of peripheral or central lesions. A common peripheral defect in infantile cerebral palsy is the retinopathy of prematurity (ROP). In the most severe stages of ROP (IV and V), visual defects may be serious enough to cause blindness. Other complex and extensive defects of visual acuity, visual fields, ocular motility, and so on are frequently observed in cerebral palsy (Lanzi *et al.*, 1998; Guzzetta *et al.*, 2001; da Costa *et al.*, 2004). However, visual impairments detected early in life in brain-injured infants may be transitory (Eken *et al.*, 1994).

Table 5. Components of cerebral palsy classification

1.	**Motor abnormalities** a) type of the motor disorder (spasticity, ataxia, dyskinesia...) b) topography (tetraplegia, hemiplegia...) c) functional skills (limitations of motor functions)	
2.	**Associated impairments** Concurrent or later developing non-motor disorders related to neurosensory and neurodevelopmental defects, seizures, and behavioural problems	
3.	**Aetiology** Identification of causes	
4.	**Timing** Presumed time of injury occurrence	
5.	**Neuroimaging findings** Cortical and white matter abnormalities, ventricular dilatation	

Defects in visual evoked potentials, brain stem auditory evoked potentials and somatosensory evoked potentials have been found predictive not only of specific impairments but also of a multi-handicap state (Laget et al., 1982; Zafeiriou et al., 2000; Kulak et al., 2006).

Developmental delay evolving towards mental retardation is a frequent finding, especially in tetraplegia. In long term follow-up, about one third of cases of cerebral palsy have severe mental retardation (Arens & Molteno, 1989; Nicholson & Alberman, 1992). Developmental delay is particularly relevant in formulating a general prognosis (involving all aspects of development including motor development). Its accurate assessment is mandatory for an appropriate management strategy.

Behavioural disorders (anxiety, overactivity, and behavioural problems including psychotic and autistic spectrum disorders), although barely yet fully identified and classified (O'Brien, 2007), are frequent in cerebral palsy, as in all other forms of childhood disability. Among the few studies reported so far, Goodman & Yude (2000) described a peculiar frequency of behavioural problems in hemiplegic cerebral palsy. They found psychiatric and behavioural problems in 50 to 60 per cent of their series: 'Fears and worries are common, particularly specific phobias, separation anxiety, and generalized anxiety. Misery was reported in some instances and is related to a depressive disorder. Conduct and oppositional defiant disorders are common. Tension and overactivity are common.' In a few cases autistic spectrum disorder has also been observed.

The association between cerebral palsy and *epilepsy* is based on common underlying mechanisms, both genetic and lesional. Epilepsy in cerebral palsy is reported with a variable incidence (in the range of 15 to 60 per cent) (Aicardi, 1994). The frequency varies according to the type of cerebral palsy, being most common in the tetraplegic form (Hagberg et al., 1975; Aicardi, 1990; Kwong et al., 1998). In hemiplegic cerebral palsy, epilepsy is reported in one third to one half of the cases (Crothers & Paine, 1988; Hadjipanayis et al., 1997; Uvebrandt, 1988). In diplegic patients, it is found less often (Hadjipanayis et al., 1997), but it appears more common in babies born at term (Kwong et al., 1998). Epilepsy is rarely present in ataxic forms of cerebral palsy (Aicardi, 1994). Cognitive impairment in cerebral palsy seems to be particularly associated with epilepsy (Süssovà et al., 1990; Vargha-Khadem et al., 1992; Kwong et al., 1998), probably because of the greater severity of the causative lesion.

The types of seizure vary in the different forms of cerebral palsy. Focal seizures are most common, often with secondary generalization. Other types of seizure (myoclonic, atonic, and so on), barely detectable in infancy without EEG monitoring, are seen in a minority of cases. The frequency of West syndrome varies significantly in the different forms of cerebral palsy (Hadjipanayis et al., 1997): 1–2 per cent in hemiplegic cerebral palsy, 13 per cent in diplegic cerebral palsy, and 27 per cent in tetraplegic cerebral palsy.

Involuntary movements and paroxysmal non-epileptic disorders (breath-holding spells, reflex anoxic attacks, vaso-vagal syncope) may mimic seizures in cerebral palsy. Video-EEG recordings may be necessary for an exact diagnosis of the epileptic nature of the disorder.

Seizures can interfere with sensory-motor and cognitive development in infantile cerebral palsy, which may lead to lack of acquisition of skills and to a gradual loss of function. Even subclinical interictal discharges may interfere with development (Deonna et al., 2000).

When seizures occur in cerebral palsy, the risk of recurrence is so high that treatment should begin promptly. Sodium valproate is probably the first choice antiepileptic drug after the neonatal period in all forms of epilepsy except West syndrome. In West syndrome vigabatrin, adrenocorticotrophic hormones, or steroids are usually given (see chapter 10).

Cerebral palsy in infancy may seriously interfere with *musculoskeletal development*, leading to impairment of the formation of bones and joints and requiring orthopaedic or surgical intervention. Problems include abnormal bone growth (reduced growth or torsional deformities of the long bones) and articulation deformities (joint dislocation or subluxation). The growing bones in infants with cerebral palsy are abnormally moulded by the unbalanced forces placed on them (contractures, abnormal postural support, and so on) (Gage, 1991), as well as by the position in which the infant is nursed (Fulford & Brown, 1976). These factors lead to femoral anteversion, coxa valgus, or tibial torsional deformity; in bilateral cerebral palsy, pes valgus is usually observed, as is equinovarus foot deformity in hemiplegic infants.

Neuroimaging

Neuroimaging complements the clinical classification of cerebral palsy, though there is not enough evidence so far to recommend any specific classification scheme. However, important information may be derived from neuroimaging about the timing of the insult, the pathogenic pathway, and the correlation with clinical features. The possible neuroimaging patterns associated with cerebral palsy may be distinguished by their (predominantly) unilateral or bilateral siting and by whether they are located in the cortex or include the basal ganglia.

Unilateral patterns include unilateral malformations (unilateral dysplasia, hemimegalencephaly), porencephaly from type IV IVH, unilateral PVL, unilateral ventricular dilatation (suggesting IVH or unilateral periventricular leukomalacia sequelae), and porencephaly extending over the cortex originating from a stroke.

Bilateral patterns include the agyria-pachygyria spectrum, schizencephaly, bilateral PVL, and central (parasagittal) cortical lesions. PVL and consequences of IVH are the most frequent types of lesion in this group, occurring in about 60 per cent of cases, and in up to 90 per cent in preterm infants (Krägeloh-Mann & Horber, 2007). The corresponding clinical syndrome is usually bilateral leg-dominated spastic cerebral palsy, but may include cases of unilateral spastic cerebral palsy.

Finally, a third group consists of cortical and/or basal ganglia lesions (about 20 per cent) (Krägeloh-Mann & Horber, 2007), suggesting a peri-/neonatal origin, proven when supported by serial neonatal ultrasound scans (Cowan et al., 2003). This group mainly involves term-born children with severe bilateral athetoid spastic cerebral palsy. In one third of the cases, there is unilateral spastic cerebral palsy, the origin of which is generally an infarct of uncertain timing. Neonatal seizures suggest a neonatal origin (Levy *et al.*, 1985). A prenatal origin, on the other hand, can be assumed in cases where the perinatal and neonatal course was uneventful (Krägeloh-Mann *et al.*, 2002).

Abnormal magnetic resonance imaging is evident in fewer than 40 per cent of cases of ataxic cerebral palsy and there may be no clear lesional changes (Krägeloh-Mann & Horber, 2007).

Brain malformations associated with cerebral palsy are relatively rare, most often occurring in full-term infants. Cerebral palsy linked to brain malformations tends to be of unilateral spastic type, caused by hemimegalencephaly, unilateral cortical dysplasia, or unilateral schizencephaly. In a minority of cases of ataxic cerebral palsy there is detectable cerebellar hypoplasia.

There is evidence of a relation between brain changes shown by neuroimaging and the quality and severity of motor disorders. Spastic cerebral palsy is apparently related to lesions of the pyramidal system (Staudt *et al.*, 2003), whereas dyskinetic cerebral palsy is linked to basal ganglia/thalamic injury (Krägeloh-Mann *et al.*, 2002). Visual impairment in brain-injured infants is associated with basal ganglia lesions (Mercuri *et al.*, 1997). As far as severity is concerned, Yokochi *et al* (1991a; 1991b) found a greater degree of functional severity in more extensive or bilateral lesions, and in combined grey and white matter injuries.

Early diagnosis

It is hard to diagnose cerebral palsy in infants under 6 months of age except in very severe forms. Thus a systematic approach is mandatory in young infants, focusing on the history (personal, maternal, obstetric, perinatal, neonatal), and trying, with the help of clinical examinations and instrumental aids, to determine the possible risk factors. In this way, infants at high risk can be identified and followed appropriately.

Risk factors

Risk factors (Table 6) are conditions significantly associated with cerebral palsy. However, in a classical study by Nelson & Ellenberg (1986), more than 60 per cent of infants with cerebral palsy did not have a high risk profile, and 97 per cent of those with a high risk profile were not affected by cerebral palsy. More recent studies with updated risk factors still show weak sensitivity and specificity in the early diagnosis of cerebral palsy, although they are important in understanding the complex mechanisms underlying the aetiopathogenic pathways leading to cerebral palsy. However, all risk factors – whether isolated or linked in a synergistic way – are useful in defining the high risk population in order to monitor them accurately during the first months of life.

Table 6. Risk factors (according to Reddihough & Collins, 2003, combined with up-to-date data)

A) Before pregnancy i) Maternal factors	• Advanced maternal age (Wu *et al.*, 2006) • Irregular menstruation or long intermenstrual intervals (Torfs *et al.*, 1990) • Unusually short or long interval between pregnancies (Pinto-Martin *et al.*, 1998; Torfs *et al.*, 1990) • Low social class (Dolk *et al.*, 2001; Dowding & Barry, 1990) • Parity of three or more (Topp *et al.*, 1997) • Previous foetal deaths (Nelson & Ellenberg, 1986; Powell *et al.*, 1988) • Abnormal maternal medical conditions (*intellectual disability*: Nelson & Ellenberg, 1986; *seizures*: Nelson & Ellenberg 1986; *thyroid disease*: Blair & Stanley 1993; Nelson & Ellenberg, 1986)
ii) Paternal and sibling factors	• Advanced paternal age (athetoid/dystonic cerebral palsy: Fletcher & Foley, 1993) • Motor deficit in a sibling (Nelson & Ellenberg, 1986).
B) During pregnancy	• Pre-eclampsia in term infants (Collins & Paneth 1998) • Antepartum haemorrhage (Stanley *et al.*, 2000) • Mutations of the factor V gene (factor V Leiden) or of the prothrombin gene favouring placental thrombosis or neonatal stroke (unilateral cerebral palsy) (Nelson & Lynch, 2004) • Multiple pregnancy, not entirely explained by their increased risk of prematurity and low birth weight (Williams *et al.*, 1996; Livinec *et al.*, 2005; Bonellie *et al.*, 2005) • Intrauterine growth retardation (Radianu *et al.*, 2007; Blair & Stanley, 1990, Uvebrandt & Hagberg, 1992; Takahashi *et al.*, 1992 ; Leitner *et al.*, 2007; Wu *et al.*, 2006) • Death of one twin in monochorionic twin pregnancies (Pharaoh & Cooke 1997; Stanley *et al.*, 2000). • Born after *in vitro* fertilization (Hvidtjorn *et al.*, 2006)
C) During labour i) Perinatal asphyxia	• Prolapsed cord, massive intrapartum haemorrhage, prolonged or traumatic delivery, dystocia due to cephalopelvic disproportion or abnormal presentation, and maternal shock (Stanley *et al.*, 2000) • Prolonged second stage of labour and emergency caesarean section (Powell *et al.*, 1988) • Premature separation of the placenta and abnormal foetal position (Torfs *et al.*, 1990) • Prolonged rupture of the membranes (Nelson & Ellenberg, 1985; Murphy *et al.*, 1995) • Meconium stained fluid (Spinillo *et al.*, 1998; Walstab *et al.*, 2002) • Tight nuchal cord (Nelson & Grether, 1998b)
ii) Intrauterine exposure to infection	• Chorioamnionitis (in the latter stages of pregnancy and during labour) in term infants (Murphy *et al.*, 1995; Nelson & Willoughby, 2000; Polivka *et al.*, 1997; Walstab *et al.*, 2002), especially when associated with PVL (Wu & Colford, 2000)
D) At birth	• Prematurity (Stanley *et al.*, 2000; Trau *et al.*, 2005; Takahashi *et al.*, 2005; Livinec *et al.*, 2005) • Low birth weight (Hagberg *et al.*, 1993; Murphy *et al.*, 1995; Stanley & Watson 1985; Torfs *et al.*, 1990) • Low placental weight (Torfs *et al.*, 1990) • Low Apgar scores (Van de Riet et al 1999; Moster et al 2001).
E) In the newborn period	• Neonatal seizures (Powell *et al.*, 1988; Torfs *et al.*, 1990; Murphy *et al.*, 1997) • Sepsis (Blair & Stanley 1993) • Respiratory disease (Powell *et al.*, 1988) • Patent ductus arteriosus, hypotension, blood transfusion, prolonged ventilation, pneumothorax, hyponatraemia, total parenteral nutrition and parenchymal damage with appreciable ventricular dilatation detected by cerebral ultrasound (Murphy *et al.*, 1997) • Hypoglycaemia (Lucas *et al.*, 1988; Stenninger *et al.*, 1998) • Hyperbilirubinaemia • Trauma

Detection of early signs of developmental abnormality

Early signs of developmental abnormality heralding the possible emergence of cerebral palsy may be detected from birth. For example, delay in the disappearance of primitive reflexes and postural reactions is a sign of CNS abnormality and may be predictive of emerging cerebral palsy. Demonstrating abnormalities in the primitive reflexes and postural reactions may provide useful information about risk status (Caputo, 1979), though the sensitivity and specificity is poor for predicting cerebral palsy, especially in the first 12 months of life (Piper *et al.*, 1988; Burns *et al.*, 1989; PeBenito *et al.*, 1989). Assessing the primitive reflexes within the context of a comprehensive neurological examination provides more reliable information. An organized schema of examination (the Primitive Reflex Profile) has been proposed to identify a possible evolution towards cerebral palsy (Caputo *et al.*, 1984; Blasco, 1994; Zafeirou, 2004). A review on the predictive value of primitive reflexes and postural reactions was published by Zafeirou (2004).

Impairment of neurological function, as assessed by neurological examination at an early age, seems to be poorly predictive of cerebral palsy, as shown by classical studies from the National Collaborative Perinatal Project (Nelson & Ellenberg, 1979; Ellenberg & Nelson, 1981). At birth and at 4 months, the percentage of children with abnormal neurological examinations who have received a diagnosis of cerebral palsy at 7 years was, respectively, 23 per cent and 33 per cent, whereas half the infants given a diagnosis of cerebral palsy at 1 year no longer had this diagnosis at 7 years.

The difficulty in predicting the evolution towards cerebral palsy may be better addressed by sequential neurological examinations together with neuroimaging and neurophysiological investigations. Dubowitz & Dubowitz (1981) proposed a neurological assessment of the preterm and full term infant aiming at following newborns at risk of neurological sequelae. They successively improved and integrated the assessment with other items including gross motor and fine motor development, as well as quality of movements as revealed by observations of general movements (Dubowitz *et al.*, 1999) (see chapter 1). A scoring system with ranges for optimal scores was introduced to allow correlations to be made between abnormal signs, the severity of the lesions, and the ongoing disability. This system has been applied to infants with hypoxic-ischaemic encephalopathy, cerebral ischaemic infarction, prematurity, and so on (see chapter 1), and has a good predictive value, especially for centres lacking in sophisticated tools such as neuroimaging (Mercuri *et al.*, 2007).

Recently, *spontaneous general movements* (see chapter 3) and their abnormalities, observed on videotape from soon after birth to 16–20 weeks' term age equivalent, have been considered capable of predicting cerebral palsy much earlier than any other tool (Cioni *et al.*, 1997; Einspieler *et al.*, 1997; Prechtl, 2001; Hadders-Algra, 2004). These are also capable of predicting the normal evolution of infants considered at risk (Prechtl, 2001). Cramped, synchronous general movements and/or the absence of normal fidgety movements of the limbs and trunk during these early weeks are predictive of cerebral palsy (Cioni *et al.*, 2000; Ferrari *et al.*, 2002; Guzzetta *et al.*, 2003). A particular abnormality of general movements (poor repertoire, 'arm movements in circle' and finger spreading) is observed in infants who later develop dyskinetic cerebral palsy (Einspieler *et al.*, 2002). In addition, abnormal fidgety movements are supposed to predict minor neurological defects (Cioni *et al.*, 2007).

More than impairment itself, functional limitations of motor day-to-day activities express the disability in cerebral palsy (Palmer, 2004). Measurements of these limitations may be evaluated by the 'motor quotient' (the ratio of motor age determined by the best motor milestone performance to that determined by chronological age); motor quotient at 8 months seems to be predictive of motor abilities at 2 years (Caputo & Shapiro, 1985).

Important tools for integrating the definition of risk factors are neuroimaging techniques (ultrasound, computed tomography, magnetic resonance imaging). Neuroimaging represents the best and the most direct indicator of the pathogenesis of cerebral palsy (Ment et al., 2002). Intraventricular and periventricular haemorrhage, white matter cystic lesions, ischaemic lesions with porencephalic sequelae, ventriculomegaly, cortical dysplasias and other brain malformations are the main conditions associated with cerebral palsy that may be detected very early on by ultrasound (Guzzetta et al., 1986; Grant & Barkovich, 1997; Rutherford et al., 1998; Wilson-Costello et al., 1998; Hack et al., 2000).

In preterm infants, although the result of ultrasound scans in the first week of life may be relevant in directing the acute treatment, the examination carried out at term age may improve the ability to predict the possible development of cerebral palsy (Ito et al., 1997). However, a lack of neonatal ultrasound changes has a poor negative predictive value (Laptook et al., 2005).

MRI may reveal congenital lesions *in utero*, although postnatal imaging provides better information and in cases of malformations the best time will be at the end of the first year or later. MRI is particularly important as a predictive tool in early investigations (Ashwal et al., 2004). Compared with ultrasound, it increases the sensitivity and specificity in predicting cerebral palsy (Mirmiran et al., 2004). Rutherford et al (2005) advise performing MRI as soon as possible in infants with abnormal ultrasound or neurological examination, as haemorrhagic and leukomalacic lesions are better detected with MRI. Diffusion-weighted imaging may identify infarcted brain matter during the ischaemic insult, though not reliably in cases of basal ganglia and thalamus injury (Ment et al., 2002; Rutherford et al., 2007).

In encephalopathic newborn infants, MRI has particular predictive value in demonstrating basal ganglia and thalamic involvement. This is associated with adverse developmental outcomes including cerebral palsy (Grant & Barkovich, 1997). In infants with focal ischaemic injuries, the extent of the initial lesion is predictive of the neurological outcome: the co-presence of involvement of the hemisphere, the basal ganglia and the posterior limb of the internal capsule is frequently associated with later hemiplegic cerebral palsy (Mercuri et al., 2001). Moreover, absence of normal signals in the posterior limb of the internal capsule in term infants with encephalopathy predicts an abnormal neurodevelopmental outcome at 1 year with high sensitivity and specificity (Rutherford et al., 1998). If the absence is asymmetrical in infants with periventricular haemorrhagic infarction, hemiplegic cerebral palsy may develop (de Vries et al., 1999).

Unfortunately, cerebral palsy is frequently caused by prenatal factors: affected neonates present no obvious abnormality at birth and will therefore not be selected for neuroimaging as a neonate.

References

Aicardi, J. (1990): Epilepsy in brain injured children. *Dev. Med. Child Neurol.* **32**, 192–202.

Aicardi, J. (1994): Epilepsy as a presenting manifestation of brain tumours and other selected brain disorders. In: *Epilepsy in children*, 2nd ed., ed. J. Aicardi, pp. 350–351. New York: Raven Press.

Alberman, E. (1984): *The epidemiology of the cerebral palsies*, pp. 27–31. Philadelphia: JB Lippincott; 1984.

Anderson, J.M., Milner, R.D.G. & Strich, S.J. (1967): Effects of neonatal hypoglycemia on the nervous system: a pathological study. *J. Neurol. Neurosurg. Psychiatry* **30**, 295–310.

Arens, L.J. & Molteno, C.D. (1989): A comparative study of postnatally acquired cerebral palsy in Cape Town. *Dev. Med. Child Neurol.* **31**, 246–254.

Arpino, C., D'Argenzio, L., Ticconi, C., Di Paolo, A., Stellin, V., Lopez, L. & Curatolo, P. (2005): Brain damage in preterm infants: etiological pathways. *Ann. Ist. Super. Sanità* **41**, 229–237.

Ashwal, S., Russman, B.S., Blasco, B.A., Miller, G., Sandler, A., Shevell, M., Stevenson, R. & Quality Standards Subcommittee of the American Academy of Neurology; Practice Committee of the Child Neurology Society (2004): Practice parameter: diagnostic assessment of the child with cerebral palsy. *Neurology* **62**, 851–863.

Avery, G.B., Fletcher, M.A. & MacDonald, M.G. (1999): *Neonatology: pathophysiology and management of the newborn*, 5th ed. Philadelphia: Lippincott Williams and Wilkins.

Barkovich, A.J., Westmark, K., Partridge, C., Sola, A. & Ferriero, D.M. (1995): Perinatal asphyxia: MR findings in the first 10 days. *Am. J. Neuroradiol.* **16**, 427–438.

Barkovich, A.J., Ali, F.A., Rowley, H.A. & Bass, N. (1998): Imaging patterns of neonatal hypoglycemia. *Am. J. Neuroradiol.* **19**, 523–528.

Bax, M.C. (1964): Terminology and classification of cerebral palsy. *Dev. Med. Child Neurol.* **6**, 295–307.

Bax, M., Goldstein, M., Rosenbaum, P., Leviton, A., Paneth, N., Dan, B., Jacobsson, B., Damiano, D. & Executive Committee for the Definition of Cerebral Palsy (2005): Proposed definition and classification of cerebral palsy, April 2005. *Dev. Med. Child Neurol.* **47**, 571–576.

Bax, M., Tydeman, C. & Flodmark, O. (2006): Clinical and MRI correlates of cerebral palsy: the European Cerebral Palsy Study. *JAMA* **296**, 1602–1608.

Beckung, E. & Hagberg, G. (2002): Neuroimpairments, activity limitations, and participation restrictions in children with cerebral palsy. *Dev. Med. Child Neurol.* **44**, 309–316.

Bekker, M.N. & van Vugt, J.M. (2001): The role of magnetic resonance imaging in prenatal diagnosis of fetal anomalies. *Eur. J. Obstet. Gynecol. Reprod. Biol.* **96**, 173–178.

Berl, M.M., Vaidya, C.J. & Gaillard, W.D. (2006): Functional imaging of developmental and adaptive changes in neurocognition. *Neuroimage* **30**, 679–691.

Blair, E. & Stanley, F. (1990): Intrauterine growth and spastic cerebral palsy. 1. Association with birth weight for gestational age. *Am. J. Obstet. Gynecol.* **162**, 229–237.

Blair, E. & Stanley, F. (1993): Aetiological pathways to spastic cerebral palsy. *Paediatr. Perinat. Epidemiol.* **7**, 302–317.

Blasco, P.A. (1994): Primitive reflexes: their contribution to the early detection of cerebral palsy. *Clin. Pediatr.* **33**, 388–397.

Bonellie, S.R., Currie, D. & Chalmers, J. (2005): Comparison of risk factors for cerebral palsy in twins and singletons. *Dev. Med. Child Neurol.* **47**, 587–591.

Bundey, S. & Griffiths, M.I. (1977): Recurrence risks in families of children with symmetrical spasticity. *Dev. Med. Child Neurol.* **19**, 179–191.

Burns, Y.R., O'Callaghan, M. & Tudehope, D.I. (1989): Early identification of cerebral palsy in high risk infants. *Aust. Paediatr. J.* **25**, 215–219.

Cabeza, R. & Nyberg, L. (2000): Imaging cognition II. An empirical review of 275 PET and fMRI studies. *J. Cogn. Neurosci.* **12**, 1–47.

Cans, C., Surman, G., McManus, V., Coghlan, D., Hensey, O. & Johnson, A. (2004): Cerebral palsy registries. *Semin. Pediatr. Neurol.* **11**, 18–23.

Cans, C., Dolk, H., Platt, M.J., Colver, A., Prasauskiene, A., Krägeloh-Mann, I., on behalf of SCPE Collaborative Group from the European Commission (2007): Recommendations from the SCPE collaborative group for defining and classifying cerebral palsy. *Dev. Med. Child Neurol.* (Suppl.) **49**, 35–38.

Capute, A.J. (1979): Identifying cerebral palsy in infancy through study of primitive-reflex profiles. *Pediatr. Ann.* **8**, 589–595.

Capute, A.J. & Shapiro, B.K. (1985): The motor quotient. A method for the early detection of motor delay. *Am. J. Dis. Child.* **139**, 940–942.

Capute, A.J., Palmer, F.B., Shapiro, B.K., Wachtel, R.C., Ross, A. & Accardo, P.J. (1984): Primitive reflex profile: a quantitation of primitive reflexes in infancy. *Dev. Med. Child Neurol.* **26**, 375–383.

Carr, L.J., Harrison, L.M., Evans, A.L. & Stephens, J.A. (1993): Patterns of central motor reorganization in hemiplegic cerebral palsy. *Brain* **116**, 1223–1247.

Cioni, G., Ferrari, F., Einspieler, C., Paolicelli, P.B., Barbani, M.T. & Prechtl, H.F.R. (1997): Comparison between observation of spontaneous movements and neurologic examination in preterm infants. *J. Pediatr.* **130**, 704–711.

Cioni, G., Bois, A.F., Einspieler, C., Ferrari, F., Martijn, A., Paolicelli, P.B., Rapisardi, G., Roversi, M.F. & Prechtl, H.F. (2000): Early neurological signs in preterm infants with unilateral intraparenchymal echodensity. *Neuropediatrics* **31**, 240–251.

Cioni, G., Einspieler, C. & Paolicelli, P. (2007): Other approaches to neurological assessment. In: *Neurological assessment in the first two years of life*, eds. G. Cioni & E. Mercuri, pp. 49–68. London: Mac Keith Press.

Collins, M. & Paneth, N. (1998): Pre-eclampsia and cerebral palsy: are they related? *Dev. Med. Child Neurol.* **40**, 207–211.

Colver, A.F. & Sethumadhavan, T. (2003): The term diplegia should be abandoned. *Arch. Dis. Child.* **88**, 286–290.

Coorssen, E.A., Msall, M.E. & Duffy, L.C. (1991): Multiple minor malformations as a marker for prenatal etiology of cerebral palsy. *Dev. Med. Child Neurol.* **33**, 730–736.

Costeff, H. (2004): Estimated frequency of genetic and nongenetic causes of congenital idiopathic cerebral palsy in west Sweden. *Ann. Hum. Genet.* **68**, 515–520.

Cowan, F., Rutherford, M., Groenendaal, F., Eken, P., Mercuri, E., Bydder, G.M., Meiners, L.C., Dubowitz, L.M.S. & de Vries, L.S. (2003): Origin and timing of brain lesions in term infants with neonatal encephalopathy. *Lancet* **361**, 736–742.

Croen, L., Grether, J., Curry, C. & Nelson, K. (2001): Congenital abnormalities among children with cerebral palsy: more evidence for prenatal antecedents. *J. Pediatr.* **138**, 804–812.

Crothers, B. & Paine, R.S. (1988): Seizures and electroencephalography. In: *The natural history of cerebral palsy. Classics in developmental medicine No. 2.*, pp. 143–157. London: Mac Keith Press.

da Costa, M.F., Salomao, S.R., Berezovsky, A., de Haro, F.M. & Ventura, D.F. (2004): Relationship between vision and motor impairment in children with spastic cerebral palsy: new evidence from electrophysiology. *Behav. Brain Res.* **149**, 145–150.

Dammann, O. & Leviton, A. (2000): Role of the fetus in perinatal infection and neonatal brain damage. *Curr. Opin. Pediatr.* **12**, 99–104.

Dammann, O., Kuba, K. & Leviton, A. (2002): Perinatal infection, fetal inflammatory response, white matter damage, and cognitive limitations in children born preterm. *Ment. Retard. Dev. Disabil. Res. Rev.* **8**, 46–50.

D'Angio, C.T., Sinkin, R.A., Stevens, T.P., Landfish, N.K., Merzbach, J.L., Ryan, R.M., Phelps, D.L., Palumbo, D.R. & Myers, G.J. (2002): Longitudinal 15-year follow-up of children born at less than 29 weeks gestation after introduction of surfactant therapy into a region: neurologic, cognitive, and educational outcomes. *Pediatrics* **110**, 1094–1102.

DeMatteo, C., Law, M., Russell, D., Pollock, N., Rosenbaum, P. & Walter, S. (1992): *QUEST: Quality of upper extremity skills test manual.* Hamilton, Ontario: Neurodevelopmental Research Unit, Chedoke Campus, Chedoke-McMasters Hospital.

Deonna, T.H., Zesiger, P., Davidoff, P., Maeder, M. & Roulet, E. (2000): Benign partial epilepsy of childhood: longitudinal neuropsychological and EEG study of cognitive function. *Dev. Med. Child Neurol.* **42**, 595–603.

de Vries, L.S., Eken, P. & Dubowitz, L.M.S. (1992): The spectrum of leukomalacia using cranial ultrasound. *Behav. Brain Res.* **49**, 1–6.

de Vries, L.S., Groenendaal, F., van Haastert, I.C., Eken, P., Rademaker, K.J. & Meiners, L.C. (1999): Asymmetrical myelination of the posterior limb, of the internal capsule in infants with periventricular haemorrhagic infarction: an early predictor of hemiplegia. *Neuropediatrics* **30**, 314–319.

Dizon-Townson, D.S., Melin, L., Nelson, L.M., Varner, M. & Ward, K. (1997): Fetal carriers of the factor V Leiden mutation are prone to miscarriage and placental infarction. *Am. J. Obstet. Gynecol.* **177**, 402–405.

Dolk, H., Pattenden, S. & Johnson, A. (2001): Cerebral palsy, low birthweight and socio-economic deprivation: inequalities in a major cause of childhood disability. *Paediatr. Perinatal. Epidemiol.* **15**, 359–363.

Dowding, V.M. & Barry, C. (1990): Cerebral palsy: social class differences in prevalence in relation to birthweight and severity of disability. *J. Epidemiol. Community Health* **44**, 191–195.

Dubowitz, L. & Dubowitz, V. (1981): *The neurological assessment of the preterm and full term infant. Clinics in developmental medicine 79.* London: Heinemann.

Dubowitz, L., Dubowitz, V. & Mercuri, E. (1999): *The neurological assessment of the preterm and full term infant. Clinics in developmental medicine 148.* London: Mac Keith Press.

Einspieler, C., Prechtl, H.F., Ferrari, F., Cioni, G. & Bos, A.F. (1997): The qualitative assessment of general movements in preterm, term and young infants – review of the methodology. *Early Hum. Dev.* **50**, 47–60.

Einspieler, C., Cioni, G., Paolicelli, P.B., Bos, A.F., Dressler, A., Ferrari, F., Roversi, M.F. & Prechtl, H.F. (2002): The early markers for later dyskinetic cerebral palsy are different from those for spastic cerebral palsy. *Neuropediatrics* **33**, 73–78.

Eliasson, A.C., Krumlinde-Sundholm, L., Rosblad, B., Beckung, E., Arner, M., Ohrvall, A.M. & Rosenbaum, P. (2006): The Manual Ability Classification System (MACS) for children with cerebral palsy: scale development and evidence of validity and reliability. *Dev. Med. Child Neurol.* **48**, 549–554.

Ellenberg, J.H. & Nelson, K.B. (1981): Early recognition of infants at high risk for cerebral palsy: examination at age four months. *Dev. Med. Child Neurol.* **23**, 705–716.

Eken, P., van Nieuwenhuizen, O., van der Graaf, Y., Schalij-Delfos, N.E. & de Vries, L.S. (1994): Relation between neonatal cranial ultrasound abnormalities and cerebral visual impairment in infancy. *Dev. Med. Child Neurol.* **36**, 3–15.

Ferrari, F., Cioni, G., Einspieler, C., Roversi, M., Bos, A., Paolicelli, P., Ranzi, A. & Prechtl, H.F. (2002): Cramped synchronized general movements in preterm infants as an early marker for later cerebral palsy. *Arch. Pediatr. Adolesc. Med.* **156**, 460–467.

Fletcher, N.A. & Foley, J. (1993): Parental age, genetic mutation, and cerebral palsy. *J. Med. Genet.* **30**, 44–46.

Floyd, H.G. (2007): Classification of cerebral palsy: neuropathologist's perspective. *Dev. Med. Child Neurol. suppl.* **49**, S19–S21.

Freud, S. (1897): Die infantile Cerebrallähmung. In: *Specielle Pathologie und Therapie*, Bd IX, Teil III, ed. H. Nothnagel, pp. 1–327. Vienna: Holder.

Friede, R.L. (1989): *Developmental neuropathology*, 2nd ed. Berlin: Springer-Verlag.

Fulford, G.E. & Brown, J.K. (1978): Position as a cause of deformity in children with cerebral palsy. *Dev. Med. Child Neurol.* **18**, 305–314.

Gage, J. (1991): Gait analysis in cerebral palsy. In: *Clinics in developmental medicine, vol. 121*, p. 122. Oxford: Blackwell Scientific Publications.

Gaillard, W.D. (2004): Functional MR imaging of language, memory, and sensorimotor cortex. *Neuroimaging Clin. North Am.* **14**, 471–485.

Garne, E., Dolk, H., Krägeloh-Mann, I., Holst Ravn, S., Cans, C. & SCPE Collaborative Group. (2008): Cerebral palsy and congenital malformations. *Eur. J. Paediatr. Neurol.* **12**, 82–88.

Glenn, O.A., Ludeman, N.A., Berman, J.I., Wu, Y.W., Lu, Y., Bartha, A.I., Vigneron, D.B., Chung, S.W., Ferriero, D.M., Barkovich, A.J. & Henry, R.G. (2007): Diffusion tensor MR imaging tractography of the pyramidal tracts correlates with clinical motor function in children with congenital hemiparesis. *Am. J. Neuroradiol.* **28**, 1796–1802.

Goodman, R. & Yude, C. (2000): Emotional, behavioural, and social consequences. In: *Clinical hemiplegia. Clinics in developmental medicine No. 150*, pp. 166–178. London: Mac Keith Press.

Graham, H.K., Harvey, A., Rodda, J., Nattrass, G.R. & Pirpiris, M. (2004): The Functional Mobility Scale (FMS). *J. Pediatr. Orthoped.* **24**, 514–520.

Grant, P.E. & Barkovich, A.J. (1997): Neuroimaging in CP: issues in pathogenesis and diagnosis. *MRDD Res. Rev.* **3**, 118–128.

Grether, J.K. & Nelson, K.B. (1997): Maternal infection and cerebral palsy in infants of normal birthweight. *JAMA* **278**, 207–211.

Gunther, G., Junker, R., Strater, R., Schobess, R., Kurnik, K., Heller, C., Kosch, A., Nowak-Göttl, U. & Childhood Stroke Study Group (2000): Symptomatic ischemic stroke in full-term neonates: role of acquired and genetic prothrombotic risk factors. *Stroke* **31**, 2437–2441.

Guzzetta, A., Mercuri, E. & Cioni, G. (2001): Visual disorders in children with brain lesions: 2. Visual impairment associated with cerebral palsy. *Eur. J. Paediatr. Neurol.* **5**, 115–119.

Guzzetta, A., Mercuri, E., Rapisardi, G., Ferrari, F., Roversi, F., Cowan, F., Rutherford, M., Paolicelli, P.B., Einspieler, C., Boldrini, A., Dubowitz, L., Prechtl, H.F. & Cioni, G. (2003): General movements detect early signs of hemiplegia in term infants with neonatal cerebral infarction. *Neuropediatrics* **34**, 61–66.

Guzzetta, A., Bonanni, P., Biagi, L., Tosetti, M., Montanaro, D., Guerrini, R. & Cioni, G. (2007): Reorganisation of the somatosensory system after early brain damage. *Clin. Neurophysiol.* **118**, 1110–1121.

Guzzetta, F., Shackelford, G.D., Volpe, S., Perlman, J.M. & Volpe, J.J. (1986): Periventricular intraparenchymal echodensities in the premature newborn: critical determinant of neurologic outcome. *Pediatrics* **78**, 995–1006.

Hack, M., Wilson-Costello, D., Friedman, H., Taylor, G.H., Schluchter, M. & Fanaroff, A.A. (2000): Neurodevelopment and predictors of outcomes of children with birth weight of less than 1000 g, 1992–1995. *Arch. Pediatr. Adolesc. Med.* **154**, 725–731.

Hadders-Algra, M. (2004): General movements: a window for early identification of children at high risk for developmental disorders. *J. Pediatr.* **145**, s12–s18.

Hadjipanayis, A., Hadjichristodoulou, C. & Youroukos, S. (1997): Epilepsy in patients with cerebral palsy. *Dev. Med. Child Neurol.* **39**, 659–663.

Hagberg, B., Hagberg, G. & Olow, I. (1975): The changing panorama of cerebral palsy in Sweden 1954-70. II: analysis of the various syndromes. *Acta Paediatr. Scand.* **64**, 193–200.

Hagberg, B., Hagberg, G. & Olow, I. (1993): The changing panorama of cerebral palsy in Sweden. VI. Prevalence and origin during the birth year period 1983–1986. *Acta Paediatr. Scand.* **82**, 387–393.

Hagberg, B., Hagberg, G., Beckung, E. & Uvebrant, P. (2001): Changing panorama of cerebral palsy in Sweden. VIII. Prevalence and origin in the birth year period 1991–94. *Acta Paediatr.* **90**, 271–277.

Hagstrom, J.N., Walter, J., Bluebond-Langner, R., Amatniek, J.C., Manno, C.S. & High, K.A. (1998): Prevalence of the factor V Leiden mutation in children and neonates with thromboembolic disease. *J. Pediatr.* **133**, 777–781.

Harum, K.H., Hoon, A.H., Kato, G.J., Casella, J.F., Breiter, S.N. & Johnston, M.V. (1999): Homozygous factor-V mutation as a genetic cause of perinatal thrombosis and cerebral palsy. *Dev. Med. Child Neurol.* **41**, 777–780.

Hayakawa, F., Okumura, A., Kato, T., Kuno, K. & Watanabe, K. (1999): Determination of timing of brain injury in preterm infants with periventricular leukomalacia with serial neonatal electroencephalography. *Pediatrics* **104**, 1077–1081.

Hemminki, K., Li, X., Sundquist, K. & Sundquist, J. (2007): High familial risks for cerebral palsy implicate partial heritable aetiology. *Paediatr. Perinat. Epidemiol.* **21**, 235–241.

High, K.A. (1998): Prevalence of the factor V Leiden mutation in children and neonates with thromboembolic disease. *J. Pediatr.* **133**, 777–781.

Himpens, E., Van den Broek, C., Oostra, A., Calders, P. & Vanhaesebrouck, P. (2008): Prevalence, type, distribution, and severity of cerebral palsy in relation to gestational age: a meta-analytic review. *Dev. Med. Child Neurol.* **50**, 334–340.

Hogeveen, M., Blom, H.J., Van Amerongen, M., Boogmans, B., Van Beynum, I.M. & Van De Bor, M. (2002): Hyperhomocysteinemia as risk factor for ischemic and hemorrhagic stroke in newborn infants. *J. Pediatr.* **141**, 429–431.

Hoon, A.H. (2005): Neuroimaging in cerebral palsy: patterns of brain dysgenesis and injury. *J. Child Neurol.* **20**, 936–939.

Hughes, I. & Newton, R. (1992): Genetic aspects of cerebral palsy. *Dev. Med. Child Neurol.* **34**, 80–86.

Hvidtjørn, D., Grove, J., Schendel, D.E., Vaeth, M., Ernst, E., Nielsen, L.F. & Thorsen, P. (2006): Cerebral palsy among children born after *in vitro* fertilization: the role of preterm delivery – a population-based, cohort study. *Pediatrics* **118**, 475–482.

Inder, T., Huppi, P., Zientara, G., Maier, S.E., Jolesz, F.A., di Salvo, D., Robertson, R., Barnes, P.D. & Volpe, J.J. (1999): Early detection of periventricular leukomalacia by diffusion-weighted magnetic resonance imaging techniques. *J. Pediatr.* **134**, 631–634.

Ingram, T.T.S. (1955): A study of cerebral palsy in the childhood population of Edinburgh. *Arch. Dis. Child* **30**, 85–98.

Ito, T., Hashimoto, K., Kadowaki, K., Nagata, N., Makio, A., Takahashi, H., Ikeno, S. & Terakawa, N. (1997): Ultrasonographic findings in the periventricular region in premature newborns with antenatal periventricular leukomalacia. *J. Perinat. Med.* **25**, 180–183.

Johnston, M.V. (2003): Brain plasticity in paediatric neurology. *Eur. J. Paediatr. Neurol.* **7**, 105–113.

Johnston, M.V. & Hagberg, H. (2007): Sex and the pathogenesis of cerebral palsy. *Dev. Med. Child Neurol.* **49**, 74–78.

Johnston, M.V., Nishimura, A., Harum, K., Pekar, J. & Blue, M.E. (2001): Sculpting the developing brain. *Adv. Pediatr.* **48**, 1–38.

Kadhim, H., Tabarki, B., DePerez, C. & Sepire, B. (2003): Cytokine immunoreactivity in cortical and subcortical neurons in periventricular leukomalacia: are cytokines implicated in neuronal dysfunction in cerebral palsy? *Acta Neuropathol.* **105**, 298–316.

Kadhim, H., Sebire, G. & Kahn, A. (2005): Causal mechanisms underlying periventricular leukomalacia and cerebral palsy. *Curr. Pediatr. Rev.* **1**, 1–6.

Kendall, G. & Peebles, D. (2005): Acute fetal hypoxia: the modulating effect of infection. *Early Hum. Dev.* **81**, 27–34.

Kostovic, I. & Judas, M. (2002): Correlation between the sequential ingrowth of afferents and transient patterns of cortical lamination in preterm infants. *Anat. Rec.* **267**, 1–6.

Krägeloh-Mann, I., Helber, A., Mader, I., Staudt, M., Wolff, M., Groenendaal, F. & DeVries, L. (2002): Bilateral lesions of thalamus and basal ganglia: origin and outcome. *Dev. Med. Child Neurol.* **44**, 477–484.

Krägeloh-Mann, I. & Horber, V. (2007): The role of magnetic resonance imaging in elucidating the pathogenesis of cerebral palsy: a systematic review. *Dev. Med. Child Neurol.* **49**, 144–151.

Kulak, W., Sobaniec, W., Solowiej, E. & Kowski, L. (2006): Somatosensory and visual evoked potentials in children with cerebral palsy: correlations and discrepancies with MRI findings and clinical picture. *Pediatr. Rehab.* **9**, 201–209.

Kwong, K.L., Wong, S.N. & So, K.T. (1998): Epilepsy in children with cerebral palsy. *Pediatr. Neurol.* **19**, 31–36.

Laget, P., Gagnard, L., Ostre, C. & d'Allest, A.M. (1982): Visual evoked potentials in children with non-hemiplegic cerebral palsy. *Adv. Neurol.* **32**, 97–107.

Lanzi, G., Fazzi, E., Uggetti, C., Cavallini, A., Danova, S., Egitto, M.G., Ginevra, O.F., Salati, R. & Bianchi, P.E. (1998): Cerebral visual impairment in periventricular leukomalacia. *Neuropediatrics* **25**, 145–150.

Laptook, A.R., O'Shea, T.M., Shankaran, S., Bhaskar, B. & NICHD Neonatal Network. Adverse neurodevelopmental outcomes among extremely low birth weight infants with a normal head ultrasound: prevalence and antecedents. *Pediatrics* **115**, 673–680.

Larroche, J.C. (1977): *Developmental pathology of the neonate.* New York: Excerpta Medica.

Leitner, Y., Fattal-Valevski, A., Geva, R., Eshel, R., Toledano-Alhadef, H., Rotstein, M., Bassan, H., Radianu, B., Bitchonsky, O., Jaffa, A.J. & Harel, S. (2007): Neurodevelopmental outcome of children with intrauterine growth retardation: a longitudinal, 10-year prospective study. *J. Child Neurol.* **22**, 580–587.

Leviton, A., Paneth, N., Reuss, M.L., Susser, M., Allred, E.N., Dammann, O., Kuban, K., Van Marter, L.J. & Pagano, M. (1999): Hypothyroxinemia of prematurity and the risk of cerebral white matter damage. *J. Pediatr.* **134**, 706–711.

Levy, S.R., Abrams, I.F., Marshall, P.C. & Rosquette, E.E. (1985): Seizures and cerebral infarction in the fullterm newborn. *Ann. Neurol.* **17**, 366–370.

Livinec, F., Ancel, P.Y., Marret, S., Arnaud, C., Fresson, J., Pierrat, V., Rozé, J.C., Escande, B., Thiriez, G., Larroque, B., Kaminski, M. for the Epipage Group. Prenatal risk factors for cerebral palsy in very preterm singletons and twins. *Obstet. Gynecol.* **105**, 134–137.

Lochshin, M.D., Druzin, M.L., Goei, S., Qamar, T., Magid, M.S., Jovanovic, L. & Ferenc, M. (1985): Antibody to cardiolipin as a predictor of fetal distress or death in pregnant patients with systemic lupus erythematosus. *N. Engl. J. Med.* **313**, 152–156.

Love, S.C. (2007): Better description of spastic cerebral palsy for reliable classification. *Dev. Med. Child Neurol. suppl.* **49**, 24–25.

Lucas, A., Morley, R. & Cole, T.J. (1988): Adverse neurodevelopmental outcome of moderate neonatal hypoglycemia. *BMJ* **297**, 304–308.

MacGillivray, I. & Campbell, D.M. (1995): The changing pattern of cerebral palsy in Avon. *Paediatr. Perinat. Epidemiol.* **9**, 146–155.

MacLennan, A. (1999): A template for defining a causal relation between acute intrapartum events and cerebral palsy: international consensus statement. *BMJ* **319**, 1054–1059.

McHale, D.P., Mitchel, S., Bundey, S., Moynihan, L., Campbell, D.A., Woods, C.G., Lench, N.J., Mueller, R.F. & Markham, A.F. (1999): A gene for autosomal recessive symmetrical spastic cerebral palsy maps to chromosome 2q24-25. *Am. J. Hum. Genet.* **64**, 526–532.

Menkes, J.H. & Flores-Sarnat, L. (2006): Cerebral palsy due to chromosomal anomalies and continuous gene syndromes. *Clin. Perinatol.* **33**, 481–501.

Ment, L.R., Bada, H.S., Barnes, P., Grant, P.E., Hirtz, D., Papile, L.A., Pinto-Martin, J., Rivkin, M. & Slovis, T.L. (2002): Practice parameter: neuroimaging of the neonate: report of the Quality Standards Subcommittee of the American Academy of Neurology and the Practice Committee of the Child Neurology Society. *Neurology* **58**, 1726–1738.

Mercuri, E., Atkinson, J., Braddick, O., Anker, S., Cowan, F., Rutherford, M., Pennock, J. & Dubowitz, L. (1997): Basal ganglia damage and impaired visual function in the newborn infant. *Arch. Dis. Child. Fetal Neonatal Ed.* **77**, F111–F114.

Mercuri, E., Cowan, F., Gupte, G., Manning, R., Laffan, M., Rutherford, M., Edwards, A.D., Dubowitz, L. & Roberts, I. (2001): Prothrombotic disorders and abnormal neurodevelopmental outcome in infants with neonatal cerebral infarction. *Pediatrics* **107**, 1400–1404.

Mercuri, E., Haataja, L., Ricci, D., Cowan, F. & Dubowitz, L. (2007): Classical neurological examination in young infants with neonatal brain lesions. In: *Neurological assessment in the first two years of life*, eds. G. Cioni & E. Mercuri, pp. 38–48. London: Mac Keith Press.

Mirmiran, M., Barnes, P.D., Keller, K., Constantinou, J.C., Fleisher, B.E., Hintz, S.R. & Ariagno, R.L. (2004): Neonatal brain magnetic resonance imaging before discharge is better than serial cranial ultrasound in predicting cerebral palsy in very low birth weight preterm infants. *Pediatrics* **114**, 992–998.

Moster, D., Lie, R., Irgens, L., Bjerkedal, T. & Markestad, T. (2001): The association of Apgar score with subsequent death and cerebral palsy: a population-based study in term infants. *J. Pediatr.* 138, 798–803.

Murakami, Y., Yamashita, Y., Matsuishi, T., Utsunomiya, H., Okudera, T. & Hashimoto, T. (1999): Cranial MRI of neurologically impaired children suffering from neonatal hypoglycaemia. *Pediatr. Radiol.* **29**, 23–27.

Murphy, C., Yeargin-Allsopp, M., Decouffle, P. & Drews, C. (1993): Prevalence of cerebral palsy among ten-year-old children in metropolitan Atlanta, 1985 through 1987. *J. Pediatr.* **123**, S13–S19.

Murphy, D.J., Sellars, S., MacKenzie, I.Z., Yudkin, P. & Johnson, A. (1995): Case-control study of antenatal and intrapartum risk factors for cerebral palsy in very preterm singleton babies. *Lancet* **346**, 1449–1454.

Murphy, D.J., Hope, P.L. & Johnson, A. (1997): Neonatal risk factors for cerebral palsy in very preterm babies: case-control study. *BMJ* **314**, 404–408.

Nagae, L.M., Hoon, A.H., Stashinko, E., Lin, D., Zhang, W., Levey, E., Wakana, S., Jiang, H., Leite, C.C., Lucato, L.T., van Zijl, P.C., Johnston, M.V. & Mori, S. (2007): Diffusion tensor imaging in children with periventricular leukomalacia: variability of injuries to white matter tracts. *Am. J. Neuroradiol.* **28**, 1213–1222.

Nelson, K.B. (2002): The epidemiology of cerebral palsy in term infants. *Ment. Retard. Dev. Disabil. Res. Rev.* **8**, 146–150.

Nelson, K.B. & Ellenberg, J.H. (1979): Neonatal signs as predictors of cerebral palsy. *Pediatrics* **64**, 225–232.

Nelson, K.B. & Ellenberg, J.H. (1985): Antecedents of cerebral palsy. I. Univariate analysis of risks. *Am. J. Dis. Child.* **139**, 1031–1038.

Nelson, K.B. & Ellenberg, J.H. (1986): Antecedents of cerebral palsy. Multivariate analysis of risk factors. *N. Engl. J. Med.* **315**, 81–86.

Nelson, K.B. & Grether, J.K. (1998): Potentially asphyxiating conditions and spastic cerebral palsy in infants of normal birth weight. *Am. J. Obstet. Gynecol.* **179**, 507–513.

Nelson, K.B. & Grether, J.K. (1999): Causes of cerebral palsy. *Curr. Opin. Pediatr.* **11**, 487–491.

Nelson, K.B. & Willoughby, R.E. (2000): Infection, inflammation and the risk of cerebral palsy. *Curr. Opin. Neurol.* **13**, 133–139.

Nelson, K.B. & Lynch, J.K. (2004): Stroke in newborn infants. *Lancet Neurol.* **3**, 150–158.

Nelson, K.B. & Chang, T. (2008): Is cerebral palsy preventable? *Curr. Opin. Neurol.* **21**, 129–135.

Nicholson, A. & Alberman, E. (1992): Cerebral palsy-an increasing contributor to severe mental retardation? *Arch. Dis. Child.* **67**, 1050–1055.

O'Brien, G. (2007): Classification of cerebral palsy: behavioural perspective. *Dev. Med. Child Neurol. suppl.* **49**, S28–S29.

Palisano, R., Rosenbaum, P., Walter, S., Russell, D., Wood, E. & Galuppi, B. (1997): Development and reliability of a system to classify gross motor function in children with cerebral palsy. *Dev. Med. Child Neurol.* **39**, 214–223.

Palmer, F.B. (2004): Strategies for the early diagnosis of cerebral palsy. *J. Pediatr.* **145**, S8–S11.

PeBenito, R., Santello, M.D., Faxas, T.A., Ferretti, C. & Fisch, C.B. (1989): Residual developmental disabilities in children with transient hypertonicity in infancy. *Pediatr. Neurol.* **5**, 154–160.

Philip, A.G., Allan, W.C., Tito, A.M. & Wheeler, L.R. (1989): Intraventricular haemorrhage in preterm infants: declining incidence in the 1980s. *Pediatrics* **84**, 797–801.

Penn, A.A., Enzmann, D.R., Hahn, J.S. & Stevenson, D.K. (1994): Kernicterus in a full term infant. *Pediatrics* **93**, 1003–1006.

Pierrat, V., Duquennoy, C., van Haastert, I.C., Ernst, M., Guilley, N. & de Vries, L.S. (2001): Ultrasound diagnosis and neurodevelopmental outcome of localised and extensive cystic periventricular leucomalacia. *Arch. Dis. Child. Fetal Neonatal Ed.* **84**, F151–F156.

Pinto-Martin, J.A., Cnaan, A. & Zhao, H. (1998): Short interpregnancy interval and the risk of disabling cerebral palsy in a low birth weight population. *J. Pediatr.* **132**, 818–821.

Piper, M.C., Mazer, B., Silver, K.M. & Ramsay, M. (1988): Resolution of neurological symptoms in high-risk infants during the first two years of life. *Dev. Med. Child Neurol.* **30**, 26–35.

Platt, M.J., Cans, C., Johnson, A., Surman, G., Topp, M., Torrioli, M.G. & Krageloh-Mann, I. (2007): Trends in cerebral palsy among infants of very low birthweight (< 1 500 g) or born prematurely (< 32 weeks) in 16 European centres: a database study. *Lancet* **369**, 43–50.

Polivka, B.J., Nickel, J.T. & Wilkins, J.R. (1997): Urinary tract infection during pregnancy: a risk factor for cerebral palsy? *J. Obstet. Gynecol. Neonat. Nurs.* **26**, 405–413.

Prechtl, H.F. (2001): General movement assessment as a method of developmental neurology: new paradigms and their consequences. The 1999 Ronnie MacKeith Lecture. *Dev. Med. Child Neurol.* **43**, 836–842.

Powell, T.G., Pharoah, P.O.D., Cooke, R.W.I. & Rosenbloom, L. (1988): Cerebral palsy in low birthweight infants. I. Spastic hemiplegia: associations with intrapartum stress. *Dev. Med. Child Neurol.* **30**, 11–18.

Radianu, B., Bitchonsky, O., Jaffa, A.J. & Harel, S. (2007): Neurodevelopmental outcome of children with intrauterine growth retardation: a longitudinal, 10-year prospective study. *J. Child Neurol.* **22**, 580–587.

Ragazzoni, A., Cincotta, M., Borgherisi, A., Zaccava, G. & Ziemann, U. (2002): Congenital hemiparesis: different functional reorganization of somatosensory and motor pathways. *Clin. Neurophysiol.* **113**, 1273–1278.

Reddihough, D.S. & Collins, K.J. (2003): The epidemiology and causes of cerebral palsy. *Aust. J. Physiother.* **49**, 7–12.

Reuss, M.L., Paneth, N., Pinto-Martin, J.A., Lorenz, J.M. & Susser, M. (1996): The relation of transient hypothyroxinemia in preterm infants to neurologic development at two years of age. *N. Engl. J. Med.* **334**, 821–827.

Robertson, C.N.M., Watt, M.J. & Yasui, Y. (2007): Changes in the prevalence of cerebral palsy for children born very prematurely within a population-based program over 30 years. *JAMA* **297**, 2733–2740.

Rosenbaum, P., Paneth, N., Leviton, A., Goldstein, M., Bax, M., Damiano, D., Dan, B. & Jacobsson, B. (2007): A report: the definition and classification of cerebral palsy April 2006. *Dev. Med. Child Neurol. (Suppl.)* **49**, 480.

Rosenbaum, P.L., Palisano, R.J., Bartlett, D.J., Galuppi, B.E. & Russell, D.J. (2008): Development of the gross motor function classification system for cerebral palsy. *Dev. Med. Child Neurol.* **50**, 249–253.

Rutherford, M.A., Pennock, J.M., Counsell, S.J., Mercuri, E., Cowan, F.M., Dubowitz, L.M. & Edwards, A.D. (1998): Abnormal magnetic resonance signal in the internal capsule predicts poor neurodevelopmental outcome in infants with hypoxic-ischemic encephalopathy. *Pediatrics* **102**, 323–328.

Rutherford, M.A., Ward, P. & Malamatentiou, C. (2005): Advanced MR techniques in the term-born neonate with perinatal brain injury. *Semin. Fetal Neonatal Med.* **10**, 445–460.

Rutherford, M., Srinivasan, L., Dyet, L., Ward, P., Allsop, J., Counsell, S. & Cowan, F. (2006): Magnetic resonance imaging in perinatal brain injury: clinical presentation, lesions and outcome. *Pediatr. Radiol.* **36**, 582–592.

Rutherford, M., Mercuri, E. & Cowan, F. (2007): Magnetic resonance imaging of the infant brain. In: *Neurological assessment in the first two years of life*, eds. G. Cioni & E. Mercuri, pp. 69–94. London: Mac Keith Press.

Salafia, C.M. & Parke, A.L. (1997): Placental pathology in systemic lupus erythematosus and antiphospholipid antibody syndrome. *Rheum. Dis. Clin. North Am.* **23**, 85–97.

Surveillance of cerebral palsy in Europe. Surveillance of cerebral palsy in Europe: a collaboration of cerebral palsy registers. *Dev. Med. Child Neurol.* **42**, 816–824.

Shapiro, B.K. (2004): Cerebral palsy: a reconceptualization of the spectrum. *J. Pediatr.* **145**, S3–S7.

Silver, R.K., MacGregor, S.N., Pasternak, J.F. & Neely, S.E. (1992): Foetal stroke associated with elevated maternal anticardiolipin antibodies. *Obstet. Gynecol.* **80**, 497–499.

Smith, R.A., Skelton, M., Howard, M. & Levene, M. (2001): Is thrombophilia a factor in the development of hemiplegic cerebral palsy? *Dev. Med. Child Neurol.* **43**, 724–730.

Spinillo, A., Capuzzo, E., Cavallini, A., Stronati, M., De Santolo, A. & Fazzi, E. (1998): Preeclampsia, preterm delivery and infant cerebral palsy. *Eur. J. Obstet. Gynecol. Reprod. Biol.* **77**, 151–155.

Stanley, F.J. & Watson, L. (1985): Methodology of a cerebral palsy register: the Western Australian experience. *Neuroepidemiology* **4**, 146–160.

Stanley, F.J., Blair, E. & Alberman, E. (2000): *Cerebral palsies: epidemiology and causal pathways*, vol. 151. London: Mac Keith Press.

Staudt, M., Pavlova, M., Böhm, S., Grodd, W. & Krägeloh-Mann, I. (2003): Pyramidal tract damage correlates with motor dysfunction in bilateral periventricular leukomalacia (PVL). *Neuropediatrics* **34**, 182–188.

Stenninger, E., Flink, R., Eriksson, B. & Sahlen, C. (1998): Long term neurological dysfunction and neonatal hypoglycaemia after diabetic pregnancy. *Arch. Dis. Child. Fetal Neonatal Ed.* **79**, F174–F179.

Stief O'Shaughnessy, E., Berl, M.M., Moore, E.N. & Gaillard, W.D. (2008): Pediatric functional magnetic resonance imaging (fMRI): issues and applications. *J. Child Neurol.* **23**, 791–801.

Anon (2002): Prevalence and characteristics of children with cerebral palsy in Europe. *Dev. Med. Child Neurol.* **44**, 633–640.

Süssovà, J., Seidl, Z. & Faber, J. (1990): Hemiparetic forms of cerebral palsy in relation to epilepsy and mental retardation. *Dev. Med. Child Neurol.* **32**, 792–795.

Takahashi, R., Uvebrant, P. & Hagberg, G. (1992): Intrauterine growth in children with cerebral palsy. *Acta Paediatr.* **81**, 407–412.

Takahashi, R., Yamada, M., Takahashi, T., Ito, T., Nakae, S., Kobayashi, Y. & Onuma, A. Risk factors for cerebral palsy in preterm infants. *Early Hum. Dev.* **81**, 545–553.

Thorarensen, O., Ryan, S., Hunter, J. & Younkin, D.P. (1997): Factor V Leiden mutation: an unrecognized cause of hemiplegic cerebral palsy, neonatal stroke, and placental thrombosis. *Ann. Neurol.* **42**, 372–375.

Tommiska, V., Heinonen, K., Lehtonen, L., Renlund, M., Saarela, T., Tammela, O., Virtanen, M. & Fellman, V. (2007): No improvement in outcome of nationwide extremely low birth weight infant populations between 1996–1997 and 1999–2000. *Pediatrics* **119**, 29–36.

Topp, M., Langhoff-Roos, J. & Uldall, P. (1997): Preterm birth and cerebral palsy. Predictive value of pregnancy complications, mode of delivery, and Apgar scores. *Acta Obstet. Gynecol. Scand.* **76**, 843–848.

Torfs, C.P., van den Berg, B.J., Oechsil, F.W. & Cummins, S. (1990): Prenatal and perinatal factors in the etiology of cerebral palsy. *J. Pediatr.* **116**, 615–619.

Uvebrandt, P. (1988): Hemiplegic cerebral palsy: aetiology and outcome. *Acta Paediatr. Scand.* (Suppl.) **345**, 65–68.

Uvebrandt, P. & Hagberg, G. (1992): Intrauterine growth in children with cerebral palsy. *Acta Paediatr.* **81**, 407–412.

Vandermeeren, Y., Sébire, G., Grandin, C.B., Thonnard, J.L., Schlögel, X. & De Volder, A.G. (2003): Functional reorganization of brain in children affected with congenital hemiplegia: fMRI study. *Neuroimage* **20**, 289–301.

Van de Riet, J.E., Vandenbussche, F.P., Le Cessie, S. & Keirse, M.J. (1999): Newborn assessment and long-term adverse outcome: a systematic review. *Am. J. Obstet. Gynecol.* **180**, 1024–1029.

Vannucci, R.C. & Vannucci, S.J. (2001): Hypoglycemic brain injury. *Semin. Neonatol.* **6**, 147–155.

Vargha-Khadem, F., Issac, E., Van der Werf, S., Robb, S. & Wilson, J. (1992): Development of intelligence and memory in children with hemiplegic cerebral palsy: the deleterious consequences of early seizures. *Brain* **115**, 315–329.

Vincer, M.J., Allen, A.C., Joseph, K.S., Stinson, D.A., Scott, H. & Wood, E. (2006): Increasing prevalence of cerebral palsy among very preterm infants: a population-based study. *Pediatrics* **118**, e11621–e11626.

Vohr, B.R., Wright, L.L., Dusick, A.M., Mele, L., Verter, J., Steichen, J.J., Simon, N.P., Wilson, D.C., Broyles, S., Bauer, C.R., Delaney-Black, V., Yolton, K.A., Fleisher, B.E., Papile, L.A. & Kaplan, M.D. (2000): Neurodevelopmental and functional outcomes of extremely low birth weight infants in the National Institute of Child Health and Human Development Neonatal Research Network. *Pediatrics* **105**, 1216–1226.

Volpe, J. (1996): Subplate neurons: missing link in brain injury of the premature infant. *Pediatrics* **97**, 112–113.

Volpe, J. (2008): *Neurology of the newborn*. Philadelphia: W.B. Saunders.

Walstab, J., Bell, R., Reddihough, D., Brennecke, S., Bessell, C. & Beischer, N. (2002): Antenatal and intrapartum antecedents of cerebral palsy – a case-control study. *Aust. NZ J. Obstet. Gynaecol.* **42**, 138–146.

Walker, I. (2000): Thrombophilia in pregnancy. *J. Clin. Pathol.* **53**, 573–580.

WHO (2001): *International classification of functioning, disability and health*. Geneva: World Health Organisation.

Wilke, M., Staudt, M., Juenger, H., Grodd, W., Braun, C. & Krägeloh-Mann, I. (2009): Somatosensory system in two types of motor reorganization in congenital hemiparesis: topography and function. *Hum. Brain Mapp.* **30**, 776–788.

Williams, K., Hennessy, E. & Alberman, E. (1996): Cerebral palsy: effects of twinning, birthweight, and gestational age. *Arch. Dis. Child. Fetal Neonatal Ed.* **75**, F178–F182.

Wilson-Costello, D., Borawski, E., Friedman, H., Redline, R., Fanaroff, A.A. & Hack, M. (1998): Perinatal correlates of cerebral palsy and other neurologic impairment among very low birth weight children. *Pediatrics* **102**, 315–22.

Wilson-Costello, D., Friedman, H., Minich, N., Fanaro, A. & Hack, M. (2005): Improved survival rates with increased neurodevelopmental disability for extremely low birth weight infants in the 1990s. *Pediatrics* **115**, 997–1003.

Winter, S., Autry, A., Boyle, C. & Yeargin-Allsopp, M. (2002): Trends in the prevalence of cerebral palsy in a population-based study. *Pediatrics* **110**, 1220–1225.

Wood, E. & Rosenbaum, P. (2000): The Gross Motor Function Classification System for cerebral palsy: a study of reliability and stability over time. *Dev. Med. Child Neurol.* **42**, 292–296.

Wu, Y.W. (2002): Systematic review of chorioamnionitis and cerebral palsy. *Ment. Retard. Dev. Disabil. Res. Rev.* **8**, 25–29.

Wu, Y.W. & Colford, J.M. (2000): Chorioamnionitis as a risk factor for cerebral palsy. A meta-analysis. *JAMA* **284**, 1417–1424.

Wu, Y.W., Croen, L.A., Shah, S.J., Newman, T.B. & Najjar, D.V. (2006a): Cerebral palsy in a term population: risk factors and neuroimaging findings. *Pediatrics* **118**, 690–697.

Wu, Y.W., Lindan, C.E., Henning, L.H., Yoshida, C.K., Fullerton, H.J., Ferriero, D.M., Barkovich, A.J. & Croen, L.A. (2006b): Neuroimaging abnormalities in infants with congenital hemiparesis. *Pediatr. Neurol.* **35**, 191–196.

Yokochi, K. (1995): Magnetic resonance imaging in children with kernicterus. *Acta Paediatr.* **84**, 937–939.

Yokochi, K., Aiba, K., Horie, M., Inukai, K., Fujimoto, S., Kodama, M. & Kodama, K. (1991a): Magnetic resonance imaging in children with spastic diplegia: correlation with the severity of their motor and mental abnormality. *Dev. Med. Child Neurol.* **33**, 18–25.

Yokochi, K., Aiba, K., Kodama, M. & Fujimoto, S. (1991b): Magnetic resonance imaging in athetotic cerebral palsied children. *Acta Paediatr. Scand.* **80**, 818–823.

Yoon, B.H., Jun, J.K., Romero, R., Park, K.H., Gomez, R., Choi, J.H. & Kim, I.O. (1997): Amniotic fluid inflammatory cytokines (interleukin-6, interleukin-1beta, and tumor necrosis factor-alpha), neonatal brain white matter lesions, and cerebral palsy. *Am. J. Obstet. Gynecol.* **177**, 19–26.

Zafeiriou, D.I. (2004): Primitive reflexes and postural reactions in the neurodevelopmental examination. *Pediatr. Neurol.* **31**, 1–8.

Zafeiriou, D.I., Andreou, A. & Karasavidou, K.(2000): Utility of brainstem auditory evoked potentials in children with spastic cerebral palsy. *Acta Paediatr.* **89**, 194–197.

Chapter 6

Congenital defects: a clinical approach

Giuseppe Zampino

Service of Epidemiology and Clinic of Congenital Defects,
Department of Paediatric Medical-Surgical Sciences and Developmental Neurosciences,
Policlinico Universitario 'A. Gemelli', Largo Gemelli 8, 00168 Rome, Italy
gzampino@alice.it

Definition

The term 'congenital defect' implies any evidence of anatomical or functional alteration during the embryonic-foetal, neonatal or postnatal periods, caused by a) an alteration in the genome, inherited or because of a new mutation; b) an unfavourable interaction between the polygenic system regulating the development of body structure and one or more damaging environmental factors at work during embryonic-foetal development; or c) an agent, external to the zygote, which alters normal embryonic-foetal development. Congenital defects include anatomical abnormalities (for example, malformations) or functional abnormalities (mental or motor deficiency, anaemia) in which the biochemical substrate may be known (in the case of a metabolic disease) or unknown.

An 'anomaly' consists of a deviation from the normal in an organ or tissue with respect to its structure, form or function. Structural anomalies can be classified in various different ways (pathogenicity, severity, pattern).

Pathogenic classification: This includes malformation, focal necrosis or 'disruption', deformation, and dysplasia.

Severity: According to their severity, anomalies are subdivided into major and minor.

Pattern: The pattern classification divides anomalies into isolated and multiple. Multiple defects are subdivided into sequence, association, and syndrome (these terms are explained below). Syndromes are a result of chromosomal abnormalities, genetic mutations, teratogenic factors, and often of unknown causes.

Malformations

Malformations are anomalies of morphogenesis of organs or parts of the body: the malformed structure does not develop normally for intrinsic (genetically determined) or extrinsic (teratogenic agents) reasons. Malformations may be divided into various subcategories according to the nature of the defective development. There are anomalies that represent incomplete stages of morphogenesis (agenesis, hypoplasia, incomplete closure or separation), others in which accessory tissue is formed (such as preauricular skin tags, polydactyly, accessory spleen), and yet others in which there are aberrant forms that never exist in any stage of normal morphogenesis (Clayton-Smith & Donnai, 2007).

Disruptions

Disruptions are defects resulting from destruction of previously normal structures. There are two main mechanisms: *amputation* of a normally developed structure or *necrosis* caused by interruption of embryonic or foetal vascularization (for example, early amniotic rupture, amniotic bands, vessel thromboses) or other causes of tissue necrosis (Higginbottom *et al.*, 1979; Cohen, 1989b).

Deformations

Deformations are anomalies of form or position and are believed to be caused by intrauterine moulding resulting from biomechanical forces that can alter the normal form and structure of the body (Dunn, 1976; Cohen, 1990b). Most deformations involve the musculoskeletal system. The pressure required to produce such moulding may be intrinsic (for example, neuromuscular imbalance within the foetus such as foetal muscle degeneration or neural tube defects), or extrinsic (for example, foetal crowding as occurs with oligohydramnios). Various forms of talipes, congenital hip dislocation, and plagiocephalies are the most frequently observed congenital deformities. Usually the prognosis is good and correction occurs spontaneously or by applying force contrary to the forces in operation during pregnancy (Graham, 1988).

Dysplasias

Dysplasias consist of abnormal cellular organization and function. They may be localized or generalized. Localized dysplasias (for example, haemangiomas or cortical dysplasias) are mostly single primary defects of development. However, generalized dysplasias such as connective tissue disorders usually appear as multiple malformation syndromes with extensive involvement of various structures (Spranger, 1985).

Major and minor anomalies

Anomalies may also be classified according to severity. It is sometimes useful to define anomalies as either *major* or *minor*. Major anomalies have significant medical and social or cosmetic consequences for the individual concerned. They are recognizable at birth in 2–3 per cent of liveborn infants. In another 2 per cent of infants, they will be detected at 5 years or more of age.

Minor anomalies are less severe anatomical, chemical or functional deviations from the 'normal' development, not life threatening and either easily repaired or of little consequence for the individual. They represent a heterogeneous group of defects without any significant health problem or cosmetic and social implications. Approximately 15 per cent of newborn babies have at least one minor anomaly, though the presence of several minor anomalies is associated with major malformations (when there are three or more minor anomalies, the risk of a major malformation is 90 per cent) (Mehes, 1985). Thus the presence of minor anomalies should alert the clinician to the presence of a major malformation. Minor anomalies may also provide clues to the timing of the damage during embryogenesis, and are an aid to diagnosis in some specific syndromes (Cohen, 1990c).

Multiple anomalies

When the infant has multiple anomalies, relations among these anomalies need to be thoroughly defined. There could be a sequence, a casual association, or a syndrome (Jones & Jones, 2007). Identifying a syndrome, an isolated anomaly, or a casual association of defects is fundamental to the care of the patient, in making a prognosis, and in genetic counselling.

Sequence

A sequence is a collection of defects caused by a primary malformation generating a cascade of effects (for example, a neural tube defect from which hydrocephalus or paresis of the lower limbs with club feet are derived). Thus a sequence may be defined as the presence of multiple anomalies secondary to a single known or presumed structural anomaly or morphogenetic error (Mastroiacovo *et al.*, 1990).

Association

'Association' is the term used to describe the occurrence of two or more features observed together more frequently than expected by chance, without a known common cause (Mastroiacovo *et al.*, 1990). A casual association occurs when two or more anomalies are present in the same subject as a casual combination with two or more different aetiologies (for example, two inherited anomalies, one from the father and one from the mother). Sometimes, it is possible to have multiple anomalies with a recurrent pattern but without evidence of a specific aetiology or sequential cascading effect (for example, the VACTERL association: Vertebral anomalies, Anal anomalies, Cardiac anomalies, T-E, Tracheo-Esophageal fistula, Renal or Radius anomalies, Limb anomalies).

Syndromes

A dysmorphic syndrome is characterized by two or more independent anomalies determined by a single cause which may be known or can be defined. The aetiological agent, when known, allows a diagnosis, as in chromosome syndromes or metabolic and genetic diseases in which the gene has been cloned. In other syndromes the diagnosis is based only on phenotype analysis (Cohen, 1989a, 1990c).

Frequency

The complex transition from a single fertilized ovum to a normally formed human depends on a series of precisely timed genetic and environmental interactions. Reproductive failure is more common than reproductive success, with fewer than half of all conceptions reaching a stage of development compatible with extrauterine life. About 15 to 20 per cent of stillborn babies have at least one major malformation, 2–5 per cent of infants at birth have a congenital defect, and 1 per cent has multiple anomalies generally consisting of polymalformative syndromes. Polymalformative syndromes cover a multitude of heterogeneous conditions (more than 2,500, with an increment of at least 50 a year). However, while congenital pathology is rather common, each condition is individually rare. The incidence of multifactorial malformations is presented in Table 1 (EUROCAT, 2005).

Table 1. Main multifactorial malformations and their incidence

Multifactorial malformations	Incidence
Heart defects	1: 140
DIV	1: 160
Fallot tetralogy	1: 3,500
Hypospadias (only male)	1: 200
Hypertrophic pyloric stenosis	1: 500
Congenital hip dysplasia	1: 1,000
Cleft lip	1: 1,700
Anencephaly	1: 2,000
Cleft palate	1: 2,000
Neural tube defects	1: 2,500
Anorectal atresia	1: 3,000
Diaphragmatic hernia	1: 3,500
Hirschprung disease	1: 5,000
Omphalocele	1: 5,000
Holoprosencephaly	1:12,000

Aetiology

In spite of progress in genetics and in particular in molecular biology, causes of the various congenital pathologies are largely unknown. Only a very minor proportion can be attributed to known teratogenic agents.

Mutations are stable and inheritable modifications of the sequence of DNA and RNA bases. New mutations occur regularly but without predictability. In most instances genetic or chromosomal mutations can be attributed to natural ionized radiation or intrinsic factors in reproduction.

In men, the frequency of some genetic mutations responsible for dominant autosomal illnesses (for example, Apert syndrome, Noonan syndrome, achondroplasia) increases with age, whereas in women there is an increase in the frequency of chromosomal anomalies (for example, Down syndrome).

So far as multifactorial congenital conditions are concerned (represented mainly by certain congenital malformations such as congenital cardiomyopathy, neural tube defects, and limb reduction defects, see Table 1), the role of genetic factors is evident. Multiple genes are involved – probably with an additive effect – along with some non-specific risk factors.

The reasons why various malformations occur are still unknown, with the possible exception of certain neural tube defects (NTD), cardiac cono-truncal and sectal defects, cleft lip and palate, and some defects in the renal apparatus. It seems that suboptimal levels of folic acid in the presence of particular genotypes – such as gene mutations which codify for methylene tetrahydrofolate reductase (MTHFR) – increase the maternal/embryonic levels of inadequately methylated homocysteine in methionine, with a negative influence on morphogenesis. Well-conducted studies have shown that supplementation with folic acid during pregnancy can reduce the risk of having a baby with one of the above-mentioned malformations (MRC Vitamin Study Group, 1991).

Teratogenic agents

The term 'teratogen' is applied to any extrinsic agent that can cause anatomical or functional damage during embryonic or foetal development. Teratogenic factors include biological agents (for example, viruses), chemicals (certain drugs), physical damage (early chorionic villus sampling), maternal biochemical anomalies (hyperglycaemia in women with insulin-dependent diabetes, hyperphenylalaninaemia in phenylketonuria), and certain intrauterine anomalies (oligohydramnios, uterine fibroma). The known human teratogens are listed in Table 2 (Briggs *et al.*, 1998; Shepard, 1998; Reprotox, 2004; Teris, 2004).

Teratogenicity is a property of an exposure taken as whole, which involves not only the physical and chemical nature of the agent but also the dose, the way it is applied, and the gestational timing. The occurrence of other exposures as well as the biological susceptibility of the mother and embryo or foetus are also factors that can determine whether a given exposure produces damage in a particular instance (Cohen, 1990a; Friedeman & Hanson, 2007). Some general concepts of teratology are summarized in Table 3.

Table 2. Teratogenic agents that cause malformations, dysmorphic syndromes, and congenital functional abnormalities

Bad habits	**Bad ambient conditions**
Alcohol abuse	Iodine deficiency
Toluene abuse	Biphenyl polychlorinated substance intake
Cocaine use	Exposure to high lead concentrations
Benzodiazepine use	Methylmercury intake
Smoking	
Marijuana use	**Diagnostic medical procedures**
	Chorionic villus sampling (< 11 weeks)
Drug treatment	
Retinoic acid	**Maternal diseases**
Antiepileptics	Insulin-dependent diabetes
Captopril and enalapril	Phenylketonuria
Cyclophosphamide	Endocrinological diseases
Diethylstilboestrol	Hyperthermia (> 39° C)
Lithium	
Androgenic hormones	**Maternal infections**
Streptomycin	Cytomegalovirus
Tetracycline	Toxoplasma Gondii
Warfarin	Rubella virus
ACE inhibitors (third quarter)	Parvovirus B19
Salicylic acid and other NSAIDs (last weeks)	Varicella-zoster virus
Aminopterin and methotrexate	Treponema pallidum
Busulfan	
Quinine	
Chloroquine	
Iodine and I^{131}	
Methimazole	
Penicillamine	
Thalidomide	
Trimethadione	
Non-drug therapy	
Overdose of X-rays (> 5–10 Rad)	

ACE, angiotensin converting enzyme; NSAID, non-steroidal anti-inflammatory drug.

Table 3. General concepts about teratology

1.	Any malformation (for example neural tube defect) may be produced by an environmental agent only if it acts before or during the primary formation. For example, as the neural tube is completely formed at 28 days of gestation, no environmental agent can modify its formation after this period.
2.	There is no teratogen that causes damage in 100 per cent of cases.
3.	Teratogens may cause: • specific syndromes such as variable association of malformations, dysmorphisms and functional alterations (produced, for example, by intrauterine infectious; retinoic acid; warfarin; alcohol) • non-specific defects, for example cardiopathy produced by maternal diabetes; valproic acid; lithium
4.	Damage severity depends on the timing of teratogenic agent exposure. Malformations are more severe in case of exposure during embryogenetic age (2–8 weeks after fertilization), whereas during foetal age (9–38 weeks after fertilization) it provokes only minor or only functional damage. In the latter case there is risk of deafness caused by foetal infectious or skeletal deformities from olygohydramnios.
5.	Variability of teratogenic effects depends on: • duration and quantity of exposure: generally, the greater the exposure to a given agent, the more severe the effect; • timing of exposure: most target tissues have specific periods of susceptibility: the stage of embryonic or foetal development at which exposure to a teratogen occurs is of critical importance in determining outcome; • variations in susceptibility of target tissues: as humans vary widely in their genetic control of drug metabolism, resistance to infection and other biochemical and molecular processes, some individuals may be at strikingly greater risk from given exposures than the whole population; • interaction among environmental exposures: it is common during pregnancy for there to be exposure to more than one agent; interactions between them may enhance or suppress the effect on the foetus.

Prevention

Prevention of human diseases can be achieved in two ways: acting on the causes, eliminating or controlling them effectively (primary prevention), and intervening in the preclinical phase of the disease – that is, before damage has occurred (secondary prevention). In relation to congenital pathology, the methods of possible primary and secondary prevention are shown in Tables 4, 5 and 6.

Table 4. Examples of primary prevention

Haemolytic disease of the newborn caused by Rh isoimmunization:	If an Rh negative women is pregnant with an Rh positive child, antibody production *vs.* Rh antigens can be blocked by administration of anti-Rh immunoglobulin within 72 h of delivery or abortion, to prevent maternal sensitization.
Defects caused by rubella virus:	Vaccination of all children, male and female, at 15 months and 12 years.
Neural tube defects:	Increased intake of folic acid from pre-conception (intake should be more than 0.4 mg per day in addition to food content).
Defects resulting from maternal insulin-dependent diabetes:	Metabolic checks from pre-conception.
Defects caused by anticonvulsive drugs:	Give lowest effective dose and avoid the most teratogenic drugs.

Table 5. Examples of secondary prevention

Disease	Early preclinical diagnosis	Treatment
PKU	Biochemical phenylalanine dosage in neonate	Diet devoid of phenylalanine
Galactosaemia	Galactitol dosage	Diet devoid of galactose
Hypothyroidism	TSH and FT3 dosage	Thyroid hormone therapy
Congenital adrenal hyperplasia	17-OH-progesterone dosage	Corticosteroid + salt therapy
Congenital dislocation of the hip	Ortolani manœuvre; ecography	Hip abduction

Table 6. Common minor anomalies

Anomaly	Explanation
Hypertelorism	Interpupillary distance longer than normal
Hypotelorism	Interpupillary distance smaller than normal
Telecanthus	Increased distance between inner corner of the eyes with a normal interpupillary distance
Epicanthus	Skin fold of the upper eyelid (from the nose to the inner side of the eyebrow) covering the inner corner of the eye
Low-set ears	Depressed positioning of the pinna which is lower than a virtual line passer by eyelid corners
Downslanting eyelid folds	Outer corner of palpebral fissures is higher than the inner corner
Brachycephaly	Front-to-back diameter of the skull shortened than normal
Single transverse palmar crease	Single crease of fingers flexion, that extends across the palm of the hand
Clinodactyly	Curvature of the fifth fingers toward the adjacent fourth fingers
Cryptorchidism	Absence of one or both testes from the scrotum

Note: the normal variability of measurements extends from the 5–10 centile to the 90–95th centile.

Diagnosis

A correct *aetiopathogenic diagnosis* has many benefits: it gives security to the family and to the physician, it can indicate the origin of the disease and permit a determination of the recurrence risk, it allows a more accurate prognosis to be made, based on the knowledge of the disease's natural history, and it also makes possible the planning of future evaluations and the setting up of therapeutic-rehabilitative strategies (Shprintzen, 1997).

Though many diagnostic tools are available, the diagnostic process in an infant with multiple congenital defects can sometimes be a long and hard road. Such difficulties concern the extreme rarity of single conditions, their wide range, and sometimes the great variability of expression of the clinical picture.

In about 60 to 70 per cent of infants with multiple anomalies, an accurate diagnosis is made sooner or later, but 30 per cent of the cases remain without diagnosis. The lack of diagnosis creates dissatisfaction in the family, makes the diagnostic process much slower, increases the number of examinations, and leads to so-called 'medical shopping'.

When an overall diagnosis is lacking, the most that can be expected is a better understanding of the nature and onset of the problems in order to provide care based on the functional diagnosis. The aims of this kind of diagnosis are:
- to establish the infant's individual profile (what the child can or cannot do);
- to define a treatment programme (what can be modified in the child) and an educative-rehabilitative programme (what can improve the child);
- to elaborate a plan of support for the family (essentially, to delineate clearly the limits of the infant's capabilities).

The clinical approach to infants with structural anomalies begins with obtaining the history and making the physical examination, to define whether the structural abnormality is a single defect or part of a multiple malformation syndrome. Diagnosis is based on clinical examination, on laboratory tests, and on a longitudinal evaluation of the evolution of the condition.

Diagnostic process

The diagnostic process in dysmorphology is similar to that in other branches of medicine but it differs in certain details:
- emphasis is on the dysmorphology and therefore on the use of specific techniques;
- a history of events occurring during pregnancy and concerning the family's genealogical tree is of particular relevance;
- awareness of syndromes, at least the most common ones, is very important.

The two basic forms of diagnostic process used by clinical geneticists are 'gestalt' and 'analytic'. Both are important and neither is sufficient on its own.

The gestalt strategy

Gestalt is a term usually applied to the process whereby people use their perceptions and judgement to develop an overall impression of something. It is often needed to fill in gaps where information may be missing. People use this type of perception all the time in recognizing objects when only parts of them are visible. It is based on everyone's capacity to recognize forms and to connect them to a single archetype even if the objects are presented in dissimilar ways. Such a process is linked to visual memory, experience, and knowledge of the phenotypic variability of various syndromes, and makes it possible to individualize all the differential elements of the phenotype so as to reach correct diagnosis (Aase, 1990). Among the classical examples of this phenotypical diagnosis are Noonan syndrome (Fig. 1), Wolf syndrome (Fig. 2), Cornelia de Lange syndrome (Fig. 3), Sotos syndrome (Fig. 4), Beckwith-Wiedemann syndrome (Fig. 5), and Rubinstein-Taybi syndrome (Fig. 6).

The analytic strategy

A second strategy is defined as analytic. The doctor assembles with care – and often according to an established and precise scheme – various pieces of data (history, objective findings, laboratory results), and analytically compiles a list of syndromes which may fit the patient under examination. In this process both sign presence and sign absence should be considered. A compilation of the syndrome list, with diagnostic features and differential evaluation, is then carried out on the basis of memory. Often, however, specialists prefer to use the 'gamut' – a sort of sign index of the syndromes (Mastroiacovo et al., 1990; Jones, 2005). Another important source of information is provided by computer programs which give access to continually

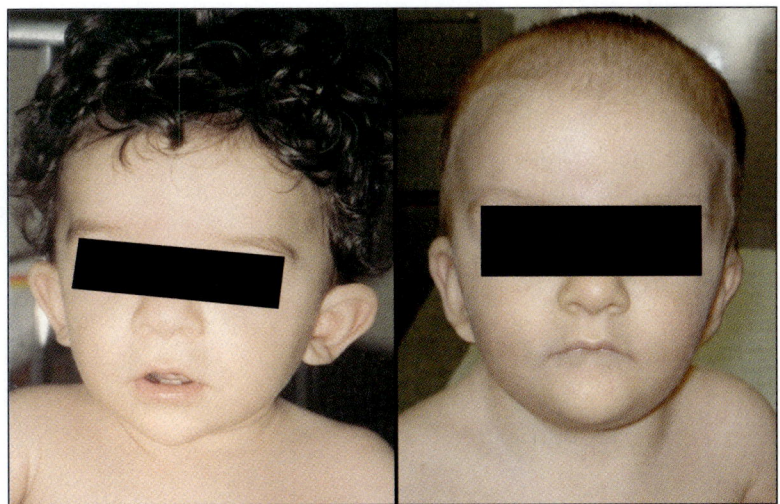

Fig. 1. Noonan syndrome: telecanthus, hypertelorism, epicanthic folds, and low-set and posteriorly rotated ears.

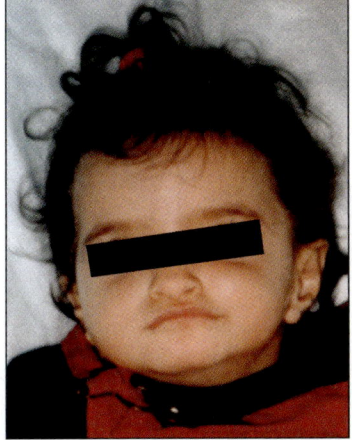

Fig. 2. Wolf syndrome: high forehead, prominent glabella, hypertelorism, epicanthus, short philtrum and downturned mouth.

updated databanks – for example, POSSUM (Bankier, 2004), the London Dysmorphology Database (Winter & Baraitzer, 2004), and OMIM (Online Mendelian Inheritance in Man) (http://www.ncbi.nlm.nih.gov/omim/). Some of these databanks even include unpublished cases or subjects that are still without a precise diagnosis.

The 'analytic' strategy is not used systematically. The attitude and experience of the specialist will result in short cuts, leaps, or a return to gestalt to reach a final conclusion.

Clinical examination

The aim of clinical examination is to detect evident anatomical anomalies (for example, malformations and deformations), milder dysmorphisms (see Table 6), evidence of visceral abnormalities, auxometric changes, and disorders of psychomotor development. As subjective evaluations often are inadequate, it is advisable to use a camera and take appropriate measurements to compare with normal standards. Even disorders of psychomotor development should always be assessed using developmental scales appropriate to the patient's age.

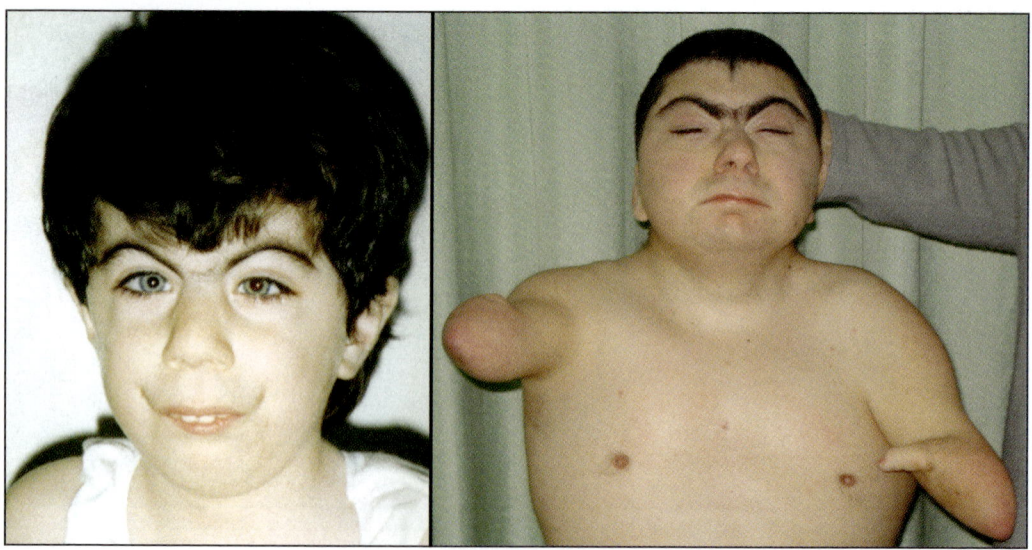

Fig. 3. Cornelia de Lange syndrome: microbrachycephaly, synophrys, arched eyebrows, depressed and broad nasal bridge, long smooth philtrum, thin upper lip, downturned corners of mouth, micrognathia, and upper extremity defect.

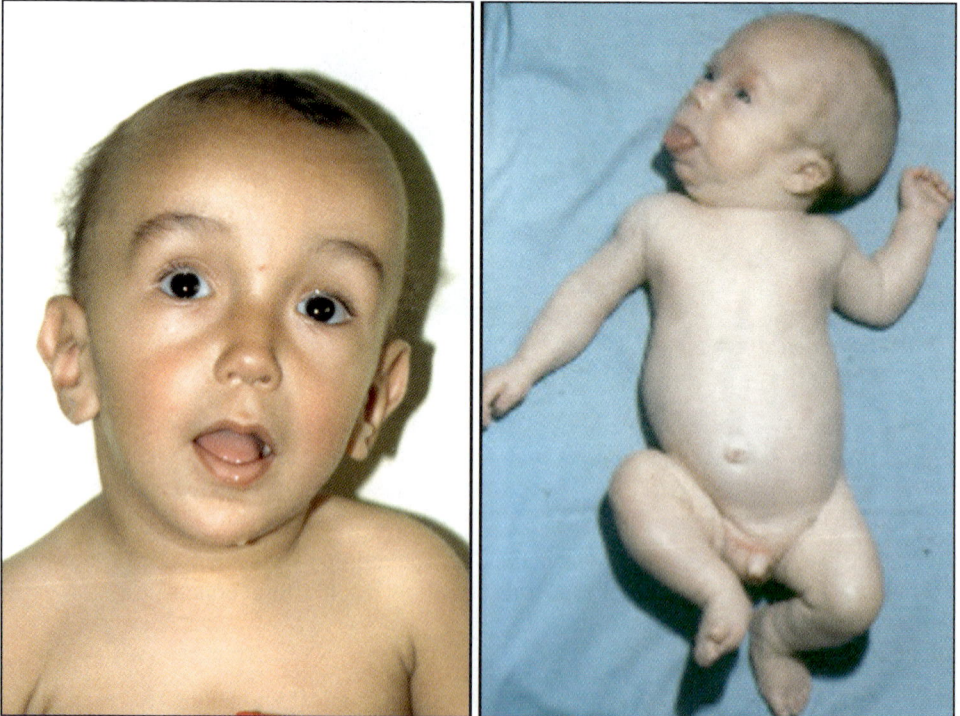

Fig. 4. Sotos syndrome: high bossed forehead, fronto-temporal hair sparsity, downslanting palpebral fissures, long narrow face, and prominent narrow jaw.

Fig. 5. Beckwith-Wiedemann syndrome: macroglossia, nevus flammeus on glabella or eyelids, and unusual fissures in lobule of external ear.

Chapter 6 Congenital defects: a clinical approach

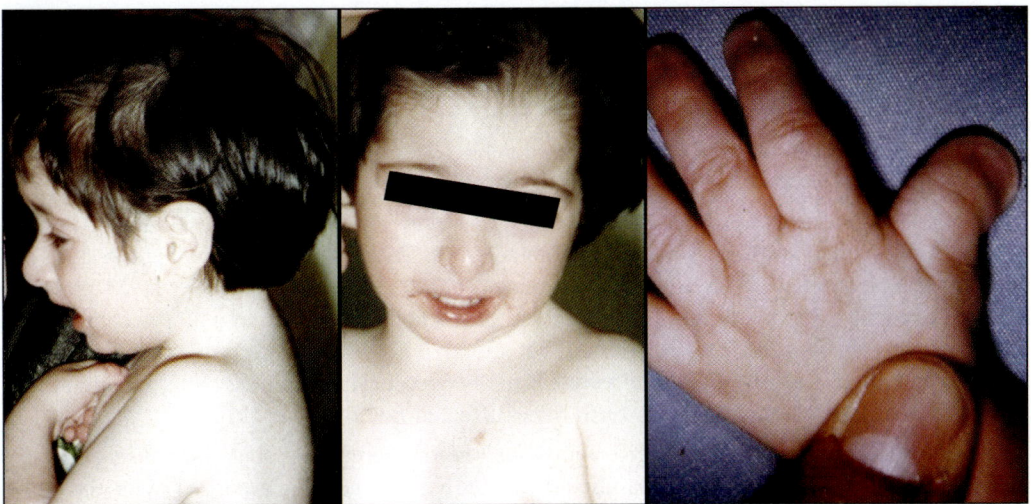

Fig. 6. Rubinstein-Taybi syndrome: prominent beaked nose with nasal septum extending below alae nasae and short columella, short philtrum, and enlarged thumb.

Family history and family tree

In the field of congenital defects, family history is the primary source of information concerning consanguinity or congenital abnormalities in the patient's family members (siblings, mother, father, grandparents, uncles, aunts, cousins). For every family member, specific questions must be asked, taking into account the patient's symptoms and clinical findings.

The most important points are:

• first and last names and any parental relationship, to ascertain the presence of a consanguineous marriage;
• place of birth, to detect a common origin of one or more family members from the same gene block;
• use of the health services (for example, surgery, admissions to hospital, eventual admission to an institution), the presence of pathological symptoms, and the timing of their appearance, in order to identify subjects affected by congenital pathologies.

Affected or suspected subjects must be personally examined, or if that is not possible it is mandatory to look at clinical documentation and photographs. All the information collected is normally summarized in a genealogical tree with standard symbols. The pedigree structure usually includes all first- and second-degree relatives spanning three or four generations (Kingston, 2007).

The history must include the latest information concerning pregnancy. For a correct diagnostic picture the following should be verified:

• obstetric complications
• drugs taken during pregnancy (which ones and for how long?)
• laboratory tests for infections (toxoplasmosis, rubella, CMV antibodies)
• results of ultrasound tests (foetal anthropometric parameters, the quantity of amniotic fluid, major malformations identified by ultrasound)
• quality of foetal movements
• any biochemical tests carried out during pregnancy.

Genealogical tree interpretation

Autosomal recessive diseases

A recessive disease is a condition in which two copies of the same gene are mutated. The affected subject is homozygous for the mutated gene. Usually an affected person has unaffected parents and each of them carries a single copy of the mutated gene.

Main characteristics of autosomal recessive diseases are: 1) the parents are clinically normal but are both heterozygous carriers of the mutated gene; 2) heterozygous parents have a 25 per cent chance of having affected children (homozygous for the mutated gene), a 25 per cent chance of having normal children (homozygous for the normal gene), and a 50 per cent chance of having children who are clinically normal but are carriers of the mutated gene (heterozygous); 3) males and females can be equally affected. Usually people with a heterozygous gene mutation learn they are carriers only after the birth of an affected homozygous child.

It is estimated that everyone is heterozygous for one or more genes that can cause clinically evident disease. However, the probability of an individual meeting a partner with the same heterozygous gene is very low, though it becomes greater if they are consanguineous or if there is genetic closeness. Recessive diseases have small phenotypic variability.

Autosomal dominant diseases

A dominant disease is a condition in which only one mutated copy of the gene is needed to generate the disorder. Thus the affected patient is heterozygous for the mutated gene.

Main characteristics of autosomal dominant diseases are: 1) one of the parents has to be affected. If the parents are normal the subject has a new spontaneous mutation or a defect of gene penetrance; 2) affected subjects have a 50 per cent chance of having affected children and a 50 per cent chance of having normal children in each pregnancy; 3) males and females are equally affected.

X-linked recessive diseases

X-linked recessive disorders are caused by mutations in genes on the X chromosome. An X-linked disease is defined as recessive when the presence of one mutated gene is not sufficient to lead to the disease in females. Males are more frequently affected than females, and the chance of passing on the disorder differs between men and women.

Main characteristics are: 1) generally only males are clinically affected; 2) female carriers have a 25 per cent chance of having affected sons, a 25 per cent chance of having normal sons, a 25 per cent of having carrier daughters, and a 25 per cent of having normal daughters; 3) the sons of a man with an X-linked recessive disorder will not be affected while the daughters will be female carriers and thus will be able to give birth to affected male offspring.

X-linked dominant diseases

X-linked dominant disorders are caused by mutations in genes on the X chromosome. 'Dominant X-linked' means a condition in which one mutated gene leads to clinical signs of disease in female as well as in male children. Only a few disorders have this inheritance pattern. Males are more frequently affected than females.

Main characteristics are: 1) affected females transfer the disease to 50 per cent of their children (male and female); 2) all daughters of affected males inherit the condition; 3) the disease is widely variable, less severe in heterozygous females than in hemizygous males and sometimes lethal in males.

Multifactorial disorders

Genetic disorders may also be complex – that is, 'multifactorial'; this means that there are probably effects of multiple gene mutations in combination with lifestyle and environmental factors. Although complex disorders are often clustered in families, they do not have a clear-cut pattern of inheritance. Thus it is difficult to determine a person's risk of inheriting or passing on these disorders. Complex disorders are also difficult to study and to treat because the specific factors that cause most of these disorders have not yet been identified.

Multifactorial aetiology is believed to account for approximately one-half of all congenital malformations, and to be relevant to many chronic disorders of adulthood and many common psychological disorders of childhood, including dyslexia, specific language impairment, and attention deficit-hyperactivity disorder (Korf et al., 2007).

Laboratory examinations

Specific laboratory examinations for studying congenital diseases include karyotyping and DNA analysis, biochemical tests for metabolic diseases, hormone tests, and immunological tests for diagnosis of prenatal infections. Indications for carrying out such tests are provided by clinical findings and family history (both of the patient, and sometimes also of other members of the family).

Cytogenetic analysis (karyotype)

Karyotype analysis is a fundamental part of the diagnostic process in infants with congenital defects, allowing identification of anomalies of chromosome number or structure that may be the cause of numerous syndromes (Schinzel, 2001). Indications for carrying out the karyotype are given in Table 6. Chromosomal analysis is usually done on circulating blood lymphocytes, but in special cases (for example, mosaicisms) it is also carried out on cutaneous fibroblasts.

Newer techniques such as telomere analysis and comparative genomic hybridization can be undertaken in patients in whom a strong suspicion of a cytogenetic abnormality remains after normal results on routine tests (de Vries et al., 2001; Shaw-Smith et al., 2004). A systematic study revealed that just over 7 per cent of children with moderate to severe mental retardation had small rearrangements involving the terminal bands (subtelomeric regions) of chromosomes (Knight et al., 1999). More recently, microarray-based comparative genomic hybridization using clones spaced at around 1-Mbp intervals is detecting abnormalities in around 20 per cent of children suspected of having a chromosome disorder but in whom karyotype analysis was negative (Shaw-Smith et al., 2004).

Metabolic study

Diagnosing diseases of metabolism is based on specific laboratory investigations, possibly revealing biochemical defects where known (see chapter 8).

DNA analysis

DNA analysis is carried out by either direct or indirect methods.

Direct analysis is done when the gene responsible for the disease is known and shows a limited number of possible mutations. There are various techniques for verifying the presence of a specific mutation in the patient under examination.

Indirect analysis is carried out when the gene has not been identified or when the identified genes have mutations that are too numerous and heterogeneous for direct analysis. Presence of a mutation can be detected from linkage analysis using particular markers called 'restriction fragment length polymorphisms' (RFLP). These fragments consist of known pieces of DNA of various lengths (present in some subjects and not in others), inherited together with the gene responsible for the disease.

Looking for these markers in the whole family, it is possible to establish presence of the mutated gene in each single individual. Using this technique it is, however, mandatory to examine several family components in order to identify the path (segregation) of the marker and of the strictly associated gene.

The most common syndromes with their relative diagnostic tests, when available, and detection rates are given in Tables 7 and 8.

Table 7. Frequent syndromes and related diagnostic tests

Syndrome	Prevalence	Test	Detection rate
Down	1/800	Karyotype	100%
Klinefelter	1/1,200	Karyotype	100%
Fragile-X	1/4,000 (M affected) 1/8000 (F affected)	CGG repetition in FMR1 (Xq27) Punctiform mutation FMR1	99% 1%
Noonan	From 1/2,500 to 1/1000	PTPN11 mutations (12q24) KRAS mutations (12q12) SOS1 mutations RAF1 mutations	50-60% 5% 10-15% 3-8%
Neurofibromatosis 1	From 1/3,000 to 1/2,500	~250 mutation of *NF1* gene (chr 17q)	70%
Turner	1/2,500	Karyotype	100%
22 Del (VCF-Di George	1/6,000	FISH test for 22q11 deletion (DGCR)	95%
Trisomy 18	1/5,000	Karyotype	100%
Tuberous sclerosis	1/5,800	Mutations in TSC1 (9q34) and TSC2 (16p13)	60–80%
VATER association	1/7,000	No test (clinical diagnosis)	
Arthrogryposis multiplex	1/10,000	No test (clinical diagnosis)	
CHARGE	1/10,000	CHD7	60-65%
Cornelia de Lange	1/10,000	NIPBL mutational analysis (5p13) SMC1L1 mutational analysis	45–50%
Facio-auriculo-vertebral	1/10,000	No test (clinical diagnosis)	
Marfan	From 1/10.000 to 1/5,000	Analysis of fibrillin 1 in fibroblasts Gene test for FBN1 (15q21.1)	> 90% 70–90% (high number of mutations)
Prader-Willi	From 1/25,000 to 1/10,000	Methylation test for 15q11-q13 region FISH test for chromosome rearrangement with rupture inside critical region	> 99% < 1%

Trisomy 13	1/10,000	Karyotype	100%
Angelman	From 1/20,000 to 1/12,000	Methylation test for 15q11-q13 Analysis of UBE3A gene Chromosome rearrangement with rupture inside critical region	78% 11% < 1%
Beckwith-Wiedemann	1/12,000	High resolution analysis of 11p15 region	10–20%
Achondroplasia	From 1/40,000 to 1/15,000	FGFR3 (4p16) mutation	98% (G1138A) 1% (G1138G)
Williams	1/20,000	FISH test for ELN (7q11) deletion	99%
Ataxia telangiectasia	1/40,000	Sequence analysis of ATM (11q22.3) gene Analysis of ATM mutation and protein truncation testing	>95% Ricerca
Thanatophoric dysplasia	1/30,000	Mutation of FGFR3	90%
Rett	From 1/20,000 to 1/10,000	Molecular analysis of MECP2 gene (Xq28)	80%
Kabuki	1/30,000	No test (clinical diagnosis)	
Smith-Lemli-Opitz	1/40,000	7-Dehydrocholesterol dosage Mutational analysis of DHCR7 gene (11q12-q13) for 6 most common mutations Sequence analysis of DHCR7 gene for punctiform mutations	100% 65% > 80%
Wolf	1/50,000	FISH test for 4p gene deletion	99%
Sotos	1/50,000	Molecular analysis of NSD1 gene (5q35) FISH test for 5q35 region	75–80% (for Japanese people) 10%
Apert	1/100,000	FGFR2 (10q26) mutation	98%
Holt-Oram	1/100,000	Analysis for TBX5 (12q24.1) mutation	>70%

FISH, fluorescence in-situ hybridization.

Table 8. Indications for karyotyping

When to request a karyotype...
- Phenotypic diagnosis of Down syndrome or in presence of phenotypic characteristics that resemble the most frequent chromosome syndromes
- In the presence of multiple malformations or dysmorphisms
- Mental retardation without a definite diagnosis
- Genital developmental anomalies, including ambiguous or hypoplastic genitalia and retardation of pubertal development
- Females with growth deficiency without a definite diagnosis
- Repetitive spontaneous abortion, dead foetus without known cause, hydropic placenta
- Relatives of a person with hereditary chromosomal rearrangements

When to request a particular examination...
- **Karyotype with diepoxybutane (DEB) or mitomycin:** instability chromosome syndrome (Fanconi syndrome, Bloom syndrome, Roberts syndrome, ataxia-telangiectasia)
- **Karyotype on fibroblasts:** in presence of somatic mosaicism (pigmentary stripes, hypomelanotic spots)
- **FISH:** Fluorescent in-situ hybridization to identify chromosomal microrearrangements invisible with other cytogenetic standard techniques
- **Telomere analysis:** in presence of multiple anomalies not included in known syndromes, with normal karyotype
- **CGH array:** in presence of multiple anomalies not included in known syndromes, with normal karyotype or known syndromic conditions in which the genetic defect was not identified

Follow-up

For an accurate diagnosis of multiple anomalies, adequate follow-up is needed. With time, the significance of many signs may become clearer, and essential symptoms which were not present in the early phase become evident. Studies have shown that during follow-up there is an increase in the number of correct diagnoses in up to 20 per cent of infants with congenital defects, including mental retardation (Curry *et al.*, 1997).

Longitudinal follow-up of an infant with a rare syndrome allows the clinical history to unfold, and is an important step in acquiring knowledge of the condition's natural history. Knowing the natural history of a particular syndrome is of great importance for the physician, for the affected subject, and for the family, allowing better management of the disease and enabling health balance sheets to be drawn up comparing the findings with 'normality' (specific growth curves, neurobehavioural profiles), as well as predicting problems which could appear later on.

Genetic counselling

Genetic consultation is a communication process undertaken when a congenital defect appears in a family, whether or not it is genetic in origin. The communication process is carried out by one or more appropriately trained health workers, with the aim of helping the affected person and his family in the following ways:

1) to help the family understand the basic biomedical concepts related to their relative's condition and its genetic nature, and to eliminate wrongly held beliefs (for example, 'any condition present at birth is hereditary', or 'when no other member of the family is affected, it cannot be genetic, repeated or transmitted', or 'a woman who has already had a normal child cannot have children with a genetic disease');

2) to prevent feelings of guilt in the mother or blame by relatives;

3) to enable the family to understand the diagnostic process, characteristics of the condition, its natural progression, possible medical treatment, any available psychosocial interventions, and the long-term outlook;

4) to show how laws of heredity can determine the condition only in some cases, and to provide recurrence risk estimates in future pregnancies and in those of other relatives;

5) to discuss reproductive options in the face of the recurrence risk, and various possible decisions to be made as a result.

Genetic counselling should be incorporated in the overall plan for the patient and the patient's family. It should be a free communication space and not limited to the discussion of future pregnancies.

Prenatal diagnosis

There are two main aims of prenatal diagnosis: 1) identification in the general population or in selected groups (for example, women of advanced reproductive age) of the presence of certain congenital defects in order to inform the couple about the timing and the most appropriate method of delivery, as well as the plan for any necessary surgical or medical treatments; 2) identification of specific congenital defects which, after genetic counselling, have an increased likelihood in a particular pregnancy. In this chapter I will deal only with the latter.

Generally, it is sufficient to remember that prenatal diagnosis provides precise answers to precise queries and it never gives a generic answer concerning the state of the foetus's health. In other words, a negative prenatal diagnosis does not mean that the infant will certainly be healthy at birth. It must also be emphasized that at present prenatal diagnosis can only rarely (for example, in the case of obstructive uropathy) allow an early diagnosis linked to the possibility of modifying the disease's natural course through suitable medical treatment.

The main techniques for prenatal diagnosis available at present are as follows:

Foetal ultrasound is carried out by vaginal probe from the first weeks of pregnancy. It is capable of identifying the most obvious anatomical defects, especially if a particular defect is sought. Recently, three-dimensional ultrasonography has been shown to be capable of detecting major and minor malformations, especially those affecting the foetal face, heart, and skeleton (Platt *et al.*, 1998)

Sampling of chorionic villi (villocentesis) is carried out after the 11th week of gestation (76 days after the last menstrual period) by transabdominal or transcervical sampling of chorionic villi (originating mainly from foetal cells from which the placenta develops). Sampling is taken at the 12th to 13th week of gestation, to minimize the risk of causing amputation of the limbs or parts of them (for example, the fingers) (Mastroiacovo & Botto, 1992). It can, however, induce spontaneous abortion in 1–2 per cent of cases (depending on the operator's expertise). Direct analysis of the villi allows both karyotype and DNA analysis. In 1 per cent of cases with cellular mosaicism the prenatal diagnosis with amniocentesis must be repeated (Shulman & Elias, 2007)

Amniocentesis is carried out from the 15th week by transabdominal sampling of the amniotic fluid, which contains foetal cells in suspension. Sampling has a risk of inducing spontaneous abortion in 0.5 to 1 per cent of cases. Analysis of the amniocytes, after cell culture lasting 2–3 weeks, aids in the study of the chromosomal disorders of the foetus, enzyme activity for diagnosing possible metabolic diseases, and DNA analysis, which can be done more rapidly and using fewer cells with polymerase chain reaction (PCR).

Chordocentesis consists of direct sampling of foetal blood for various purposes (for example, karyotype after ultrasound study of malformations), including evaluation of the foetus's immunological response to maternal infections contracted during pregnancy. It can be carried out after the 18th week of gestation. The sampling risk is at present around 1–2 per cent of foetal loss.

Treatment

A dysmorphic syndrome is not a disease; it is a condition, a way of being. Syndromes are chronic and rare conditions. Frequently there is no precise diagnosis. They are recognizable at birth or in the first years of life and are characterized by various congenital anomalies of morphogenesis. They are often accompanied by developmental disorders. Care of the malformative syndromes is complex because many organs and systems may be involved.

The fundamental characteristic of a chronic condition is its impact on quality of the life of the child and the child's family, and therefore treatment needs to integrate both strictly medical care and psychosocial help.

The difficult rarity of malformative syndromes results in specific problems of health care. Diagnosis is and often delayed, and treatment is complicated. Guidelines for clinical management are available for some of the commoner syndromes (Cassidy & Allason, 2005; Firth *et al.*,

2005), but in most rare syndromes there is a lack of any clear protocol-based treatment or monitoring, and little in the way of guidelines and clinical experience. Finally, the ability of the child and the family to come to terms with the condition is poor unless they can share their experiences with families of similar patients.

Assistance models

The basic principles of good care of children with chronic and rare conditions are as follows. There needs to be multidisciplinary assistance (medical, paramedical, psychological, social and scholastic). Assistance provided should link hospital structures (the multidisciplinary team of specialists) with community structures. It should have an individual basis directed to the particular child and his family and be responsive to their individual needs, depending on the clinical and functional diagnosis of the abilities and characteristics of the child, psychological and socioeconomic resources of family, and available resources in the vicinity of the child's home (access to rehabilitation services, groups of volunteers, and so on). Every child with a syndrome has particular difficulties and needs, though these are sometimes common to others in the community.

References

Aase, J.M. (1990): *Diagnostic dysmorphology*. New York: Plenum Medical Book Co.

Bankier, A. (2004): POSSUM (dysmorphology database and photos library): CD ROM, version 5.7. Melbourne: The Murdoch Institute for Research in to Birth Defects. Available at http://www.possum.net.au

Briggs, G.G., Yaffe, S.J. & Freeman, R.K. (1998): *Drugs in pregnancy and lactation: a reference guide to fetal and neonatal risk*, 5th edition. Baltimore: Williams and Wilkins.

Cassidy, S.B. & Allason, J.E. (2005): *Management of genetic syndromes*, 2nd edition. New York: Wiley-Liss.

Clayton-Smith, J. & Donnai, D. (2007): Human malformations. In: *Principles and practice of medical genetics*, 5th edition, ed. A.E. Emery & D.L. Rimoin, pp. 361–373. New York: Churchill Livingstone.

Cohen, M.M. (1989a): Syndromology: an updated conceptal overview. III. Syndrome delineations. *Int. J. Oral Maxillofac. Surg.* **18**, 281–285.

Cohen, M.M. (1989b): Syndromology: an updated conceptal overview. IV. Perspectives on malformation syndromes. *Int. J. Oral Maxillofac. Surg.* **18**, 286–290.

Cohen, M.M. (1990a): Syndromology: an updated conceptual overview. VII. Aspects of teratogenesis. Int. J. Oral Maxillofac. Surg. **19**, 26–32.

Cohen, M.M. (1990b): Syndromology: an updated conceptual overview. VIII. Deformations and disruptions. *Int. J. Oral Maxillofac. Surg.* **19**, 33–37.

Cohen, M.M. (1990c): Syndromology: an updated conceptual overview. IX. Facial dysmorphology. *Int. J. Oral Maxillofac. Surg.* **19**, 81–88.

Curry, C.J., Stevenson, R.E., Aughton, D., Byrne, J., Carey, J.C., Cassidy, S., Cunniff, C., Graham, J.M., Jones, M.C., Kaback, M.M., Moeschler, J., Schaefer, G.B., Schwartz, S., Tarleton, J. & Opitz, J. (1997): Evaluation of mental retardation: recommendations of a Consensus Conference. *Am. J. Med. Genet.* **72**, 468–477.

de Vries, B.B.A., White, S.M., Knight, S.J.L., Regan, R., Homfray, T., Young, I.D., Super, M., McKeown, C., Splitt, M., Quarrell, O.W., Trainer, A.H., Niermeijer, M.F., Malcolm, S., Flint, J., Hurst, J.A. & Winter, R.M. (2001): Clinical studies on submicroscopic subtelomeric rearrangements. A checklist. *J. Med. Genet.* **38**, 145–150.

Dunn, P.M. (1976): Congenital postural deformities. *Br. Med. Bull.* **32**, 71–76

EUROCAT (2005): 1980-2003: Prevalence data. Available at: http://www.Eurocat.ulster.ac.uk/pubdata/tables.html

Firth, H.V., Hurst, J.A. & Hall, J.G. (2005): *Oxford desk references: clinical genetics*. Oxford: Oxford University Press.

Friedeman, J.M. & Hanson, J.W. (2007): Clinical teratology. In: *Principles and practice of medical genetics*, 5th edition, ed. A.E. Emery & D.L Rimoin, pp. 900–930. New York: Churchill Livingstone.

Graham, J.M. (1988): In: *Smith's recognizable pattern of human deformation*, 2nd edition. Philadelphia: WB Saunders.

Higginbottom, M.C., Jones, K.L., Hall, B.D. & Smith, D.W. (1979): The amniotic band disruption complex: timing of amniotic rupture and variable spectra of consequent defects. *J. Pediatr.* **95**, 544–549.

Jones, K.L. (2005): In: *Smith's recognizable patterns of human malformation*, 6th edition. Philadelphia: WB Saunders.

Jones, K.L. & Jones, M.C. (2007): A clinical approach to the dysmorphic child. In: *Principles and practice of medical genetics*, 5th edition, ed. A.E. Emery & D.L. Rimoin, pp. 889–899. New York: Churchill Livingstone.

Kingston, H.M. (2007): Genetic assessment and pedigree analysis. In: *Principles and practice of medical genetics*, 5th edition, ed. A.E. Emery & D.L. Rimoin, pp. 518–535. New York: Churchill Livingstone.

Knight, S.L., Regan, R. & Nicod, A. (1999): Subtle chromosomal rearrangements in children with unexplained mental retardation. *Lancet* **354**, 1676–1681.

Korf, B.R., Rimoin, D.L., Connor, J.M. & Pyeritz, R.E. (2007): Nature and frequency of genetic disease. In: *Principles and practice of medical genetics*, 5th edition, ed. A.E. Emery & D.L. Rimoin, pp. 49–52. New York: Churchill Livingstone.

Mastroiacovo, P., Dallapiccola, B., Andria, G., Camera, G. & Lungarotti, M.S. (1990): *Difetti congeniti e sindromi malformative*. Milan: McGraw Hill Libri Italia.

Mastroiacovo, P. & Botto, L.D. (1992): Safety of chorionic villus sampling. *Lancet* **340**, 1034.

Mehes, K. (1985): Minor malformations in the neonate: utility in screening infants at risk of hidden major defects. *Prog. Clin. Biol. Res.* **63C**, 45–49.

MRC Vitamin Study Group (1991): Prevention of neural tube defects: results of the Medical Research Council vitamin study. *Lancet* **338**, 131-XXX.

OMIM, Online Mendelian Inheritance in Man (2000): McKusick-Nathans Institute for Genetic Medicine, Johns Hopkins University (Baltimore, MD) and National Center for Biotechnology Information, National Library of Medicine, Bethesda, MD. Available at: http://www.ncbi.nlm.nih.gov/omim/

Platt, L.D., Santulli, T. & Carlson, D.E. (1998): Three dimensional ultrasonography in obstetrics and gynecology: preliminary experience. *Am. J. Obstet. Gynecol.* **178**, 1199.

Reprotox (2004): Available at: http/reprotox.org/

Schinzel, A. (2001): *Catalog of chromosome aberrations in a man*, 2nd edition. Berlin: Walter deGruyter. Available at: http://www.research-projects.unizh.ch/med/unit42200/area313/p772.htm

Shaw-Smith, C. & Redon, R. (2004): Microarray based comparative genomic hybridisation (array-CGH) detects submicroscopic chromosomal deletions and duplications in patients with learning disability/mental retardation and dysmorphic features. *J. Med. Genet.* 41, 241–248.

Shepard, T.H. (1998): *A catolog of teratogenic agents*, 9th edition. Baltimore: Johns Hopkins University Press.

Shprintzen, R.J. (1997): *Genetics syndromes and communication disorders*. San Diego: Singular Publishing Group.

Shulman, L.P. & Elias, S. (2007): Techniques for prenatal diagnosis. In: *Principles and practice of medical genetics*, 5th edition, ed. A.E. Emery & D.L. Rimoin, pp. 679–702. New York: Churchill Livingstone.

Spranger, J. (1985): Pattern recognition in bone dysplasias. *Prog. Clin. Biol. Res.* **200**, 315–42.

Teris (2004): Available at: http://depts.washington.edu/-terisweb/teris/

Winter, R.M. & Baraitzer, M. (2004): London dysmorphology database CD ROM, version 3. London: London Medical Databases. Available at: http:/www.lmdatabases.com/about_lmd.htlm

Chapter 7

Early intervention

Giovanni Cioni*°, Giulia D'Acunto* and Paola Bruna Paolicelli*

*Department of Developmental Neurosciences, IRCCS Stella Maris, via dei Giacinti 2, 56128 Calambrone Pisa, Italy;
°Division of Child Neurology and Psychiatry, University of Pisa, via dei Giacinti 2, 56128 Calambrone Pisa, Italy
cioni@inpe.unipi.it

Introduction

The concept of early intervention was introduced into clinical management some decades ago but its importance has increased considerably in the last 20 to 30 years, thanks to new methods of intervention and greater systematic use in clinical practice.

Stimulation programmes were historically addressed to disadvantaged children to promote optimal development by providing them with education, health care, social services, and parental support. Several studies have shown the efficacy of these programmes, with substantial cognitive and social benefits (Denhoff, 1981; Shonkoff & Hauser-Cram, 1987; Kruskal *et al.*, 1989).

A greater push for intervention programmes has been created by the increasing number of surviving preterm infants with brain lesions and motor, cognitive and behavioural disabilities (Bhutta *et al.*, 2002; Doyle *et al.*, 2004). In fact, the survival rate for extremely low birthweight preterm babies has been increasing while the disability rate has remained constant. Up to 50 per cent of these infants later show developmental disabilities and disorders (5–15 per cent cerebral palsy) (Tin *et al.*, 1997; Vohr *et al.*, 2005).

In the current literature three main at-risk populations have been identified for early intervention:

i) high-risk children as a result of low socioeconomic status and limited home environmental stimulation;
ii) children with disorders causing developmental delay (for example, Down syndrome, sensory impairment);
iii) children at biological risk because of conditions that could lead to developmental disorders (for example, preterm birth, low birthweight, asphyxia).

According to Blauw-Hospers & Hadders-Algra (2005), early intervention consists of ''*multidisciplinary services provided to children from birth to 5 years of age to promote child health and well-being, enhance emerging competencies, minimize developmental delay, remediate existing or emerging disabilities, prevent functional deterioration, and promote adaptive parenting and overall family functioning*'. An interesting discussion by the authors explores the meaning of the adjective 'early', which may be interpreted as meaning either 'early in life' or 'early in the expression of the condition', with important consequences for the onset age of stimulation, clinical conditions, and intervention goals.

In the first case, there is the advantage of intervening during a period of great brain plasticity; however, the intervention is applied to large high-risk child populations without establishing precise stimulation goals aimed at resolving individual specific developmental dysfunctions or disorders. This is because these are generally not yet evident or may even never show up during life. In this case early intervention can be considered a 'prevention programme' and its primary focus is to facilitate the acquisition of developmental skills and to inhibit or minimize the long-term effects of specific developmental risk factors. Services are given before the diagnosis of developmental delay or neurological impairment.

Conversely, an intervention beginning when a specific dysfunction is fully expressed has the advantage of being directed at that dysfunction and is only applied to a selected child population. However, it risks being applied excessively late relative to brain plasticity. Interventions meant to improve specific areas of difficulties or minimize their effects on functioning and independence, directed at children with a diagnosis of delay or disorder, can rightly be called 'rehabilitation'.

We can conclude that according to the previous definition, 'early intervention' includes both prevention and rehabilitation, and may be interpreted as two different phases of the same process for those children who, at a latter age, show a specific neurodevelopmental dysfunction that requires particular therapeutic programmes (physical, speech, cognitive, educational, behavioural).

Traditionally, the term 'rehabilitation' refers to the 'recovery of a lost function that had been previously acquired'. This holds true for adults, but it is difficult to adapt this definition to infants who develop many functions only later on in life. During infancy, the use of (re)habilitation would be more correct because it would refer to the possibility of 'becoming able to do something' by developing new not yet acquired functions (for example, being able to move around, thanks to the acquisition of independent walking).

Depending on when they are applied, stimulation programmes may be categorized as *neonatal intervention programmes*, focused on the environment, infant and parents, and mainly designed to minimize the stress on infants in neonatal intensive care (NICU), and *postnatal intervention programmes*, which begin soon after discharge or in the first year of life, with or without an in-patient hospital component, aimed at enhancing infant development.

The actual structure of intervention programmes varies greatly and may be designed to help parents learn about child development and milestones, gain an understanding of behavioural cues, cooperate in physical therapy, promote early educational programmes, or enhance the parent-infant relationship. Health professionals – such as doctors, psychologists, physiotherapists, nurses, occupational therapists, and speech therapists – are generally involved, operating in multidisciplinary teams.

Early intervention services may focus on infant development, on parent-infant relationships, or both. Child-focused programmes are generally carried out at centres or schools and involve children in a programme built to promote developmental acquisition and school readiness. Family-focused programmes involve family participation at centres or through home visits. These interventions are directed at improving parenting skills and relationships. By optimizing caregiving behaviour, parent-child interactions are facilitated and subsequent child development is enhanced. Parents are effective agents for maximizing the developmental performance of their children. They play an essential role as active participants in early intervention and are involved in identifying goals and specific needs (Humphry, 1989; Simeonsson *et al.*, 1995; Majnemer, 1998).

A recent Cochrane review (Spittle *et al.*, 2007) suggests that interventions with components that focus on the parent-infant relationship have a greater impact on cognitive skills for infant and preschool subjects than interventions focused only on infant development or parental support. Although interventions focused solely on infant development had the greatest impact on motor development, the effect was not significant and the studies were of low quality.

Family-centred care

According to a more traditional biomedical viewpoint, the interest of clinicians has generally been centred on the sick individual, so therapy is guided towards those treatments that are most useful in directly obtaining improvements in pathological and physical conditions. No relevance has ever been given to unavoidable emotional, psychological and social problems affecting individuals with diseases or disabilities, especially chronic disorders.

Recent reports suggest there have been important modifications in the approach to health care, changing its main objective. This is now shifting from providing treatment to supporting and improving the individual as a whole, thus ensuring a better all-round quality of life.

The International Classification of Functioning, Disability and Health (ICF) (WHO, 2001) has included biological and social perspectives of disablement to represent more fully the impact of health conditions on the quality of life and participation in society of the individual. The five dimensions proposed by the ICF are given in Figure 1. As can be seen they are in continual mutual interaction in the disabling process model.

Target population	Where implemented	Reference	Description	Results in the early-stimulation group
Low income		Majnemer 1998	Meta-analysis	"Head start" programs started in 1965 in the US; several hundred thousend children/year; decreases in school dropout rates, crimes rates, and welfare service use; long-term support needed to maintain effects.
Known disease		Hines et Bernet 1996		Improved cognitive function, better adjustement
Down syndrome				Improvements in fine motor skills and self-sufficiency
Cerebral palsy		Parette et Hourcade 1984	Meta-analysis, 18 studies	Quantitative motors assessments: limited effects; no qualitative assessments or evaluation of other functions.
Preterm, VLBW	Hospital – combined	Als 1994 USA, Sweden	NIDCAP: individualized care for VLBW babies in NICUs; nurses deliver stimulation and adjust the program with the parents every 10 days.	Confirmation of results noted in 1986; improvements in respiratory and nutritional disorders, better weight gain, and shorter hospital stay. At 9 months corrected age, improvements in motor and cognitive Bayley scores.
	Hospital-home transition	Acherbach 1993 USA	Vermont Mother – Infant Transaction Program: Once a day on the last 7 days in the NICU, by the nurses, then four sessions at home over 3 months.	No short-tem effects but better cognitive performance between 3 and 9 years of age.
	Post-hospitalisation – combined	Field 1980	Program for low-income teen-aged mothers with preterm babies.	Marked benefits. At 4 months, improvements in growth, mother-child interactions, and Derwer scores; mothers had more realistic expectations At 8 months, improved mental Bayley scores, decrease in reported behavioural disorders.
		Ross 1984	Regular visits by nurse-occupational therapist	After 1 year, improved Bayley scores and decreased behavioural disorders

NIDCAP, Newborn Individualized Developmental Care and Assessment Program; VLBW, Very Low Birth Weight; NICU, Neonatal Intensive Care Unit.

Fig. 1. Main controlled studies of early stimulation programmes for various populations (Bonnier, 2008).

In the ICF, an important change in terminology has been introduced: 'handicap' is replaced by 'participation restriction' and 'disability' by 'activity limitation'. 'Disability' now refers to the negative aspect of functioning – that is, both activity limitation on an individual level and participation restriction on a social level. Environmental factors – such as the physical, social and attitudinal environment in which people live – have been included in the model as they may influence the effect on the person of the impairment or activity limitation.

The ICF can be a good framework in the formulation of problems from different dimensions and could also serve as a bridge between professionals and families (Beckung & Hagberg, 2002). Great relevance has been attributed to family-centredness, as the family is considered to be a system of constant primary support in emotional and social relationships, particularly during infancy and childhood.

The family is considered to be the ecological system of child development in which parents and family, as primary caregivers, play a vital role in ensuring the health and well-being of children. The child grows up and performs in the family context and here learns and selects social behaviours; the family has a key role in promoting the child's developmental potential. Families are increasingly recognized as knowledgeable consumers and effective agents for maximizing the developmental performances of their children (Majnemer, 1998).

The family must to be considered as a general system ruled by the main principle of the general system theory (Von Bertalanffy, 1968) – that is, the importance of seeing any system as a whole in which the different parts have continual mutual interaction and influence. Thus, in the health care field, the family represents one of the most important sources of support and insight for behaviour and copying strategies (Bamm & Rosenbaum, 2008). Severe illnesses and injuries are regarded as stressful events not only for the individual but also for the family; they break the subtle equilibrium of the family system and create an inevitable distortion of family dynamics. Thanks to its characteristics as an ecological system, the family has the ability to reorganize and adapt to new circumstances in order to reduce stress; this process differs in every family.

Family-centred care is an approach to the planning, delivery, and evaluation of health care based on a partnership between health professionals and patient families (Council on Children with Disabilities, 2007). It is a current and very widespread model of early intervention, rehabilitation and other health problems, not only in childhood but also for adults.

As reported in the definitions proposed by the Canadian Center for Childhood Disability Research and by the Institute for Family-Centred Care, the main concepts of this health care model for both children and adults are the central role of the parents as experts in their child's needs, and the importance of partnership between parents and providers of services.

In family-centred health care, great importance is given to the development of true collaborative relations between families and health care providers who furnish services that have to meet all physical, emotional, and social needs. Communication between families and professionals is a key-point in creating a collaborative and significant contribution in the health care process. Families are disadvantaged with respect to professionals because they are not experts in health care (but they are experts in their own children), although they generally desire to be involved in care-giving and decision-making. Therefore, communication should be open, comprehensive, culturally sensitive, sincere and continuous, in an atmosphere of mutual respect. In this process, time availability is needed but what is more important is emotional availability by professionals in paying attention to parental problems and needs. Only through consideration and understanding of every physical, emotional, cultural and social problem can real encouragement and support for the family be possible, thus ensuring the child's well-being.

Great efforts are now being devoted to demonstrating the efficacy and utility of this new model of health care by means of valid and reliable measures (King et al., 1996; Campbell et al., 2003; Bamm & Rosenbaum, 2008). However, the development of measures that quantify human interactions is especially difficult as they must take into account the presence of many subjective factors (King et al., 1996; Mead & Bower 2000).

From observation to rehabilitation

A family-centred approach is a fundamental part of early intervention for preterm infants in the NICU. A model of caring, coined Developmental Care, was proposed by Als in 1986 to assist and help parents of these fragile infants (Als, 1986).

Preterm birth represents a very stressful event for the family and this may have a negative influence on parental ability to sustain the child's development. Families and providers have emphasized the stressful, difficult, and emotional nature of NICU admission (Harrison, 1993; Holditch-Davis, 2000).

Preterm infants (in particular if they were born at low gestational age and of low birth weight) are at high risk not only for neurodevelopmental disabilities but also for distortions in their early interactions.

Environmental conditions in the NICU are often not favourable for promoting early interactions with parents (especially with the mother), and moreover parents do not feel confident in handling infants so weak, fragile, and different from those they eagerly awaited during pregnancy. Parents need some sort of help and support to understand their feelings and behaviours, and to learn how to handle their little babies in order to promote the child's developmental potential.

To assist their presence in the NICU, parents must be welcomed as essential partners in the care of their baby – the concept of parents as 'visitors' must be eliminated (Lawhon, 2002). Several reports are available confirming the positive impact of family-centred care in the NICU in reducing stress levels and creating more parenting confidence (Griffin, 2006; Kaaresen et al., 2006; Cooper et al., 2007).

Supporting parents does not stop when children are discharged from hospital, but continues during follow-up services aimed at monitoring their development and detecting any early abnormal neurological signs. During this observation period, an attentive exchange between parents and professionals should occur; the former must be able to describe their problems and ask professionals questions, whereas the latter must be able not only to communicate examination results but also to listen and respond to the parents' problems.

Nowadays the early diagnosis of brain damage is easier, thanks to sophisticated techniques mainly based on brain imaging (ultrasound, magnetic resonance imaging, computed tomography) which allow clinicians to identify a lesion soon after birth and follow its evolution. Fortunately, not all the infants with clear brain lesions will develop neurological dysfunction such as cerebral palsy or mental retardation. Clinicians need instruments such as neurological examination (Haataja et al., 1999), Prechtl's method for neurological assessment (Einspieler et al., 2004), and developmental assessment scales (Bayley, 1993; Griffiths, 1996). To be included in specific rehabilitation programmes, these instruments have to be suitable, specific, and useful for the early identification of infants with neurological dysfunction.

Communication of diagnosis plays a crucial role not only for the parents but also for the physician involved. It is obviously a stressful event that may alter parent-child interaction and may also be detrimental for physician-family relationships. The manner of communicating 'bad news' – namely 'news that dramatically alters the future perspectives of the patient' (Buckman, 1992) – depends on individual sensibility, emotional feelings and personal experience and is not something that is learned at school. Diagnostic communication is not a one-time event but it has a gradual developmental course, starting with NICU admission and continuing right up to the time when the pathological or dysfunctional diagnosis is well defined.

Adequate communication of the diagnosis is the first real step in family caretaking because it establishes a relationship between the parents and the physician, with a positive influence on child-family interactions that is constructive for child growth and development.

The transmission of diagnosis often induces a strong reaction in parents, who compare the baby 'imagined' and desired during pregnancy with the 'real' one; this may generate a narcissistic wound with consequent feelings of despair, rejection, shame and an overwhelming sense of guilt.

The process of accepting the diagnosis is a not simple one and parents need time to think it over and consider its implications. They generally need support and counselling for the elaboration and the acceptance of a diagnosis.

Neurological prognosis is often rooted in the uncorrectable nature of the diagnosis, for example in cases of cerebral palsy. It is often hard to provide a functional prognosis, as it may be influenced by several different factors (the age of the child, the degree of cerebral plasticity, any associated disorders) and environmental influences (interaction with the parents, environmental stimulation).

The prognosis for the acquisition of adaptive functions is strictly bound to the developmental dimensions of child disabilities. The moment of diagnostic communication plays a central role in creating a therapeutic alliance between parents and professionals.

Rationale of early intervention

The concept of early intervention is justified by the high plasticity of the developing brain at an early age, so that an early intervention can be considered as a 'neuroprotective' strategy that stimulates brain development during this important phase (Bonnier, 2008).

The developing brain is particularly plastic when neural multiplication and migration have been largely completed but arborization of dendrites and axons and the processes of synaptogenesis are still occurring very rapidly (Kolb et al., 2001).

These phenomena occur normally between 2 to 3 months before and 6 to 8 months after term age, brain plasticity and capacity for recovery being relatively high in this age period (Hadders-Algra, 2001). Myelination is developing at this time and neuronal death from apoptosis is more frequent than at any other time (Evrard et al., 1997); it has been demonstrated that up to 70 per cent of the neurons in the human cortex undergo apoptosis between the 28th week of gestation and term (Rabinowicz et al., 1996).

The human brain shows maximum plasticity during infancy and early childhood. In particular, cortical circuits are sensitive to experiences during well defined intervals of early postnatal development called 'critical periods' (Hubel & Weisel, 1970; Berardi et al., 2000). After the critical period, brain plasticity is reduced, becoming more rigid and less adaptable. The plasticity of the brain is thought to allow us to adapt our behaviour in the light of experiences, to acquire new tasks, to remember past events, and to recognize objects.

A critical period can be considered as a time window during which a specific function normally develops if conditions are favourable, but at the same time it represents a sensitive period – that is, a time window during which abnormal conditions can modify the structure or the function of a cortical region (Bonnier, 2008).

Early intervention offers the possibility of a positive influence on child development during critical periods, thanks to early experience-dependent neuroplasticity. For this reason, the importance of starting intervention programmes as soon as possible is generally emphasized.

Neuroplasticity represents the basic neurophysiological rationale for the possibility of inducing positive and stable changes in the organization of adaptive functions, and these changes are the most imperative targets of early rehabilitation.

Animal models have shown that plasticity allows a reorganization of cortical maps after early brain injuries. Normally cerebral plasticity implies a reprogramming of spared neural tissue – that is, a reorganization of the remaining cortico-subcortical networks and their descending fibres (Carr *et al.*, 1993; Chu *et al.*, 2000). The earlier the brain lesion occurs, the better the processes of functional recovery appear to be, because early neuroplasticity is greater in cortical regions not involved in brain damage which may eventually assume the functions normally carried out by the damaged regions.

The neuroanatomical mechanisms proposed to explain the process of neuroplasticity are represented by the following: i) 'functional substitution', which implies the transfer of a certain function to a different vacant cortical region; ii) the possibility of using the 'neuronal redundancy' which is so prevalent in the developing brain; iii) 'neuronal repairing' by means of axonal regeneration, increased fibre sprouting, and reactive synaptogenesis. Recent neurophysiological evidence has shown that neuroplasticity is correlated with the activation of several cellular and molecular mechanisms that determine the production of neurotrophins (for example, nerve growth factor, NGF) and the changes in gene expression responsible for the synthesis of proteins that play a role in plastic brain processes.

As confirmed by many reports in animal paradigms, experience-dependent neuroplasticity – often studied by means of environmental enrichment (see below) – relies on the activation of these mechanisms. Striking brain changes are induced, mainly in the visual cortex and the hippocampus, in both infants and adults (Fagiolini *et al.*, 1994; Cancedda *et al.*, 2004; Engineer *et al.*, 2004; Sale *et al.*, 2004; Nithianantharajah & Hannan, 2006; Tropea *et al.*, 2006; Champagne *et al.*, 2008). Results of recent research on the visual cortex in adult rats affected by amblyopia have shown the possibility of reactivate plasticity in adulthood as well; this represents a valid argument for revising the concept of critical periods (Sale *et al.*, 2007). These results present important opportunities for the treatment of this type of pathology.

Programmes proposed for early intervention in infants at risk of developmental disability, such as the Newborn Individualized Developmental Care and Assessment Program (NIDCAP) (Als, 1986) and infant massage (Field, 2002), are based on the concept of enriching the environmental experiences.

Standardized programmes of early intervention: scientific evidence of their effect

Several early intervention programmes for infants at risk of developmental dysfunction and disability have been proposed in recent years, but clear evidence of their efficacy in improving neurodevelopmental outcome for those children remains scarce. Randomized controlled studies and meta-analyses are needed to verify the effectiveness of these programmes. However, these would consume significant economic resources and occupy the time of the health services. In the rest of this chapter we will describe some of the most commonly used and evaluated programmes, listing them as in the recent review by Bonnier (2008) according to when they are applied during neonatal and postnatal intervention programmes (Fig. 2).

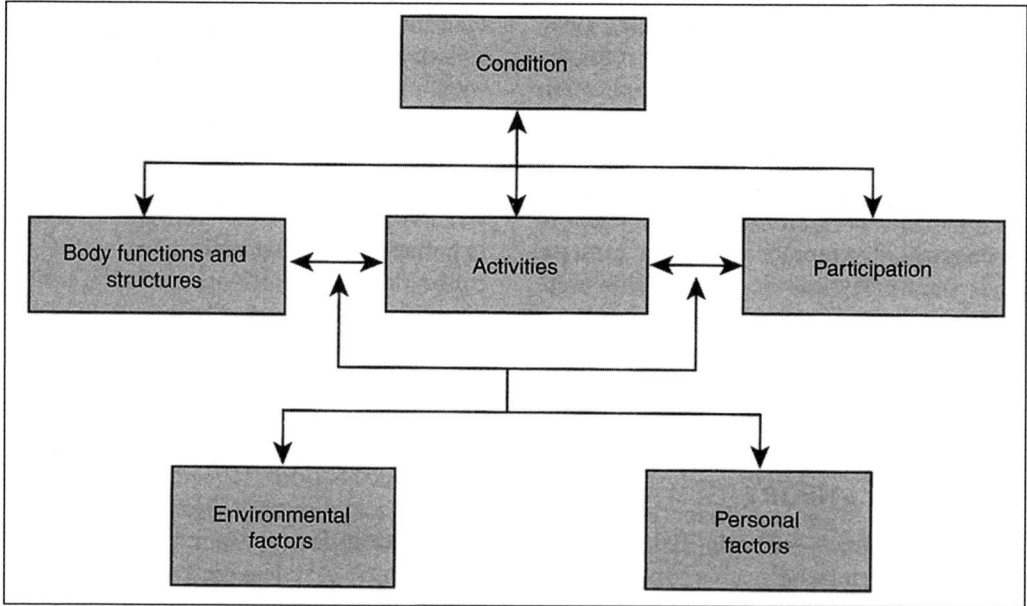

Fig. 2. Interaction between the components of the International Classification of Functioning, Disability and Health (WHO, 2001).

Early intervention programmes in neonatal period

Early intervention programmes in the neonatal period have been dedicated to preterm infants and they are applied soon after birth in the NICU. They target the child, the family, or both (McCarton et al., 1995).

The environment of the NICU, so different from the intrauterine environment, may have a negative impact on neurodevelopmental outcome in the preterm infant. The infant's sensory experiences in the NICU – including exposure to bright lights, loud sounds, and frequent disturbing interventions – has been assumed to have negative effects on the immature brain, with alterations in subsequent development (Field, 1990; Als et al., 1994; Buehler et al., 1995; Anand & Scalzo, 2000; Kleberg et al., 2002). Taking into account the importance of experience on animal brain plasticity, particularly during critical periods, Als proposed an intervention called Developmental Care, aimed at minimizing the negative impact and stress of environmental exposure on brain development in NICU at such a critical time (Als, 1986). Developmental care is a broad category of interventions mainly based on positioning, clustering of nursery activities, modification of external stimuli and individualized developmental care interventions.

The Newborn Individualized Developmental Care and Assessment Program (NIDCAP) is without any doubt the best known and most used early intervention programme in the NICU. It is particularly common and widespread in the USA and Sweden.

Newborn Individualized Developmental Care and Assessment Program (NIDCAP)

Als (1986) integrated findings from other scientific disciplines with those from developmental psychology and formulated a new form of caregiving, which places the focus on respect for the very tiny human being. She has developed a theory for family-centred, developmental supportive care – the so-called 'synactive theory' – which describes the infant as an organism consisting of five subsystems: autonomic-physiological; motor; state organizational; attentional-interactive; and self-regulatory. These systems are described as interactive – that is, the functional state of one system profoundly influences the others. Thus the stability and efficient functioning of one of these systems affects the functions of the other systems in a positive fashion. For example, helping an infant to calm down (reduce movements) results in better autonomic function, with improved respiration and oxygen saturation, which in turn promotes the infant's ability to interact socially with parents or caregivers. The five subsystems interact synergistically.

Based on this theoretical construct, Als has developed a programme of intervention known as NIDCAP. The programme consists of weekly observations of the infant before, during, and after caregiving procedures – for example, feeding, diaper change, blood sample collection, repositioning and so on. Behavioural and physiological changes are monitored in 2-minute periods. Subsequently the observer evaluates the infant in terms of its present ability to organize and modulate the five subsystems, and notes signals of wellbeing and self-regulation as well as signs of sensitivity and stress. These observations provide information concerning how well the environment, caregivers and family members are attuned to the current needs of the infant and whether the intervention is suitable for each child-parent combination. For a trained observer this entire procedure requires 3 to 4 hours.

Based on this procedure, recommendations on caregiving designed to support individual infant development are formulated. Such recommendations may include details on how to adjust the infant's physical environment by reducing sound, light, and activity levels; how to make it easier for the infant to assume a foetal position by means of placing a nest in the incubator, thus facilitating self-soothing regulatory behaviour; how to concentrate caregiving to certain limited periods in order to allow for prolonged sleep; and how to help the parents recognize their infant's needs and encourage their early participation in caregiving.

Als and other groups have reported positive effects of NIDCAP with respect to short term outcome (for example, a reduced requirement for assisted ventilation, fewer intracranial haemorrhages, faster weight gain, shorter hospital stay, and better behavioural scores at the time of discharge) (Als, 1986; Becker *et al.*, 1991; Als *et al.*, 1994; Buehler *et al.*, 1995; Fleisher *et al.*, 1995; Brown & Heermann, 1997; Westrup *et al.*, 2000), as well as improvement in parent-infant interaction and early child development (Als, 1986; Als *et al.*, 1994; Kleberg *et al.*, 2002; Westrup *et al.*, 2004).

Functional and brain structural differences between low risk preterm infants who had NIDCAP intervention and a standard care group have been published (Als *et al.*, 2004). In particular, the NIDCAP group showed better neurobehavioural functioning, increased EEG coherence between brain regions (indicating a change in connectivity between brain regions), and MRI findings suggesting more advanced white matter maturation.

However, Symington & Pinelli (2006) in a recent Cochrane Review concluded that *'these interventions may have some benefits on the outcomes of the preterm infants but there continues to be conflicting evidence among the multiple studies. Before a clear direction for practice can be supported, evidence demonstrating more consistent effects of these interventions on short and long-term clinical outcomes is needed. The economic impact of the implementation and maintenance of developmental care practice should be considered by clinical institutions'*. Therefore, high quality randomized trials are still required to support the favourable effects of developmental care and NIDCAP.

Multisensory intervention

Massage therapy is an early stimulation programme included in many intervention programmes, based on external stimuli such as vestibular, auditory, visual, tactile, and kinaesthetic stimulations, used alone or in various multisensory combinations, in order to make up for the lack of tactile stimuli that preterm infants would otherwise experience in the intrauterine environment or with postnatal mothering care (Montagu, 1978). Massage therapy was introduced in the NICU primarily with the aim of improving weight gain, in particular in low birthweight subjects during their hospital admission, and, as a consequence, to obtain an earlier hospital discharge (Field, 2002).

The term 'massage' refers to any form of tactile skin stimulation performed by human hands. There are differences in technique – for example, in the pressure applied and the sequences in which each body part is stimulated. The type of massage used in NICU is gentle, slow stroking, and involves all parts of the body.

In the model proposed by the American group (Field *et al.*, 1986; Scafidi *et al.*, 1990), preterm infants receive 15-minute massages three times a day for 10 days while staying in the incubator, and each stimulation session consists of three standardized 5-minute phases. Tactile stimulation is given during the first and third phases, while kinaesthetic stimuli are applied during the middle phase. Massage therapy begins with the infant in a prone position followed by a middle supine phase, and a final prone one. Gentle stroking is carried out with warm hands following a well defined and sequenced methodology.

Other kinds of stimulation may be concurrent, such as visual, vestibular, and auditory stimuli, as suggested by many studies.

Gentle, 'minimal' touch is another technique applied by nurses who place their hands on the infants gently as they sleep. The hands should not move or stroke the skin, and are removed after 15 or 20 minutes. Several studies using this intervention have shown positive effects on weight gain, behavioural reactions, postnatal complications, and hospital discharge (Rice, 1977; Field *et al.*, 1987; Scafidi *et al.*, 1993; Wheeden *et al.*, 1993; Scafidi & Field, 1997). Hormonal changes, in particular decreased blood cortisol, have also been reported in massaged preterm infants (Schanberg & Field, 1987; Acolet *et al.*, 1993).

A recent approach called 'positive touch' has been proposed by Bond (2002). This method is primarily practiced by parents and involves various types of infant touch interaction including handling, holding, kangaroo care (or skin-to-skin contact care) and massage.

In a recent Cochrane Review by Vickers *et al.* (2004) it was reported that massage intervention improved daily weight gain and reduced the length of hospital stay, although there were methodological concerns about the blindness of the observers on this outcome. There was also some evidence that massage intervention has a slight positive effect on postnatal complications and weight at 4 to 6 months. However, serious concerns about the methodological quality of the studies included, particularly with respect to the selective reporting of outcomes, has weakened the credibility of these findings. In conclusion, according to the authors, evidence that massage therapy for preterm infants is beneficial for developmental outcomes is weak and does not warrant wider use of this intervention. Where massage is currently practiced by nurses, consideration should be given to whether it is a cost-effective use of time. Further research should assess the effects of massage interventions on clinical outcome measures, such as medical complications or the length of hospital stay, and on care process outcome, such as caregiver or parental satisfaction.

Early intervention programmes in the postnatal period

According to Blauw-Hospers & Hadders-Algra (2005) the objectives of early interventions are multiple (see above). As in the neonatal period, these programmes may be focused on the child, on the family, or both. Intervention programmes that are aimed at enhancing the parent-infant relationship by focusing on making parents aware of infant cues and teaching them appropriate and timely responses to infant needs seem to give the greatest benefit in cognitive and social development (Melnyk et al., 2001). As an example, we will describe the Vermont Mother-Infant Transition Program, one of the best known programmes with a long follow-up of results.

Vermont Mother-Infant Transition Program (MIPT)

Vermont Mother-Infant Transition Program proposed by Nurcombe et al. (1984) was designed to optimize caregivers' interactions by enhancing the mothers' adaptations to their low birth-weight infants. Emphasizing changing the mother's attitude, sensitivity, and behaviour towards her child, the MIPT has the following aims:

- to enable the mother to appreciate her baby's specific behavioural and temperamental characteristics;
- to make her aware of her infant's cues, especially those that signal stimulus overload, distress, and readiness for interaction;
- to teach her to respond appropriately to those cues in order to facilitate mutually satisfying interactions.

The MIPT is implemented by NICU nurses who work with the mother and the infant in seven daily sessions during the week before hospital discharge, plus four home sessions at 3, 14, 30, and 90 days after discharge (Nurcombe et al., 1984; Rauh et al., 1988; Rauh et al., 1990; Achenbach et al., 1993).

Techniques include demonstration, verbal instruction, and practical experience. The nurse encourages the mother to feel confident and comfortable with her baby. Each in-hospital session deals with a different aspect of infant functioning, such as self-regulation and interaction, behavioural signs of distress, and predominant conditions and techniques necessary for bringing about the quiet alert state which is most responsive to social interaction. In the last two in-hospital sessions, the nurse helps the mother to achieve sensitivity and responsiveness in her daily caretaking and prepares her for life at home.

Home visits involve discussions regarding mutual enjoyment through play and understanding of temperamental patterns. The final visit reviews all the recent changes the mother has noticed in her child and the mother is then presented with a log book of the child's development. There is no other intervention after the 90-day home visit.

The effects of MITP on development have been evaluated in a group of treated children vs. a control group at different ages up to school age. The results showed that benefits are delayed, become significant after 3 years and remain until 9 years of age (Achenbach et al., 1993). These findings raise important questions not only about the optimal duration of follow-up studies but also about the mechanisms whereby early intervention acts.

Other programmes

Many other early intervention programmes have been proposed, varying widely with respect to starting age, intervention frequency, type of stimulation, intervention focus, duration of the stimulation, duration of follow-up, and the measurement tools used to evaluate outcomes (Blauw-Hospers & Hadders-Algra, 2005; Spittle *et al.*, 2007). Some studies applied prevention programmes aimed at thwarting neurodevelopmental delays or dysfunctions, whereas in others, rehabilitation programmes directed at specific motor, cognitive or language disorders are proposed.

In the first group, the theoretical construct of early intervention includes teaching parents about infant development and milestones (Barrera *et al.*, 1986; Bao *et al.*, 1999; Ohgi *et al.*, 2004; Cameron *et al.*, 2005), understanding behavioural cues (Nurcombe *et al.*, 1984; Melnyk *et al.*, 2001; Cameron *et al.*, 2005), early educational intervention (Bao *et al.*, 1999), and enhancement of infant-parent relationships (Field *et al.*, 1980; Resnick *et al.*, 1988; Melnyk *et al.*, 2001; Cameron *et al.*, 2005). In the second group of studies, physical therapy or language therapy has been used (Goodman *et al.*, 1985; Piper *et al.*, 1986; Yigit *et al.*, 2002; Cameron *et al.*, 2005). The aim of intervention programmes varies, but it is mainly directed at improving cognitive or motor development, or both.

The place where the programmes is carried out also varies. Generally, observers make periodic home visits during which the child is observed and advice is given to the parents. Conversely, when early intervention includes specific programmes directed at functional recovery (for example, physical therapy) the infants are treated by therapists in a specialized centre.

A recent Cochrane review by Spittle *et al.* (2007) concluded that the great heterogeneity between types of early intervention makes it difficult to compare the results of various studies in order to establish the real effectiveness of early intervention programmes in children at developmental risk. On the basis of the studies included, they reported a significant impact of early intervention in preterm children on cognitive development at school age, but little evidence of the effect of early post-discharge programmes on motor development.

Blauw-Hospers & Hadders-Algra (2005) also reported no significant effects on motor development in children at high risk of disabilities when physiotherapy (in particular passive handling techniques) was applied. On the other hand, some evidence of effectiveness on motor development was found in programmes in which parents learn how to promote infant development or in others that included some specific motor training programmes, such as treadmill locomotion training.

Evidence of the effects of environmental enrichment model in animal paradigms

As mentioned in previous sections, research on development and plasticity of the central nervous system (CNS) increasingly uses the model of environmental enrichment. The latter has revealed unexpected effects of the environment on cognitive functions, behaviour and aging processes, providing information on a cellular and molecular basis (van Praag *et al.*, 2000; Nithianantharajah *et al.*, 2006). Although the vast majority of studies based on environmental enrichment protocols have been carried out in animals, some evidence on their application in humans is now available (Vickers *et al.*, 2004).

We will now summarize the evidence obtained from the animal paradigms, underlying the main effects of environmental enrichment on the CNS and discussing the related molecular mediators. We will then present the potential applications in humans, particularly during infancy.

The first observations about the effects of enrichment were made almost serendipitously at the end of the forties by the Canadian neuropsychologist Donald Hebb (1949). From time to time he used to take one or two rats from their laboratory cages and bring them home for some weeks as pets for his children. He noticed that these rats would gradually become more curious, less frightened, and more prone to explorative behaviour. In particular, he observed that once these rats were brought back to the laboratory, their performance in several behavioural tests was better than those of rats that had never left their usual cages. These pioneering observations inspired various studies on the rat, done principally at Berkeley University, where a group of neuroscientists, coordinated by Mark Rosenzweig, demonstrated how the experience of what they called an 'enriched environment' led to a significant and consistent improvement in tasks involving cognitive functions, especially learning and memory (Rosenzweig *et al.*, 1978).

The exposure to a complex environment is obtained by raising rats in numerous groups, in larger than standard cages, equipped with stairs, tunnels, various coloured objects, frequently changed nesting materials which enhance exploratory behaviour, and running wheels for spontaneous exercise. It was shown that one of the most significant effects of environmental enrichment involve hippocampal-dependent performance, such as spatial memory (evaluated with a Morris water maze), both through direct performance improvement (active effect) and through a reduction in progressive cognitive decline normally associated with the aging process (protective effect) (Rampon *et al.*, 2000; Bartoletti *et al.*, 2004). At the same time, several studies showed the influence of environmental enrichment on emotional reactions and stress, supporting its potential anxiolytic effect, mediated, for instance, by preventing enhancement of cortisol levels in response to induced stress (a low intensity electric shock) (Benaroya-Milshtein *et al.*, 2004).

Further experimental evidence showed that the improvement in behavioural performance in environmentally enriched animals is accompanied by anatomical modifications of the cerebral cortex – for example, an increase in cortical weight and thickness, increased neuronal cellular bodies and cell body dimensions, and dendritic structural modifications (enhanced arborization in the pyramidal cells of layers II, IV, and V in the occipital cortex, increased dendritic length and arborization field, and an increase in synaptic spine length by up to 10 per cent in basal dendrites) (Globus *et al.*, 1973; Greenough & Volkmar, 1973; Green *et al.*, 1983).

Another structure highly sensitive to environmental enrichment is the hippocampus, where modifications similar to those reported for the cortex were found, involving pyramidal cells of CA1 and CA3 areas and the dentate gyrus (Walsh *et al.*, 1969; Walsh & Cummins, 1979; Rosenzweig & Bennett, 1996; Rampon *et al.*, 2000).

Despite the large amount of data collected for the adult animal model, the possibility that the complex stimulation provided by environmental enrichment had effects on the early stages of CNS development has been explored only relatively recently. Taking visual system development as a paradigm of nervous system development, it was shown that exposure to environmental enrichment from birth in the rat prevented the effects of dark rearing on cortical visual development (Bartoletti *et al.*, 2004). This suggested that there are factors contributing to the development of the visual cortex through which environmental enrichment establishes its effects that are not under the direct control of visual experience. Other studies in the rat showed that rearing the animal in environmentally enriched conditions leads to a significant acceleration of visual system development, revealed at behavioural, neurophysiological and molecular level (Cancedda et al., 2004; Landi et al., 2007). In particular, these animals, compared to controls reared in standard conditions, exhibit earlier eye opening and faster visual acuity development.

Some of the principal changes observed in enriched rats were first evident at very early ages (7 to 15 days from birth), when pups still spend almost all the time in the nest. The precocity of these events makes a direct effect of environmental enrichment on the pups unlikely; it has thus been hypothesized that environmental enrichment encourages a higher level of maternal care toward pups (in terms of physical contact, licking and grooming behaviour, and so on) that would act as an indirect mediator of the enrichment effects on visual system development. It was soon demonstrated that the increased licking behaviour and physical contact experienced by environmentally enriched pups is accompanied in the first week of life by higher levels of brain-derived neurotrophic factor (BDNF), a decisive neurotrophin for visual cortex plasticity in the early stages of development during a specific critical period (Cancedda et al., 2004; Sale et al., 2004).

A recent study underlines the key role of insulin-like growth factor 1 (IGF-1) in mediating the effects of environmental enrichment on visual system development. In particular, it provokes an increase in IGF-1-positive neurones in the visual cortex. Increasing the IGF-1 levels in the visual cortex of non-enriched rats by means of osmotic minipumps leads to an acceleration of visual acuity development, while blocking the action of IGF-1 on the visual cortex in enriched animals with IGF-1 receptor antagonists blocks the action of IGF-1 on the development of visual acuity (Ciucci et al., 2007). The effect of IGF-1 on the enhancement of neuronal activity had been demonstrated previously (Carro et al., 2000), as had its role in several pre- and postnatal events that guide central nervous system development, such as cell proliferation control, glycogenesis, neurogenesis, neuronal survival, differentiation, synaptogenesis, and myelination (Aberg et al., 2000; D'Ercole et al., 2002).

In adulthood, the IGF-1 role as a mediator of the effects of physical exercise has been largely proven, both in terms of a neuroprotective effect against neuronal death, and through the promotion of hippocampal plasticity, learning and memory (Carro et al., 2000; Cotman & Berchtold, 2002). Running induces IGF-1 uptake from specific neuronal groups, increasing electrical activity and hippocampal IGF-1 expression. Higher levels of IGF-1 in the visual cortex of environmentally enriched rats could exercise their effect on neurons through IGF-1 receptors, leading to an increase in spontaneous neuronal activity, in the production of activity-dependent factors and neurotrophins, and in the activation of activity-dependent metabolic pathways such as ERK/CREB, which are important for visual cortical development and plasticity (Berardi et al., 2003).

Application of the environmental enrichment model in children: infant massage

Infant massage, described in the previous sections, could be a valid model of environmental enrichment in humans for two main reasons: it represents a well known and widely used technique in Neonatal Intensive Care Units (NICU) and, as already mentioned above, data in rodents show that pups reared in an enriched environment receive in their first days of life a greater amount of tactile stimulation, through maternal licking, grooming and physical contact, thus suggesting that tactile stimulation represents a crucial component in early environmental enrichment. Smooth massage performed on preterm (<37 weeks) or low birthweight infants (<2500 g) has some positive effects on development and behaviour (Vickers et al., 2004). Massage has an effect in both countering the stress-inducing stimuli of the NICU (bright light, constant noise, and so on) and providing an additional amount of tactile stimulation, thus constituting an instrument capable of assisting growth and development in these selected newborns. However, as reported above, clinical evidence of the effect of the massage in preterm development is still weak. Preliminary data resulting from a recent study in preterm infants (Fig. 3) show that massage increases IGF-1 blood levels and leads to an acceleration of visual system maturation and to a modification of electroencephalographic activity (Guzzetta et al., 2009).

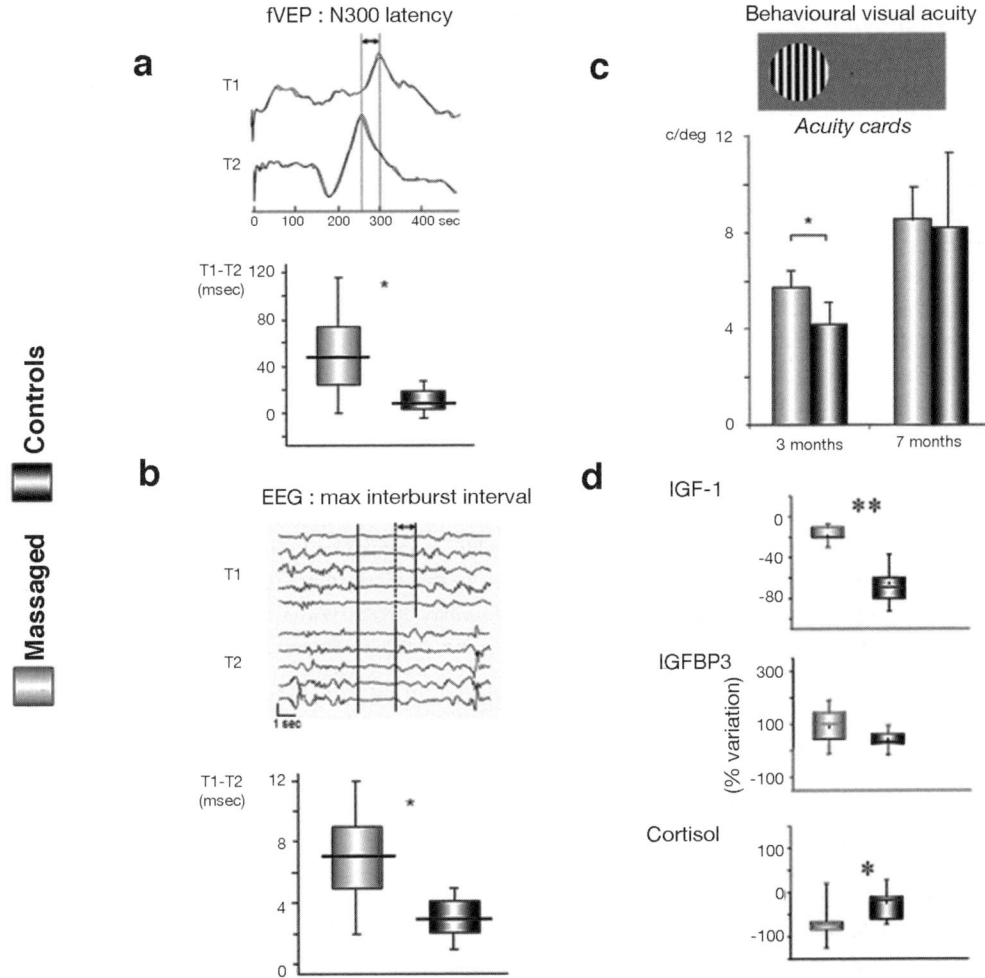

Fig. 3. (a) Difference between pre- and post-massage assessment of N300 latency (fVEP). Boxes indicate median (black horizontal line), interquartile values and range. Massaged infants show greater differences between T2 and T1. (b) Difference between pre- and post-massage assessment of maximum inter-burst interval (EEG). Massaged infants show greater differences between T2 and T1. (c) Behavioural visual acuity measured in cycles/degree by means of the Vital-Durand acuity cards at 3 and 7 months corrected age. Bars indicate mean values and standard error of the mean. Significant differences were found at 3 months, with acuities greater in massaged infants than in controls, but not at 7 months. (d) Variation between pre- and post-massage assessment of blood IGF-1, IGFBP3 and cortisol (T2-T1/T1). Massaged infants showed a small decrease of IGF-1, a larger decrease in cortisol, and no significant difference for IGFBP3. (*$p \leq 0.1$; ** $p \leq 0.01$). (Guzzetta et al. 2009, modified). EEG, electroencephalogram; IGF, insulin-like growth factor; IGFBP, IGF binding protein.

It is reasonable that IGF-1 could play a role as a mediator of the effects of therapeutic massage on visual development in infants, as in rats. This could occur through an acceleration of the maturation of the intracortical inhibitory circuits that shape the receptive fields of the visual cortex (Sillito, 1975; Hensch et al., 1998; Ciucci et al., 2007). Recently, the presence of lower plasma levels of IGF-1 and IGF-1 binding protein in premature subjects has been correlated with an increased incidence of retinopathy of prematurity (ROP) (Hellstrom et al., 2003; Lofqvist et al., 2006; Lofqvist et al., 2007). Therapeutic massage, causing an increase in plasma IGF-1 and to a lesser extent IGF binding protein-3, could have a clinical application in preterm infants, especially between 30 and 35 weeks of postmenstrual age when typically ROP is induced (Hellstrom et al., 2003).

The effect of massage is not limited to the visual system, as shown by a significant difference in EEG power between massaged neonates and controls (Guzzetta, A. et al., unpublished data). There is evidence that such changes in the EEG in preterm infants approaching term are a positive phenomenon, probably related to an increase in synaptic density and connectivity (Scher et al., 1994; Scher et al., 1997). Recently, a direct link has been shown between environmental enrichment, synaptic plasticity, and the spectral power of slow wave activity, sustaining the concept that the sleep EEG is strongly influenced not just by the length of the previous waking period, but also in general by its quality (Huber et al., 2007; Faraguna et al., 2008). This study maintains the idea that therapeutic massage favours the maturation of bioelectrical cerebral activity through a process similar to that occurring *in utero* in term neonates, probably by attenuating the discrepancy between the intrauterine and the extrauterine environment.

In conclusion, preliminary data support the view that infant massage represents a model of environmental enrichment in the human that shares significant characteristics with animal models. Effects of infant massage are observed at the electrophysiological, behavioural, and molecular level. The visual system seems particularly sensitive to environmental enrichment effects, even when the enrichment is not directly focused on increasing visual stimulation.

Future studies will clarify the clinical application of infantile massage and related techniques and the consistency of their effects on the mechanisms of adaptive cerebral plasticity.

Conclusions

Despite much interest by clinicians and the wealth of publications in the international literature, so far scarce evidence has been provided on the effectiveness of early intervention programmes. The most important problems underlined by meta-analyses are the great heterogeneity between the aims and the types of intervention and the low methodological quality of the studies conducted up to now, mainly relating to the selection of subjects and the blinding of the observers.

More high quality randomized trials and longer follow-up periods are needed to evaluate the benefits of early intervention programmes on the clinical outcome and to justify the economic impact of these programmes.

Promising results from animal models have improved our understanding of the cellular and molecular effects of environmental stimulation on neuroplasticity under normal and pathological conditions. These results may provide a stimulus for the improved application of these programmes in terms of the aims of the intervention, the type of neurological dysfunction assessed, the type of stimulation given, and the age at which stimulation is begun.

References

Aberg, M.A., Aberg, N.D., Hedbacker, H., Oscarsson, J. & Eriksson, P.S. (2000): Peripheral infusion of IGF-I selectively induces neurogenesis in the adult rat hippocampus. *J. Neurosci.* **20**, 2896–2903.

Achenbach, T.M., Howell, C.T., Aoki, M.F. & Rauh, V.A. (1993): Nine-year outcome of the Vermont Intervention Program for low birth weight infants. *Pediatrics* **91**, 45–55.

Acolet, D., Modei, N., Giannakoulopoulos, X., Bond, C., Clow, A. & Glover, V. (1993): Changes in plasma cortisol and catecholamine concentrations in response to massage in preterm infants. *Arch. Dis. Child.* **68**, 29–31.

Als, H. (1986): A synactive model of neonatal behavioral organization. *Phys. Occup. Ther. Pediatr.* **6**, 3–35.

Als, H., Lawhon, G., Duffy, F.H., McAnulty, G.B., Gibes-Grossman, R. & Blickman, J.G. (1994): Individualized developmental care for very low-birth-weight preterm infant: medical and neurofunctional effects. *JAMA* **272**, 853–858.

Als, H., Duffy, F.H., McAnulty, G.B., Rivkin, M.J., Vajapeyam, S., Mulkern, R.V., Warfield, S.K., Huppi, P.S., Butler, S.C., Conneman, N., Fischer, C. & Eichenwald, E.C. (2004): Early experience alters brain function and structure. *Pediatrics* **113**, 846–857.

Anand, K.J.S. & Scalzo, F.M. (2000): Can adverse neonatal experiences alter development and subsequent behaviour? *Biol. Neonat.* **77**, 69–82.

Bamm, E.L. & Rosenbaum, P. (2008): Family-centered theory: origins, development, barriers, and support to implementation in rehabilitation medicine. *Arch. Phys. Med. Rehabil.* **89**, 1618–1624.

Bao, X., Sun, S. & Wei, S. (1999): Early intervention promotes intellectual development of premature infants: a preliminary study. *Chin. Med. J.* **112**, 520–523.

Barrera, M.E., Cunningham, C.E. & Rosenbaum, P. (1986): Low birth weight and home intervention strategies: preterm infants. *Dev. Behav. Pediatr.* **7**, 361–366.

Bartoletti, A., Medini, P., Berardi, N. & Maffei, L. (2004): Environmental enrichment prevents effects of dark-rearing in the rat visual cortex. *Nat. Neurosci.* **7**, 215–216.

Bayley, N. (1993): *Bayley scales of infant development*, 2nd edition (BSID-II). San Antonio: The Psychological Corporation.

Becker, P.T., Grunwald, P.C., Moorman, J. & Stuhr, S. (1991): Outcomes of developmentally supportive nursing care for very low birth weight infants. *Nurs. Res.* **40**, 150–155.

Beckung, E. & Hagberg, G. (2002): Neuroimpairments, activity limitations, and participation restriction in children with cerebral palsy. *Dev. Med. Child Neurol.* **44**, 309–316.

Benaroya-Milshtein, N., Hollander, N., Apter, A., Kukulansky, T., Raz, N., Wilf, A., Yaniv, I. & Pick, C.G. (2004): Environmental enrichment in mice decreases anxiety, attenuates stress responses and enhances natural killer cell activity. *Eur. J. Neurosci.* **20**, 1341–1347.

Berardi, N., Pizzorusso, T., Ratto, G.M. & Maffei, L. (2003): Molecular basis of plasticity in the visual cortex. *Trends Neurosci.* **26**, 369–378.

Berardi, N., Pizzorusso, T. & Maffei, L. (2000): Critical periods during sensory development. *Curr. Opin. Neurobiol.* **10**, 138.

Bhutta, A.T., Cleves, M.A., Casey, P.H., Cradock, M.M. & Anand, K.J.S. (2002): Cognitive and behavioural outcomes of school-aged children who were born preterm. *JAMA* **288**, 728–737.

Blauw-Hospers, C.H. & Hadders-Algra, M. (2005): A systematic review of the effects of early intervention on motor development. *Dev. Med. Child Neurol.* **47**, 421–432.

Bond, C. (2002): Positive touch and massage in the neonatal unit: a British approach. *Semin. Neonatol.* **7**, 477–486.

Bonnier, C. (2008): Evaluation of early stimulation programs for enhancing brain development. *Acta Paediatr.* **97**, 853–858.

Brown, L.D. & Heermann, J.A. (1997): The effect of developmental care on preterm infant outcome. *Appl. Nurs. Res.* **10**, 190–197.

Buckman, R. (1992): *How to break bad news: a guide for health care professionals*. Baltimore: Johns Hopkins University Press.

Buehler, D.M., Als, H., Duffy, F.H., McAnulty, G.B. & Liederman, J. (1995): Effectiveness of individualized developmental care for low-risk preterm infants: behavioural and electrophysiologic evidence. *Pediatrics* **96**, 923–932.

Cameron, E.C., Maehle, V. & Reid, J. (2005): The effects of an early physical therapy intervention for very preterm, very low birth weight infants: a randomized controlled clinical trial. *Pediatr. Phys. Ther.* **17**, 107–119.

Campbell, K., Gan, C., Snider, A. & Cohen, S. (2003): Measuring what young people think about clinical service [abstract]. *Can. Psychol.* **44**, 26.

Cancedda, L., Putignano, E., Sale, A., Viegi, A., Berardi, N. & Maffei, L. (2004): Acceleration of visual system development by environmental enrichment. *J. Neurosci.* **24,** 4840–4848.

Carr, L.J., Harrison, L.M., Evans, A.L. & Stephens, J.A. (1993): Patterns of central motor reorganization in hemiplegic cerebral palsy. *Brain* **116,** 1223–1247.

Carro, E., Nunez, A., Busiguina, S. & Torres-Aleman, I. (2000): Circulating insulin-like growth factor I mediates effects of exercise on the brain. *J. Neurosci.* **20,** 2926–2933.

Champagne, D.L., Bagot, R.C., van Hasselt, F., Ramakers, G., Meaney, M.J., de Kloet, E.R., Joëls, M. & Krugers, H. (2008): Maternal care and hippocampal plasticity: evidence for experience-dependent structural plasticity, altered synaptic functioning, and differential responsiveness to glucocorticoids and stress. *J. Neurosci.* **28,** 6037–6045.

Chu, D., Huttenlocher, P.R., Levin, D.N. & Towle, V.L. (2000): Reorganization of the hand somatosensory cortex following perinatal unilateral brain injury. *Neuropediatrics* **31,** 63–69.

Ciucci, F., Putignano, E., Baroncelli, L., Landi, S., Berardi, N. & Maffei, L. (2007): Insulin-like growth factor 1 (IGF-1) mediates the effects of enriched environment (EE) on visual cortical development. *PLoS ONE* **2,** e475.

Cooper, L.G., Gooding, J.S., Gallagher, J., Sternesky, L., Ledsky, R. & Berns, S.D. (2007): Impact of a family-centered care initiate on NICU care, staff and families. *J. Perinatol.* **27,** 32–37.

Cotman, C.W. & Berchtold, N.C. (2002): Exercise: a behavioural intervention to enhance brain health and plasticity. *Trends Neurosci.* **25,** 295–301.

Council on Children with Disabilities (2007): Role of the medical home in family-centered early intervention services. *Pediatrics* **120,** 1153–1158.

D'Ercole, A.J., Ye, P. & O'Kusky, J.R. (2002): Mutant mouse models of insulin-like growth factor actions in the central nervous system. *Neuropeptides* **36,** 209–220.

Denhoff, E. (1981): Current status of infant stimulation or enrichment programs for children with developmental disabilities. *Pediatrics* 67, 32–37.

Doyle, L.W., for The Victorian Infant Collaborative Study Group (2004): Evaluation of neonatal intensive care for extremely low birth weight infants in Victoria over two decades. I. Effectiveness. *Pediatrics* **113,** 505–509.

Einspieler, C., Prechtl, H.F.R., Bos, A., Ferrari, F. & Cioni, G. (2004): *Prechtl's method on the qualitative assessment of general movements in preterm, term and young infants.* Clinics in Developmental Medicine No. 167. London: Mac Keith Press.

Engineer, N.D., Percaccio, C.R., Pandya, P.K., Moucha, R., Rathbun, D.L. & Kilgard, M.P. (2004): Environmental enrichment improves response strength, threshold, selectivity, and latency of auditory cortex neurons. *J. Neurophysiol.* **92,** 73–82.

Evrard, P., Marret, S. & Gressens, P. (1997): Environmental and genetic determinants of neural migration and post migratory survival. *Acta Paediatr.* (Suppl.) **422,** 20–26.

Fagiolini, M., Pizzorusso, T., Berardi, N., Domenica, L. & Maffei, L. (1994): Functional postnatal development of the rat primary visual cortex and the role of visual experience: dark rearing and monocular deprivation. *Vision Res.* **34,** 709–720.

Faraguna, U., Vyazovskiy, V.V., Nelson, A.B., Tononi, G. & Cirelli, C. (2008): A causal role for brain-derived neurotrophic factor in the homeostatic regulation of sleep. *J. Neurosci.* **28,** 4088–4095.

Field, T. (1990): Alleviating stress in newborn infants in the intensive care unit. *Clin. Perinatol.* **17,** 1–9.

Field, T. (2002): Preterm infant massage therapy studies: an American approach. *Semin. Neonatol.* **7,** 487–494.

Field, T., Widmayer, S.M., Stringer, S. & Ignatoff, E. (1980): Teenage, lower class, black mothers and their preterm infants: an intervention and developmental follow-up. *Child Dev.* **51,** 426–436.

Field, T., Schanberg, S., Scafidi, F., Bauer, C.R., Vega-Lahr, N., Garcia, R., Nystrom, J. & Kuhn, C.M. (1986): Tactile/kinesthetic stimulation effects on preterm neonates. *Pediatrics* **77,** 654–658.

Field, T., Scafidi, F. & Schanberg, S. (1987): Massage of preterm newborn to improve growth and development. *Pediatr. Nurs.* **13,** 385–387.

Fleisher, B.E., VandenBerg, K. & Constantinou, J. (1995): Individualized developmental care for very low birthweight premature infants improves medical and neurodevelopmental outcome in neonatal intensive unit. *Clin. Pediatr.* **10,** 523–529.

Globus, A., Rosenzweig, M.R., Bennett, E.L. & Diamond, M.C. (1973): Effects of differential experience on dendritic spine counts in rat cerebral cortex. *J. Comp. Physiol. Psychol.* **82,** 175–81.

Goodman, M., Rothberg, A.D., Houston-McMillan, J.E., Cooper, P.A., Cartwright, J.D. & van der Velde, M.A. (1985): Effect of early neurodevelopmental therapy in normal and at-risk survivors of neonatal intensive care. *Lancet* ii, 1327–1330.

Green, E.J., Greenough, W.T. & Schlumpf, B.E. (1983): Effects of complex or isolated environments on cortical dendrites of middle-aged rats. *Brain Res.* **264**, 233–240.

Greenough, W.T. & Volkmar, F.R. (1973): Pattern of dendritic branching in occipital cortex of rats reared in complex environments. *Exp. Neurol.* **40**, 491–504.

Griffin, T. (2000): Family-centered care in the NICU. *J. Perinat. Neonat. Nurs.* **20**, 98–102.

Griffiths, R. (1996): *The Griffiths mental development scales from birth to 2 years, manual*, 1996 revision (revised by M. Huntley). Henley, UK: Association for Research in Infant and Child Development, Test Agency.

Guzzetta, A., Baldini, S., Bancale, A., Baroncelli, L., Ciucci, F., Ghirri, P., Putignano, E., Sale, A., Viegi, A., Berardi, N., Boldrini, A., Cioni, G. & Maffei, L. (2009): Massage accelerates brain development and the maturation of visual function. *J Neurosci.* **29**, 6042-6051.

Haataja, L., Mercuri, E., Regev, R., Cowan, F., Rutherford, M., Dubowitz, V. & Dubowitz, L. (1999): Optimality score for the neurological examination of the infant at 12 and 18 months. *J. Pediatr.* **135**, 153–161.

Hadders-Algra, M. (2001): Early brain damage and the development of motor behaviour in children: clues for therapeutic intervention. *Neural Plast.* **8**, 31–49.

Harrison, H. (1993): The principles for family-centered neonatal care. *Pediatrics* **92**, 643–650.

Hebb, D.O. (1949): *The organisation of behaviour*. New York: John Wiley.

Hellstrom, A., Engstrom, E., Hard, A.L., Albertsson-Wikland, K., Carlsson, B., Niklasson, A., Löfqvist, C., Svensson, E., Holm, S., Ewald, U., Holmström, G. & Smith, L.E. (2003): Postnatal serum insulin-like growth factor I deficiency is associated with retinopathy of prematurity and other complications of premature birth. *Pediatrics* **112**, 1016–1020.

Hensch, T.K., Fagiolini, M., Mataga, N., Stryker, M.P., Baekkeskov, S. & Kash, S.F. (1998): Local GABA circuit control of experience-dependent plasticity in developing visual cortex. *Science* **282**, 1504–1508.

Holditch-Davis, D. (2000): Mother's stories about their experiences in the neonatal intensive care unit. *Neonat. Netw.* **19**, 13–21.

Hubel, D.H. & Weisel, T.N. (1970): The period of susceptibility to the physiological effects of unilateral eye closure in kitten. *J. Physiol. (Lond.)* **206**, 419–436.

Huber, R., Tononi, G. & Cirelli, C. (2007): Exploratory behavior, cortical BDNF expression, and sleep homeostasis. *Sleep* **30**, 129–139.

Humphry, R. (1989): Early intervention and the influence of the occupational therapist on the parent-child relationship. *Am. J. Occup. Ther.* **43**, 738–742.

Kaaresen, P.I., Ronning, J.A., Ulvund, S.E. & Dahl, L.B. (2006): A randomized, controlled trial of the effectiveness of an early-intervention program in reducing parenting stress after preterm birth. *Pediatrics* **118**, 9–19.

King, S.M., Rosenbaum, P. & King, G.A. (1996): Parent's perceptions of caregiving: development and validation of a measure of process of care. *Dev. Med. Child Neurol.* **38**, 757–772.

Kleberg, A., Westrup, B., Stjernqvist, K. & Lagercrantz, H. (2002): Indications of improved cognitive development at one year of age among infants born very prematurely who received care based on the Newborn Individualized Developmental Care and Assessment Program (NIDCAP). *Early Hum. Dev.* **68**, 83–91.

Kolb, B., Brown, R., Witt-Lajeunesse, A. & Gibb, R. (2001): Neural compensations after lesion of the cerebral cortex. *Neural Plast.* **8**, 1–16.

Kruskal, M.O., Thomasgard, M.C. & Shonkoff, J.P. (1989): Early intervention for vulnerable infants and their families: an emerging agenda. *Semin. Perinatol.* **13**, 506–512.

Landi, S., Sale, A., Berardi, N., Viegi, A., Maffei, L. & Cenni, M.C. (2007): Retinal functional development is sensitive to environmental enrichment: a role for BDNF. *FASEB J.* **21**, 130–139.

Lawhon, G. (2002): Facilitation of parenting the premature infant within the newborn intensive care unit. *J. Perinat. Neonat. Nurs.* **16**, 71–82.

Lofqvist, C., Andersson, E., Sigurdsson, J., Engström, E., Hård, A.L., Niklasson, A., Smith, L.E. & Hellström, A. (2006): Longitudinal postnatal weight and insulin-like growth factor I measurements in the prediction of retinopathy of prematurity. *Arch. Ophthalmol.* **124**, 1711–1718.

Lofqvist, C., Chen, J., Connor, K.M., Smith, A.C., Aderman, C.M., Liu, N., Pintar, J.E., Ludwig, T., Hellstrom, A. & Smith, L.E. (2007): IGFBP3 suppresses retinopathy through suppression of oxygen-induced vessel loss and promotion of vascular regrowth. *Proc. Natl. Acad. Sci. USA* **104**, 10589–10594.

Majnemer, A. (1998): Benefits of early intervention for children with developmental disabilities. *Semin. Pediatr. Neurol.* **5**, 62–69.

McCarton, C.M., Wallace, I.F. & Bennett, F.C. (1995): Preventive interventions with low birth weight premature infants: an evaluation of their success. *Semin. Perinatol.* **19**, 330–340.

Mead, N. & Bower, P. (2000): Patient-centredness: a conceptual framework and review of the empirical literature. *Soc. Sci. Med.* **51**, 1087–1100.

Melnyk, B.M., Alpert-Gillis, L., Feinstein, N.F., Fairbanks, E., Schultz-Czarniak, J., Hust, D., Sherman, L., LeMoine, C., Moldenhauer, Z., Small, L., Bender, N. & Sinkin, R.A. (2001): Improving cognitive development of low birth-weight premature infants with the COPE program: a pilot study of the benefit of early NICU intervention with mothers. *Res. Nurs. Health* **24**, 373–389.

Montagu, A. (1978): *Touching: the human significance of the skin*. London: Harper & Row.

Nithianantharajah, J. & Hannan, A.J. (2006): Enriched environments, experience-dependent plasticity and disorders of the nervous system. *Nat. Rev. Neurosci.* **7**, 697–709.

Nurcombe, B., Howell, D.C., Rauh, V., Teti, D.M., Ruoff, P. & Brennan, J. (1984): An intervention program for mothers of low-birthweight infants: preliminary results. *J. Am. Acad. Child Psychiatry* **23**, 319–325.

Ohgi, S., Fukuda, M., Akiyama, T. & Gima, H. (2004): Effect of an early intervention programme on low birthweight infants with cerebral injuries. *J. Paediatr. Child Health* **40**, 689–695.

Piper, M.C., Kunos, V.I., Willis, D.M., Mazer, B.L., Ramsay, M. & Silver, K.M. (1986): Early physical therapy effects on the high-risk infant: a randomized controlled trial. *Pediatrics* **78**, 216–224.

Rabinowicz, T., de Courten-Myers, G.M., Petetot, J.M. & Xi, G. (1996): Human cortex development: estimates of neuronal numbers indicate major loss late during gestation. *J. Neuropathol. Exp. Neurol.* **55**, 320–328.

Rampon, C., Tang, Y.P., Goodhouse, J., Shimizu, E., Kyin, M. & Tsien, J.Z. (2000): Enrichment induces structural changes and recovery from nonspatial memory deficits in CA1 NMDAR1-knockout mice. *Nat. Neurosci.* **3**, 238–244.

Rauh, V.A., Achenbach, T.M., Nurcombe, B., Howell, C.T. & Teti, D.M. (1988): Minimizing adverse effects of low birthweight: four-year results of an intervention program. *Child Dev.* **59**, 544–553.

Rauh, V.A., Nurcombe, B., Achenbach, T. & Howell, C. (1990): The Mother-Infant Transaction Program: the content and implication of an intervention for the mothers of low-birthweight infants. *Clin. Perinatol.* **17**, 31–45.

Resnick, M.B., Armstrong, S. & Carter, R.L. (1988): Developmental intervention program for high risk premature infants: effects on development and parent-infant interaction. *J. Dev. Behav. Pediatr.* **9**, 73–78.

Rice, R.D. (1977): Neurophysiological development in premature neonates following stimulation. *Dev. Psychol.* **13**, 69–76.

Rosenzweig, M.R. & Bennett, E.L. (1996): Psychobiology of plasticity: effects of training and experience on brain and behaviour. *Behav. Brain Res.* **78**, 57–65.

Rosenzweig, M.R., Bennett, E.L., Hebert, M. & Morimoto, H. (1978): Social grouping cannot account for cerebral effects of enriched environments. *Brain Res.* **153**, 563–576.

Sale, A., Putignano, E., Cancedda, L., Landi, S., Cirulli, F., Berardi, N. & Maffei, L. (2004): Enriched environment and acceleration of visual system development. *Neuropharmacology* **47**, 649–660.

Sale, A., Maya Vetencourt, J.F., Medini, P., Cenni, M.C., Baroncelli, L., De Pasquale, R. & Maffei, L. (2007): Environmental enrichment in adulthood promotes amblyopia recovery through a reduction of intracortical inhibition. *Nat. Neurosci.* **10**, 679–681.

Scafidi, F., Field, T., Schanberg, S., Bauer, C., Tucci, K., Roberts, J. & Kuhn, C. (1990): Massage stimulates growth in preterm infants: a replication. *Infant Behav. Dev.* **13**, 167–188.

Scafidi, F., Field, T. & Schanberg, S.M. (1993): Factors that predict which preterm infants benefit most from massage therapy. *J. Dev. Behav. Pediatr.* **14**, 176–180.

Scafidi, F. & Field, T. (1997): Brief report: HIV exposed newborn show inferior orientating and abnormal reflexes on Brazelton Scale. *J. Pediatr. Psychol.* **22**, 105–112.

Schanberg, S.M. & Field, T. (1987): sensory deprivation stress and supplemental stimulation in the rat pup and preterm human neonate. *Child Dev.* **58**, 1431–1447.

Scher, M.S., Sun, M., Steppe, D.A., Banks, D.L., Guthrie, R.D. & Sclabassi, R.J. (1994): Comparisons of EEG sleep state-specific spectral values between healthy full-term and preterm infants at comparable postconceptional ages. *Sleep* **17**, 47–51.

Scher, M.S., Steppe, D.A., Sclabassi, R.J. & Banks, D.L. (1997): Regional differences in spectral EEG measures between healthy term and preterm infants. *Pediatr. Neurol.* **17**, 218–223.

Shonkoff, J.P. & Hauser-Cram, P. (1987): Early intervention for disabled infants and their families: a quantitative analysis [review]. *Pediatrics* **80**, 650–658.

Sillito, A.M. (1975): The contribution of inhibitory mechanisms to the receptive field properties of neurones in the striate cortex of the cat. *J. Physiol. (Lond.)* **250**, 305–329.

Simeonsson, R.J., Edmondson, R., Smith, T., Carnahan, S. & Bucy, J.E. (1995): Family involvement in multidisciplinary team evaluation: professional and parent perspectives. *Child Care Health Dev.* **21**, 199–215.

Spittle, A.J., Orton, J., Doyle, L.W. & Boyd, R. (2007): Early developmental intervention programs post hospital discharge to prevent motor and cognitive impairments in preterm infants. *Cochrane Database Syst. Rev.*, Apr. 18, CD005495.

Symington, A. & Pinelli, J. (2006): Developmental care for promoting development and preventing morbidity in preterm infants. *Cochrane Database Syst. Rev.*, Apr. 19, CD001814.

Tin, W., Wariyar, U. & Hey, E. (1997): Changing prognosis for babies of less than 28 weeks' gestation in the north of England between 1983 and 1994. Northern Neonatal Network. *BMJ* **314**, 107–111.

Tropea, D., Kreiman, G., Lyckman, A., Mukherjee, S., Yu, H., Horng, S. & Sur, M. (2006): Gene expression changes and molecular pathways mediating activity-dependent plasticity in visual cortex. *Nat. Neurosci.* **9**, 660–668.

Van Praag, H., Kempermann, G. & Gage, F.H. (2000): Neural consequences of environmental enrichment. *Nat. Rev. Neurosci.* **1**, 191–198.

Vickers, A., Ohlsson, A., Lacy, J.B. & Horsley, A. (2004): Massage for promoting growth and development of preterm and/or low birth-weight infants. *Cochrane Database Syst. Rev.* (2), CD000390.

Vohr, B.R., Wright, L.L., Poole, W.K. & McDonald, S.A. (2005): Neurodevelopmental outcomes of extremely low birth weight infants <32 week's gestation between 1993 and 1998. *Pediatrics* **116**, 635–643.

Von Bertalanffy, L. (1968): *General system theory*. New York: Braziller.

Walsh, R.N. & Cummins, R.A. (1979): Changes in hippocampal neuronal nuclei in response to environmental stimulation. *Int. J. Neurosci.* **9**, 209–212.

Walsh, R.N., Budtz-Olsen, O.E., Penny, J.E. & Cummins, R.A. (1969): The effects of environmental complexity on the histology of the rat hippocampus. *J. Comp. Neurol.* 137, 361–366.

Westrup, B., Kleberg, A., von Eichwald, K., Stjernqvist, K. & Lagercrantz, H. (2000): A randomized, controlled trial to evaluate the effects of the Newborn Individualized Developmental Care and Assessment Program in a Swedish setting. *Pediatrics* **105**, 66–72.

Westrup, B., Bohm, B., Lagercrantz, H. & Stjernqvist, K. (2004): Preschool outcome in children born very prematurely and cared for according to the Newborn Individualized Developmental Care and Assessment Program (NIDCAP). *Acta Paediatr.* **93**, 498–507.

Wheeden, A., Scafidi, F., Field, T., Ironson, G., Valdeon, C. & Bandstra, E. (1993): Massage effects on cocaine-exposed preterm neonates. *J. Dev. Behav. Pediatr.* **14**, 318–322.

WHO (2001): *International classification of functioning, disabilities and health*. Geneva: World Health Organisation.

Yiğit, S., Kerem, M., Livanelioğlu, A., Oran, O., Erdem, G., Mutlu, A., Turanli, G., Tekinalp, G. & Yurdakök, M. (2002): Early physiotherapy intervention in premature infants. *Turk J Pediatr.* **44**, 224-229.

Chapter 8

Metabolic disorders

Enrico Bertini[*] and Carlo Dionisi-Vici[°]

[*] *Unit of Molecular Medicine for Neuromuscular and Neurodegenerative Disorders;*
[°] *Unit of Metabolic Disorders, Bambino Gesù Children's Research Hospital, Piazza S. Onofrio 4, 00165 Rome, Italy*
ebertini@tin.it

Inborn errors of metabolism can be classified in three groups (Saudubray *et al.*, 2006). *Group 1* includes *inborn errors of intermediary metabolism* that give rise to an acute or chronic intoxication. This group encompasses aminoacidopathies, organic acidurias, urea cycle disorders, sugar intolerances, metal disorders and porphyrias. Clinical expression can be acute or systemic or can involve a specific organ, and can strike in the neonatal period or later and intermittently from infancy to late adulthood. Most of these disorders are treatable and require the emergency removal of the toxin by special diets, extracorporeal procedures, cleansing drugs or vitamins. *Group 2* includes *inborn errors of intermediary metabolism that affect the cytoplasmic and mitochondrial energetic processes.* Cytoplasmic defects encompass those affecting glycolysis, glycogenosis, gluconeogenesis, hyperinsulinisms, and creatine and pentose phosphate pathways. Mitochondrial defects include respiratory chain disorders, Krebs cycle and pyruvate oxidation defects, and disorders of fatty acid oxidation and ketone bodies. *Group 3* involves *cellular organelles* and *includes lysosomal, peroxisomal, glycosylation,* and *cholesterol synthesis defects.*

Each of these groups of disorders requires a distinctive methodology to detect the clinical features and metabolic markers for diagnostic assessment.

Inborn errors of intermediary metabolism

Inborn errors of intermediary metabolism generally give rise to an acute or chronic intoxication. This group encompasses aminoacidopathies, organic acidurias, urea cycle disorders, sugar intolerances, metal disorders and porphyrias. It includes disorders that lead to an acute or progressive intoxication from the accumulation of toxic compounds proximal to the metabolic block. The following disorders can be clustered in this group: inborn errors of amino acid catabolism (phenylketonuria, maple syrup urine disease, homocystinuria, tyrosinaemia, and so on), most organic acidurias (methylmalonic, propionic, isovaleric), congenital urea cycle defects, sugar intolerances (galactosaemia, hereditary fructose intolerance), metal intoxication (Wilson disease, Menkes disease, haemochromatosis), and the porphyrias. All these conditions share clinical similarities: they do not interfere with the embryofetal development and they present with a symptom-free interval and clinical signs of 'intoxication', which may be acute (vomiting, coma, liver failure, thromboembolic complications) or chronic (failure to thrive, developmental delay, ectopia lentis, cardiomyopathy). In the branched chain amino acid disorders (phenylketonuria, maple syrup urine disease, methylmalonic acidaemia, propionic acidaemia, isovaleric acidaemia, and multiple carboxylase deficiency) the neurological manifestations are characterized by coma. In glutaric aciduria type II, urea cycle disorders, and triple H syndrome (hyperornithinaemia-hyperammonaemia-homocitrullinuria), in addition to coma there may be abnormal movements such as dystonia, and spastic paraplegia during follow-up. Seizures may appear, particularly with vitamin-B6-responsive seizure disorder, pyridox(am)ine-5?-phosphate oxidase deficiency, biotin deficiency, folinic-acid-responsive seizures, congenital magnesium malabsorption, and multiple carboxylase deficiency. Seizures with microcephaly appear in 3-phosphoglycerate dehydrogenase deficiency and in the cerebral glucose carrier GLUTI deficiency.

Circumstances that can provoke acute metabolic attacks include catabolism, fever, intercurrent illness and food intake. Clinical expression is often both late in onset and intermittent.

Most of these disorders are treatable in the acute stage and require the emergency removal of the toxin by special diets, extracorporeal procedures or 'cleansing' drugs (carnitine, sodium benzoate, penicillamine, vitamins, and so on). Nutritional treatment is the backbone of the management in this group. It includes approaches aimed at depleting the toxic substrate that accumulates or at replacing the crucial metabolic product that is deficient. Breast milk can still play an important role in these special diets.

Another subgroup that might be considered among the aminoacidopathies is related to a deficiency in the biosynthesis of a given substance that is critical to the intermediary metabolism such as an organic acid (creatine) or an aminoacid (glutamine, serine) or some neurotransmitters (dopamine, serotonin, GABA). Each of these disorders may be detected by searching for the defective biological marker in the CSF or blood.

Most of these disorders are generally managed by metabolic units. The paediatric neurologist is helpful for undertaking EEG monitoring and managing epilepsy. For a more detailed description of these conditions see the review by Fernandes *et al.* (2006).

Inborn errors of intermediary metabolism that affect the cytoplasmic and mitochondrial energetic processes

Inborn errors of intermediary metabolism have symptoms due at least in part to a deficiency in energy production or utilization within the liver, myocardium, muscle, brain or other tissues. This group can be divided into mitochondrial and cytoplasmic energy defects. Mitochondrial defects are the most severe. They encompass the congenital lactic acidaemias (defects of pyruvate transporter, pyruvate carboxylase, pyruvate dehydrogenase, and the Krebs cycle), and mitochondrial respiratory chain disorders, which are in general not amenable to treatment with the exception of coenzyme Q10 biogenesis, pyruvate dehydrogenase deficiency and pyruvate carboxylase deficiency, and the fatty acid oxidation and ketone body defects, which are partly treatable.

Cytoplasmic energetic processes

Cytoplasmic energetic process defects encompass those affecting glycolysis, glycogenosis, gluconeogenesis, hyperinsulinisms, and creatine and pentose phosphate pathways. Most of these disorders, particularly the glycogenoses, are treatable and are summarized in Table 1. The characteristic neurological manifestation are myopathy, cardiomyopathy, myoglobinuria, muscle pain, hepatomegaly, and ketotic hypoglycaemia. Some glycogenoses with a predominantly myopathic picture share a differential diagnosis with other myopathic disorders manifesting with increased creatine kinase or myoglobinuria. For more details on these disorders see a review by Yoon & Shin (2006).

Table 1. Summary of glycogenoses

Type	Deficient enzyme	Gene symbol
I (von Gierke)		
Ia	Glucose 6-phosphatase	G6PC
Ib	G6P translocase (T1)	SLC37A4
Ic	Phosphotranslocase (T2)	NPT4 (?)
Id	Glucose translocase (T3)	?
II (Pompe)		
Infantile (Pompe disease)	Lysosomal-glucosidase	GAA 1
Childhood	"	"
Juvenile	"	"
Adult	"	"
III (Cori disease)		
IIIa (liver and muscle form)	Amylo-1,6-glucosidase	AGL
IIIb (liver form)	"	"
IIIc (muscle form)	"	"
IV (Andersen disease)		
Infantile form	Branching enzyme	GBE1
(Liver)	Branching enzyme	"
(Neuromuscular)	"	"
Juvenile or adult form (liver, muscle)	"	"
Polyglucosan body disease (APBD)	"	"
V (McArdle disease)		
Adult form	Muscle phosphorylase	PYGM
Infantile form	"	"
VI (Hers disease)	Liver phosphorylase PYGL	PYGL
VII (Tarui disease)		
Severe form	Phosphofructokinase	PFKM
Mild form	"	"
Phosphorylase activation system defects		
VIII (VIa/IXA)	Phosphorylase kinase (liver PBK)	
(XLG I/II)	α-subunit of PBK	PHKA2 X (multisystem)
Autosomal recessive	β-subunit of PBK	PHKB
IXB	γ or δ subunit of PBK (?)	PHKG
IXC	Cardiac muscle PBK?	?
IXD (adult form)	Muscle PBK	PHKA1
(Severe muscle form)		PHKA1(?), PHKG1(?)
X (multisystem)	Protein kinase (?)	?
GSD 0	Glycogen synthase (liver)	GYS2
	Glycogen synthase (muscle)	GYS1

Mitochondrial cytopathies

Mitochondrial cytopathies with deficiency of respiratory chain enzymes will be summarized in more detail owing to the pleiotropism of clinical symptoms (Table 2), the complexity of clinical assessment, and the variability in the genetic causes. This makes it difficult to determine their true prevalence, but recent studies have documented a minimum birth prevalence of 13.1/100,000 (1/7,634) for oxidative phosphorylation disorders with onset at any age. This clearly remains an underestimate but it indicates that oxidative phosphorylation disorders can be regarded as the most common group of inborn errors of metabolism.

Mitochondria have their own distinct DNA. Each mitochondrion contains several circular double-stranded DNA copies that are normally 16,569 base pairs in length. Each copy contains 37 genes that code for several respiratory chain structural proteins and for mitochondrial DNA transcription and translation factors (22 tRNAs).

Mitochondrial DNA abnormalities were first linked to human disease in 1988. In that year, Leber's hereditary optic neuropathy and several progressive muscle disorders were found to be caused by mutations in mitochondrial DNA (Holt et al., 1988; Wallace et al., 1988). Aerobic metabolism depends on the hundreds of mitochondria that every cell in the body contains. Cellular dysfunction results when the proportion of mutated mitochondrial DNA strands exceeds a threshold level.

Because the sperm does not contribute mitochondria to the zygote, mutations of mitochondrial DNA are classically inherited only from the mother (maternal inheritance). Mitochondria have their own distinct DNA. The proportion of mutated mitochondria can differ widely from one oocyte to another. Consequently, siblings can have widely varying symptoms and disease severity. Similarly, the proportion of mutant mitochondrial DNA differs from cell to cell in an embryo, so different daughter cell lines can have widely varying levels of cell dysfunction.

Table 2. Summary of the main symptoms of mitochondrial cytopathies

Affected organ	Symptoms
Central nervous system	Apnoea, lethargy, hypotonia, coma in the neonatal period, hypotonia, psychomotor regression, cerebellar ataxia, stroke-like episodes, myoclonus, seizures, dementia, spasticity, headache, hemiparesis in infants and children, leucodystrophy, myoclonus
Muscle	Myopathy, poor head control, limb weakness, myalgia, exercise intolerance, rhabdomyolysis
Liver	Liver enlargement, hepatocellular dysfunction
Heart	Cardiomyopathy, heart block
Kidney	Proximal tubulopathy, nephrotic syndrome, renal failure, tubulointerstitial nephritis
Gut	Vomiting, diarrhoea, villous atrophy, colonic pseudo-obstruction, exocrine pancreas dysfunction
Endocrine	Diabetes mellitus, growth hormone deficiency, hypoparathyroidism, hypothyroidism
Bone marrow	Sideroblastic anaemia, neutropenia, thrombocytopenia
Ear	Hearing loss
Eye	Progressive external ophthalmoplegia, pigmentary retinal degeneration, ptosis, diplopia, cataract
Skin	Mottled pigmentation, discoloration, acrocyanosis, vitiligo, cutis marmorata, anhidrosis and jaundice. Trichothiodystrophy, hirsutism, alopecia, alopecia with brittle hair. Symmetrical cervical lipomas

Somewhat later it became evident that defects in chromosomal DNA can also cause mitochondrial disease, because chromosomal DNA supplies most of the proteins necessary for mitochondrial DNA replication and expression. These conditions are inherited by a Mendelian trait in an autosomal dominant or autosomal recessive fashion (Zeviani et al., 1989; Moraes et al., 1991).

Providing an overview of mitochondrial encephalomyopathies, we will keep with the concept that the term 'mitochondrial encephalomyopathy' or 'mitochondrial cytopathy' refers to defects of oxidative phosphorylation of the mitochondrial respiratory chain, excluding other mitochondrial disorders related to different mitochondrial functions such as iron homeostasis, β-oxidation, and so on. The clinical presentation of these disorders is extraordinarily heterogeneous, because any tissue can be affected, in isolation or multisystemically. Symptoms may begin at any age, but the first symptoms are observed before 1 month of age in more than a third of cases and before the age of 2 years in 80 per cent of cases (Munnich et al., 1992).

Tissues that are highly energy-dependent are more frequently affected, such as brain, skeletal muscle, heart, and kidney. Skeletal muscle is the most commonly affected tissue, suggesting that these are somatic mutations – that is, spontaneous events that arose in myoblasts or in myoblast precursors after germ layer differentiation. Pure myopathy, dominated by exercise intolerance with or without myoglobinuria, is generally highly evocative of a mitochondrial encephalomyopathy. Exercise intolerance is a common complaint, which – if the patient has no objective weakness, increased serum creatine kinase (CK) levels, or abnormal electromyography (EMG) – is often dismissed as 'psychogenic' or mislabelled as 'chronic fatigue syndrome' or 'fibromyalgia rheumatica'. Many patients with mutations in mtDNA protein coding genes fall into this group, and the lack of maternal inheritance further deflects the physician from thinking about a mitochondrial cytopathy. It is important, when faced with these puzzling patients, to consider the possibility of a mitochondrial disease and at least to obtain a resting lactate value. Myoglobinuria, and especially recurrent myoglobinuria, is commonly associated with a block in the utilization of one or other of the two major sources of energy for muscle contraction, glycogen and fatty acids (DiMauro & Haller 1999). Another peculiar symptom that may occur in a mitochondrial encephalomyopathy is sideroblastic anaemia or megaloblastic anaemia, generally associated with complex I deficiency.

The fact that tissues other than muscle can be selectively affected suggests that we should keep an open mind about the possibility that somatic mutations of mtDNA protein coding genes may be involved in other tissue-specific disorders, such as cardiomyopathies and encephalopathies.

A multisystemic presentation affecting multiple tissues is highly evocative of a mitochondrial encephalomyopathy; however, it is important that the clinician confirms the clinical suspicion by searching for persistent or fluctuating increases in lactate in blood, urine, or cerebrospinal fluid, or by magnetic resonance spectroscopy. If lactate is not increased, further attempts to obtain molecular genetic confirmation are not recommended.

The diagnostic approach to mitochondrial encephalomyopathies is complicated and needs multiple forms of expertise: muscle morphology, neuroradiology, biochemistry (enzymology, chemical analysis), and genetics.

In muscle morphology, *ragged-red fibres* (RRF) – the histochemical hallmark of massive mitochondrial proliferation in muscle – are typically seen in patients with mtDNA mutations that impair overall mitochondrial protein synthesis, such as mutations in tRNA or rRNA genes, single or multiple deletions, or mtDNA depletion. The most frequent and well known phenotypes are MELAS (mitochondrial encephalomyopathy, lactic acidosis and stroke-like episodes),

MERRF (myoclonic epilepsy with ragged red fibres), Pearson syndrome, Kearn-Sayre syndrome, and progressive external ophthalmoplegia. Conversely, RRF are absent in muscle biopsies from patients with mutations in mtDNA protein coding genes, such as the NARP/MILS mutations in the ATPase 6 gene, or the various mutations in genes encoding complex 1 subunits (ND genes) associated with Leber's hereditary optic neuropathy (LHON).

Genetics

Mitochondrial diseases can result from mitochondrial DNA (mtDNA) mutations or mutations in nuclear genes. mtDNA is more often subject to mutations because it is more susceptible to damage by reactive oxygen species resulting from the low efficiency of its repair systems, lack of protection by histones, and its unique structural characteristics favouring mutations (DiMauro, 1999).

Point mutations in mtDNA are generally transmitted by maternal inheritance; however, point mutations in protein coding genes may arise *de novo* and cause sporadic disorders. Moreover, severe large scale deletions of mtDNA rearrangements are rarely segregated through generations and frequently arise sporadically.

Nuclear DNA mutations have increasingly been identified as being responsible for respiratory chain defects (DiMauro, 1999). Two of the four most common causes of Leigh syndrome, a devastating neurodegenerative disease of infancy or childhood, are specific respiratory chain defects: complex I deficiency, and reduction in cyclo-oxygenase (COX) caused by SURF-I deficiency (Tiranti *et al.*, 1999). Both conditions are inherited as autosomal recessive traits. The product of *SURF-I* is a mitochondrial protein which appears to act at the third stage in the four-step process of COX assembly.

The other two common causes of Leigh syndrome are pyruvate dehydrogenase complex (PDHC) deficiency and the *T8993G* mutation in the mtDNA ATPase 6 gene. PDHC deficiency is usually inherited as an X-linked dominant trait while the *T8993G* mutation is the most common cause of maternally inherited Leigh syndrome (MILS).

In addition to *SURF-I*, other COX assembly genes have been studied, and pathogenic mutations were found in the *SC02* gene in three infants with fatal infantile cardiomyopathy and encephalopathy, but without the typical neuropathological features of Leigh syndrome (DiMauro, 1999). The *SC02* gene encodes a copper binding protein that must play a crucial role in the assembly of COX, which contains two copper atoms. This essential function, coupled with northern blot evidence that the SC02 protein is expressed predominantly in heart and muscle, explains both the clinical phenotype and the extremely low levels of COX activity found in heart and muscle.

A special group of mendelian mitochondrial diseases reflects the gradual loss of autonomy of the mitochondrial genome, which now depends heavily on factors encoded by nuclear genes for some of its essential functions, including transcription, translation and replication. Disorders of intergenomic signalling are caused by mutations in nuclear genes that, directly or indirectly, control mtDNA number, function or integrity.

The first examples of such faulty 'dialogue' between the two genomes were provided by patients with autosomal dominant progressive external ophthalmoplegia and multiple mtDNA deletions in muscle, instead of the single type of mtDNA rearrangement that characterizes patients with Kearns-Sayre syndrome or sporadic progressive external ophthalmoplegia (DiMauro, 1999).

Another disorder of intergenomic communication – resulting in tissue specific paucity of mtDNA copies ('mtDNA depletion') – has been described in infants with severe congenital myopathy or hepatopathy (Moraes *et al.*, 1991). There are milder myopathic forms of mtDNA depletion and the clinical spectrum may involve both the central and the peripheral nervous systems. Several genetic defects have been characterized for conditions related to mtDNA depletion though others remain elusive. A defect of polymerase-γ (POLG) has been reported in children with Alpers syndrome and mtDNA depletion and in adults affected by neuropathy and ataxia inherited as an autosomal recessive trait (Naviaux & Nguyen, 2004); dominant polymerase-γ deficiency has also been found in adult patients with autosomal dominant progressive external ophthalmoplegia. Another example of a disorder of intergenomic signalling is an autosomal recessive form of progressive external ophthalmoplegia known by the acronym 'MNGIE' – mitochondrial neurogastrointestinal encephalomyopathy – dominated by gastrointestinal problems (chronic diarrhoea, intestinal pseudo-obstruction) leading to cachexia and early death. The gene was characterized by Nishino *et al.* in 1999 as thymidine phosphorylase (*TP*). *TP* is widely expressed in human tissues, including some that are selectively involved in MNGIE, such as the gastrointestinal system, brain, and peripheral nerves. Additional symptoms and signs include ptosis and ophthalmoplegia, peripheral neuropathy, and leucoencephalopathy. In contrast to the autosomal dominant forms of progressive external ophthalmoplegia, which are largely confined to muscle, the autosomal recessive forms with multiple mtDNA deletions tend to be multisystemic (DiMauro, 1999). Muscle biopsy shows COX-negative RRF, biochemical evidence of COX deficiency, and molecular evidence of multiple mtDNA deletions, sometimes associated with mtDNA depletion (DiMauro, 1999).

We will now summarize the main clinical presentations of mitochondrial cytopathies, dividing them systematically by the different tissues predominantly involved.

Symptoms of mitochondrial cytopathies

Myopathy

Myopathy is a frequent feature in mitochondrial cytopathy although rarely symptomatic in the first 2 years of life. It is responsible for muscle weakness with myalgia and exercise intolerance (DiMauro, 1999). Sometime rhabdomyolysis can be the principal symptom. Limb weakness may be associated with chronic progressive external ophthalmoplegia. The main features of this syndrome are ptosis, limitation of eye movements, and diplopia. While progressive external ophthalmoplegia may be isolated, it is often part of Kearn-Sayre syndrome, characterized by the association of progressive external ophthalmoplegia, pigmentary retinopathy, ataxia, and heart block occurring before 20 years of age (Berenberg *et al.*, 1977).

Central nervous system

Symptoms that predominantly or exclusively involve the central nervous system may occur, in various combinations. They comprise psychomotor retardation, seizures, stroke, sensorineural hearing loss, optic atrophy, ataxia, myoclonus, peripheral neuropathy, and dementia. Several clinico-pathological entities – such as Kearn-Sayre syndrome, MELAS, MERRF, Leigh syndrome (Rahman *et al.*, 1996; Huntsman *et al.*, 2005) (Fig. 1D, 1E), and Alpers syndrome (Horvath *et al.*, 2006) (Fig. 1A, 1B, 1C) – have been described according to their clinical presentations. There are several reports of patients with overlap syndromes such as Kearn-Sayre syndrome plus MELAS, Kearn-Sayre syndrome plus MERRF, progressive external ophthalmoplegia plus MERRF, or MERRF plus MELAS.

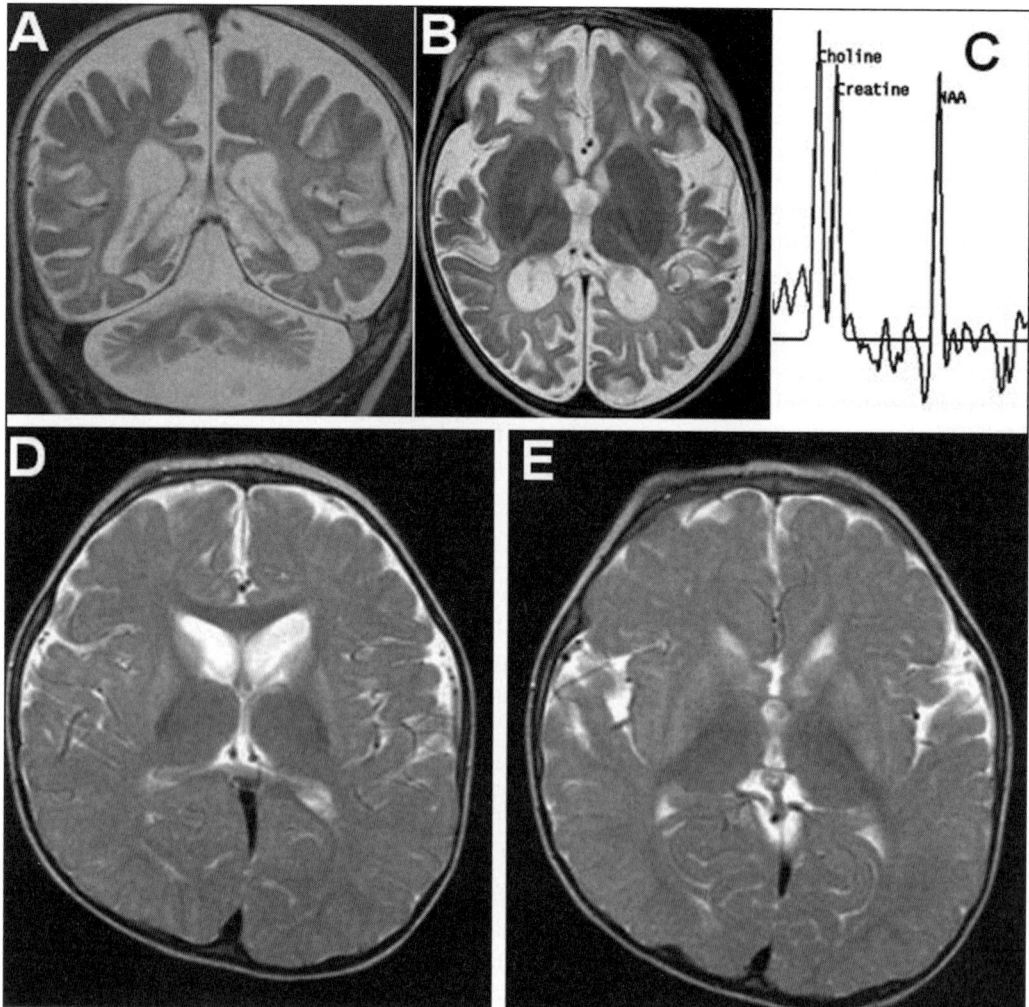

Fig. 1. Some characteristic MRI and MRS features of mitochondrial cytopathies. (A), (B) T2-weighted images of a 3-year-old girl with a 2-year history of Alpers syndrome. (C) MRS shows a lactate peak. (D), (E) T2-weighted image of a child with Leigh syndrome caused by a defect in SUCLA2. MRI, magnetic resonance imaging; MRS, magnetic resonance spectroscopy.

Recently, new neurological syndromes have been related to mutations in autosomal recessive genes which affect the mRNA translation machinery and in which biochemical assessment of muscle biopsies for the mitochondrial respiratory chain enzymes is frequently normal or not helpful in producing genetic confirmation. These disorders often start in the first 2 years of life. Mutations affecting elongation factors are responsible for agenesis of the corpus callosum with dysmorphism and fatal neonatal lactic acidosis (Miller et al., 2004), encephalomyopathy and hypertrophic cardiomyopathy (Smeitink et al., 2006), lactic acidosis, diffuse cystic leucoencephalopathy, polymicrogyria, liver involvement and early death (Valente et al., 2007). In addition, mutations affecting mitochondrial amino-acyl-tRNA synthetase give rise to autosomal recessive leucoencephalopathy with brain stem and spinal cord involvement and raised lactate levels (aspartyl-tRNA synthetase) (Scheper et al., 2007) or autosomal recessive ponto-cerebellar atrophy with lactic acidosis (Edvardson et al., 2007).

Kidney

Renal disease is more often reported in children than in adults. The most frequent renal manifestation is proximal tubulopathy with a de Toni-Debré-Fanconi syndrome. Other renal presentations have been reported, including glomerular disease with a nephrotic syndrome and chronic tubulointerstitial nephropathy (Nialdet & Rotig, 1997).

The de Toni-Debré-Fanconi syndrome is characterized by impairment of proximal tubular reabsorption, leading to urinary losses of amino acids, glucose, proteins, phosphate, uric acid, bicarbonate, potassium and water. A renal Fanconi syndrome has been reported as the most frequent renal disorder in mitochondrial cytopathy (Niaudet & Rotig 1997). Proximal tubular losses are often moderate, with some patients showing only hyperaminoaciduria. Others present with plasma acidosis, impaired tubular phosphate reabsorption, moderate glycosuria, hypercalciuria and tubular proteinuria.

The first symptoms may develop in the neonatal period and before the age of 2 years in most patients. Renal biopsy shows more or less severe non-specific anomalies of the tubular epithelium with dilatations or obliterations by casts, dedifferentiation, or atrophy. Some tubular cells show cytoplasmic vacuolization. Giant mitochondria are often observed ultrastructurally. Extrarenal symptoms are generally present in all patients with mitochondrial encephalomyopathies: myopathy or other neurological symptoms, hepatic dysfunction, Pearson syndrome, cardiac involvement or diabetes mellitus, hearing loss, or growth retardation. Some patients may have signs of proximal tubular acidosis with hypercalciuria. A 'Bartter-like' phenotype has rarely been reported (Emma *et al.*, 2006).

Glomerular disease has been observed in a few patients with mitochondrial cytopathy. Patients are affected by a nephrotic syndrome where renal biopsy showed focal and segmental glomerular sclerosis (Niaudet & Rotig, 1997). One patient had a decrease in glomerular filtration rate at 9 years of age. Patients in addition had myopathy, ophthalmoplegia, pigmentary retinopathy, hearing loss, and hypoparathyroidism. More recently, nephrotic syndrome and segmental glomerular sclerosis have been related to disorders of the coenzyme Q10 biogenetic genes (López *et al.*, 2006; DiMauro *et al.*, 2007; Diomedi-Camassei *et al.*, 2007).

Renal disease in patients with mitochondrial cytopathies may also consist of tubulointerstitial nephritis. Six patients with chronic renal insufficiency without proximal tubular losses have been reported (Niaudet & Rotig, 1997). Renal biopsy in patients showed diffuse interstitial fibrosis with tubular atrophy and sclerosed glomeruli within the area of interstitial fibrosis. All patients developed extrarenal symptoms including hearing loss, cardiomyopathy, myopathy, ataxia, developmental delay, ophthalmoplegia, and diabetes mellitus.

Gut

Gastrointestinal symptoms include recurrent vomiting, colonic pseudo-obstruction or untreatable diarrhoea. Gastrointestinal symptoms are particularly frequent in a condition called mitochondrial neurogastrointestinal encephalomyopathy (MNGIE) or POLIP (polyneuropathy, ophthalmoplegia, leucoencephalopathy, and intestinal pseudo-obstruction), an autosomal recessive disease clinically defined by gastrointestinal dysmotility, cachexia, ptosis, ophthalmoparesis, peripheral neuropathy, white matter changes in brain magnetic resonance imaging, and mitochondrial abnormalities. Loss-of-function mutations in the thymidine phosphorylase gene induce pathological accumulations of thymidine and deoxyuridine, which in turn cause mitochondrial mtDNA defects (depletion, multiple deletions, and point mutations).

Another condition where gastrointestinal symptoms are prominent is ethylmalonic encephalopathy, a rare metabolic disorder with an autosomal recessive mode of inheritance that is clinically characterized by neuromotor delay, hyperlactic acidaemia, recurrent petechiae, orthostatic acrocyanosis, and chronic diarrhoea. Increased urinary levels of ethylmalonic acid and methylsuccinic acid are the main biochemical features of the disorder (Hirano et al., 2006; Tiranti et al., 2006).

Villous atrophy syndrome has been recognized as an mtDNA rearrangement defect. A complex-III deficiency was found in the muscle of affected patients. Southern blot analysis showed evidence of heteroplasmic mtDNA rearrangements that involved deletion and deletion duplication. Two different mutations were described in the two children reported. In one patient, a deletion spanning 3380 base pairs encompassed three genes for complex I and three transfer ribonuclease genes. The deletion in the second patient was larger (Cormier-Daire et al., 1994).

Heart

Hypertrophic cardiomyopathy is the most commonly reported type of cardiomyopathy associated with mitochondrial respiratory chain disorders (Yaplito-Lee et al., 2007). Cardiac hypertrophy in these disorders is thought to result from an increased oxidative stress, and its pathogenic mechanism to involve cross-talk between several cellular signalling pathways as well as several transcription factors. Supraventricular tachycardia (Wolf-Parkinson-White) has rarely been reported in association with hypertrophic cardiomyopathy.

Dilated cardiomyopathy is nearly as common as hypertrophic cardiomyopathy, and a change in pattern (an 'undulating cardiomyopathy' type) can be observed (Yaplito-Lee et al., 2007). Dilated cardiomyopathy is thought to result from acute oxidative stress caused by a surge in reactive oxygen species, inducing damage to the mitochondrial DNA, as shown in a mouse model.

Cardiac conduction disturbances have been reported in Kearn-Sayre syndrome with large mitochondrial DNA deletions (Anan et al., 1995).

Repeat cardiac assessment as part of monitoring disease progression is warranted in patients with confirmed mitochondrial oxidative phosphorylation (OXPHOS) disorders, even in the absence of clinical cardiac symptoms. Patients with OXPHOS defects who present with primary cardiac manifestations have a poorer outcome.

Endocrine system

Besides common MELAS syndromes, patients may develop endocrine disorders such as neuroendocrine dysfunction with growth hormone deficiency, hypothalamopituitary hypothyroidism, hypogonadotropic hypogonadism, hypoparathyroidism, diabetes, and short stature (Stark & Roden, 2007).

Kearn-Sayre syndrome, a form of mitochondrial myopathy, is also associated with a variety of endocrine and metabolic abnormalities, in particular growth hormone deficiency (short stature), hypogonadism, diabetes mellitus, thyroid disease, hyperaldosteronism, hypomagnesaemia, and calcification abnormalities. These patients can also show features of Pearson's syndrome – a rare, often fatal disorder of infancy characterized by impaired bone marrow, exocrine pancreatic, hepatic and renal function, and adrenal insufficiency (Bruno et al., 1998).

Finally, a few patients with diabetes mellitus have mitochondrial disorders. Patients with Kearn-Sayre syndrome, MELAS syndrome, and Wolfram syndrome may develop diabetes (DiMauro, 1999). The MELAS mtDNA – involving substitution of guanine for arginine at position 3243 of tRNA leu(UUR) – has been described in several families with maternally transmitted diabetes as well as in sporadic cases with insulin-dependent or non-insulin-dependent diabetes (Kadowaki et al., 1994). This mutation was also reported in a family with maternally inherited cardiomyopathy, diabetes mellitus, sensorineural deafness, and renal failure that was not related to diabetes mellitus (DiMauro, 1999). It may be postulated that mutations of mtDNA in pancreatic β cells contribute to the development of diabetes mellitus.

Liver

Hepatic manifestations of mitochondrial disorders range from hepatic steatosis, cholestasis, and chronic liver disease with insidious onset to neonatal liver failure, which is often associated with neuromuscular symptoms, multisystem involvement, and lactic acidaemia. The liver disease is usually progressive and eventually fatal. Current medical therapy of mitochondrial hepatopathies is largely ineffective and the prognosis is usually poor. These conditions include primary disorders, in which the mitochondrial defect is the primary cause of the liver disorder, and secondary disorders, in which a secondary insult to mitochondria is caused either by a genetic defect that affects non-mitochondrial proteins or by an acquired (exogenous) injury to mitochondria. Examples of secondary mitochondrial hepatopathies include Reye syndrome, Wilson disease, and valproic acid hepatotoxicity (Lee & Sokol, 2007). Primary mitochondrial diseases can be further divided into those caused by mutations affecting mtDNA genes and those caused by mutations in nuclear genes that encode mitochondrial respiratory chain proteins or cofactors.

Several specific molecular defects in nuclear genes (*SCO1*, *BCS1L*, *POLG*, *DGUOK*, and *MPV17*, and deletion or rearrangement of mitochondrial DNA) have been identified in recent years.

Four male siblings with mitochondrial cytochrome c oxidase deficiency due to compound heterozygosity for mutations in the *SCO1* gene have been reported. They were predominantly affected by hepatic failure in infancy, lactic acidosis, and neurodevelopmental delays. One patient died at age 2 months, a second at the age of 5 days. Histopathological studies of the liver showed swollen hepatocytes with microvesicular lipid vacuoles and panlobular steatosis. A muscle biopsy sample showed an accumulation of lipid droplets. *SCO1* mutations are associated with COX deficiency and SCO1 is a COX assembly nuclear gene. The *SCO1* gene, located at chromosome 17p13.1, is believed to encode a protein functioning as a copper chaperone that transfers copper from Cox17p, a copper-binding protein of the cytosol and mitochondrial intermembrane space, to the mitochondrial COX subunit II.

A mutation in *BCS1L* has been found to be associated with mitochondrial neonatal liver failure. Deficient activity of complex III of the respiratory chain has been reported in the liver (Lee & Sokol, 2007), fibroblasts, or muscle in affected infants, who have hepatic failure, lactic acidosis, renal tubulopathy, and varying degrees of encephalopathy. Three mutations in *BCS1L* were demonstrated in three affected families. Subsequently, it was confirmed that mutations in *BCS1L* were associated with fatal complex III deficiency and liver failure in two siblings. *BCS1L* is a nuclear gene encoding proteins involved in the assembly of respiratory complex III (Lee & Sokol, 2007).

The mitochondrial deoxynucleoside salvage pathway is regulated by nuclear encoded enzymes, including dGK and TK2 (Lee & Sokol, 2007). Human dGK phosphorylates deoxyguanosine and deoxyadenosine, whereas TK2 phosphorylates deoxythymidine, deoxycytidine, and deoxyuridine. It has been proposed that an imbalance of this mitochondrial dNTP pool is responsible for both the hepatocerebral and myopathic forms of mitochondrial cytopathy. Mutations in two genes involved in this pathway have been identified in patients with mitochondrial cytopathy: deoxyguanosine kinase (*DGUOK*) in the hepatocerebral form and *TK2* in the myopathic form (Lee & Sokol, 2007).

Mandel et al. (2001), using homozygosity-mapping in three consanguineous kindreds affected by hepatocerebral mitochondrial cytopathy, mapped this disease to chromosome 2p13, which encompasses the gene *DGUOK* encoding dGK. A single-nucleotide deletion (204delA) within the coding region of *DGUOK* was identified. The reduction in enzymatic activities of mitochondrial respiratory chain complexes containing mtDNA-encoded subunits (complexes I, III, and IV but not complex II, which is solely encoded by nuclear genes) was demonstrated in the liver but not in muscle, showing the tissue-specific nature of this disorder. However, Salviati et al. (2002) screened the frequency of *DGUOK* mutations in 21 patients with hepatocerebral mitochondrial cytopathy and noted that *DGUOK* mutations were present in only 14 per cent, suggesting this was not the only gene responsible for mitochondrial cytopathy in the liver. Patients with DGUOK mutations present with lactic acidosis, hepatomegaly, hypoglycaemia, jaundice, and encephalopathy with hypotonia, hyperreflexia, and nystagmus, and oculogyric crises.

Two other nuclear genes have recently been linked to the hepatocerebral form of mitochondrial cytopathy (Naviaux & Nguyen, 2004; Spinazzola et al., 2006) – *POLG* and *MPV17*. Mutations in DNA *POLG*, which is confined to mitochondria but encoded by a nuclear gene, have now been described in infants with mitochondrial cytopathy and in older children with Alpers-Huttenlocher disease. Most of the cases with mitochondrial cytopathy in early childhood are associated with at least one mutation in the linker region of *POLG* and one in the polymerase domain. More recently, Spinazzola and colleagues. (Spinazzola et al., 2006) used a novel integrative genomics approach to discover mutations in the nuclear gene *MPV17* in three families affected by the hepatocerebral form of mitochondrial cytopathy. This gene encodes an inner mitochondrial membrane protein of uncertain function.

Mutations in *POLG* have recently been shown to be common in patients with Alpers-Huttenlocher syndrome. The mtDNA polymerase g (POLG) is essential for mtDNA replication and repair. Polymerase g is composed of a 140-kDa catalytic (α) subunit that contains DNA polymerase, 3-5 exonuclease, and dRP (deoxyribose phosphate) lyase activities and a 55-kDa accessory (β) subunit that functions as a processivity and DNA binding factor.

In Alpers-Huttenlocher syndrome, children are usually normal at birth, with some developmental delay in infancy, often with hypotonia and bouts of vomiting. The seizure disorder usually has an abrupt onset with accompanying progressive atrophy of the brain (Fig. 1A, 1B). Lactate is frequently high on *in vivo* MRS (Fig. 1C). Clinical and laboratory signs of liver disease often appear later; biochemical evidence of liver disease is sometimes present before the onset of seizures. EEG and visual evoked potentials are abnormal. Most patients die before the age of 3 years. Less frequently, a late presentation occurs, even up to 25 years of age. Some patients also have visual disturbances. Liver pathology – including fatty changes, abnormal bile duct architecture, and fibrosis – is unrelated to anticonvulsant therapy. Neuropathology shows severe cortical neurodegeneration and astrocytosis.

A deficiency in mitochondrial POLG activity and mtDNA depletion was first reported in a patient with Alpers-Huttenlocher syndrome in 1999 (Naviaux & Nguyen, 2004). These investigators reported that in two unrelated pedigrees with this syndrome, each affected child harboured a homozygous mutation in exon 17 of *POLG* that led to a Glu873Stop mutation just upstream of the polymerase domain of the protein. In addition, each affected child was heterozygous for the G1681A mutation in exon 7, which led to an Ala467Thr substitution in POLG, within the linker region of the protein. Biochemical examination of muscle and fibroblasts for abnormally reduced activity of mitochondrial respiratory enzymes is generally normal in Alpers-Huttenlocher syndrome, while abnormal results are obtained in the liver. Thus liver biopsy for biochemical examination for abnormally reduced activity of mitochondrial respiratory enzymes and for mtDNA depletion should be recommended as the first step in the diagnosis of this condition, although some patients can be negative with this test.

Vu et al. (2001) first demonstrated mtDNA depletion in liver biopsies from two patients with Navajo neurohepatopathy, which was consistent with the hypothesis that a nuclear gene might be responsible for this autosomal recessive disease. Navajo neurohepatopathy is an autosomal recessive multisystem disorder prevalent in the Navajo population of the southwestern USA. Patients with this condition present with liver disease, severe sensory and motor neuropathy, corneal anaesthesia and scarring, cerebral leucoencephalopathy, failure to thrive, and recurrent metabolic acidosis with intercurrent illness. A genome-wide scan, carried out with 400 DNA microsatellite markers, showed mapping of the disease to chromosome 2p24.1. The gene was *MPV17* (Karadimas et al., 2006), involved in mtDNA maintenance and in the regulation of OXPHOS and which is localized to the inner mitochondrial membrane. The sequencing of *MPV17* in six patients with Navajo neurohepatopathy from five families in 2006 demonstrated the same homozygous disease-causing R50Q mutations in exon 2 in all patients, confirming a founder effect in this disease. Thus it is now clear that Navajo neurohepatopathy is indeed a form of mtDNA depletion with a unique clinical presentation in Navajos.

Prospective longitudinal multicentre studies will be needed to address the gaps in our knowledge in these rare liver diseases. The role of liver transplantation in patients with liver failure remains poorly defined because of the systemic nature of the disease that does not respond to transplantation.

Blood

Haematological manifestations of mitochondrial cytopathies include aplastic, megaloblastic, and sideroblastic anaemia, leucopenia, neutropenia, thrombocytopenia, and pancytopenia. In isolated cases either permanent or recurrent eosinophilia has been observed. Haematological abnormalities may occur together with syndromic or non-syndromic mitochondrial cytopathies. Syndromic mitochondrial cytopathies, in which haematological manifestations predominate, are the Pearson syndrome (pancytopenia), Kearns-Sayre syndrome (anaemia), Barth syndrome (neutropenia), and the autosomal recessive mitochondrial myopathy, lactic acidosis and sideroblastic anaemia syndrome (MLASA) (Fernandez-Vizarra et al., 2007). The association of Pearson syndrome and a specific deletion in mtDNA was first reported in 1990 by Rotig et al. (1990). It is now established that mtDNA rearrangements are present in all patients with Pearson syndrome, with large deletions (4,000–5,000 base pairs) predominating in three quarters of the reported cases. The most common deletion is located between nt 8,488 and nt 13,460. The proteins affected by this deletion include respiratory chain enzymes (complex I is the most severely affected), two subunits of complex V, one subunit of complex IV, and five transfer RNA genes. Other mtDNA deletions of differing lengths are associated with clusters of the characteristic clinical manifestations.

Another rare form of mitochondrial cytopathy is X-linked sideroblastic anaemia with ataxia (XLSA/A) – a rare syndromic form of inherited sideroblastic anaemia associated with spinocerebellar ataxia, due to mutations in the mitochondrial ATP-binding cassette transporter Abcb7 (Pondarre et al., 2007).

Anaemia has been described in isolated cases of Leigh's syndrome, MERRF syndrome, and Leber's hereditary optic neuropathy. Anaemia, leucopenia, thrombocytopenia, eosinophilia, or pancytopenia can frequently also be found in non-syndromic mitochondrial cytopathies with or without involvement of other tissues. Therapy of blood cell involvement in MID comprises application of antioxidants, vitamins, iron, bone marrow stimulating factors, or substitution of cells.

Skin

Reviewing the literature of skin disorders associated with mitochondrial encephalomyopathies, the most frequent sign is lipoma. Symmetrical cervical lipomas are a presenting feature of Ekbom's syndrome of cervical lipomas associated with myoclonic epilepsy, MERRF, and mutations in the mtDNA tRNA LysUUR 8344A-G (Bodemer *et al.*, 1999).

Excluding lipomas, skin findings that have been reported in several other patients include discoloration, hirsutism, and anhidrosis. Pigment alterations consistent with poikiloderma have been found in some, along with acrocyanosis and vitiligo. Acrocyanosis has been reported in Pearson syndrome, and the presence of episodic acrocyanosis is part of the syndromic association of ethylmalonic encephalopathy, a devastating infantile metabolic disorder affecting the brain, gastrointestinal tract and peripheral vessels. The gene responsible of the ethylmalonic encephalopathy is *ETHE1* (Tiranti *et al.*, 2006) and the principal signs of the syndrome are recurrent petechiae, orthostatic acrocyanosis and chronic diarrhoea.

Other discolorations of the skin have been reported, such as periorbital darkening, generalized hyperpigmentation associated with adrenal insufficiency, cutis marmorata, and jaundice in patients with the hepatocerebral form of mitochondrial DNA depletion syndrome (MDDS) caused by mutations in the nuclear-encoded mitochondrial deoxyguanosine kinase gene *DGUOK* (Mandel *et al.*, 2001) or in the MPV17 gene (Spinazzola *et al.*, 2006).

Another characteristic finding of mitochondrial encephalomyopathies is hirsutism or hypotrichosis which has been reported in patients with Pearson syndrome and quite frequently in severe Leigh syndrome with encephalomyopathy, cytochrome-c-oxidase deficiency and mutations in the *SURF-1* gene. Alopecia, alopecia with brittle hair, and trichothiodystrophy have also been reported (Bodemer *et al.*, 1999).

Disorders involving cellular organelles and including lysosomal, peroxisomal, glycosylation, and cholesterol synthesis defects

Peroxisomal disorders

The peroxisomes are small, ubiquitous, cellular organelles that play an important role in oxygen, lipid, and glucose metabolism. More than 50 biochemical pathways have been characterized within peroxisomes. Some of the major peroxisomal functions are peroxisomal oxidation and respiration, the regulation of adipose cell number, the transport and cellular uptake of lipids, intracellular balance between free and bound fatty acids, conversion of fatty acids to their activated CoA form, penetration of fatty acids into membrane-delineated organelles, microsomal?-oxidation, β-oxidation and ketogenesis, and the formation of glycerol for triglyceride synthesis, cholesterol synthesis, as well as sex steroid metabolism, plasmalogen biosynthesis, insulin sensitivity, catabolism of purines and D-amino acids, L-α-hydroxy acids, and urates, and the metabolism of a diverse group of xenobiotics (Wanders & Waterham, 2006).

There are at least 24 identified disorders caused by inherited peroxisomal defects (Baumgartner *et al.*, 1998; Moser & Raymond 1998; Moser, 1999) and biological markers for diagnosis are numerous (Table 3).

Table 3. Summary of peroxisomal disorders

Disorder	Symptoms	Morphology of peroxisomes	Molecular disorder
Peroxisomal biogenesis disorder with loss of multiple peroxisomal functions			
• Classical ZS • NALD • Infantile Refsum disease	Facial dysmorphia, developmental delay, delayed closure of fontanelle, seizure, cortical dysplasia,	Absent or mosaicism	Caused by mutations in any of several different genes involved in peroxisome biogenesis: peroxin-1 (PEX1; 602136), peroxin-2 (PEX2; 170993), peroxin-3 (PEX3; 603164), peroxin-5 (PEX5; 600414), peroxin-6 (PEX6; 601498), peroxin-12 (PEX12; 601758), peroxin-14 (PEX14; 601791), and peroxin-26 (PEX26; 608666)
Peroxisome biogenesis disorder with loss of at least two peroxisomal functions • RCDP (classic and atypical phenotype) • Unclassified peroxisomal biogenesis disorder	Ichthyosiform lesions Limb defects	Enlarged Present or absent	PEX7 gene (601757), which encodes the peroxisomal type 2 targeting signal (PTS2) receptor Deficiency of plasmalogens in phospholipids from red cells and deficient activity of the enzyme DHAPAT
Loss of a single peroxisomal function			
• RCDP	Ichthyosiform, limb defects*, alopecia	Normal	Isolated DHAPAT or alkyl-DHAP XCDP2; XCDP1 synthase
• XCDP2 CHILD#	Ichthyosiform Follicular atrophoderma Limb defects	Normal	Abnormal sterol metabolism with increased 8-dehydrocholesterol and cholest-8(9)en- 3β-ol deficiency 3β-hydroxysteroid-Δ8, Δ7-isomerase
• CHILD#	Ichythosiform*	Decreased	DHAPAT and catalase decreased
• X-linked adrenoleucodystrophy *Clinical forms:* Childhood form Juvenile form Adult cerebral form Adult Addison only Adrenomyeloneuropathy	Hyperpigmentation. Progressive neurological disorder, spastic paraplegia, peripheral neuropathy, sphincter disturbances, limb and truncal ataxia, hypogonadism	Present	ALD protein
• Pseudo-NALD		Enlarged	Acyl-CoA oxidase
• Bifunctional enzyme deficiency	Facial dysmorphia	Abnormal	Bi(tri)functional enzyme deficiency.
• Pseudo-Zellweger syndrome	Facial dysmorphia	Enlarged	Peroxisomal 3-oxoacyl-CoA thiolase
• Mevalonic aciduria	Morbilliform rash Oedema	NA	Mevalonate kinase
• Trihydroxycholestanoic acidaemia	Facial dysmorphia	NA	Branched chain acyl-CoA oxidase
• Classic Refsum disease	Ichthyosiform*	NA	Phytanoxyl-CoA hydroxylase
• Glutaric aciduria type III		Normal	Peroxisomal glutaryl-CoA oxidase
• Hyperoxaluria type I	Livedo racemosa-like erythema of the limbs	Smaller	Alanine glyoxylate aminotransferase
• Acatasaemia	Ulcers/gangrene	Normal	Catalase

#With X-linked dominant inheritance, the ichthyosiform eruption follows Blaskho's line because of random inactivation of one X chromosome.
• Often with a more psoriasiform with an associated inflammatory component.
ALD, adrenoleucodystrophy; CDP, chondrodysplasia punctata; CHILD, congenital hemidysplasia with ichthyosiform erythroderma and limb defects; CoA, coenzyme A; DHAP, dihydroxyacetone phosphate; DHAPAT, dihydroxyacetone phosphate acyltransferase; NA, not available; NALD, neonatal adrenoleucodystrophy; RCDP, rhizomelic chondrodysplasia punctata; ZS, Zellweger syndrome; X, X chromosome; X1, X-linked recessive; X2, X-linked dominant; XCDP2, X-linked dominant chondrodysplasia punctata.

Until recently peroxisomal disorders were listed under three main clinical syndromes: Zellweger syndrome, neonatal adrenoleucodystrophy, and infantile Refsum disease. Polymalformations (Fig. 2A–D) occur in classic Zellweger syndrome, as well as in rhizomelic (autosomal recessive) chondrodysplasia punctata (RCDP), X-linked dominant chondrodysplasia punctata (Conradi-Hunermann-Happle syndrome) or X-linked recessive chondrodysplasia punctata, and congenital hemidysplasia with ichthyosiform erythroderma and limb defects (CHILD) syndrome (Baumgartner et al., 1998; Moser & Raymond 1998). Neurological manifestations predominate in neonatal adrenoleucodystrophy, and hepatodigestive manifestations in infantile Refsum disease (Baumgartner et al., 1998). However, with expansion in our understanding of the biochemical phenotypes within the spectrum of peroxisomal disorders, it has become obvious that there is little or no relation between the clinical and biochemical phenotypes (Baumgartner et al., 1998) (Table 4).

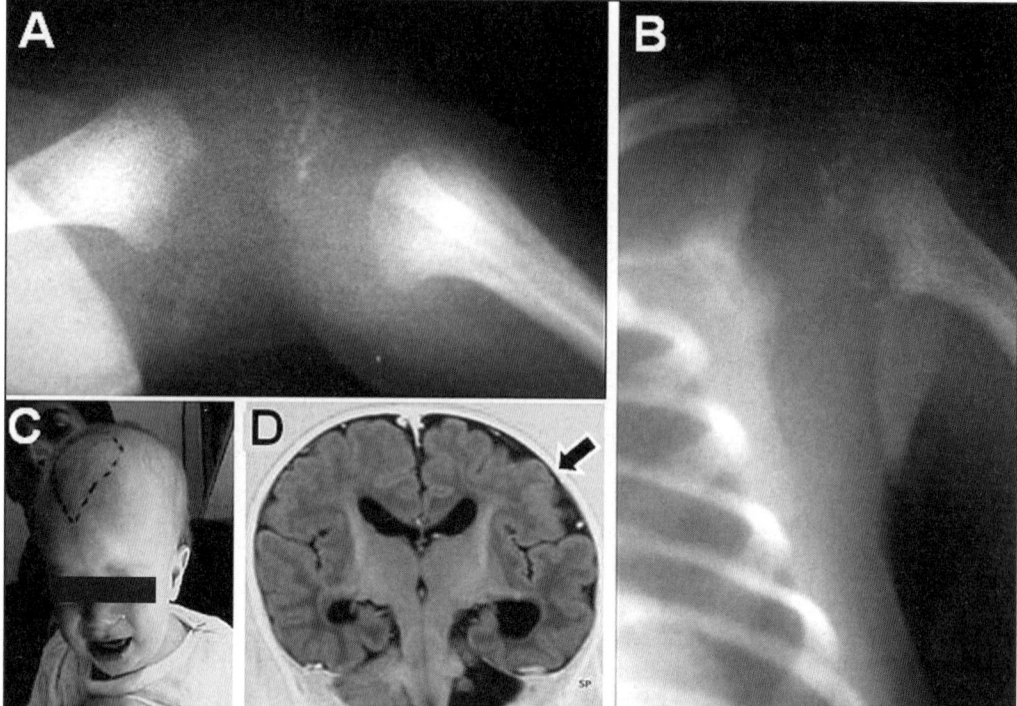

Fig. 2. Some characteristic of peroxisomal disorders. (A), (B) Stippled epiphyses (in shoulder and acetabular regions). (C) A child with Zellweger syndrome with macrocephaly and a large fontanelle. (D) The child in (C) had epilepsy associated with focal cortical dysplasia (arrow).

Table 4. Biochemical assays for the diagnosis of peroxisomal disorders

Biological material	Assay
Plasma	VLCFAs; phytanic and pristanic acids; THCA and DHCA; pipecolic acid, plasmalogens, and PUFAs including DHA, 8-dehydrocholesterol and cholest-8(9)-en-3b-ol
Urines	Organic acids and pipecolic acid
Red blood cells	Plasmalogens and PUFAs including DHA
Fibroblasts	Plasmalogen biosynthesis, DHAPAT, and alkyl-DHAP synthase particle-bound catalase; VLCFAs, β-oxidation, and phytanic acid oxidation; immunoblotting β-oxidation proteins
Liver	Cytochemical localization of peroxisomal proteins, trilamellar inclusions, and insoluble lipid

CA, cholic acid; CDCA, chenodeoxycholic acid; DHA, docosahexaenoic acid; DHAP, dihydroxyacetone phosphate; DHAPAT, dihydroxyacetone phosphate acyltransferase; DHCA, dihydroxycholestanoic acid; PUFAs, polyunsaturated fatty acids; THCA, trihydroxycholestanoic acid; VLCFAs, very long chain fatty acids.

RCDP, CDPX2, autosomal recessive chondrodysplasia punctata, and CHILD syndrome are the syndromes most commonly associated with significant cutaneous manifestations (Table 3), and each is related to one or more of the various peroxisomal-related biochemical abnormalities in Table 4 or the morphological abnormalities listed in Table 3. Conversely, the same biochemical defects, or even the same genetic complementation group, can be associated with different clinical phenotypes – that is, classic Zellweger syndrome and infantile Refsum disease and a form of CDPX2 and CHILD syndrome (Moser, 1999). Thus a newer classification of peroxisomal disorders has been proposed, based on the extent of peroxisomal dysfunction (Table 3). However, this biochemical classification is not helpful for evaluating the clinical symptoms. Peroxisomal disorders are classified genetically as those in which the organelle is not formed normally – disorders of peroxisome biogenesis – and those that involve a single peroxisomal enzyme (Moser, 1999). Twelve peroxisome biogenesis disorders have been defined, and molecular defects have been identified in most of them, all involving defects in protein import mechanisms (Moser, 1999). Cytoplasmic polyribosomes synthesize peroxisomal matrix proteins, which are imported post-translationally. Factors required for this import of peroxisomal proteins are called peroxins (Moser, 1999).

Chondrodysplasia punctata is a pattern of abnormal punctate calcification of dystrophic epiphyseal cartilage and certain other cartilaginous structures. Peroxisomal disorders are the most common associations. However, chondrodysplasia punctata is seen with other genetic conditions – for example, ganglosidosis, mucolipidosis II, and trisomy 21 – and can be acquired *in utero* secondary to warfarin embryopathy, phenacetin, fetal alcohol syndrome, and hydantion (Lawrence et al., 1989).

Chondrodysplasia punctata is a consistent finding in a group of peroxisomal disorders, especially those with characteristic but variable cutaneous manifestations (Moser, 1999). Qualitative and quantitative peroxisomal dysregulation is demonstrated in most cases of RCDP, CDPX2, autosomal dominant chondrodysplasia punctata, and CHILD syndrome, and specific genetic defects have been identified in RCDP and in some patients with CDPX2 and CHILD syndrome (Moser, 1999).

The phenotypic expression of the known peroxin disorders and enzymatic defects appears to vary with the nature of the mutation. In general, the severe forms manifest as classical Zellweger syndrome, while milder phenotypes present as neonatal adrenoleucodystrophy and infantile Refsum disease, and are associated with mutations that do not abolish function completely or are associated with mosaicism. Thus, with the continued identification of a specific molecular defect, hopefully there will not only be better genetic counselling and better estimates of prognoses, but also improved understanding of the divergent and overlapping spectrum of clinical findings in these diseases.

Other associated clinical findings vary but include cataracts, short stature, dysmorphic facies, a variety of skeletal malformations, and an ichthyosiform erythroderma in the neonatal period.

CDPX2 has a relatively good prognosis and frequently shows asymmetrical bone defects, cataracts, and skin lesions, while RCDP is more severe, being a bilateral and diffuse disease normally leading to death within the first year of life.

CHILD syndrome is characterized by unilateral ichthyosiform erythroderma which, unlike CDPX2, is often inflammatory with psoriasiform hyperplasia, though most cases show a similar X-linked dominant inheritance following Blashko's lines. Additional clinical findings in patients with CHILD syndrome include ipsilateral limb reduction defects and, in some cases, ipsilateral internal organ defects. Partial resolution of the cutaneous manifestations may occur in CHILD syndrome, but it is not as characteristic as in CDPX2, and internal organ involvement is not characteristic of CDPX2.

A relevant neurological disorder is adrenoleucodystrophy or the spastic paraplegia variant called adrenomyeloneuropathy, although this disease never has its onset in the first 2 years of life (for a summary see Table 3).

Lysosomal diseases

Lysosomal storage disorders are a group of over 50 inherited diseases, which have a combined incidence of 1:7,700 to 1:8,275 live births (Meikle *et al.*, 1999, Dionisi-Vici *et al.*, 2002). Each disorder is caused by the dysfunction of either a lysosomal enzyme or a lysosome associated protein involved in enzyme activation, enzyme targeting, or lysosomal biogenesis (Table 5).

Table 5. Human lysosomal disorders: pathophysiological classification

A: Defective enzyme activity (missing or defective protein, defects of activator or protective protein)	Hexosamindase A and B; GM1 and GM2 AB variant; fucosidosis; mucopolysaccharidoses; sphingolipidoses; glycoproteinoses (ADP-ribose protein hydrolase); mucolipidoses I and IV; glycogenosis type 2; galactosialidosis; acid lipase deficiency
B: Enzyme misplacement (lysosomal biogenesis)	Mucolipidoses II and III
C: Transport defects	Cystinosis; sialic acid storage diseases
D: Unknown	Ceroidlipofuscinoses; Chediak-Higashi syndrome

GM1, GM2, gangliosidoses.

The most frequent cause by far is the absence of an enzyme needed for degradation. This lack of enzyme activity can be caused by mutations leading to absence of the protein or to defective enzyme protein, by defects of activators needed for the degradation of some sphingolipids, or by defects of protective stabilizing proteins or peptide sequences. The largest group of lysosomal disorders is related to deficiencies of hydrolases involved in the degradation of heteroglycans, presenting as mucopolysaccharidoses, sphingolipidoses, glycoproteinoses, and mucolipidosis I and IV (Tables 6, 7, and 8).

The second type of lysosomal disease results from defective synthesis of the specific carbohydrate recognition marker (the mannose-6-phosphate receptor system) as shown in mucolipidosis II and III (Table 6). Research on these disorders has increased our basic knowledge about the carbohydrate recognition marker.

The third group is likely to comprise transport defects through the lysosomal membrane. Examples in the human are cystine storage in cystinosis and N-acetylneuraminic acid storage in Salla disease (Table 7).

There remain diseases which from morphological observations are probably caused by a lysosomal dysfunction but for which the biochemical and pathophysiological defects have not yet been established (Table 9). The different forms of the large group of ceroidolipofuscinosis and the Chediak-Higashi syndrome are among these diseases (Table 9).

Table 6. Lysosomal storage disorders: mucopolysaccaridosis and mucolipidosis

Disease	Enzyme deficiency	Storage material	Screening test	Diagnostic test	Prenatal diagnosis	Symptoms
MPS						
MPS I (Hurler, Scheie)	Iduronidase	DS, HS	Urine GAGs	WBC	CVB	Umbilical and inguinal herniae, coarse face, organomegaly, MR, multiple bone dysostosis
MPS II (Hunter)	Iduronate-2-sulphatase	DS, HS	Urine GAGs	Plasma	CVB2 As	
MPS III (Sanfilippo)						Same as above
IIIA	Heparin-N sulphatase	HS	Urine GAGs	WBC	CVB	
IIIB	N-acetyl-glucosaminidase	HS	Urine GAGs	Plasma	CVB	
IIIC	Acetyl CoA glucosamine N-acetyl-transferase	HS	Urine GAGs	WBC	CVB	
IIID	N-acetyl-glucosamine-6-sulphatase	HS	Urine GAGs	WBC	CVB	
MPS IV (Morquio) IVA						
IVB	Galactose-6-sulphatase	KS	Urine GAGs	WBC	CVB	Hydrops fetalis reported
	β-galactosidase	KS	Urine GAGs	WBC	CVB	
MPS VI (Maroteaux-Lamy)	Galactosamine-4-sulphatase	DS	Urine GAGs	WBC	CVB	Endocardial fibroelastosis
MPS VII (Sly)	β-glucuronidase	HS, DS	Urine GAGs	WBC	CVB	Hydrops fetalis is common
MPS IX	Hyaluronidase	HA	None	Cultured cells	Unknown	
Mucolipidoses						
ML I (sialidosis I and II)	Neuraminidase	SA	Urine sialic acid	Cultured cells	Cultured cells	Coarse face organomegaly, MR, multiple bone dysostosis endocardial fibroelastosis. Congenital form: hydrops, ascites, stillbirth. Neonatal presentation common
ML II (I Cell)	Transferase	Many urine oligos	Plasma	Cultured cells or AF		
ML III (pseudo Hurler)						
IIIA	As ML II	Many urine oligos	Plasma	Cultured cells or AF		Course face, MR multiple bone dysostosis
IIIC	Transferase δ-sub-unit	Many urine oligos	Plasma	Cultured cells or AF		
ML IV	Unknown	Unknown	None	Histology	Histology CVB	Corneal clouding

AF, amniotic fluid; CVB, chorionic villus biopsy; DS, dermatan sulphate; GAGs, glycosaminoglycans; HA, hyaluronic acid; HS, heparin sulphate; IVA, isovaleric acidaemia; KS, keratin sulphate; MR, mental retardation; oligos, oligosaccharides; plasma, plasma enzyme assay; SA, sialic acid; WBC, white blood cell enzyme assay.

Table 7. Lysosomal storage disorders: sphingolipidoses

Disease	Enzyme deficiency	Storage material	Screening test	Diagnostic test	Prenatal diagnosis	Symptoms
GM1-gangliosidosis	β-Galactosidase	KS, oligos, glycolipids	Urine oligos	WBC	CVB	Common: dysmorphism, organomegaly, hydrops fetalis (see Table 10)
GM2-gangliosidosis: Tay-Sachs	β-Hexosaminidase A	Globoside, oligos, glycolipids	None	WBC	CVB	
Sandhoff	β-Hexosaminidase A and B	GM2-gang: oligos	None	WBC	CVB	
GM2-gangliosidosis	GM2 activator GM2-gangliosidosis	Glycolipids	None	Cultured cells	Unknown	
Globoid cell leucodystrophy: Krabbe	Galacto-cerebrosidase	Galacto-sylceramide	None	WBC	CVB	Hypertonia, irritability, twitching
MLD	Arylsulphatase A	Sulphatides	None	WBC	CVB	Leucodystrophy
MLD: saposin B activator (sap B)	Sulphitides	GM1-gang: glycolipids	None	Sulphatide loading of cultured cells or DNA	CVB	Leucodystrophy
Fabry disease	α-Galactosidase A	Galactosyl-sphingo-lipids, oligos	None	WBC	CVB	See text
Gaucher disease	β-Glucosidase	Gluco-ceramide	None	WBC	CVB	Severe type II disease
Gaucher disease: saposin C	As above	None	Unknown	Unknown	CVB	Ichthyosis, organomegaly, hydrops, ataxia, ophthalmoplegia, MR
Farber disease	Ceramidase	Ceramide	None	WBC	CVB	Diffuse joint swelling and hoarseness can appear as early as 2 weeks of age Hydrops also reported
Niemann-Pick A and B	Sphingomyelinase	Sphingo-myelin	None	WBC	CVB	Prolonged jaundice and hydrops reported in type A

AF, amniotic fluid; CVB, chorionic villus biopsy; DS, dermatan sulphate; GAGs, glycosaminoglycans; gang, gangliosidosis; HA, hyaluronic acid; HS, heparin sulphate; KS, keratin sulphate; MR, mental retardation; oligos, oligosaccharides; plasma, plasma enzyme assay; SA, sialic acid; WBC, white blood cell enzyme assay.

Table 8. Lysosomal storage disorders: accumulation of glycoproteins, lipids, and glycogen

Disease	Enzyme deficiency	Storage material	Screening test	Diagnostic test	Prenatal diagnosis	Symptoms
Glycoproteinoses						
α-Mannosidosis	α-Mannosidase	α-Mannosides	Urine oligos	WBC	CVB	See Table 10
β-Mannosidosis	β-Mannosidase	β-Mannosides	Urine oligos	WBC	CVB	
Fucosidosis	Fucosidase	Fucosides, glycolipids	Urine oligos	WBC	CVB	
Aspartyl-glucosaminuria	Aspartyl-glucosaminidase	Aspartyl-glucosamine	Urine oligos	WBC	CVB	
Schindler disease	α-galactosidase B	N-acetyl-galactosamide, glycolipids	Urine oligos	WBC	CVB	?
Glycogen						
Pompe disease	α-glucosidase	Glycogen	ECG characteristic	Enzyme assay	CVB	Myopathy, CMP can occur ?
Lipid						
Wolman disease and CESD	Acid lipase	Cholesterol esters	None	WBC	CVB	Hydrops fetalis
Niemann-Pick C	*NPC1* gene	Cholesterol, sphingolipids	Filipin staining of cultured cells	Cholesterol esterification studies	CVB	Neonatal liver disease common, ataxia, vertical ophthalmoplegia, hydrops fetalis
Monosaccharide aminoacids and monomers						
ISSD	Sialic acid transporter	Sialic acid, glucuronic acid	Urine oligo	Cultured cells	AF	Hydrops fetalis common
Salla disease	As ISSD	As ISSD	As ISSD	As ISSD		
Cystinosis	Cystine transporter	Cystine	Renal tubular disease	WBC cystine	Cultured cells	
Cobalamin F disease	Cobalamin transporter	Cobalamin	MMA, Homocystinuria	Cultured cells	Cultured cells	Combined methylmalonic aciduria and homocystinuria
Danon disease	Lamp-2	Cytoplasmic debris and glycogen	Muscle biopsy	WBC	CVB	Myopathy, CMP

AF, amniotic fluid; CESD, cholesterol ester storage disease; CMP, cardiomyopathy; CVB, chorionic villus biopsy; DS, dermatan sulphate; GAGs, glycosaminoglycans; HA, hyaluronic acid; HS, heparin sulphate; ISSD, infantile sialic acid storage disease; KS, keratin sulphate; MMA, methylmalonic acidaemia; MR, mental retardation; oligos, oligosaccharides; plasma, plasma enzyme assay; SA, sialic acid; WBC, white blood cell enzyme assay.

Table 9. Lysosomal storage disorders: accumulation of S-acylated proteins and multiple enzyme deficiency

Disease	Enzyme deficiency	Storage material	Screening test	Diagnostic test	Prenatal diagnosis	Symptoms
S-acylated proteins						
Ceroid lipofuscinosis (CLN, Batten's disease)						
CLN 1 (infantile)	Palmitoyl protein thioesterase	Saposins	Histology	Cultured cells and DNA	DNA	MR, epilepsy, myoclonus, progressive cerebral atrophy
CLN 2 (late infantile)	Pepstatin-insensitive carboxypeptidase	Subunit C mitochondrial ATP synthase	Histology	Cultured cells and DNA	DNA	
CLN 3 (juvenile)	Membrane protein	As CLN 2	Histology	DNA	DNA	
CLN 4 A (adult, Kuf disease)	Unknown	As CLN 2	Histology	Histology	Unknown	
CLN 5 (late infantile, Finnish variant)	Membrane protein	As CLN 2	Histology	DNA	DNA	
CLN 6 (late infantile variant)	Unknown	As CLN 2	Histology	Histology	DNA	
CLN 7 (late infantile variant)	MFSD8 transporter protein	Unknown	Histology	Histology	DNA	
CLN 8 (progressive epilepsy with mental retardation, EPMR)	Membrane protein	As CLN 2	Histology	Histology	DNA	
Multiple enzyme deficiencies						
Multiple sulphatase deficiency	Multiple sulphatase enzymes	Sulphatides, glycolipids, GAGs	Urine GAGs	WBC and Plasma Enzyme Assays	CVB	Dysmorphism, hydrocephalus, heart disease, hydrops fetalis
Galactosialidosis	Neuraminidase and β-galactosidase protective protein	Oligos, sialic acid	Urine oligos	Cultured cells	Cultured cells	Hydrops, oedema, proteinuria, hernias, telangiectasia

AF, amniotic fluid; CMP, cardiomyopathy; CVB, chorionic villus biopsy; DS, dermatan sulphate; GAGs, glycosaminoglycans; HA, hyaluronic acid; HS, heparin sulphate; KS, keratin sulphate; MR, mental retardation; oligos, oligosaccharides; plasma, plasma enzyme assay; SA, sialic acid; WBC, white blood cell enzyme assay.

These defects lead to the accumulation of substrate that would normally be degraded in the endosome-lysosome system. In severely affected patients, this ultimately leads to the chronic and progressive deterioration of affected cells, tissues and organs. Most lysosomal storage disorders display a broad spectrum of clinical manifestations, which have previously been identified as clinical subtypes (such as the Hurler/Scheie definition of mucopolysaccharidosis: mucopolysaccharidosis I and the infantile-, juvenile-, and adult-onset forms of Pompe disease). Some of the clinical symptoms that are observed in multiple lysosomal storage disorders (for example, most of the mucopolysaccharidoses) include bone abnormalities, organomegaly, coarse hair/facies (Table 10), and central nervous system dysfunction (Meunzer & Neufeld, 2001). Each disease has a broad spectrum of clinical presentation, ranging from attenuated to severe forms. At the severe end of the clinical spectrum, the onset of pathology tends to be rapid and progressive or may be congenital, as non-immune hydrops fetalis. With the advent of molecular biology/genetics and the characterization of many of the genes associated with lysosomal storage disorders, it is now recognized that the range of clinical severity may in part be ascribed to different mutations within the same gene. However, genotype-phenotype correlations are not always informative.

Many aspects of lysosomal diseases are still poorly understood. There remain a large number of questions. One of these is: what produces the different phenotypical expressions of the same enzyme defect? For instance, the same enzyme, α-hyaluronidase, is defective in two different diseases – Hurler and Scheie mucopolysaccharidosis – both with similar skeletal symptoms, but the first with severe brain damage, the second without any. It is most likely that the explanation of such differences will come from molecular genetics. An important question is why and how a lysosomal storage process causes a disease; this question will be answered by biochemists and biologists. These are related problems. The first concerns the specificity of a disease caused by a certain storage product. What we need is more insight into the biochemical sequelae causing damage to cells and organs and leading to a disease. The other unsolved questions are what happens to the stored material: what is its final destination, how does it get there, does it affect endocytosis, is it undergoing exocytosis, does it affect the function of other cells or organelles? These questions can be answered only by continuous research and collaboration among biochemists, cell biologists, geneticists and clinicians.

Coarse facies (Fig. 3A) together with organomegaly (Fig. 3B) and skeletal dysostosis are the most recurrent symptoms in lysosomal storage disorders (Table 10). A peculiar skin lesion is angiokeratoma corporis diffusum, characteristic of Fabry disease, an X chromosomal recessive disorder (α-galactosidase deficiency with deposition of ceramide trihexoside in various internal organs including kidney and heart). Typical cutaneous manifestations are erythematous-telangiectatic papules on the periumbilical skin, lower abdomen, and buttocks (angiokeratomas). The strategy for assessing the diagnosis of a lysosomal storage disorder is summarized in Table 11. For a comprehensive review on lysosomal disorders see the paper by Scriver *et al.* (2001).

Only three treatment methods are of potential use for lysosomal diseases. Removal of toxic material is the rationale for the treatment of cystinosis with cysteamine. When treatment is started early, the progress of the disease can be halted. Cystinosis and Fabry's disease are diseases for which renal transplantation may be considered in the event of renal failure. Enzyme replacement might be a technique of special interest for the treatment of lysosomal diseases, because the lysosomal enzymes contain a carbohydrate recognition marker for which receptors are expressed on the cell surface pathway to the desired destination, the lysosome. However, practical realization of this concept is at present difficult for most lysosomal storage disorders. Despite these problems, there have been many efforts to apply enzyme replacement for the treatment of human lysosomal diseases. All the earlier trials with discontinuous treatment have been unsatisfactory, because either the enzyme concentration was low, such as in plasma, or the side effects were not acceptable, such as after repeated buffy coat transfusions, or simply

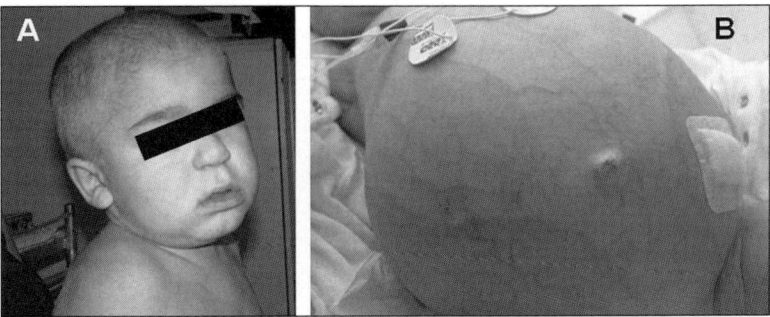

Fig. 3. Frequent features of lysosomal disorders. (A) A child with a typical gargoyl facies. (B) A child affected with Nieman-Pick type A with organomegaly.

Table 10. Conditions of lysosomal deficiency associated with coarse facies

Disorders	Age at onset when first visible and symptoms	Other relevant associated symptoms
Generalized GM1 disease: +230500, β-galactosidase deficiency, chr. 3p21.33	Neonatal	Hydrops fetalis, ascites, oedema, failure to thrive, hypotonia, joint stiffness, osteoporosis, hirsutism
Sialidosis type II: #256550, neuraminidase, chr. 6p21.3	Neonatal	
Galactosialidosis (early infancy): +256540, β-galactosidase + neuraminidase deficiency=cathepsin A, chr. 20q13.1	Neonatal	Bone changes, cherry red spot, corneal opacities, neurological deterioration, perinuclear cataracts, hepatosplenomegaly
Sly syndrome, MPS VII: +253220, beta-glucuronidase deficiency, chr. 7q21.11.	Neonatal	I-cell disease or mucolipidosis II:
#252500, GNPTA, chr. 12q23.3	Neonatal	Fucosidosis type I:
+230000, alpha-fucosidase def., chr.1p34	Early infancy (3–12 months)	Seizures, myoclonus, spasticity, mental retardation, leucodystrophy Salla disease or sialuria Finnish type:
#604369, SLC17A5, 6q14-q15	Early infancy (3–12 months)	Hurler syndrome (MPS type IH):
#607014, alpha-L-iduronidase, 4p16.3	Early infancy (3–12 months)	Inguinal hernias, ear, nose and throat infections, hirsutism Austin disease:
#272200, sulphatase-modifying factor-1 gene, chr. 3p26	1–2 years	Coarse face, Leucodystrophy, Failure to thrive, Hepatosplenomegaly, Bone changes, Mental regression, Quadriplegia, Vacuolated lymphocytes
Mannosidosis: #248500, α-mannosidosis, 19cen-q12	1–2 years	Hypertrichosis, low anterior hairline Anterior hair whorl, heavy eyebrows macrocephaly, flat occiput, deafness angiokeratoma, mental retardation
#248510, β-mannosidosis, 4q22-q25 Maroteaux-Lamy (MPS VI): +253200, arysulphatase B, chr. 5q11-q13	1–2 years	Normal intelligence, macrocephaly, hearing loss, glaucoma, corneal clouding, mild hirsutism
Hunter syndrome (MPS II): +309900, iduronate sulphatase deficiency, Xq28	2–6 years	Developmental delay, mental regression Scaphocephaly, macrocephaly, hearing loss, recurrent otitis media
Aspartylglucosaminuria: +208400, N-aspartyl-beta-glucosaminidase chr. 4q32-q33	2–6 years	Developmental delay, mental regression
Pseudo-Hurler polydystrophy or mucolipidosis IIIA: #252600, α/β-subunits precursor of GLcNAc-phosphotransferase, 12q23.3	2–6 years	Developmental delay, mental regression, short stature, corneal clouding, mild retinopathy
Sanfilippo syndrome A (MPS IIIA): #252900, N-sulphoglucosamine sulphohydrolase, chr. 17q25.3 Sanfilippo syndrome B (MPS IIIB) #252920, N-alpha-acetylglucosaminidase, chr. 17q21	2–6 years	Slight coarse face, abnormal behaviour, hearing loss, mild hepatomegaly, synophrys hirsutism, coarse hair

chr., chromosome; GM1, GM2, gangliosidoses; MPS, mucopolysaccharidosis

Table 11. Strategy for the detection of lysosomal storage diseases

Possible lysosomal disorder (association of organomegaly +/- CNS damage) ▼ Blood smear: lymphocyte vacuoles (foamy lymphocytes) ▼ Tissue biopsy: intracellular storage vacuoles (e.g., liver, kidney, nerve tissue, bone marrow) ▼ ▼
Analysis of storage tissue   **Enzymology** • Histological differentiation by staining procedures   • Lymphocytes, fibroblasts • Isolation and chemical analysis of storage material   **Genetic analysis** • EM-cytochemistry; immunocytochemistry; cell fractionation with co-purification of lysosomes/storage material (research)

CNS, central nervous system; EM, electronmicroscopy.

because of the technical problems to be overcome to gain the amount of enzyme needed for treatment. However, the use of enzyme preparations for intravenous application is being further developed. Molecular genetics allows the biosynthesis of large amounts of the missing enzymes. They can be modified to neoglycoproteins by adding carbohydrates, which can direct the enzymes to targeted organs. Another promising technique is to form more stable hydrolase-albumin complexes linked to antibodies that are directed to surface antigens of the targeted organ, though continuous enzyme replacement from transplanted organs seems to be more feasible (Table 12). Bone marrow transplantation might be a viable treatment method for some lysosomal diseases. It has been shown that after transplantation, a previously absent enzyme activity can be detected in organs such as the liver, spleen and kidneys. But for all diseases with central nervous system involvement, the blood-brain barrier seems to limit this approach. It is presently under discussion whether this is completely true, because microglia cells, which comprise 5 per cent of the brain cells, may be derived from bone marrow stem cells. If this proves correct, a very early bone marrow transplant might even benefit those with lysosomal diseases with central nervous system involvement. However, bone marrow transplantation (Table 13) has already been attempted as an experimental, sometimes desperate, trial. The presentation of data and the discussion of the results is very controversial and a definite recommendation cannot be given.

Table 12. Enzyme replacement for the treatment of lysosomal disorders: different options and open problems

Methods
A: *Discontinuous therapy*
   1. Plasma infusion
   2. Leucocyte transfusion (buffy coat)
   3. Purified enzymes from urine, plasma, spleen and placenta
B: *Continuous therapy*
   1. Organ transplantation
   2. Bone marrow transplantation

Problems
• Continuous supply of enzyme necessary
• Ligand properties of enzyme versus receptor specificity of target organ
• One enzyme form may not reach all tissues affected
• Blood-brain barrier?

Table 13. Bone marrow transplantation in human lysosomal diseases

Mucopolysaccharidoses		Sphingolipidoses
MPS I	(Hurler)*	Metachromatic Leucodystrophy*
MPS II	(Hunter)	M. Niemann-Pick*
MPS IIIA, B	(Sanfilippo)	M. Krabbe*
MPS IV	(Morquio)	M. Gaucher*
MPS VI	(Maroteaux-Lamy)*	

*Animal model available.

Glycosylation, and cholesterol synthesis defects

Defects of N-glycosylation

Congenital disorders of glycosylation (CDG) result from defects in the assembly, transfer, and processing of N-linked oligosaccharides. The CDGs are divided into groups I and II. Defective genes are lettered in chronological order of their discovery. Type I CDGs are defined by mutations in steps leading to the assembly and transfer of the lipid-linked oligosaccharide chain from the carrier lipid to potential N-glycosylation sites on newly synthesized proteins in the endoplasmic reticulum. Approximately 40 genes are needed to carry out the first stage. Type II CDG defects are defined as those that involve the sequential, highly ordered removal and addition of individual sugars on protein-bound N-linked sugar chains. More than 20 additional genes are required for this stage. All the CDGs are autosomal recessive disorders.

Clinical and genetic features, together with the enzymatic defects, are summarized in Table 14. Symptoms may be multisystemic but the most frequent are drug-resistant epilepsy, unexplained stroke, and developmental delay, mental retardation, and cerebellar atrophy.

Most CDG patients can be diagnosed by a simple blood test to analyse the glycosylation transfer status (Tf). Abnormal Tf is detected by isoelectric focusing, or by electrospray ionization mass spectrometry. Once CDG is diagnosed, further biochemical and genetic testing is required to determine the type.

There is no specific therapy for CDG, except for CDG-Ib and some CDG-IIc patients. Current treatment for CDG patients is supportive and the treatment of symptoms and sequelae. The effective therapy for CDG-Ib is oral mannose. CDG-Ib presents with protein losing enteropathy, coagulopathy and liver disease without neurological involvement. These patients have significant gastrointestinal problems, but are neurologically and intellectually normal. Fucose supplements have been used to treat patients with CDG-IIc who have a defective GDP-fucose transporter. Infections cease and health improves. Unfortunately, fucose does not improve or reverse the developmental delay. For more detailed review consult (Jaeken & Matthijs, 2007).

Cholesterol synthesis defects

Eight distinct inherited disorders have been linked to different enzyme defects in the isoprenoid/cholesterol biosynthetic pathway following the finding of abnormally increased levels of intermediate metabolites in patients, and confirmed by the demonstration of disease-causing mutations in genes encoding the implicated enzymes. Patients affected by these disorders are characterized by multiple morphogenic and congenital anomalies including internal organ,

Table 14. Disorders of N-glycosylation

Type	Enzyme Defect (Gene Name)	Features
CDGIa	Phosphomannomutase II (PPM2)	Developmental delay, hypotonia, esotropia, lipodystrophy, cerebellar hypoplasia/atrophy, stroke-like episodes, seizures
CDGIb	Phosphomannose isomerase (MPI)	Hepatic fibrosis, protein losing enteropathy, coagulopathy, hypoglycaemia
CDGIc	Glucosyltransferase I Dol-P-Glc: Man9GlcNAc2-PP-Dol glucosyltransferase (ALG6)	Moderate developmental delay, hypotonia, esotropia, epilepsy
CDGId	Dol-P-Man: Man5GlcNAc2-PP-Dol mannosyltransferase (ALG3)	Profound psychomotor delay, optic atrophy, acquired microcephaly, iris colobomas; hypsarrhythmia
CDGIe	Dol-P-Man synthase I GDP-Man: Dol-P mannosyltransferase (DPM1)	Profound psychomotor delay, severe developmental delay, optic atrophy, epilepsy, hypotonia, mild dysmorphism, coagulopathy
CDGIf	MPDU1/Lec35 (MPDU1)	Short stature, ichthyosis, psychomotor retardation, pigmentary retinopathy
CDGIg	Dol-P-Man: Man7GlcNAc2PP-Dol mannosyltransferase (ALG12)	Hypotonia, facial dysmorphism, psychomotor retardation, acquired microcephaly, frequent infections
CDGIh	Glucosyltransferase II: Dol-P-Glc:Glc1Man9GlcNAc2-PPDol glucosyltransferase (ALG8)	Hepatomegaly, protein losing enteropathy, renal failure, hypoalbuminaemia, oedema, ascites
CDGIi	Mannosyltransferase II: GDP-Man: Man1GlcNAc2-PP-Dol mannosyltransferase (ALG2)	Normal at birth; developmental delay, hypomyelination, intractable seizures, iris colobomas, hepatomegaly, coagulopathy
CDGIj	UDP-GlcNAc: dolichol phosphate N-acetylglucosamine 1- phosphate transferase (DPAGT1)	Severe developmental delay, hypotonia, seizures, microcephaly, exotropia
CDGIk	Mannosyltransferase I: GDP-Man: GlcNAc2-PP-Dol mannosyltransferase (ALG1)	Severe psychomotor retardation, hypotonia, acquired microcephaly, intractable seizures, fever, coagulopathy, nephrotic syndrome, early death
CDGIL	Mannosyltransferase Dol-P-Man: Man6 and 8GlcNAc2-PP-Dol mannosyltransferase (ALG9)	Severe microcephaly, hypotonia, seizures, hepatomegaly
CDGIIa	GlcNAc-transferase 2 (GnT II) (MGAT2)	Developmental delay, dysmorphism, stereotypies, seizures
CDGIIb	Glycosidase I (GLS1)	Dysmorphism, hypotonia, seizures, hepatomegaly, hepatic fibrosis (death at 2.5 months)
CDGIIc	GDP-fucose transporter (SLC35C1/FUCT1)	Recurrent infections, persistent neutrophilia, developmental delay, microcephaly, hypotonia (normal Tf)
CDGIId	β1,4 Galactosyltransferase (B4GALT1)	Hypotonia (myopathy), spontaneous haemorrhage, Dandy-Walker malformation
CDGIIe	Conserved oligomeric Golgi complex subunit 7 (COG7)	Fatal in early infancy; dysmorphism, hypotonia, intractable seizures, hepatomegaly, progressive jaundice, recurrent infections, cardiac failure.
CDGIIf	CMP-sialic acid transporter (SLC35A1)	Thrombocytopenia, no neurological symptoms, normal Tf, abnormal platelet glycoproteins

Tf, tissue factor.

skeletal, and skin abnormalities, underlining an important role for cholesterol in human embryogenesis and development. The aetiology of the underlying pathophysiology may involve multiple affected processes due to lowered cholesterol or the increased teratogenic levels of the intermediate sterol precursors, or both.

Two disorders – classic mevalonic aciduria (MIM 251170) and the hyperimmunoglobulinaemia D and periodic fever syndrome (HIDS) (MIM 260920) – are caused by a deficiency of the enzyme mevalonate kinase, albeit to different degrees owing to specific mutations in the *MVK* gene. Patients with mevalonic aciduria may present with motor disability starting in childhood and cerebellar atrophy. Patients with the mevalonic aciduria presentation show high levels of mevalonic acid in plasma and urine, while those with the HIDS presentation have low to moderate levels of mevalonic acid. Levels in these disorders are generally low normal. Patients with mevalonate kinase deficiency characteristically present with recurrent episodes of high fever associated with abdominal pain, vomiting and diarrhoea, (cervical) lymphadenopathy, hepatosplenomegaly, arthralgia and skin rash, and, in severe cases, with additional symptoms such as mental retardation, failure to thrive, ataxia, cerebellar atrophy, hypotonia and dysmorphic features (Drenth *et al.*, 1994).

The remaining six enzyme defects exclusively affect sterol synthesis and involve four autosomal recessive and two X-linked dominant inherited syndromes. In general, patients affected by these defects present with multiple congenital, developmental and morphogenic anomalies, including internal organ, skeletal and skin abnormalities, and a marked delay in psychomotor development.

The most common defect of cholesterol biosynthesis is autosomal recessive Smith-Lemli-Opitz syndrome (SLOS; MIM 270400), a multiple malformation syndrome caused by 3β-hydroxysterol Δ^7-reductase deficiency (mutations in the *DHCR7* gene at 11q13). The deficiency results in low cholesterol and increased levels of 7-dehydrocholesterol (cholesta-5,7-dien-3β-ol) and its isomer 8-dehydrocholesterol (cholesta-5,8(9)-dien-3β-ol) in plasma, cells and tissues from these patients. Patients with SLOS often present with a large and variable spectrum of morphogenic and congenital anomalies, including dysmorphic craniofacial features, microcephaly, multiple internal organ, limb/skeletal, and urogenital malformations, (intrauterine) growth and mental retardation, and behavioural problems.

Desmosterolosis (MIM 602398) and lathosterolosis (MIM 607330) are two autosomal recessive cholesterol biosynthesis defects with a rather similar clinical presentation to SLOS, but for each of which so far only two patients have been reported. Desmosterolosis is caused by mutations in the *DHCR24* gene at 1p31.1-p33 causing a deficiency of 3β-hydroxysterol Δ^{24}-reductase, resulting in low cholesterol and raised levels of desmosterol. Lathosterolosis is caused by mutations in the *SC5D* gene (at 11q23.3) causing a deficiency of 3β-hydroxysterol Δ^5-desaturase, resulting in low cholesterol and raised levels of lathosterol in plasma, tissue and cultured cells.

Autosomal recessive Greenberg skeletal dysplasia (MIM 215140), also known as HEM skeletal dysplasia, is rare severe cholesterol biosynthesis defect leading to early death *in utero*. Affected fetuses are characterized by fetal hydrops, short-limb dwarfism with an unusual 'moth-eaten' appearance of the shortened long bones, bizarre ectopic ossification centres and disorganization of chondro-osseous histology. The defect is caused by mutations in the *LBR* gene at 1q42 causing a deficiency of the lamin B receptor which functions as the 3β-hydroxysterol Δ^{14}-reductase, resulting in raised levels of cholesta-8,14-dien-3β-ol and cholesta-8,14,24-trien-3β-ol in tissues or cultured cells.

For the two X-linked dominant inherited disorders, Conradi-Hünermann-Happle syndrome (CDPX2; MIM 302960) and CHILD syndrome (MIM 308050), see the section on peroxisomal disorders. For details on these disorders, consult Waterham, 2006.

References

Anan, R., Nakagawa, M., Miyata, M., Higuchi, I., Nakao, S., Suehara, M., Osame, M. & Tanaka, H. (1995): Cardiac involvement in mitochondrial diseases. A study on 17 patients with documented mitochondrial DNA defects. *Circulation* **91**, 955–961.

Baumgartner, M.R., Poll-The, B.T., Verhoeven, N.M., Jakobs, C., Espeel, M., Roels, F., Rabier, D., Levade, T., Rolland, M.O., Martinez, M., Wanders, R.J. & Saudubray, J.M. (1998): Clinical approach to inherited peroxisomal disorders: a series of 27 patients. *Ann. Neurol.* **44**, 720–730.

Berenberg, R.A., Pellock, J.M., DiMauro, S., Schotland, D.L., Bonilla, E., Eastwood, A., Hays, A., Vicale, C.T., Behrens, M., Chutorian, A. & Rowland, L.P. (1977): Lumping or splitting? 'Ophthalmoplegia-plus' or Kearns-Sayre syndrome? *Ann. Neurol.* **1**, 37–54.

Rahman, S., Blok, R.B., Dahl, H.H., Danks, D.M., Kirby, D.M., Chow, C.W., Christodoulou, J. & Thorburn, D.R. (1996): Leigh syndrome: clinical features and biochemical and DNA abnormalities. *Ann. Neurol.* **39**, 343–351.

Bodemer, C., Rötig, A., Rustin, P., Cormier, V., Niaudet, P., Saudubray, J.M., Rabier, D., Munnich, A. & de Prost, Y. (1999): Hair and skin disorders as signs of mitochondrial disease. *Pediatrics* **103**, 428–433.

Bruno, C., Minetti, C., Tang, Y., Magalhães, P.J., Santorelli, F.M., Shanske, S., Bado, M., Cordone, G., Gatti, R. & DiMauro, S. (1998): Primary adrenal insufficiency in a child with a mitochondrial DNA deletion. *J. Inherit. Metab. Dis.* **21**, 155–161.

Cormier-Daire, V., Bonnefont, J.P., Rustin, P., Maurage, C., Ogler, H., Schmitz, J., Ricour, C., Saudubray, J.M., Munnich, A. & Rötig, A. (1994): Mitochondrial DNA rearrangement with onset as chronic diarrhea with villous atrophy. *J. Pediatr.* **124**, 63–70.

DiMauro, S. Mitochondrial encephalomyopathies: back to mendelian genetics. *Ann. Neurol.* **45**, 693–694.

DiMauro, S. & Haller, R.G. (1999): Metabolic myopathies: substrate use defects. In: *Muscle diseases*, ed. A.H.V. Schapira & R.C. Griggs, pp. 225–249. Boston: Butterworth-Heinemann.

DiMauro, S., Quinzii, C.M. & Hirano, M. (2007): Mutations in coenzyme Q10 biosynthetic genes. *J. Clin. Invest.* **117**, 587–589.

Diomedi-Camassei, F., Di Giandomenico, S., Santorelli, F.M., Caridi, G., Piemonte, F., Montini, G., Ghiggeri, G.M., Murer, L., Barisoni, L., Pastore, A., Muda, A.O., Valente, M.L., Bertini, E. & Emma, F. (2007): COQ2 nephropathy: a newly described inherited mitochondriopathy with primary renal involvement. *J. Am. Soc. Nephrol.* **18**, 2773–2780.

Dionisi-Vici, C., Rizzo, C., Burlina, A.B., Caruso, U., Sabetta, G., Uziel, G. & Abeni, D. (2002): Inborn errors of metabolism in the Italian pediatric population: a national retrospective survey. *J. Pediatr.* **140**, 321–327.

Drenth, J.P., Haagsma, C.J. & van der Meer, J.W. (1994): Hyperimmunoglobulinemia D and periodic fever syndrome. The clinical spectrum in a series of 50 patients. International Hyper-IgD Study Group, *Medicine (Baltimore)* **73**, 133–144.

Edvardson, S., Shaag, A., Kolesnikova, O., Gomori, J.M., Tarassov, I., Einbinder, T., Saada, A. & Elpeleg, O. (2007): Deleterious mutation in the mitochondrial arginyl-transfer RNA synthetase gene is associated with pontocerebellar hypoplasia. *Am. J. Hum. Genet.* **81**, 857–862.

Emma, F., Pizzini, C., Tessa, A., Di Giandomenico, S., Onetti-Muda, A., Santorelli, F.M., Bertini, E. & Rizzoni, G. (2006): 'Bartter-like' phenotype in Kearns-Sayre syndrome. *Pediatr. Nephrol.* **21**, 355–360.

Fernandes, J., Saudubray, J.M., van Den Berghe, G. & Walter, J.H., eds (2006): *Inborn metabolic diseases: diagnosis and treatment*, 4th edition, pp. 177–188. Heidelberg: Springer Verlag.

Fernandez-Vizarra, E., Berardinelli, A., Valente, L., Tiranti, V. & Zeviani, M. (2007): Nonsense mutation in pseudouridylate synthase 1 (PUS1) in two brothers affected by myopathy, lactic acidosis and sideroblastic anaemia (MLASA). *J. Med. Genet.* **44**, 173–180.

Hirano, M., Nishino, I., Nishigaki, Y. & Martí, R. (2006): Thymidine phosphorylase gene mutations cause mitochondrial neurogastrointestinal encephalomyopathy (MNGIE). *Intern. Med.* **45**, 1103.

Holt, I.J., Harding, A.E. & Morgan Hughes, J.A. (1988): Deletions of muscle mitochondrial DNA in patients with mitochondrial myopathies. *Nature* **331**, 717–719.

Horvath, R., Hudson, G., Ferrari, G., Fütterer, N., Ahola, S., Lamantea, E., Prokisch, H., Lochmüller, H., McFarland, R., Ramesh, V., Klopstock, T., Freisinger, P., Salvi, F., Mayr, J.A., Santer, R., Tesarova, M., Zeman, J., Udd, B.,

Taylor, R.W., Turnbull, D., Hanna, M., Fialho, D., Suomalainen, A., Zeviani, M. & Chinnery, P.F. (2006): Phenotypic spectrum associated with mutations of the mitochondrial polymerase gamma gene. *Brain* **129**, 1674–1684.

Huntsman, R.J., Sinclair, D.B., Bhargava, R. & Chan, A. (2005): Atypical presentations of Leigh syndrome: a case series and review. *Pediatr. Neurol.* **32**, 334–340.

Jaeken, J. & Matthijs, G. (2007): Congenital disorders of glycosylation: a rapidly expanding disease family. *Annu. Rev. Genomics Hum. Genet.* **8**, 261–278.

Kadowaki, T., Kadowaki, H., Mori, Y., Yasuda, K., Kadowaki, H., Mori, Y., Hagura, R., Akanuma, Y. & Yazaki, Y. (1994): A subtype of diabetes mellitus associated with a mutation of mitochondrial DNA. *N. Engl. J. Med.* **330**, 962–968.

Karadimas, C.L., Vu, T.H., Holve, S.A., Chronopoulou, P., Quinzii, C., Johnsen, S.D., Kurth, J., Eggers, E., Palenzuela, L., Tanji, K., Bonilla, E., De Vivo, D.C., DiMauro, S. & Hirano, M. (2006): Navajo neurohepatopathy is caused by a mutation in the MPV17 gene. *Am. J. Hum. Genet.* **79**, 544–548.

Lawrence, J.J., Schlesinger, A.E., Kozlowski, K., Poznanski, A.K., Bacha, L., Dreyer, G.L., Barylak, A., Sillence, D.O. & Rager, K. (1989): Unusual radiographic manifestations of chondrodysplasia punctata. *Skel. Radiol.* **18**, 15–19.

Lee, W.S. & Sokol, R.J. (2007): Mitochondrial hepatopathies: advances in genetics and pathogenesis. *Hepatology* **45**, 1555–1565.

López, L.C., Schuelke, M., Quinzii, C.M., Kanki, T., Rodenburg, R.J., Naini, A., Dimauro, S. & Hirano, M. (2006): Leigh syndrome with nephropathy and CoQ10 deficiency due to decaprenyl diphosphate synthase subunit 2 (PDSS2) mutations. *Am. J. Hum. Genet.* **79**, 1125–1129.

Mandel, H., Szargel, R., Labay, V., Elpeleg, O., Saada, A., Shalata, A., Anbinder, Y., Berkowitz, D., Hartman, C., Barak, M., Eriksson, S. & Cohen, N. (2001): The deoxyguanosine kinase gene is mutated in individuals with depleted hepatocerebral mitochondrial DNA. *Nat. Genet.* **29**, 337–340.

Meikle, P.J., Hopwood, J.J., Clague, A.E. & Carey, W.F. (281): Prevalence of lysosomal storage disorders. *JAMA* **281**, 249–254.

Meunzer, J. & Neufeld, E.F. (2001): In: *The metabolic and molecular basis of inherited disease*, 8th edition, ed. C.R. Scriver, A.L. Beaudet, W.S. Sly & D. Vaile, pp. 3421–3452. New York: McGraw-Hill.

Miller, C., Saada, A., Shaul, N., Shabtai, N., Ben-Shalom, E., Shaag, A., Hershkovitz, E. & Elpeleg, O. (2004): Defective mitochondrial translation caused by a ribosomal protein (MRPS16) mutation. *Ann. Neurol.* **56**, 734–738.

Zeviani, M., Bonilla, E., DeVivo, D.C. & DiMauro, S. (1989): Mitochondrial diseases. *Neurol Clin.* **7**, 123-156. Review.

Moraes, C.T., Shanske, S., Tritschler, H.-J., Aprille, J.R., Andreetta, F. & Bonilla, E. (1991): MtDNA depletion with variable tissue expression: a novel genetic abnormality in mitochondrial diseases. *Am. J. Hum. Genet.* **48**, 492–501.

Moser, H.W. (1999): Genotype-phenotype correlations in disorders of peroxisome biogenesis. *Mol. Genet. Metab.* **68**, 316–327.

Moser, H.W. & Raymond, G.V. (1998): Genetic peroxisomal disorder: why, when, and how to test. *Am. Neurol. Assoc.* **44**, 713–715.

Munnich, A., Rustin, P., Rotig, A., Chretien, D., Bonnefont, J.P., Nuttin, C., Cormier, V., Vassault, A., Parvy, P., Bardet, J., *et al.* (1992): Clinical aspects of mitochondrial disorders. *J. Inher. Metab. Dis.* **15**, 448–455.

Naviaux, R.K. & Nguyen, K.V. (2004): POLG mutations associated with Alpers' syndrome and mitochondrial DNA depletion. *Ann. Neurol.* **55**, 706–712.

Niaudet, P. & Rotig, A. (1997): The kidney in mitochondrial cytopathies. *Kidney Int.* **51**, 1000–1007.

Nishino, I., Spinazzola, A. & Hirano, M. (1999): Thymidine phosphorylase gene mutations in MNGIE, a human mitochondrial disorder. *Science* **283**, 689–692.

Pondarre, C., Campagna, D.R., Antiochos, B., Sikorski, L., Mulhern, H. & Fleming, M.D. (2007): Abcb7, the gene responsible for X-linked sideroblastic anemia with ataxia, is essential for hematopoiesis. *Blood* **109**, 3567–3569.

Rötig, A., Cormier, V., Blanche, S., Bonnefont, J.P., Ledeist, F., Romero, N., Schmitz, J., Rustin, P., Fischer, A., Saudubray, J.M. *et al.* (1990): Pearson's marrow-pancreas syndrome. A multisystem mitochondrial disorder in infancy. *J Clin Invest.* **86**, 1601-1608.

Salviati, L., Sacconi, S., Mancuso, M., Otaegui, D., Camaño, P., Marina, A., Rabinowitz, S., Shiffman, R., Thompson, K., Wilson, C.M., Feigenbaum, A., Naini, A.B., Hirano, M., Bonilla, E., DiMauro, S. & Vu, T.H. (2002): Mitochondrial DNA depletion and dGK gene mutations. *Ann. Neurol.* **52**, 311–317.

Saudubray, J., Sedel, F. & Walter, J. (2006): Clinical approach to treatable inborn metabolic diseases: an introduction. *J. Inherit. Metab. Dis.* **29**, 261–274.

Scheper, G.C., van der Klok, T., van Andel, R.J., van Berkel, C.G., Sissler, M., Smet, J., Muravina, T.I., Serkov, S.V., Uziel, G., Bugiani, M., Schiffmann, R., Krägeloh-Mann, I., Smeitink, J.A., Florentz, C., Van Coster, R., Pronk, J.C.

& van der Knaap, M.S. (2007): Mitochondrial aspartyl-tRNA synthetase deficiency causes leukoencephalopathy with brain stem and spinal cord involvement and lactate elevation. *Nat. Genet.* **39,** 534–539.

Scriver, C.R., Beaudet, A.L., Sly, W.S. & Vailem D., eds. (2001): *The metabolic and molecular basis of inherited disease*, 8th ed. New York: McGraw-Hill.

Smeitink, J.A., Elpeleg, O., Antonicka, H., Diepstra, H., Saada, A., Smits, P., Sasarman, F., Vriend, G., Jacob-Hirsch, J., Shaag, A., Rechavi, G., Welling, B., Horst, J., Rodenburg, R.J., van den Heuvel, B. & Shoubridge, E.A. (2006): Distinct clinical phenotypes associated with a mutation in the mitochondrial translation elongation factor EFTs. *Am. J. Hum. Genet.* **79,** 869–877.

Spinazzola, A., Viscomi, C., Fernandez-Vizarra, E., Carrara, F., D'Adamo, P., Calvo, S., Marsano, R.M., Donnini, C., Weiher, H., Strisciuglio, P., Parini, R., Sarzi, E., Chan, A., DiMauro, S., Rötig, A., Gasparini, P., Ferrero, I., Mootha, V.K., Tiranti, V. & Zeviani, M. (2006): MPV17 encodes an inner mitochondrial membrane protein and is mutated in infantile hepatic mitochondrial DNA depletion. *Nat. Genet.* **38,** 570–575.

Stark, R. & Roden, M. (2007): Mitochondrial function and endocrine diseases. *Eur. J. Clin. Invest.* **37,** 236–248.

Tiranti, V., Jaksch, M., Hofmann, S., Galimberti, C., Hoertnagel, K., Lulli, L., Freisinger, P., Bindoff, L., Gerbitz, K.D., Comi, G.P., Uziel, G., Zeviani, M. & Meitinger, T. (1999): Loss-of-function mutations of SURF-1 are specifically associated with Leigh syndrome with cytochrome c oxidase deficiency. *Ann. Neurol.* **46,** 161–166.

Tiranti, V., Briem, E., Lamantea, E., Mineri, R., Papaleo, E., De Gioia, L., Forlani, F., Rinaldo, P., Dickson, P., Abu-Libdeh, B., Cindro-Heberle, L., Owaidha, M., Jack, R.M., Christensen, E., Burlina, A. & Zeviani, M. (2006): ETHE1 mutations are specific to ethylmalonic encephalopathy. *J. Med. Genet.* **43,** 340–346.

Valente, L., Tiranti, V., Marsano, R.M., Malfatti, E., Fernandez-Vizarra, E., Donnini, C., Mereghetti, P., De Gioia, L., Burlina, A., Castellan, C., Comi, G.P., Savasta, S., Ferrero, I. & Zeviani, M. (2007): Infantile encephalopathy and defective mitochondrial DNA translation in patients with mutations of mitochondrial elongation factors EFG1 and EFTu. *Am. J. Hum. Genet.* **80,** 44–58.

Vu, T.H., Tanji, K., Holve, S.A., Bonilla, E., Sokol, R.J., Snyder, R.D., Fiore, S., Deutsch, G.H., Dimauro, S. & De Vivo, D. (2001): Navajo neurohepatopathy: a mitochondrial DNA depletion syndrome? *Hepatology* **34,** 116–120.

Wallace, D.C., Singh, G., Lott, M.T., Hodge, J.A., Schurr, T.G., Lezza, A.M., Elsas, L.J. & Nikoskelainen, E.K. (1988): Mitochondrial DNA mutation associated with Leber's hereditary optic neuropathy. *Science* **242,** 1427–1430.

Wanders, R.J. & Waterham, H.R. (2006): Biochemistry of mammalian peroxisomes revisited. *Annu. Rev. Biochem.* **75,** 295–332.

Waterham, H.R. (2006): Defects of cholesterol biosynthesis. *FEBS Lett.* **580,** 5442–5449.

Yaplito-Lee, J., Weintraub, R., Jamsen, K., Chow, C.W., Thorburn, D.R. & Boneh, A. (2007): Cardiac manifestations in oxidative phosphorylation disorders of childhood. *J. Pediatr.* **150,** 407–411.

Shin, Y.S. (2006): Glycogen storage disease: clinical, biochemical, and molecular heterogeneity. *Semin. Pediatr. Neurol.* **13,** 115–120.

Chapter 9

Brain tumours

Luca Massimi, Gianpiero Tamburrini and Concezio Di Rocco

*Division of Paediatric Neurosurgery, Hospital Policlinico A. Gemelli,
Largo A. Gemelli 8, 00168, Rome, Italy*
lmassimi@email.it

Central nervous system (CNS) tumours are among the most common neoplasms in childhood, representing the principal cause of oncological mortality along with lymphoid-haematopoietic system tumours (children) and neuroblastomas (infants). Once considered rare and hard to treat, infantile brain tumours (IBTs) are currently an important issue in paediatric neurosciences. Modern neuroimaging tools provide earlier and more reliable diagnosis, accounting for the apparently increasing overall incidence of these tumours. The large numbers of newly diagnosed cases and the advances in the field of molecular biology and immunohistochemistry have led to the identification of infant-specific neoplasms, such as desmoplastic infantile ganglioglioma, atypical teratoid/rhabdoid tumour, and pilomixoid astrocytoma. IBTs differ significantly from similar tumours in older age groups with respect to their biological and clinical behaviour, location, treatment, outcome and prognosis. In spite of the improvement in the biological, pathological, imaging and therapeutic knowledge, their management remains challenging. However, current progress in neurosurgical and anaesthesiological care and the development of more effective chemotherapeutic and radiotherapeutic protocols allow infants to receive more adequate treatment than in the past.

Definition

There is no explicit agreement on the definition of 'infantile' brain tumours. Such a divergence depends in part on the vagueness of the term 'infant' (from the Latin *infans*, that is 'not speaking person'). Infant is actually defined as 'a baby, often more specifically a child of 12 months old or less or, by some criteria, 2 years old or less'. In neuro-oncology, however, children with brain tumours (especially malignant neoplasms) are usually grouped into those under 3 years and over 3 years because of difference in management and, especially, prognosis. Uncertainties in the definition are further increased by the dissimilar classification criteria adopted in the different centres, which may refer to the patient's age at the time of the clinical onset or at the time of diagnosis.

Some writers draw a distinction between congenital and acquired tumours during infancy. A historical classification (Solitare & Krigman, 1964) proposed three distinct subgroups of congenital tumours: i) 'definitely congenital' – that is, tumours presenting or producing symptoms at birth; ii) 'probably congenital' – presenting or producing symptoms within the first week of life; and iii) 'possibly congenital' – presenting or producing symptoms during the first 2 months of life. Advances in prenatal and neonatal diagnosis have led to an extension of this original classification (Jellinger & Sunder-Plassman, 1973) as follows: 'definitely connatal' – tumours producing symptoms within the first 2 weeks of life; 'probably connatal' – tumours first seen within the first year of life; and 'possibly connatal' – tumours seen in infants beyond 1 year of age. Some investigators still refer to Collins law, stating that all intracranial tumours diagnosed up to the 9th month of life should be included in the category of congenital brain tumours, while others put the cut-off age at 18 months. Craniopharyngiomas, medulloblastomas, intracranial teratomas, and hamartomas are known to have a possible congenital origin but they do not necessarily produce symptoms at an early age. This suggests that some paediatric neoplasms might be congenital even when their clinical manifestations do not occur until after infancy.

In this chapter, the term 'IBTs' will be used to indicate all the brain tumours occurring within the second year of life, and the words 'congenital' and 'neonatal' will refer to the tumours diagnosed prenatally, at birth, or within the first 2 to 4 weeks of life, except when stated otherwise.

Epidemiology

The incidence of paediatric brain tumours has increased significantly in the last 20 years, mainly as a result of the advances in, and the expanded use of, new diagnostic techniques, but also, possibly, because of changing environmental factors. CNS tumours are reported to have overtaken acute lymphoblastic leukaemia as the most common neoplasm in children, with an incidence of 2.5 to 3.3 paediatric patients per 100,000 per year, representing about one fifth of all paediatric cancers and the most common cause of cancer deaths in children (24 per cent of all cancer-related deaths).

IBTs account for 10 to 20 per cent of all paediatric brain tumours (Rickert, 1998). Their incidence of approximately 5/100,000/year is higher than that reported for all the remaining paediatric age groups (4/100,000/year), according to a recent US statistical report (CBTRUS, 2008). No significant differences are found among different geographical areas, while a moderate male predominance is usually reported (males *vs.* females: 54.2 *vs.* 45.8 per cent). Characteristically, two peaks of age are observed, one under the first month of life and the second toward the end of the first year (9 to 12 months).

The most commonly encountered histotypes are, in decreasing order of frequency, astrocytomas, medulloblastomas, ependymomas, choroid plexus tumours, primitive neuroectodermal tumours (PNETs), teratomas, craniopharyngiomas, sarcomas, meningiomas, gangliogliomas and neuroblastomas. In the analysis of their paediatric series of 340 children and meta-analysis of 10,582 childhood brain tumours, Rickert and Paulus (Rickert & Paulus, 2001) confirmed that astrocytomas were the most common tumours throughout infancy (42 per cent), childhood (41 to 45 per cent) and adolescence (> 50 per cent). Pilocytic astrocytoma was found to be the single most frequent brain tumour in the 3 to 14 years age group, though high grade astrocytomas were predominant in the youngest and oldest children in this age group. During infancy, the incidence of pilocytic astrocytoma (13.3 per cent) is exceeded by that of malignant astrocytomas (17.8 per cent), ependymomas (17.8 per cent), and medulloblastomas (15.6 per cent). Malignant IBTs actually account for about one quarter of all malignant brain tumours in childhood. High grade tumours represent more than half of all infant brain neoplasms (55 per cent), reaching a value of 77 per cent in children less than 1 year old. Medulloblastoma is the most common infant malignant tumour, followed by high grade ependymoma, malignant glioma, and PNET. While the incidence of medulloblastoma remains quite stable through the different age periods (15 per cent during infancy, 20 per cent during childhood, 10 per cent during adolescence), anaplastic ependymoma is prevalent in infants (8.7 per cent) and adolescents (8.9 per cent) compared with children (1.8 per cent). A halfway trend is shown by malignant gliomas (17.8 per cent in infants, 11 per cent in children, 21.7 per cent in adolescents).

According to the descriptions of clinical series, infants with IBTs are usually split into three subgroups: < 12 months, 12 to 24 months, and 24 to 36 months. In the first year of life, there is no difference in the sex incidence (M/F: 1); malignant tumours are highly prevalent (77 per cent), medulloblastoma/PNETs being the most common histotype (23 per cent), with a preponderance of supratentorial over infratentorial location (ratio, 3.5). During the second year, a male prevalence develops (M/F: 1.5), the supratentorial space is less predominant (ratio, 1.5), the prevalence of malignant forms falls to 36 per cent, and astrocytomas and ependymomas become the most common tumours (24 per cent each). Finally, between the second and the third year, a further reduction in the supratentorial location is found (ratio, 1.2), as well as a further reduction in the malignant histotypes (25 per cent), astrocytomas being the most frequent tumours (21 per cent); the M/F ratio is near 1.2.

A further distinction divides congenital and neonatal tumours. Approximately 10 per cent of the perinatal tumours arise in the brain and about 5 per cent of all childhood brain tumours occur within the first six months of life. The incidence of congenital/neonatal tumours is relatively low, ranging from 1.1 to 3.6 per 100,000 newborns and accounting for 0.5 to 2 per cent of all CNS paediatric tumours (but for 5 to 12 per cent of all neonatal cancers) (Carstensen et al., 2006). Such tumours account for between 0.04 and 0.18 per cent of the overall mortality during the first year of life and between 5 and 20 per cent of the cancer mortality in the fetal and neonatal period. No significant difference in the sex prevalence is recorded. Almost a half of the neonatal tumours are composed of poorly differentiated tissues (immature teratoma, PNET, medulloblastoma). Teratoma is the most common histotype, representing 25 to 30 per cent of the total (up to 50 to 55 per cent in some series) and 0.5 per cent of all intracranial neoplasms; its incidence decreases progressively in older children. The second most common oncotype is low grade glioma (13 to 20 per cent), followed by PNET (15 to 20 per cent), medulloblastoma (10 per cent), high grade glioma (10 per cent), choroid plexus tumour (5 to 10 per cent), craniopharyngioma (3 to 5 per cent), germinoma (1 to 5 per cent), ependymoma (1 to 5 per cent), and other rarer neoplasms (overall 5 to 10 per cent).

Table 1 summarizes the main epidemiological differences between infants and older children.

Aetiological considerations

In spite of the epidemiological studies and the continuous progress in molecular biology, the aetiological and biological background of primitive IBTs remain poorly understood. Only two factors, ionizing radiation and heritable syndromes, show a clear correlation with brain tumour oncogenesis, though these are responsible for only a minority of the diagnosed cases. Radiation-induced brain tumours represent a well known disease in adults as well as in children and, though only a few cases have been detected so far, irradiation is the only recognized exogenous cause of primitive IBTs. Studies in this field show a clear correlation between high-dose ionizing exposure (maternal or fetal) and nerve sheath tumours, meningiomas and malignant

Table 1. Epidemiological differences between infantile brain tumours and other paediatric brain tumours

Age group	Male sex prevalence (%)	Supratentorial location (%)	Main histotype	Prevalence (%)	WHO III+IV (%)
Perinatal age (0–2 months)	50–55	58–65	Astrocytoma	20	54–60
			Ependymoma	10	
			Choroid plexus tumour	7	
			DIG	1.5	
			DNET	/	
			Medulloblastoma	8	
			ST PNET	3	
			AT/RT	2	
			Craniopharyngioma	5	
			Pituitary adenoma	/	
			Germ cell tumour	1	
			Teratoma	30–55	
Infancy (2 months to 2 years)	65–68	60–65	Astrocytoma	42	53–55 (> 70 in the first year)
			Ependymoma	18	
			Choroid plexus tumour	2	
			DIG	4.5	
			DNET	/	
			Medulloblastoma	15.5	
			ST PNET	2.2	
			AT/RT	7	
			Craniopharyngioma	4.5	
			Pituitary adenoma	/	
			Germ cell tumour	/	
			Teratoma	5	
Childhood (3–11 years)	60–62	40–45	Astrocytoma	47	50
			Ependymoma	7	
			Choroid plexus tumour	0.6	
			DIG	/	
			DNET	1.2	
			Medulloblastoma	20	
			ST PNET	2.3	
			AT/RT	0.5	
			Craniopharyngioma	7	
			Pituitary adenoma	/	
			Germ cell tumour	1.2	
			Teratoma	1.2	

Adolescence (12–18 years)	55–58	65–66	Astrocytoma	50	45
			Ependymoma	11.5	
			Choroid plexus tumour	0.8	
			DIG	/	
			DNET	/	
			Medulloblastoma	10	
			ST PNET	1.1	
			AT/RT	/	
			Craniopharyngioma	3.5	
			Pituitary adenoma	3	
			Germ cell tumour	5.5	
			Teratoma	1.5	

AT/RT, atypical teratoid/rhabdoid tumour; DIG, desmoplastic infantile ganglioglioma; DNET, dysembryoplastic neuroepithelial tumour; ST PNET, supratentorial primitive neuroectodermal tumour; WHO, World Health Organization grading.

gliomas (Davis, 2007). The role of low-dose irradiation, on the other hand, is harder to assess. Accurate investigations on the impact of non-ionizing radiation exposure in children seem to exclude significant risks for brain cancer at the levels experienced in the home environment. Future studies should provide an answer about the possible cumulative effect of low-dose exposure in infants.

A higher incidence of brain tumours in infancy has been observed among family members and siblings with cerebral neoplasms or other diseases of the nervous system, associated congenital anomalies, birth defects, genetic and malformative factors. In their series of 50 patients with malignant IBTs, Garré and coworkers (Garré et al., 2006) found genetic conditions in 22 per cent of the cases, thus confirming that some syndromes predispose to the occurrence of brain tumour in infants. This association has been reported for neurofibromatosis types I and II (NF-1, NF-2), tuberous sclerosis, von Hippel-Lindau syndrome, Li-Fraumeni syndrome, Gorlin syndrome, Turcot syndrome, Cowden syndrome, and Klinefelter syndrome. Familial brain tumours, however, account only for a small proportion of all IBTs. The most common familial syndromes and their associated IBTs are reported in Table 2.

The geographic prevalence of some histological types reported in different retrospective studies led to the consideration of racial or environmental effects, or both, in the pathogenesis of intracranial tumours in infants. A higher prevalence of some tumours in specific geographic areas has been reported – for example, a high incidence of teratomas in the Japanese or Taiwanese infant population. Nevertheless, similar figures have also been described in other countries far removed from eastern Asia, such as Mexico and Germany. Analogous data were reported for craniopharyngioma, which was found to have a particularly high incidence in Asia as well as in Africa and central America. The same considerations are applicable to most of the observational studies on this subject, in which deep analysis of the population characteristics is not possible. Therefore, a definite cause-effect correlation between race and paediatric brain tumour oncogenesis has not yet been identified. The higher incidence of paediatric brain tumours detected in some developed countries, indeed, is thought to result from different diagnostic facilities and better cancer registry practices in these countries compared with less developed ones, rather than from different racial characteristics and socioeconomic levels.

Table 2. Familial syndromes and infantile brain tumours

Syndrome	Altered genes and loci	Associated brain tumours
Neurofibromatosis-I	NF1 (17q11)	Neurofibroma, astrocytoma, optic pathways glioma
Neurofibromatosis-II	NF2 (22q12)	Neurofibroma, VIII cranial nerve schwannoma, meningioma, astrocytoma, ependymoma
Tuberous sclerosis complex	TSC1 (9q34) TSC2 (16p13)	Subependymal giant cell astrocytoma, cortical tuber, hamartoma
Von Hippel-Lindau	VHL (3p25-26)	Haemangioblastoma (cerebellum, retina)
Li-Fraumeni	TP53 (17p13)	PNET, astrocytoma, choroid plexus tumour
Gorlin	PTC (9q22)	Desmoplastic medulloblastoma
Turcot	APC (5q21) hMLH1 (3p21) hPMS2 (7p22)	Medulloblastoma Glioblastoma
Cowden	PTEN (10q23)	Gangliocytoma
Klinefelter	XXY	Germ cell tumour

PNET, primitive neuroectodermal tumour.

Recent investigations focused on other more specific predisposing factors. For instance, some studies have explored the association between high fetal/neonatal weight and the development of leukaemia and various paediatric tumours, including astrocytoma and neuroblastoma. Owing to the increased cell turnover, fat babies have high levels of insulin-like growth factor I, and its possible role in predisposing to IBTs has been hypothesized. On the other hand, an increased vitamin intake during pregnancy and early childhood appears to be related to a lower paediatric brain tumour incidence. A recent study evaluated the association between immune function and certain adult tumours (Wigertz et al., 2007). The investigators found an inverse relation between some types of non-asthmatic allergy (hay fever, eczema, food allergy) and brain glioma. These preliminary results should encourage similar investigations in infants.

The limitations found when examining possible ethnic influences are also encountered when investigating environmental factors, where the results are often inconclusive or contradictory. None of the proposed risk factors – for example, parental smoking and alcohol assumption, pesticides, electromagnetic fields, trauma – has proved to be significantly correlated with brain tumorigenesis. Other parental factors – such as high maternal or paternal age, infertility, exposure to or ingestion of toxic substances, chemotherapeutic agents, nitrites/nitrates, anticonvulsant drugs, and antiemetic drugs (especially during pregnancy) – have been proposed as predisposing to congenital or infant tumours, but no clear correlation has been demonstrated. Among carcinogens, nitrates are the most studied. However, neither the risk relating to the rubber industry nor that linked to dietary exposure has proven to be a factor in brain tumour development. Among numerous other potential neurocarcinogens (for example, ethylene oxide, chloroethane, and diphenhydramine hydrochloride), only the relation between acrylamide and brain tumours has been addressed specifically and no association was found (Marsh et al., 2007). Similarly, the role of infections occurring during pregnancy – such as toxoplasmosis (possibly linked to glioma) and chicken pox (with a suggested link to medulloblastoma) – remains inconclusive.

Cytogenetics and molecular genetics

As tumour development is thought to be influenced by both genetic predisposition and the environmental background, many genetic studies are now focusing on infants because their young age makes the role of environmental factors less likely to be important. The term 'molecular epidemiology' has been introduced because of the flood of studies revealing new tumour oncogenes and oncosuppressor genes. The correlation between genetic alterations and oncogenesis, however, is evident only within families with inheritable syndromes or in patients with constitutional chromosomal abnormalities. The most frequent genetic alterations in primary IBTs are summarized in Tables 3 and 4.

Medulloblastoma is the best studied IBT. The most common cytogenetic alteration is a loss of genetic material from the short arm of chromosome 17 (17p deletion), as well as duplication of its long arm (isochromosome 17q), occurring in 30 to 50 per cent of the cases (Biegel, 1999). Such an alteration is not specific for medulloblastoma but with this tumour the frequency is much higher than with any other histotype. Among the genes localized to the usual breakpoint of chromosome 17 – that is, 17p13.3 – the suppressor gene HIC-1 is thought to be inactivated by the 17p deletion. Moreover, loss of 17p13.3 is associated with amplification of the c-myc oncogene product (MYCC) which predicts a poor response of medulloblastoma to therapy. For these reasons, although the effects of 17p deletion are still uncertain, they are associated with a worse prognosis. Other frequent cytogenetic alterations include unbalanced translocations or deletions of chromosomes 8, 9q, 10q, 11p, 11q, and 16q, which implies a role of different oncosuppressor genes in the initiation or progression of medulloblastoma. Loss of 9q (deletion or mutation of PTCH gene) is responsible for the development of the non-sporadic *desmoplastic medulloblastoma* which is part of the Gorlin syndrome (also known as nervoid basal cell carcinoma syndrome). This syndrome is characterized by multiple basal cell carcinomas, palmar and plantar pits, keratocysts of the jaw, and skeletal abnormalities. The 9q deletion, however, also occurs in about 10 per cent of sporadic desmoplastic medulloblastomas. Differently, mutation of APC gene (5q21), which regulates β-catenin and typifies the Turcot syndrome (inherited polyposis coli), is not found among sporadic medulloblastomas. Among the molecular alterations linked to this tumour, high expression of the products of the oncogene erbB-2 is the most common, being found in 84 per cent of the cases (MacDonald *et al.*, 2003). One such product is HER2, a receptor for epidermal growth factor: the prognosis is poor when expression of this product is increased. On the other hand, high expression of trkC, observed in 48 per cent of medulloblastomas, is associated with a more favourable outcome (5-year survival, 89 per cent, compared with 46 per cent in low expression cases); trkC, a receptor for neurotrophin-3, regulates the cell growth, differentiation, and apoptosis in the developing cerebellum.

A further genetic alteration in medulloblastoma is monosomy 22. This has been found in about 10 per cent of medulloblastomas and *PNETs* as a primary change. Despite the similar histological features, PNETs do not share genetic alterations with medulloblastoma except for monosomy 22 and rearrangements of chromosome 11, both observed in pinealoblastoma, and homozygous deletions of DMBT1 gene (10q), observed in supratentorial PNETs. Little is known about the genetic anomalies in supratentorial PNETs but a few other chromosomal deletions (1q, 16p, 19p) have been identified (Inda *et al.*, 2005).

Monosomy 22 is also found in *atypical teratoid/rhabdoid tumour* (AT/RT). Genetic analyses detected a rhabdoid gene in chromosome band 22q11.2 (22q deletion is observed in 85 per cent of cases of AT/RT). The function of this gene, known as hSNF5/INI1 (INI1), is still uncertain, though a role as tumour suppressor has been hypothesized. INI1 is part of the

Table 3. Most common biological alterations in primitive malignant infantile brain tumours

Gene and/or protein alterations	Histotype and rate	Clinical correlation
erbB-2 (HER2)	Medulloblastoma (84%)	High expression → unfavourable outcome
TrkC	Medulloblastoma (48%)	Low expression → unfavourable outcome
C-MYC	Medulloblastoma/PNET (42%)	High expression → unfavourable outcome
17p deletion, i17q (HIC-1)	Medulloblastoma (35–50%)	Deletion → unknown significance; putative tumour suppressor gene locus
β-Tubulin class III expression	Medulloblastoma (15–20%)	MB differentiation in neuronal cells: indicator of lower aggressiveness
PTCH	Medulloblastoma (8–10%)	Mutation → development of sporadic and non-sporadic desmoplastic MB
17q deletion	PNET (60%)	Putative tumour suppressor gene locus
13q14 deletion	Pinealoblastoma (93%)	Expression of trilateral retinoblastoma
Loss of heterozygosity 10q	Glioblastoma (70%)	Tumour development
Loss of heterozygosity 10p	Glioblastoma (47%)	Tumour development
Loss of heterozygosity 22q	Glioblastoma (41%)	Tumour development
9p deletion	Malignant glioma (40%)	Putative tumour suppressor gene locus
EGFR amplification	Malignant glioma (36%)	Worse prognosis
$p16^{INK4a}$ deletion	Malignant glioma (31%)	Promoter methylation (late progression)
TP53 mutation (p53)	Malignant glioma (28%)	Tumour progression (secondary glioblastoma)
PTEN mutations	Malignant glioma (25%)	Phosphatase activation (cell migration)
22q11 deletion (hSNF5/INI1 gene); 22 monosomy	AT/RT (85%), medulloblastoma (10%)	Altered expression of SWI/SNF protein (oncosuppressor protein)
+7, +11, +12, +15, +18, +20 (hyperdiploid chromosomes)	Choroid plexus carcinoma (30–40%)	Hyperdiploid state indicative of tumour aggressiveness 22q11 deletion (hSNF5/INI1 gene) Choroid plexus carcinoma Altered expression of SWI/SNF protein (oncosuppressor protein)

AT/RT, atypical teratoid/rhabdoid tumour; EGFR, epidermal growth factor receptor; MB, medulloblastoma; PNET, primitive neuroectodermal tumour.

chromatin remodelling complex (the SWI/SNF complex) which is believed to cause ATP-dependent conformational changes in the nucleosome, altering histone-DNA binding. Mutations of this gene cause premature truncation of the protein, resulting in the development of most rhabdoid tumours regardless of their site. The INI1 mutation is present in extracranial rhabdoid infantile tumours (for example, kidney rhabdoid tumour), and occasionally in choroid plexus carcinomas, thus constituting the genetic basis for the so-called 'rhabdoid tumour predisposing

Table 4. The most common biological alterations in primitive benign infantile brain tumours

Gene and/or protein alterations	Histotype and rate	Clinical correlation
7, 8, 11 structural abnormalities	Pilocytic astrocytoma (50%)	Significance unknown
C to T transition (C169) in a CpG dinucleotide (NF2 gene)	NF2-related meningeal tumours (50%)	Presentation of the disease in infancy
+7, +12, and +20 (hyperdiploid chromosomes)	Choroid plexus papilloma (30–40%)	Hyperdiploidy indicative of atypical papillomas
Reelin signalling and tuberin/insulin growth receptor pathways	Ganglioglioma (30%)	Cellular division control proteins
22q11d13 breakpoint or 22 monosomy	Ependymoma (28%)	Putative tumour suppressor gene locus

syndrome'. Once misdiagnosed by pathologists as medulloblastoma, PNET, or choroid plexus carcinoma – owing to the presence of primitive neuroepithelial elements and similar histological features – AT/RT can be now differentiated from these neoplasms by immunohistochemical analysis. Immunostaining for INI1 is usually retained in choroid plexus carcinomas and medulloblastoma/PNETs but absent in AT/RT.

A mutation in the NF2 gene, found in patients affected by neurofibromatosis type II harbouring *ependymomas*, has not been confirmed in sporadic forms of this tumour (not associated with NF2). Interestingly, the correlation between NF2 gene mutation (22q12) and ependymomas involves spinal cord ependymomas (in 43 per cent of the cases) but not intracranial ones. Other cytogenetic alterations concern monosomy 22 and numerous possible deletions (1p, 4q, 6q, 9p, 17p, 19q, 20q, and 22q) occasionally found in both 'benign' and anaplastic ependymomas (Biernat Żawrocki, 2007). Current investigation are focusing on 6q and on some translocations of chromosome 9 that are increasingly detected in paediatric ependymomas and could be involved in their development. Loss of chromosome 9, in particular, is found in 40 per cent and 100 per cent of World Health Organization (WHO) grade II and III clear cell ependymomas, respectively.

Genetic studies specifically devoted to *choroid plexus tumours* are limited in number. The information results mainly from occasional observations such as the above mentioned INI1 mutation in choroid plexus carcinoma or the constitutional (X;17) (q12; p13) translocation described in a patient with Ito's hypomelanosis and choroid plexus papilloma. Additional abnormalities are represented by hyperdiploid karyotypes composed of 51, 52, or 56 chromosomes per cell with extra copies of chromosomes 7, 11, 12, 15, and 18, according to the different studies (Biegel, 1999).

Many of the genetic studies on *brain gliomas* refer to investigations on adult patients because the genetic alterations found in low grade astrocytomas (which are typical of the younger aged patients) are so rare, and because of the complex genetic pattern of abnormalities in glioblastoma, which is the most common histotype in adults. Cytogenetic studies on *juvenile pilocytic astrocytoma* have generally shown normal karyotypes except for some cases of trisomy 7 and 8 or sporadic structural chromosomal abnormalities, the meaning of which remains uncertain (though probably correlated with tumour recurrence). In contrast, *high grade gliomas* show a variety of numerical and structural chromosomal changes other than molecular alterations. Apart from gains of chromosome 7 and loss of chromosome 10, prevalent in adults, the structural chromosomal changes of malignant gliomas (chromosomes 1, 7, 9, 17, and 22) are also found in children. The same observation applies to mutations of p53, p16, and PTEN genes that are found in WHO grades III–IV gliomas of all ages, suggesting similar molecular patterns of tumour development regardless of age (Ohgaki & Kleihues, 2007). Epidermal growth factor receptor (EGFR) amplification, on the other hand, is involved in the development of primary adult glioblastomas and is very rare or absent in the paediatric population.

Special mention must be made of TP53 mutations. TP53 (17p13.1) is a tumour suppressor gene encoding a 53 kDa protein (p53) which appears to play an important role in several cellular processes, including the cell cycle, cell differentiation, cell death, response to DNA damage, and neovascularization; it is therefore called 'The Guardian of the Genome'. TP53 is the most mutated gene in human cancer (mainly in breast and colorectal malignancies); it also represents the genetic basis of the Li-Fraumeni syndrome, one of the better known inherited cancer-predisposing syndromes. TP53 mutation is found in glioblastoma (WHO grade IV) as well as in anaplastic astrocytomas (WHO III) and even in grade II astrocytomas. Although it also occurs in primary glioblastomas (28 per cent), TP53 mutation plays a crucial role in the development of secondary glioblastoma from low grade diffuse or fibrillary astrocytoma (65 per cent). TP53 mutation is involved in the telomere maintenance function. As known, telomeres are eroded after every cell division and are repaired by a telomere maintenance system including a telomerase or an alternative lengthening of the telomere pathway (ALT). It has been found that an early mutation of TP53 during tumorigenesis – corresponding to early loss of p53 protein – can facilitate the selection of the ALT phenotype for telomere maintenance. Such an association has important clinical significance, as ALT identifies a subtype of glioblastomas with a significantly more favourable prognosis that occurs in infants and children (Hakin-Smith *et al.*, 2003). TP53 mutation seems to have prognostic value only in youngest patients, in whom survival time is doubled in the presence of the ALT phenotype compared with the TP53-telomerase phenotype association. On the other hand, accumulation of p53 protein in the nuclei of perinatal glioblastoma cells is associated with a worse prognosis. In the series by Pollack and colleagues (Pollack *et al.*, 1997), the mean progression-free survival time of infants with p53 overexpression was 5.5 months compared with 25 months in those without p53 accumulation.

Anatomical location

In contrast to tumours occurring in older children, IBTs have a significant predilection for the supratentorial (ST) compartment. According to the Cooperative ISPN Survey (Di Rocco *et al.*, 1991), supratentorial IBTs accounted for 65.4 per cent of the 840 collected cases and infratentorial (IT) tumours for 29.6 per cent. This anatomical distribution is found in other series (Di Rocco *et al.*, 1993; Rickert *et al.*, 1997; Sala *et al.*, 1999). In their 20-year review of paediatric CNS tumour series, Rickert and colleagues (Rickert *et al.*, 1997) reported an ST/IT ratio varying from 1.5 to 9.0. The supratentorial location shows the highest incidence among the 0 to 12 month old patients (70 to 78 per cent), then progressively decreasing in frequency among those in the 12 to 24 month group and the 24 to 36 month group (30 to 35 per cent). If the analysis of the anatomical distribution is restricted to malignant tumours, however, the infratentorial location becomes prevalent owing to the high incidence of medulloblastoma and ependymoma. Diverse tumours may show different distributions according to topography and age. Pilocytic astrocytoma, for example, occurs more often in the supratentorial space in infants (ST/IT ratio = 3.8) compared with children more than 2 years old (ST/IT = 0.5), while ependymoma is preferentially located in the infratentorial compartment (ST/IT in infants = 0.5, *vs.* 0.4 in older aged children).

The predilection for the midline and ventricular/periventricular structures is another distinctive aspect of IBTs (Table 5). The suprasellar-chiasmatic-hypothalamic region in the supratentorial compartment and the cerebellar vermis-fourth ventricle region in the infratentorial space are the areas most commonly involved. The large majority of lateral tumours are supratentorial while those located along the midline are preferentially infratentorial. In the series by Sala and colleagues (Sala *et al.*, 1999), lateral tumours were supratentorial in 90 per cent of the cases while midline tumours occurred in only 30 per cent of the cases. Such a distribution results from the occurrence of tumours taking their origin from lateral regions, such as ependymomas, choroid plexus tumours, supratentorial PNETs, and gliomas. Among the hemispheric locations, the frontal lobe appears to be the more commonly affected. In the infratentorial compartment, the preferential distribution along the midline results from the occurrence of medulloblastoma, ependymoma and brain stem gliomas, while juvenile pilocytic astrocytoma, which typically occurs in the cerebellar hemisphere, is relatively rare.

There is no definite explanation for the prevalent location of IBTs along the midline and the ventricular structures. The old theory that most infantile neuroectodermal tumours originate from the phylogenetically older structures of the CNS remains the most accepted hypothesis. Accordingly, the proximity with secondary germinal areas – where substantial cell proliferation occurs in the first 6 months of extrauterine life – and the neoplastic transformation of physiologically proliferating primitive cell populations would explain the midline/periventricular location, the patients' young age, and the frequent finding of mixed populations and immature/aggressive tumours in this subset of patients.

Table 5. Intracranial distribution of the main infantile brain tumours

Location	Anatomical region	Pertinent tumours
Supratentorial (lateral)	Cerebral hemispheres	PNET, astrocytoma, DIG > ependymoma°, teratoma° > AT/RT, mesenchymal tumours°
Supratentorial (lateral)	Lateral ventricles/periventricular area	Ependymomas, choroid plexus tumour, PNET > teratoma°, astrocytoma
Supratentorial (midline)	Third ventricle	Ependymoma, choroid plexus tumour > astrocytoma, teratoma > craniopharyngioma°
Supratentorial (midline)	Suprasellar region	Optic hypothalamic glioma, craniopharyngioma, teratoma/germ cells tumour
Supratentorial (midline)	Pineal region	Teratomas/germ cells tumour, PNET > astrocytoma > pineal parenchymal tumour
Infratentorial (lateral)	Cerebellar hemispheres	Astrocytoma > MB/PNET > AT/RT > ependymoma°
Infratentorial (lateral)	Cerebello-pontine angle	AT/RT, ependymoma° > astrocytoma°, MB/PNET°, schwannoma/meningioma (NF-2)
Infratentorial (midline)	Vermis	MB/PNET > astrocytoma
Infratentorial (midline)	IV ventricle	Ependymoma > MB/PNET°, astrocytoma°
Infratentorial (midline)	Brain stem	Astrocytoma >> MB/PNET°, ependymoma°

° Tumours not strictly originating from these areas but frequently extending into or infiltrating them.
AT/RT, teratoid/rhabdoid tumour; DIG, desmoplastic infantile ganglioglioma; MB, medulloblastoma; PNET, primitive neuroectodermal tumour.

Another typical feature of brain tumours in infants is their tendency to involve more than one intracranial compartment. In neonates, for example, the tumour mass can occupy more than one third of the intracranial volume in up to 75 per cent of the cases. The mean IBT diameter at diagnosis ranges from 40 to 45 mm. The frequent origin of IBTs from multiple cell lineages and the higher compliance of the 'elastic' skull during the first months of life may explain this finding.

Clinical presentation

Because of the elasticity of the skull and the adaptability of the still immature and developing brain, IBTs usually present with non-specific signs and symptoms, such as vomiting, lethargy, and headache. Furthermore, the cranio-cerebral plasticity allows the tumour mass to enlarge progressively to reach a huge size before these signs or symptoms become apparent. Such features explain the peculiar clinical picture of IBTs and their possibly delayed diagnosis.

Perinatal period and neonates

Advances in prenatal neuroimaging techniques and their increased availability is steadily improving the prenatal diagnosis of congenital intracranial tumours. These techniques allow detection and differentiation of intracranial masses and the associated maternal and fetal signs such as polyhydramnios, breech presentation, macrocrania, hydrocephalus and fetal hydrops.

The tumour and its related anomalies may produce premature labour, dystocia and cephalopelvic disproportion. A caesarean section is required in cases of huge tumour dimensions and macrocephaly, with or without hydrops. Large tumour size may also be associated with stillbirth. Among the 250 congenital brain neoplasms reviewed by Isaacs (Isaacs, 2002), 21 per cent of the patients were stillborn. The highest incidence was detected among teratomas (25 of 74 cases, 34 per cent), followed by PNETs (11 of 33 cases, 33 per cent) and astrocytomas (6 of 47, 13 per cent).

Macrocephaly is the most common postnatal sign, being observed in 30 per cent of the cases. It results from the chronic intracranial hypertension caused by the tumour mass effect or from the possibly associated hydrocephalus, or both. Hydrocephalus often complicates perinatal neoplasms (in 15 to 60 per cent of the cases) as a result of obstruction of the cerebrospinal fluid (CSF) pathways by the tumour or secondary haemorrhages. The neonatal signs and symptoms of raised intracranial pressure consist of a bulging fontanelle, separation of the cranial sutures, venous engorgement of the scalp and face, sunset sign, vomiting, irritability, poor feeding, and lethargy. These features, however, can be relatively subtle owing to the widening of the cranial sutures (Table 6). A clear intracranial hypertension syndrome is evident only in cases of rapidly growing tumours or during the late phases of the clinical history of slowly enlarging neoplasms.

Another finding often correlated with perinatal neoplasms is tumour haemorrhage. This results either from spontaneous bleeding in the tumour tissues, especially in malignant and rapidly evolving tumours such as medulloblastoma, glioblastoma and PNET (where there is active and anarchic vascular proliferation due to isoforms of vascular endothelial growth factors), or from the change in pressure forces on the fetal head during delivery, or both. The incidence of haemorrhage ranges from 3 to 20 per cent (mean, 14–18 per cent), a rate significantly higher than in children and adults. Tumour haemorrhage is a major clinical problem as it can produce hydrocephalus or even death. Severe anaemia can be the main clinical feature in low birthweight newborns.

Table 6. Clinical features of intracranial hypertension in newborns and infants

Patient category	Acute onset IH*	Progressively developing IH
Newborns and infants with open sutures	Marked bulging of the fontanelle Diastasis of the sutures Inconsolable crying Vomiting Irritability Cushing's triad (late)°	Macrocrania Bulging fontanelle Reduced feeding Caput medusae Suture diastasis (late) Sunset sign (late) Vomiting/irritability (late) Lethargy (late)
Infants with fused sutures	Asthenia Hyporeactivity Headache Vomiting Focal neurological deficit Cushing's triad (late)°	Headache Vomiting Papilloedema Strabismus and diplopia Psychomotor regression Behaviour changes

* Rapid increase in intracranial pressure: haemorrhage, acute and severe hydrocephalus, rapidly growing tumours with massive oedema.
° Bradycardia, arterial hypertension, irregular breathing (expression of brain stem damage).
IH, intracranial hypertension.

Associated congenital anomalies are quite common, being reported, for example, in 11.5 per cent of the 230 cases reviewed by Wakai and colleagues (Wakai et al., 1984). Cleft lip and cleft palate are the most frequently encountered. Teratoma is the most common associated tumour (anencephaly, cleft palate, proptosis). Other anomalies are included in the familial syndromes discussed above in the section on epidemiology.

The presenting neurological signs of perinatal tumours are flaccidity, hypotonia, seizures, hemiparesis, cranial nerve palsy, and eye signs (strabismus, nystagmus, exophthalmos, ptosis, sunset eyes, doll's eyes). These signs usually appear late because of the high compliance of the developing brain. Neurological signs may help in localizing the tumour mass and are mainly found with infratentorial tumours.

Fever has been reported in association with congenital tumours, probably resulting from the deposition of necrotic debris or blood in the CSF following tumour necrosis or haemorrhage.

To summarize, the four-part classification of Volpe (1995) is as follows: i) severe macrocephaly resulting from huge tumours and causing cephalopelvic disproportion, dystocia, stillbirth and premature labour; ii) increased head circumference and bulging fontanelle as consequence of hydrocephalus; iii) neurological deficits related to the mass and its location (epilepsy, hemiparesis, cranial nerve palsy, signs of raised intracranial pressure); iv) sudden onset of intracranial haemorrhage.

Infants

The clinical picture in infants older than 2 months in part overlaps that reported for neonates. Studies specifically devoted to this age subgroup showed that raised intracranial pressure syndrome is the most common clinical feature, being present in 40 to 75 per cent of the cases (Rickert et al., 1997; Di Rocco et al., 2007). Macrocrania is again the most frequent sign (64 to 82 per cent), followed by vomiting (39 to 52 per cent), other 'cranial' signs (bulging fontanelle, suture diastasis, caput medusae) and neurologically related signs (lethargy, irritability, sixth cranial nerve palsy). Some associated findings, such as papilloedema or regression of motor skills, can be better appreciated in infants than in neonates, and symptoms of increased intracranial pressure are more evident, especially in infants with fused cranial sutures. Table 6 summarizes the main clinical aspects of intracranial hypertension according to the different age subgroups. In older infants, neurological deficits are more evident, occurring more often and earlier than in neonates. Seizures represent the most common clinical finding after raised intracranial pressure (12 to 20 per cent of cases), followed by psychomotor retardation (16 per cent), nystagmus (9 to 16 per cent), cranial nerve palsies (5 to 12 per cent), and ataxia (10 per cent). Visual symptoms and failure to thrive complete the spectrum of symptoms. Finally, hydrocephalus affects a significant percentage of these children (78 to 90 per cent).

Infants with brain tumours are often completely asymptomatic when referred to hospital (for example, following an incidental finding on neuroimaging done for other reasons) or when admission is precipitated by intercurrent events (fever, head injuries). The clinical picture is influenced by the tumour location. Infants harbouring a posterior cranial fossa neoplasm show a combination of signs and symptoms resulting from the mass effect of the tumour against the cerebellum and the brain stem, and from the almost invariably associated hydrocephalus. Generally, the clinical history tends to be shorter in infants with midline tumours than in those with laterally placed masses. The typical presentation is with headache and vomiting (70 to 75 per cent of the cases) in otherwise well children. Physical examination shows papilloedema and diplopia in 15 to 20 per cent of the cases. In other instances, the clinical picture is more specific, with cerebellar or brain stem deficits. Cerebellar signs include gait problems, truncal ataxia, dysmetria, vertigo, dysarthria, nystagmus (to the side of the lesion) or more subtle signs such as unsteadiness, tremor and incoordination of the upper or lower extremities. Brain stem involvement is revealed by pyramidal signs (one third of the cases), rarely complicated by severe hemiparesis or tetraparesis and cranial nerve dysfunction (hypoacusia, tinnitus, strabismus, facial palsy, wheeziness, dysphagia, dysphonia). Torticollis (head tilt away from the lesion) is an important localizing sign, mainly found in infants affected by medulloblastoma (45 per cent). In rare circumstances, the patient is referred to hospital as an emergency because of cerebellar herniation or brain stem compression (severe nuchal pain, opisthotonus, marked pyramidal signs, alteration in consciousness), or because of extremely raised intracranial pressure (stuporous or comatose state, bradycardia, increased systemic blood pressure).

Tumours of the cerebral hemispheres and lateral ventricles are frequently revealed by intracranial hypertension (40 to 80 per cent of the cases). A typical distinctive finding is skull asymmetry or the presence of a bulging skull mass caused by tumour growth within one hemicranium. Focal deficits such as motor weakness, visual field loss (homonymous hemianopia), sensory impairment or extrapyramidal signs are highly localizing when detectable. However, infants with hemispheric tumours often present with subtle and poorly specific signs such as personality change, behaviour disturbance, and deterioration in motor or speech performance. Seizures occur in about 40 per cent of the cases, often as isolated symptoms. The whole epilepsy spectrum is represented.

The clinical features of neoplasms arising from the optic-chiasmatic-hypothalamic or suprasellar regions depend on the involvement of the optic pathways and impairment of the hypothalamic-pituitary axis. The main ocular and visual signs are exophthalmos (50 per cent of the cases with optic pathway astrocytomas), ptosis, conjunctival redness, strabismus, and impaired ocular movements (because of tumours growing within the orbital cavity). Visual signs and symptoms usually consist of optic atrophy (60 per cent), papilloedema (20 per cent), papillary blurring (20 per cent), visual loss (late clinical history), and visual field defects. Hypothalamic involvement is revealed by intracranial hypertension caused by anterior third ventricle obstruction, or by signs of hypothalamic dysfunction. A specific manifestation in infants is failure to thrive (25 per cent of the cases) characterizing the so-called diencephalic syndrome. Infants with this syndrome usually harbour large optic-hypothalamic gliomas and present with emaciation and loss of subcutaneous fat, normal height and muscle mass, normal appetite, hyperactivity, and nystagmoid eye movements. Another hypothalamic syndrome is known as 'bobble-head doll syndrome' (or spasmus nutans), and consists of head bobbing, head tilt, and nystagmus. The spectrum of endocrinology deficits is wide. The most common single hormone deficit is of growth hormone, followed by thyroid hormones, vasopressin, and cortisol. Hypopituitarism or panhypopituitarism are not uncommon. Some of the typical hypothalamic postsurgical deficits – such as electrolytic imbalance, abnormal alimentary behaviour (anorexia or obesity), thermoregulation disorders, and jet-lag syndrome – may be present at diagnosis. On the other hand, precocious puberty and hormone hyperfunction syndromes (gigantism, Cushing disease, and so on) are exceptional in infants, as they are caused mainly by secreting pituitary gland adenomas which are very rare at this age.

IBTs originating from the pineal gland region can compress the aqueduct of Sylvius and the posterior portion of the third ventricle and infiltrate the mesencephalon. In the former, the main consequences are hydrocephalus, occurring in 85 per cent of the cases, and subsequent intracranial hypertension. Infiltration of the mesencephalon produces an ocular movement disorder, namely Parinaud syndrome (in 50 per cent of the cases). The main signs of this syndrome are upward gaze paralysis (rarely downward paralysis), nystagmus rectractorius, and convergence paralysis; when present, transient or permanent papillary dilatation, ptosis, bilateral auditory loss and ataxia indicate extensive intraparenchymatous tumour infiltration. Oculomotor nerve paralysis is considered a further sign of midbrain infiltration, though it probably depends more on raised intracranial pressure. In case of huge pineal tumours, hemiparesis (invasion of the internal capsule), hemi-sensory syndrome with or without hemi-hyperalgesia (thalamic invasion), disturbance of the mnesic function (fornix disruption), cerebellar syndrome (posterior cranial fossa invasion), or endocrine deficits (infiltration of the hypothalamus) become evident. Precocious puberty can occur as result of pineal region tumours. This would be the effect of i) the tumour compressing the posterior part of the diencephalon, with subsequent disinhibition of the hypothalamic median eminence (gonadotropin secretion); or ii) disruption of the pineal gland, with consequent lack of secretion of antigonadotropins; or iii) secretion of β-HCG by the tumour itself (chorioncarcinoma, mixed tumours).

Neuroimaging

Ultrasound

Ultrasonography is the most readily available and widespread diagnostic technique for the antenatal diagnosis of brain tumours. Its advantages are as follows: it has quite high sensitivity and specificity; there is no radiation; there is little discomfort for the mother; it only takes a short time to do; and it is cheap. It has recently been shown that dedicated neurosonography can provide similar results to magnetic resonance imaging (MRI) in the prenatal diagnosis of fetal brain anomalies (Malinger et al., 2004).

Neurosonography continues to play a significant role in the postnatal period, being useful in the follow-up of neonates and younger infants with open fontanelles. Ultrasound is currently used to obtain very early images after birth, especially if computed tomography (CT) or MRI are not readily available; to detect possible complications after treatment, reducing the need for CT or MRI; to monitor the evolution of hydrocephalus; and to carry out ultrasound-assisted procedures. Limitations of ultrasound result from the lower contrast resolution and the operator-dependent nature of the technique. During pregnancy, moreover, impaired visualization of the anterior cerebral hemispheres because of reverberations from the overlying maternal organs, a poor sonographic window when there is decreased amniotic fluid, and variations in fetal position represent further limitations.

On ultrasound, IBTs usually appear as large hyperechogenic (if mainly solid) or hypoechogenic (if mainly cystic) masses, possibly showing hyperechogenic spots (haemorrhagic areas) or internal shadowing (calcifications). The distortion of the brain architecture is usually well appreciated, as are the possibly associated findings (such as loss of brain substance).

Computed tomography

CT is widely used thanks to its high resolution, the possibility of obtaining images in all three planes, the very short examination times (10 to 15 seconds for a single standard brain investigation with modern machines), the high sensitivity in visualizing dense tissues such as bone, calcium and blood, and the relatively low cost. The main limitation is the exposure to radiation. Further limitations are the lower resolution power for brain structures compared with MRI and possible allergic effects related to the use of iodinated contrast medium.

CT is used for IBTs when a quick examination is required, such as when a huge mass or severe hydrocephalus cause a sudden and rapid neurological deterioration. A further indication is to avoid sedation or general anaesthesia (required for MRI) in very young children. A specific indication for CT is the detection of tumour calcification. As it shows greater sensitivity for demonstrating calcium, CT is often carried out in addition to MRI when scanning for possible calcific neoplasms such as craniopharyngiomas, teratomas, low grade astrocytomas, glioneuronal tumours, and meningiomas. For the same reason, CT is the gold standard for investigating possible bone defects (for example, skull erosion due to large intracranial tumours), thanks to the ability to obtain very thin slices and three-dimensional (3D) reconstructions. 3D reconstructions are also used in angiographic sequences: the high definition power of 3D angio-CT allows the relationship between a brain tumour and the surrounding vessels to be clarified, contributing to preoperative planning. A rare application of CT in infants concerns neuronavigation and stereotaxy. In the former, CT is employed preoperatively to enable a reconstruction to be created by dedicated software for frameless intraoperative guidance. MRI is preferred for most intracranial procedures except in cases requiring greater bone definition (for example, in maxillo-cranial reconstruction of a sellar tumour to be approached endoscopically). Stereotaxy is less and less used, as frameless techniques and endoscopy allow better and quicker approaches for tumour biopsy.

CT measures the attenuation of X-rays by Hounsfield units (HU). Compared with grey (30–40 HU) and white matter (20–35 HU), the tissues with low attenuation power are defined as hypodense (fat, –35 HU; CSF, 5 HU; oedema, 10–14 HU), while those with high attenuation power are defined as hyperdense (blood clot, 75–80 HU; calcium, 100–300 HU; bone, 600 HU). Accordingly, the appearance of brain tumours can be as follows:

- *isodense* – moderate to high cellularity: medulloblastoma, PNET, ependymoma, atypical teratoid/rhabdoid tumour (AT/RT)

- *hypodense* – cellularity poor and tumour rich in interstitial water: low grade astrocytoma
    cystic tumour: low grade astrocytoma, desmoplastic infantile ganglioglioma (DIG),
    craniopharynioma
    necrotic tumour: malignant histotypes
    fatty tumour: teratoma, lipomas

- *hyperdense* – calcified: teratoma, low grade tumour, craniopharyngioma, and/or
    haemorrhagic: teratoma, PNET, ependymoma, and/or
    hypervascularized: choroid plexus tumour, meningioma, glioblastoma.

The enhancement after administration of contrast medium is the result of rupture of the brain-blood barrier, as occurs in most solid brain tumours or in the solid portion of mixed tumours. Necrotic neoplasms typically show a characteristic enhancement of the peripheral portion of the tumour (vital and vascularized compared with the central, necrotic zone). Note that extracerebral structures, such as the choroid plexuses and the pituitary gland (adenohypophysis) are normally enhanced.

Magnetic resonance imaging

MRI is the gold standard neuroimaging technique both for diagnosis and follow-up of IBTs. The very high contrast resolution, the multiplanarity, the increasing number of tissue-specific sequences, the use of paramagnetic contrast medium (very low allergic risk), and increasing availability make MRI almost indispensable for a correct diagnosis. This technique normally provides the greatest detail with regard to tumours (size, morphology, location, differential diagnosis), their growth pattern (infiltrative or expansive), and the condition of the surrounding neural and vascular structures (infiltration, distortion, gliosis, necrosis, haemorrhage). Moreover, the tumour-associated findings are very highly defined. The most important of these are:

- *hydrocephalus*, presenting as mono-, bi-, tri- or tetra-ventricular dilatation as a result of the obstruction of the CSF pathways by tumour, brain oedema, secondary haemorrhage and, theoretically, CSF hypersecretion in case of choroid plexus tumours. Transependymal CSF adsorption (having the same characteristics as brain oedema but localized in the periventricular region) indicates an acute or uncompensated hydrocephalus;
- *tumour-related mass effect*, detectable as ventricular compression, distortion of the neighbouring structures, contralateral shift of the midline, bulging of the skull, and cerebral or cerebellar herniations;
- *perilesional vasogenic oedema*, appearing as a hypointense area (T1-weighted images) or a hyperintense area (T2-weighted images) surrounding the tumour and indicating a rupture of the brain-blood barrier. This sign is most commonly associated with malignant tumours (rapid and infiltrative growth);
- *tumour seeding*, visible as abnormal leptomeningeal enhancement or as secondary tumour localization (leptomeningeal, parenchymal or intraventricular nodules), or both.

Tumour seeding is a strongly negative prognostic factor, usually associated with malignant IBTs, though it cannot be excluded in cases of 'benign' tumours such as low grade astrocytoma. Tumour diffusion is favoured by infiltrative growth and, in particular, by the CSF circulation. The most common secondary localizations of IBTs occur throughout the CSF pathways. A typical location of brain tumour metastases is along the leptomeninges of the spinal cord, especially with fourth ventricular neoplasms and with the effect of gravity ('drop metastases'). Because of these features, MRI plays a fundamental role not only in tumour diagnosis but also in the differential diagnosis, staging, preoperative and pre-radiation planning, postoperative follow-up, and surveillance imaging during and after adjuvant treatment.

Limitations of MRI are the length of time it takes and the discomfort for the patient. In infants (and sometimes also in adults) this results in the need for sedation or anaesthesia to enable the examination to be done. In addition, MRI scans cannot be carried out in patients who have internal metallic bodies or prostheses (unless of compatible materials, such as titanium), they are still expensive, and capillary diffusion has not yet been achieved.

Standard MRI is currently carried out through 1.5 Tesla or 3 Tesla systems. The slice thickness is usually 5 mm (reduced to 3 mm for acquiring images of the pituitary gland and orbits). Brain tumour standard protocols are based on axial-coronal-sagittal T1-weighted images (T1) for the anatomical details (for example, sagittal views allow better appreciation of the midline structures). Axial-coronal-(sagittal) T2-weighted images (T2) and fluid-attenuated inversion recovery (FLAIR) are used to assess the tumour characteristics (cellularity, oedema, cysts). Axial-coronal-sagittal T1 after contrast medium administration is used to detect possible brain-blood barrier rupture and to study tumour enhancement. Other sequences can be added according to the tumour characteristics, such as T2 gradient-echo sequences (sensitive to the breakdown products of haemoglobin) to investigate previous tumour haemorrhages; angiographic sequences to study the relation between tumour mass and neighbouring vessels and to evaluate the tumour blood supply; or contrast-enhanced volumetric T1 images for image-guided surgery (neuronavigation).

Specific MRI protocols for children have recently been proposed (Saunders *et al.*, 2007). These consist of a reduced number of basal sequences (axial T2, coronal FLAIR, coronal, and sagittal T1) to reduce the examination times without affecting the specificity. Moreover, explicit sequences for infants can be used, such as dual-echo short-tau inversion recovery or T2 turbo spin echo to better visualize the grey/white matter differentiation (usually poor in infants because of the higher water content and the stage of myelination), or rapid T2 pulse sequences to overcome the limits of fetal motion during prenatal MRI.

Recent developments have strongly enhanced the sensitivity and specificity of MRI for tumour diagnosis, making it very useful for preoperative assessment and surgical planning. Its uses can be summarized as follows:

• *Functional MRI*: based on blood oxygen level dependent (BOLD) contrast to detect changes in regional deoxyhaemoglobin concentration. This may significantly influence therapeutic planning in patients with resectable tumours localized close to eloquent brain areas. As it requires collaboration by the patient, it cannot be used in infants.

• *MRI spectroscopy*: frequently accompanying standard MRI, this technique quantifies the various different molecules composing the brain tissues. The most important are: *creatine*, an energy metabolism molecule indicating the overall condition of the tissue; *N-acetyl-aspartate*, a neuronal marker which decreases in cases of neuronal stress or death; *choline*, a marker of membrane turnover which increases in the presence of cell proliferation (tumours); *myo-inositol*, a sugar present within the glial cells which increases when there is glial proliferation (low grade gliomas, metastases) or activation (gliosis); *lactate*, which increases when there is anaerobic metabolism (ischaemia, seizures); and *lipids*, which indicate cellular necrosis (high grade tumours). These markers provide quite non-specific information, except in the following instances:

i) For differentiating between high grade tumours (↑ choline and lipids, ↑ apparent diffusion coefficient (ADC) (see below)) and cerebral abscesses (↓ ADC, ↑ free amino acids);

ii) For differentiating between the presence of malignant tumour (↑ choline and lipids) and radiation necrosis (↑ lipids, ↓ N-acetyl-aspartate, choline and creatine);

iii) For assessing glial tumour infiltration (↑ choline and myo-inositol, ↓ N-acetyl-aspartate) *vs.* vasogenic oedema (normal metabolic profile).

• *Diffusion-weighted imaging (DWI)*: based on the molecular mobility, this measures the apparent diffusion coefficient (tissues with higher densities show a lower ADC by impeding molecular mobility). By integrating standard MRI and spectroscopy, it can help in the differential diagnosis between tumours and abscesses (see above), between cytotoxic oedema

(ADC reduction) and vasogenic oedema (ADC increase), and between tumour (very high ADC augmentation) and radionecrosis (moderate ADC augmentation). It is also valuable in assessing the response to therapy (an early increase in ADC during therapy would indicate cell necrosis while a drop in ADC values within the neoplasm area would indicate tumour regrowth).

- *Diffusion tensor imaging (DTI) and tractography*: this technique exploits the preferential movement of water protons along the long axis of the axons (in white matter the water diffusion is anisotropic as movement perpendicular to the long axis of the axons is prevented by the myelin, while that along the long axis is favoured). DTI provides information on the white matter status (tumour infiltration *vs.* oedema) which is of paramount importance for correct radiotherapy planning (irradiation volume). The 3-D reconstructions (tractography) allow visualization of the main white matter tracts (for example, the corticospinal tracts, cerebellar peduncles, medial lemniscus, arcuate fascicle, corpus callosum and commissural fibres), thus significantly contributing to preoperative planning.

- *Perfusion imaging*: this combines several perfusion-weighted imaging methods to provide a non-invasive and consistent marker for tumour angiogenesis and capillary permeability – two important markers of tumour malignancy (especially in gliomas).

- *Intraoperative MRI*: currently available in a few centres, this consists of an MRI machine placed within a dedicated operating theatre. It provides significant help in the real-time assessment of the surgical excision of the tumour.

The specific MRI features of the main IBTs are discussed later in the chapter.

Other neuroimaging techniques

Thanks to the high resolution of angio-MRI and angio-CT, cerebral angiography is now used only in selected IBTs, namely when an accurate definition of the relation between tumour and brain vessels is mandatory. Such an instance occurs, for example, in cases of huge suprasellar tumours (craniopharyngiomas, teratomas or optic pathway gliomas) which can be adherent to or encase the arteries of the circle of Willis, and in extra-axial tumours (meningiomas), superficial tumours (DIG), or critically located tumours (pineal region) which can compress, infiltrate, or encase the venous sinuses. The best indication for cerebral angiography is represented by the preoperative study of a possibly hypervascularized tumour (for example, choroid plexus tumours, meningiomas). Evaluation of the degree of tumour vascularization (afferent and efferent vessels) and preoperative tumour embolization result in a safer surgical procedure.

The role of functional neuroimaging in IBTs is limited. A useful clinical application of positron emission tomography (PET) is in evaluating anaplastic transformation, tumour recurrence, and tumour differentiation resulting from radiotherapy- or chemotherapy-induced brain damage (Chen, 2007). A high uptake of the PET marker ^{18}F-FDG usually indicates a high grade tumour; an increased uptake in a previously low grade tumour points to malignant transformation. Tumour recurrence or tumour differentiation from normal brain tissue can be achieved using different tumour-imaging markers, such as amino acid PET tracers, as their increased uptake indicates the presence of a tumour compared with the low uptake shown by the normal brain tissues.

Pathology

Challenges and classification

The pathology of primitive IBTs is a complex topic. First, cerebral tumours show exclusive features eluding any comparison with visceral and connective tissues, and often present macroscopic and microscopic findings that barely resemble brain tissue. Second, the increasingly sophisticated immunohistochemical and molecular approaches used for tumour diagnosis, classification and grading require specialized pathologists and laboratories. Third, IBTs show significant differences from tumours seen in children and adults, so that specialists devoted to paediatric neuropathology are required. The common adult CNS tumours – such as glioblastoma, anaplastic astrocytoma, meningioma, metastases, pituitary tumours, and schwannomas – are rare in infants (apart from malignant gliomas), while the histotype distribution in the infantile population includes several neoplasms almost exclusively found in this age group, such as pilocytic and pilomixoid astrocytomas, embryonal neuroepithelial tumours, AT/RT, and mixed neuronal-glial tumours.

A further problem concerns tumour classification. The need for a universally accepted classification and grading of brain tumours is felt by all the specialists in neuro-oncology in order to define more specific epidemiological studies, standardize histopathological and radiological approaches, and undertake more effective clinical trials. Consequently, brain tumour classification is still a matter of discussion and the object of continuous update. Initial classifications were based on the concept of 'the cell of origin', presuming that brain tumours developed from modifications of normal brain cells. This hypothesis led to the naming of most brain tumours as currently applied – for example, neoplasms arising from astrocytes: astrocytomas; neoplasms arising from ependymal cells: ependymomas. Nevertheless, normal cells are rarely subject to transformation and, when this occurs, they do not necessarily recapitulate their ancestry. In many instances, indeed, IBTs are composed of primitive, undifferentiated, pleomorphic, or anaplastic cells that do not resemble any specific cell of origin. Subsequently, current classifications consider both the possible histogenesis (such as tumours of neuroepithelial tissue) and the anatomical location (for example, tumours of the sellar region).

The WHO brain tumour classification is the most widely accepted. It was first published in 1979 (Zülch, 1979) and reflected the above-mentioned limitations relating to histogenesis as well as the rather primitive diagnostic tools that were available then. The second edition (Kleihues et al., 1993) opened a new era of CNS histopathology thanks to the introduction of immunohistochemistry, with significantly better definition of cerebral tumours, further enhanced by the acquisition of genetic profiles by the time of the third edition (Kleihues & Cavenee, 2000). The 2000 edition also incorporated concise but specific sections on tumour epidemiology, clinical and imaging features, and prognosis. Some of the most important changes compared with the 1993 version concerned IBTs: medulloblastoma was listed separately from the other PNETs, the 'large cell' medulloblastoma variant was included, AT/RT was added as a distinct disease, and desmoplastic infantile ganglioglioma was added among the mixed neuroglial tumours. Moreover, some infantile and paediatric tumour-like lesions were removed (epidermoid and dermoid cysts, colloid cysts, Rathke cleft cysts, neuroglial cysts) while in other cases the grading was modified (choroid plexus carcinoma received grade III instead of grade IV, central neurocytoma grade II instead of grade I). The fourth and most recent edition of the WHO classification (Louis et al., 2007) resulted from the international consensus of 75 experts (25 invited pathologists and geneticists plus 50 other contributors). It provides an update of the 2000 classification, as new entities have been added, and new variants with different age distribution, location, genetics and clinical features are included. Some new entities occur in the paediatric age range (angiocentric glioma, atypical choroid plexus papilloma, rosette-forming glioneuronal tumour of the fourth ventricle), and most of the new variants concern infants (pilomyxoid astrocytoma, anaplastic medulloblastoma, medulloblastoma with extensive nodularity). The main IBTs according to the 2007 WHO classification are given in Tables 7 and 8.

Histology, immunohistochemistry and molecular pathology

The pathological diagnostic process can be divided into three main steps: analysis of the histological and cytological features of the tumour; immunohistochemical and molecular characterization; and tumour grading. The first step allows one to establish whether the tumour samples are compatible with a neoplasm arising from the CNS and to orientate further investigations. This crucial analysis is carried out using standard histological staining, such as haematoxylin/eosin. The information obtained relates to tumour cell density and morphology, the nucleus to cytoplasm ratio, the presence of abnormal tumour vessels, necrosis, cystic areas, and calcification. Possible infiltration by the tumour into the surrounding normal tissues is also assessed. These data permit the formulation of an initial hypothesis on the tumour group and its grading. 'Malignant' brain tumours have a high cell density, frequent mitoses, a high nucleus to cytoplasm ratio, anaplasia, necrosis, neoangiogenesis, and infiltration; 'benign' tumours have well-differentiated cells with abundant cytoplasm and scarce mitoses, cystic and calcified portions, and no angiogenesis or necrosis.

Immunohistochemistry and molecular pathology analyses are aimed at identifying possible phenotypic and nuclear tumour markers. A positive immunohistochemical stain for the glial fibrillary acid protein (GFAP), for example, suggests a glioma, a PNET with neuroepithelial derivation or, more generally, a gliotic reaction. Immunostaining for synaptophysin (a neuronal marker) indicates a possible neurofibroma, a glio-neuronal tumour, or a PNET with neuronal differentiation. Increasing numbers of markers are being identified and a certain overlap among the different histotypes is present. The most useful markers are given in Table 9.

Immunohistochemistry and molecular pathology are currently also used as research tools to expand the knowledge of oncogenesis and the response of tumours to therapy. A recent study (Kurmasheva & Houghton, 2007) reported on the possible dysregulated growth factor pathways in paediatric cancers. With CNS tumours, the cytokines most often involved are as follows, in order of frequency: epidermal growth factor (EGF), found in glioblastoma (EGFR), medulloblastoma (erbB-2) and ependymoma (erbB-2/4); insulin-like growth factor 1 (IGF-1), found in glioblastoma and medulloblastoma; IGF-2, found in neuroblastoma and rhabdomyosarcoma; basic fibroblast growth factor (bFGF), found in glioblastoma and neuroblastoma; platelet-derived growth factor (PDGF), found in glioblastoma; vascular endothelial growth factor (VEGF), found in neuroblastoma; and hepatocyte growth factor/scatter factor (HGF/SF), found in glioblastoma.

A decisive application of nuclear marker immunohistochemistry is the assessment of tumour proliferation. The traditional method of estimating tumour proliferation was to calculate the mitotic index on standard histological slides. This was affected by difficulties in estimating the mitotic index correctly in low grade tumours (with scarce mitoses) and by possible differences in the length of the various cell cycle phases among the proliferating cells. For that reason, the method has been replaced by alternative immunohistochemical techniques measuring nuclear proliferation markers, such as the incorporation of bromodeoxyuridine or the expression of

Table 7. Infantile brain tumours and grade according to the 2007 WHO classification (part I)

Tumour derivation class	Subgroup	Histotype	Grade
Neuroepithelial tumours	Astrocytic tumours	Pilocytic astrocytoma	I
		Pilomixoid astrocytoma	II
		Subependymal giant cell astrocytoma	I
		Diffuse astrocytoma	II
		Pleomorphic xanthoastrocytoma	II
		Anaplastic astrocytoma	III
		Glioblastoma	IV
		Gliomatosis cerebri	IV
	Ependymal tumours	Subependymoma	I
		Myxopapillary ependymoma	I
		Ependymoma	II
		Anaplastic ependymoma	III
	Choroid plexus tumours	Choroid plexus papilloma	I
		Atypical choroid plexus papilloma	II
		Choroid plexus carcinoma	III
	Neuronal and neuroglial tumours	Dysplastic cerebellar gangliocytoma	I
		Desmoplastic infantile ganglioglioma	I
		Dysembryoplastic neuroepithelial tumour	I
		Gangliocytoma	I
		Ganglioglioma	I
		Anaplastic ganglioglioma	III
		Central neurocytoma	II
		Extraventricular neurocytoma	II
		Cerebellar liponeurocytoma	II
		Papillary glioneuronal tumour	I
		Rosette-forming glioneuronal tumour	I
		Paraganglioma	I
	Pineal region tumours	Pineocytoma	I
		Pineal parenchymal tumour of intermediate differentiation	II/III
		Pinealoblastoma	IV
		Papillary tumour of the pineal region	II/III
	Embryonal tumours	Medulloblastoma	IV

		CNS PNET
		    CNS neuroblastoma
		    CNS ganglioneuroblastoma
		    Medulloepithelioma
		    Ependymoblastoma
			IV

		Atypical teratoid/rhabdoid tumour	IV
Tumours of cranial and paraspinal nerves	Tumours of cranial and paraspinal nerves	Schwannoma (neurinoma)	I
		Neurofibroma	I
		Perineurioma	I/II/III
		Malignant peripheral nerve sheath tumour	II/III/IV

PNET, primitive neuroectodermal tumour.

Table 8. CNS tumours and grade according to the 2007 WHO classification (part II)

Tumour derivation class	Subgroup	Histotype	Grade
Tumours of the meninges	Tumours of the meningothelial cells	Meningioma	I
	Other meningeal neoplasms	Haemangioblastoma	I
Germ cell tumours	Germ cell tumours	Germinoma	IV
		Embryonal carcinoma	IV
		Yolk sac tumour	IV
		Choriocarcinoma	IV
		Teratoma	I–III
		Mixed germ cell tumour	IV
Tumours of the sellar region	Tumours of the sellar region	Craniopharyngioma	I
		Granular cell tumour	I
		Pituicytoma	I
		Spindle cell oncocytoma of the adenohypophysis	I
Metastatic tumours	Metastatic tumours	Metastatic tumours	IV

Table 9. CNS tumours and their main cellular and nuclear markers

Brain tumours	Markers
Medulloblastoma/PNET	GFAP, S-100, neurofilament, synaptophysin, cytokeratin, NeuN, HER-2, c-myc, TrkC, p53
Gliomas	GFAP, S-100, vimentin, nestin, p53, EGFR, *PTEN*
Ependymomas	GFAP, vimentin, EMA, cytokeratin
Neuronal tumours	Neurofilament, synaptophysin, chromogranin, NeunN, NSE, CD34
Teratoma	SMA, cytokeratin, synaptophysin
Germ cell tumours	PLAP
Chorioncarcinoma	β-HCG
Yolk sac tumour, embryonal carcinoma	α-FP
AT/RT	INI1, vimentin, actin, SMA
Craniopharyngioma	Cytokeratin, nuclear β-catenin
Pituitary adenoma	Pituitary peptides, chromogranin, cytokeratin
Meningioma	EMA, cytokeratin, PAS, CEA
Schwannoma, neurofibroma	Neurofilament, S-100, VEGF
Chordoma	Cytokeratin, S-100, CEA

AT/RT, atypical teratoid/rhabdoid tumour; CEA, carcinoembryonic antigen; EGFR, epidermal growth factor; EMA, epithelial membrane antigen; GFAP, glial fibrillary acid protein; NeuN, neuronal nuclei; NSE, neuron-specific enolase; PAS, periodic acid-Schiff; PLAP, placental alkaline phosphatase; PNET, primitive neuroectodermal tumour; SMA, smooth muscle actin; VEGF, vascular endothelial growth factor.

proliferating cell nuclear antigen. The currently most used technique is based on the expression of Ki-67 nuclear antigen detected by MIB-1 antibody. The MIB-1 monoclonal antibody allows one to detect the Ki-67 epitopes on a nuclear protein present in a portion of the cells in the G1, S, G2, and M phases of the cell cycle, thus being a reliable indicator of tumour proliferative activity (Fig. 1). The Ki-67 labelling index has important value for brain tumour grading and prognosis.

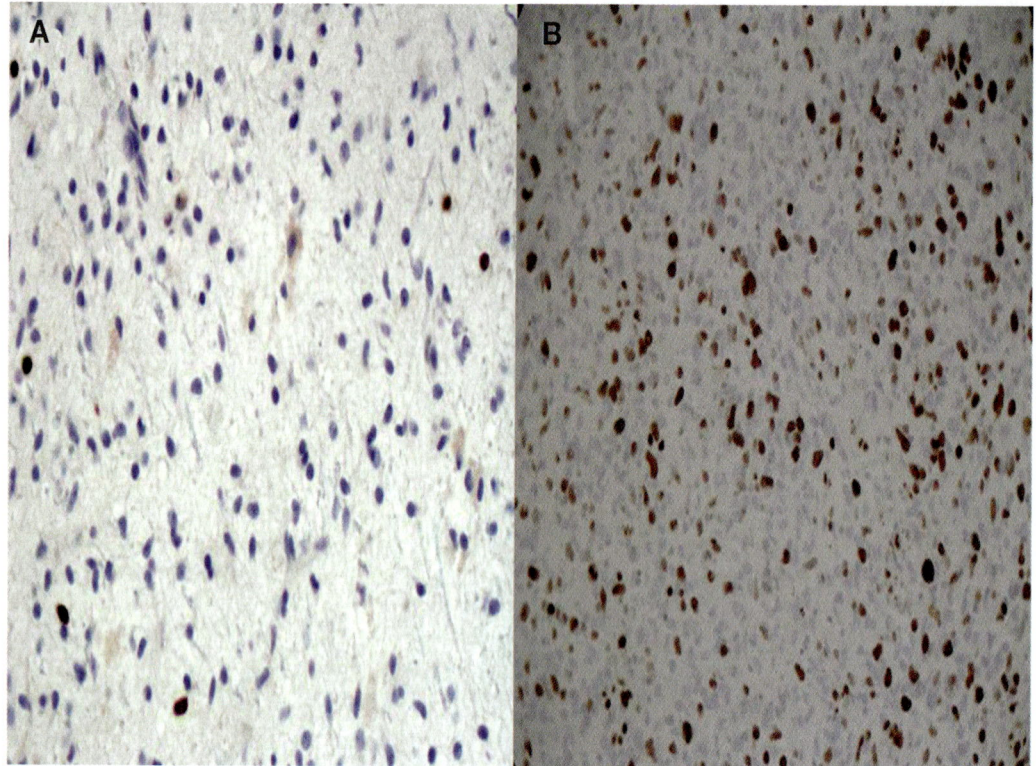

Fig. 1. MIB-1 immunostaining for Ki-67 (brown). Comparison between pilocytic astrocytoma (A, low proliferation index) and glioblastoma pattern (B, very high proliferation index).

When the immunohistochemical information has been acquired, the tumour can be identified and its grade assigned. The WHO grading system uses a scale of malignancy once employed only for astrocytomas. This considers four main variables: nuclear atypia, high proliferative index, neoangiogenesis, and necrosis, as follows:

• Grade I: none of the four features is present. WHO grade I tumours have a low proliferative activity and can be cured by surgery alone (for example, pilocytic astrocytoma, DIG, craniopharyngioma, choroid plexus papilloma);

• Grade II: one of the four features is present. WHO grade II lesions are infiltrative, may recur despite the low proliferative potential, and may progress into more malignant neoplasms (for example, diffuse astrocytoma, ependymoma);

• Grade III: two of the four features are present. WHO grade III tumours show evidence of malignancy, such as nuclear anomalies and a high mitotic activity, and often require adjuvant treatment (for example, anaplastic astrocytoma, choroid plexus carcinoma, anaplastic ependymoma);

- Grade IV: three or four of the four features are present. WHO grade IV tumours have high proliferative activity, with necrosis and signs of severe anaplasia. They are prone to infiltrate the surrounding tissues and to disseminate along the CSF pathways. They necessarily need adjuvant treatment (for example, glioblastoma, medulloblastoma/PNET, AT/RT).

By definition, in tumours showing areas with different characteristics or in mixed neoplasms, the grade is assigned according to the most malignant area, though this may not be the most widely represented. A possible bias in tumour grading may result from partial histological analysis of the tumour sample. This can occur in cases of small biopsy samples or partially resected tumours with different components.

Management: general considerations

The pre-hospital diagnostic phase of IBTs is often critical. As infants show a high degree of adaptability towards a growing intracranial mass, they tend to have a relatively long and asymptomatic clinical history but eventually develop acute symptoms and sudden worsening. It is important to define the duration of clinical signs and symptoms so as to assess the residual brain and skull compliance. If necessary, an intravenous injection of corticosteroids and osmotic agents should be given and the child urgently referred to hospital. The child's family and clinical history needs to be reviewed, looking for possible associated syndromes, affected family members, and clinical findings revealing multicentric tumours.

Although requiring anaesthesia, MRI is the best neuroimaging study if an IBT is suspected. Spinal MRI should always be carried out when a malignant brain tumour is diagnosed, even if it is supratentorial, to exclude possible tumour seeding. The diagnostic work-up includes EEG and video-EEG recordings, ophthalmological evaluation (ocular fundus, visual acuity, and visual fields if possible), and hormonal and tumour markers, depending on tumour location.

IBTs are complex and rare diseases. The average number of IBTs observed at a single institution is relatively small, ranging from 0.7 to 4.6 per year. Thus an infant with a brain tumour should be referred to a centre specialized in paediatric neuro-oncology and treatment should be planned by an expert multidisciplinary team. Most of the criteria involved in treatment decisions are similar to those considered in older children (histology, tumour location and extent, staging), but some are specific to infants (for example, inherited syndromes, clinical status).

Limitations on the treatment of IBTs are related to the young age of the patients and to the tumour itself. The developing and not yet fully myelinized brain is a contraindication to irradiation therapy because of the risk of endocrine dysfunction and severe late cognitive sequelae. The risk of drug neurotoxicity (mental retardation, leucoencephalopathy) is greater than in older children. Infants (especially neonates) have significantly different amounts of extracellular water (45 per cent of body weight at birth, 20 per cent by 3 years) and total body water (80 per cent of body weight at birth, 50 to 55 per cent in older children and adolescents), so that the distribution of chemotherapeutic agents may be unforeseen. The metabolism of drugs is also different: glomerular filtration and urine concentration are lower, gastric emptying time slower, some hepatic enzymatic pathways may be poorly functioning or absent, and the binding power of some blood proteins may be lower. All these factors can result in an unexpectedly high tissue concentration of drugs, especially with high-dose chemotherapy. Furthermore, for technical reasons, peripheral blood stem cells collection may be difficult in children less than 6 months old or less than 10 kg in weight. The infant's circulating blood volume is significantly lower than in older children, thus making surgery particularly risky. In addition, metabolic homeostasis during surgery is more difficult to maintain and temperature regulation requires the avoidance of sudden heat losses during the operation. Finally, the limitations related to the tumour (huge size, critical location, easy bleeding, biological aggressiveness) contribute significantly to making the management of these tumours particularly challenging.

IBTs with benign biological behaviour are usually managed by surgery alone. An exception is optic-hypothalamic low grade glioma in children affected by neurofibromatosis type I, which usually show a benign course. In this case, surgery is limited to a biopsy (if required) and to the treatment of the possibly associated hydrocephalus, while the tumour is managed by a wait-and-see policy; when necessary, the current primary treatment is chemotherapy and, in cases of late progression, radiotherapy (Massimi et al., 2007). Infantile low grade optic-hypothalamic astrocytomas, however, can have an unexpectedly malignant course, thus requiring surgery (tumour debulking) and adjuvant treatment. Another exception is totally or mainly cystic craniopharyngiomas which can be managed by intracystic drug injection.

Until the mid-1980s, malignant IBTs were treated by surgery followed by radiation. Afterwards, because of the poor results in terms of both long term survival and neurotoxicity, chemotherapy was introduced as the main adjuvant treatment. The enormous progress in drug development now allows the use of chemotherapy in children under 2 years of age for 1–2 years after surgery, therefore deferring radiotherapy. The complete treatment protocol (surgery + chemotherapy + radiotherapy) is associated with the best overall survival rates in the most malignant IBTs.

Highly chemosensitive and radiosensitive tumours, such as germ cell tumours, are managed differently. Children harbouring these neoplasms usually undergo tumour biopsy (which can be avoided in cases of secreting tumours thanks to the use of biomarkers) followed by chemo- and radiotherapy. Surgery is done only in cases of residual tumour or tumour progression.

Surgery

Indications

Surgery remains the principal treatment for IBTs. According to the tumour size and location, the surgical treatment aims at obtaining a histological diagnosis, acutely relieving increased intracranial pressure, treating the associated hydrocephalus, and excising the tumour mass. Only specific types of tumour can be cured by surgery alone.

The first step in surgery is to provide samples for pathological examination. IBTs are often malignant or critically located so that adjuvant treatment is frequently required. Correct histological characterization is mandatory to establish the optimal treatment protocol and formulate the prognosis. The tumour samples are usually taken during the surgical removal of the lesion. In the following instances, however, a tumour biopsy can be planned as the sole (at least initially) surgical step:

1) tumour masses not surgically amenable (holocranial teratomas, bithalamic gliomas, diffuse brain stem gliomas, gliomatosis cerebri);
2) optic-hypothalamic gliomas in patients with NF-1 (see above);
3) germ cell tumours (see above);
4) tumour-like masses or lesions with uncertain imaging;
5) tumour masses in infants not able to tolerate a direct surgical approach (tiny babies, very poor clinical condition, operation not accepted by the family).

In all these cases (except for number 5), the tumour biopsy can be carried out through the standard open surgical access (craniotomy). Modern neurosurgery, however, tends to favour mini-invasive approaches, such as endoscopy or stereotaxy. Neuroendoscopy is indicated for tumours arising from or extending into the cerebral ventricles (single burr hole approach) or located within the sellar/suprasellar region (transnasal transphenoidal approach). The transventricular approach is very useful in infants (mini-invasive, short duration) and can be facilitated by the associated hydrocephalus (that can be treated endoscopically at the same time as the biopsy). In contrast, the transphenoidal approach has a quite limited application in infants owing to the undersized anatomical pathways (minute nostrils, small and not yet pneumatized sphenoidal sinus, narrow operating field). Also stereotaxy is quite limited in infants as the stereotactic frame positioning requires a reasonably thick skull. Nowadays, this technique has been replaced by neuronavigation which allows a frameless image-guided tumour biopsy to be carried out regardless of the location of the neoplasm.

The second purpose of surgery is to provide rapid cranial decompression in tumours exerting a major mass effect. This is the case of huge tumours with large cystic components, such as teratoma, craniopharyngioma, DIG, optic-hypothalamic astrocytoma, or rapidly growing malignant masses (such as AT/RT, medulloblastoma, PNET, or anaplastic ependymoma). In all these cases, associated hydrocephalus or haemorrhage significantly contributes to the intracranial hypertension. Surgical decompression is obtained, if possible, by tumour excision and haematoma evacuation. A CSF diversion procedure is carried out to reduce hydrocephalus and attenuate the intracranial hypertension. In the most severe cases, brain oedema and swelling require a decompressive craniectomy to be done.

The treatment of hydrocephalus is the traditional role of surgery for IBTs, dating from the time when these tumours were considered inoperable. Tumour-associated hydrocephalus is mainly obstructive, being mono-, bi-, tri-, or tetra-ventricular depending on the tumour location. Exceptionally, a hypersecretive (choroid plexus tumour) and a non-resorptive aetiology (haemorrhage) coexist. Hydrocephalus is most frequent in tumours of the posterior cranial fossa and pineal region, because these tumours threaten the patency of the narrowest CSF pathway, the aqueduct of Sylvius. In 30 to 50 per cent of the cases, hydrocephalus resolves after tumour removal (Tamburrini et al., 2008). Persistent hydrocephalus is treated by CSF shunting (transient perioperative external ventricular drainage or permanent internal shunt) or endoscopy. The current trend favours endoscopy, which has the advantages of CSF shunting (mini-invasive neurosurgery, short surgery time, high success rate, low risk, low cost) but does not require prosthetic materials. The most extensive procedure is endoscopic third ventriculostomy (ETV), consisting of opening the floor of the third ventricle to restore the CSF circulation in cases of obstruction of the aqueduct of Sylvius or of the fourth ventricular foramina. ETV gives the best results in the neoplastic obstructive hydrocephalus unless CSF reabsorption through the arachnoid spaces is impaired (spreading leptomeningeal tumours, previous CSF infection, or brain irradiation). Endoscopic fenestration of the septum pellucidum allows cure of monoventricular hydrocephalus and obviates a double shunt in cases of biventricular hydrocephalus.

Approaches

The most important role of surgery remains tumour excision. Its aim should be the radical removal of the tumour mass, but this goal may be not achievable because of the large size of IBTs, infiltration of eloquent areas, and the small circulating blood volume of the infant. Of the 886 cases in the International Society for Paediatric Neurosurgery survey (Di Rocco et al.,

1991), only 389 (43.9 per cent) underwent total tumour removal. In 290 cases (32.7 per cent) partial tumour removal could be achieved, while in 85 cases (9.5 per cent) only a biopsy was taken. Similar results have been reported by other investigators, with overall rates of total tumour resection of between 27 and 58 per cent, subtotal/partial resection between 17 and 46 per cent, and biopsy between 5 and 20 per cent (Di Rocco et al., 1993; Rickert et al., 1997; Wakai et al., 1984). A safer method to remove tumours in infants is to carry out a multi-step operation (Di Rocco et al., 2007). This allows the young patient to have the tumour progressively excised with a reduced operative risk and a decreased rate of postoperative complications. Radical surgery is curative alone in most of the low grade tumours. Radical surgery in combination with chemotherapy and radiotherapy is associated with a better prognosis in grade II–IV neoplasms.

Tumours of the posterior cranial fossa are approached through a midline suboccipital craniotomy (or craniectomy) when located within the fourth ventricle, the cerebellar vermis/hemispheres, or the posterior brain stem. Either a prone or a sitting position is used, according to choice. Tumours located more laterally can be reached with a paramedian or a retrosigmoid craniotomy (cerebello-pontine angle) or by a subtemporal approach (midbrain), while those located anterior to the brain stem (exophytic astrocytoma, chordoma) require more complex and narrower surgical routes (transnasal or transoral transclival approaches). The brain stem, cranial nerves, posterior arteries of the circle of Willis, and the vertebro-basilar system are the most delicate structures to deal with.

Pineal region neoplasms are removed either by a suboccipital transtentorial approach (unilateral occipital craniotomy) or by a supracerebellar infratentorial approach (midline suboccipital craniotomy). The former is indicated for large tumours extending far from the midline, the latter for smaller midline or mainly infratentorial tumours. The veins of Galen's system represent the main limitation for surgery of the pineal region.

Supratentorial tumours of the cerebral hemispheres or the lateral ventricles are approached through a corresponding craniotomy (for example, frontal craniotomy for a frontal mass) and a transcortical route for deeply located tumours. Neoplasms arising from or extending into the third ventricle can be reached by the interhemispheric transcallosal approach. In both cases, the neurosurgeon must spare as much normal tissue as possible while preserving the eloquent cortical areas.

Optic-hypothalamic and suprasellar tumours are usually reached through a fronto-temporal (pterional) craniotomy, by opening the Sylvian fissure. Dissection of the Sylvian fissure may be particularly hard in infants because of the degree of adherence between the temporal and frontal lobes, so a subfrontal route is often necessary to gain access to the tumour. The main structures to be dealt with are the anterior branches of the circle of Willis, the carotid artery, the optic nerve and third cranial nerve, the optic chiasm, and the pituitary stalk. Suprasellar midline tumours (craniopharyngiomas) can also be approached by a subfrontal route or using a bicoronal craniotomy, according to preference. In tumours extending into the third ventricle, opening of the lamina terminalis may be required. Entirely sellar or sellar/suprasellar (small craniopharyngiomas, Rathke's cleft cysts and, exceptionally in infants, pituitary adenomas) can be managed by a transphenoidal approach, which, however, has limited application in infants.

All these operative approaches are currently achieved using microscopic magnification. Recently, moreover, endoscopic instrumentation (endoscopically-assisted neurosurgery) has been developed which improves the view of the operating field and allows safer and more radical tumour excision. Endoscopy may also be useful in the preliminary acute treatment of tumours with large cystic components. In this instance, a mini-invasive endoscopic approach can be carried out to fenestrate the tumour cyst, thus reducing the intracranial hypertension and gaining time for the direct surgical approach to the solid portion of the tumour.

Complications

There is no qualitative difference between infants undergoing neurosurgery for brain tumours and older patients with regard to preoperative and postoperative complications. However, some complications have a higher incidence in infants. As expected, the haemorrhagic risk is very high and represents the most important limitation during a neurosurgical procedure. The circulating blood volume is about 90 ml/kg in newborns and 80 ml/kg in infants, meaning that a child weighing 10 kg has no more than 800 ml of circulating volume. This is a very small amount compared with older children and adults (70 ml/kg), so that even small intraoperative blood losses become critical for the patient. This problem is further complicated by the huge size and rich vascularity that often characterizes IBTs. Haemorrhagic losses can be reduced by preoperative tumour embolization in selected cases, and by meticulous intraoperative haemostasis. Perioperative autologous blood donation, intraoperative isovolaemic haemodilution, and intraoperative blood recovery may help in reducing the risk of haemotransfusion, although these need to be used with particular care in infants.

Another common postoperative complication is represented by subdural fluid collections (hygroma or haematoma) as a consequence of cranio-encephalic disproportion. Because of its elasticity, the infant's skull grows abnormally to compensate for the presence of the intracranial tumour and, when the mass is removed, the empty space between brain and bone is filled by CSF. This collection may remain asymptomatic and disappear over the time. However, because of possible tearing of some bridging veins, it may result in a chronic (or even acute) subdural haematoma, thus requiring an additional surgical procedure.

Infants have very fragile neurological structures, resulting from the still incomplete myelination and the small size of the structures. The risk of neurological injury during surgery is thus increased. On the other hand, however, recovery after neurological damage is better and more rapid in infants than in their older counterparts thanks to brain plasticity.

The risk of infection is increased because of the physiologically reduced immune response. In addition, the risk of postoperative CSF leakage is increased as the thin bones and the poorly developed overlying soft tissues form an inadequate barrier to prevent the escape of CSF.

Chemotherapy

Indications

The goals of chemotherapy for IBTs have changed over the past 40 years and its indications have become increasingly extended (Kellie, 1999). During the 1960s and 1970s, based on evidence of the chemosensitivity of some brain tumours, chemotherapy was used as adjuvant treatment, mainly in children with medulloblastoma, together with radiotherapy. In infants, because of the risk of severe late complications of radiotherapy, chemotherapy was developed to allow deferral of radiotherapy and a reduction in the dose. Results during the 1980s allowed radiotherapy to be postponed by 12 to 24 months; subsequently, intensification of conventional chemotherapy and the development of new protocols allowed prolonged courses of chemotherapy to be given, and radiotherapy to be delayed beyond 2 years or even avoided. The trend during the 1990s and up to the present has been to develop chemotherapy protocols specifically devoted to infants and to broaden the spectrum of treatable IBTs. Current evidence suggests that outcome is improved by using high dose chemotherapy combined with low dose radiotherapy, or by integrating systemic chemotherapy with intrathecal chemotherapy and early radiotherapy, or both.

The main role of chemotherapy is in the adjuvant treatment of malignant IBTs, to prolong the disease-free survival, possibly delaying radiotherapy, and to improve the overall survival rates. IBTs that benefit from chemotherapy are medulloblastoma and PNETs, for which several chemotherapeutic agents (cisplatin, carboplatin, vincristine, etoposide, cyclophosphamide, procarbazine, thiotepa, methotrexate) in different combinations and regimens are currently available.

The results of some clinical trials show that infants with medulloblastoma can be cured by radical surgery and chemotherapy without radiotherapy (Kalifa & Grill, 2005). In contrast, irradiation is usually required to control supratentorial PNETs.

AT/RT necessarily needs both chemotherapy (platinum derivatives and alkylating agents, often integrated with intrathecal chemotherapy) and radiotherapy for its treatment, although prolonged survival without radiotherapy has been reported in some patients.

Malignant gliomas in infants seem to have a better outcome than in older children, chemotherapy being capable of achieving about a 50 per cent overall survival at 5 years, without radiotherapy in half these cases.

Ependymomas are not very chemosensitive so chemotherapy is used primarily to delay radiotherapy for as long as possible. Radical surgery remains the best therapeutic option for ependymomas, especially for supratentorial tumours, while infratentorial tumours are prone to recur and to require radiotherapy for their control.

In spite of an improvement in the survival rate after chemotherapy in some cases, the role of chemotherapy in the treatment of choroid plexus carcinoma has not yet been defined, the prognosis of this tumour mainly depending on radical surgical excision. Second-look surgery is the best option in cases of regrowth/recurrence. Chemotherapy can be very useful as neoadjuvant therapy in huge choroid plexus carcinomas (and papillomas) to reduce their size and vascularization before surgery.

Chemotherapy is not reserved entirely for malignant IBTs. It may also be indicated for low grade tumours if their location is critical (optic-hypothalamic, (bi)-thalamic and brain stem astrocytomas), if they regrow or recur, or if they are disseminated. In cases of tumour metastases at the time of diagnosis, neoadjuvant chemotherapy remains the best option, regardless of tumour grading, both to assess the chemosensitivity of the tumour and to make surgery and radiotherapy more feasible.

Main protocols

Conventional chemotherapy is applied using different protocols, depending on the tumour characteristics and the oncologist's experience. The first protocol designed specifically for infants was that based on mechloretamine-oncovin-procarbazine-prednisone (MOPP) (Ater *et al.*, 1997). The introduction of platinum derivatives (carboplatin, cisplatin) initiated a new generation of protocols for IBTs, such as the updated version of the first Paediatric Oncology Group (Baby POG 1) (Duffner *et al.*, 1999) and the Children's Cancer Group (CCG) (Geyer *et al.*, 1994). Infants also benefit from the standard protocols available for low grade gliomas (Reddy & Packer, 1999), which include several drugs given in different combinations (vincristine/cyclophosphamide, vincristine/carboplatin, cisplatin/vepeside, carboplatin/procarbazine).

Intrathecal chemotherapy is used to increase the drug delivery to the CNS and is a valid option in cases of CSF tumour dissemination. The chemotherapeutic agent (methotrexate) is administered by lumbar puncture or by a ventricular catheter connected to a subcutaneous reservoir. The best known protocol using intraventricular methotrexate was proposed by the German Cooperative Group (Infants HIT 92) (Rutkowski et al., 2005).

High dose chemotherapy (or myeloablative chemotherapy) consists of aggressive regimens that are increasingly widely applied in high risk children (tumour progression, inoperable tumour remnants, dissemination at diagnosis), but also for front-line consolidation or even for induction treatment (usually following a few standard-dose cycles). The autologous bone marrow transplantation needed by patients undergoing high dose chemotherapy is usually safe and effective. Specific protocols have been designed for infants, such as the baby protocol of the Société Française D'Oncologie Pediatrique (BB-SFOP) (Kalifa et al., 1992) and the 'Head Start II' protocol for infantile disseminated medulloblastoma (Chi et al., 2004).

Complications

Acute complications of chemotherapy are well known, being found with most of the currently used chemotherapeutic agents. They consist mainly of myelotoxicity (neutropenia and thrombocytopenia), with a subsequent increased risk of infection and haemorrhage, skin rash, alopecia, liver toxicity, and electrolytic imbalance. Their management in infants – especially with regard to infections, thrombocytopenia and electrolytic disturbances – may be particularly challenging.

More specific acute and late complications involve certain groups of drugs. Alkylating agents (cyclophosphamide, ifosfamide, procarbazine, thiotepa, busulfan, carmustine, lomustine) can have several organ-specific complications; these may affect the gonads (hypogonadism, infertility), bladder (cystitis, fibrosis, dysfunctional voiding, secondary cancer), kidney (nephrotoxicity), lung (fibrosis), eye (cataracts), bone (secondary cancer), and bone marrow (secondary tumours such as treatment-related acute myelogenous leukaemia and myelodysplastic syndrome). Cisplatin typically causes ototoxicity (sensorineural high frequency hearing loss) in addition to nephropathy and neuropathy. Methotrexate is known to cause liver damage (cirrhosis) and osteoporosis, while its role in producing leucoencephalopathy if given intrathecally is still debated. Vincristine may be neurotoxic and hepatotoxic; etoposide can induce acute myelogenous leukaemia/myelodysplastic syndrome; and, finally, corticosteroids may cause cataracts, osteopenia and osteoporosis.

A problem still under debate concerns the possible late neurotoxicity of chemotherapy. Some chemotherapeutic agents (in particular, platinum compounds) are known to induce neurotoxicity in the form of cognitive disorders, seizures or motor deficits caused by leucoencephalopathy, cerebral infarctions and neuropathy. These complications, however, could also result from the additional effects of concomitant radiotherapy and surgery, or from the tumour growth itself. Moreover, the exact mechanisms of chemotherapy-induced neurological toxicity remain largely unknown, though a combination of genetic risk factors for the development of cancer, the development of cognitive problems, and sensitivity to the effects of chemotherapy (for example, low efficiency of DNA repair, deregulated immune response) could be involved.

Radiotherapy

Indications and current strategies

Virtually, all the unresectable or partially resected CNS tumours may be an indication for radiotherapy. Radiation has been proved to control both low grade and high grade brain tumours. Germ cell tumours are the most radiosensitive, followed by medulloblastoma, AT/RT, PNET, and high grade gliomas. In these tumours, radiotherapy is used as adjuvant treatment, as first line therapy or, more often, following chemotherapy, according to the different oncological protocols. Radiotherapy represents the first therapeutic option in cases of unresectable or poorly resectable low grade gliomas, such as diffuse pontine astrocytoma, bi-thalamic gliomas, and optic-hypothalamic astrocytomas. It is also used to control recurrent or regrowing low grade astrocytomas located elsewhere, and craniopharyngioma (using conventional radiotherapy or radiosurgery). Finally, radiotherapy is increasingly used for ependymomas (both grade II and III), even after radical surgical removal, to improve the long term control of this chemo-resistant disease (Merchant & Fouladi, 2005).

All these considerations are applicable to children, adolescents and adults but not to infants owing to the high risk of radiation-induced neurotoxicity (see below). For this reason, most of the infants harbouring one of the above-mentioned tumours are usually managed by surgery or chemotherapy or both, possibly followed by second look surgery or further chemotherapy in order to delay radiotherapy for as long as possible. Recently, thanks to the development of new regimens and technologies, radiotherapy is being used in infants with rapidly progressing tumours (AT/RTs, medulloblastoma/PNETs, ependymomas), with good initial results both in terms of disease control and late toxicity (Massimino *et al.*, 2000).

The first modification to standard radiotherapy that allows its application in infants is a reduction in treatment volumes. In the past, large irradiation volumes were used to reduce the risk of treatment failure at the tumour margins. For example, gliomas were irradiated using margins placed 2–3 cm around the tumour, while in infratentorial ependymomas and medulloblastomas, the whole posterior cranial fossa received the high boost dose. Currently, owing to the increasing availability of MRI and modern techniques of radiotherapy, the tumour and the tumour bed can be accurately delineated and the volumes significantly reduced, especially when dealing with sensitive structures like the optic nerves and chiasm, the cochlea and the pituitary gland. Several investigators have reported a very low or negligible risk of marginal failure with margins ranging from 0.8 to 1.5 cm and a 54 Gy conventional boost dose (Merchant *et al.*, 2004).

Another improvement in radiotherapy application consists of a reduction in the treatment dose. This is a direct result of the development of effective chemotherapy protocols. In the past, medulloblastoma was managed by surgery and radiotherapy, with a 36 Gy dose to the whole cranio-spinal axis. After the introduction of chemotherapy, the cranio-spinal dose fell to 23.4 or even 18 Gy, with similar survival rates and a reduction in neurocognitive side effects.

The last and most important development in radiotherapy resulted from the introduction of modern 3D conformal techniques, such as stereotactic radiosurgery, intensity-modulated radiotherapy, and proton beam radiotherapy (Knab & Connell, 2007). Conformal radiotherapy allows high doses to be distributed within the targeted tissues but reduces the dose given to the surrounding normal tissues. Stereotactic radiosurgery is delivered by highly focal, precise beams (linear accelerator or radioactive source-base system), the patient's head being fixed with a head fixation system to reduce its movements. The entire dose can be given as a single step or in multiple daily fractions (fractionated stereotactic radiotherapy). The advantage of stereo-radiotherapy is that it further reduces the treatment volumes. Intensity-modulated radiotherapy is based on the possibility of varying the intensity of the radiation beam according to the shape and location of the tumour. It is indicated for tumours close to critical structures. To ensure low doses to the critical structures, this method requires that a large volume of normal brain is exposed to low levels of radiation (referred to as the integral dose), thus increasing the risk of second malignancies. Finally, proton beam radiotherapy currently represents the ultimate development. Owing to the unique energy absorption profile of protons in tissues, this allows the whole dose to be concentrated within the target, with little or no radiation beyond it. Proton beam radiotherapy thus significantly reduces the post-treatment sequelae and is the ideal type of radiotherapy for IBTs, especially when they are large and irregular. The main disadvantage of this technique is its limited availability.

Complications

Neurotoxicity following radiotherapy can present with neurocognitive dysfunction, psychological and behavioural disturbances, stroke, seizures, hearing loss, endocrine dysfunction, and second malignancies. Neurocognitive deficits are undoubtedly the most important late complication in infants, affecting 20 to 60 per cent of long term survivors, according to the patient's age and the radiotherapy doses and volumes. Overall, children receiving irradiation are reported to show a 2 to 4 point IQ decline per year after radiotherapy (Spiegler *et al*., 2004). Infants are considered to show the worst outcome, as a child of 3 years or less is predicted to have a mean final IQ decline 12 points greater than a 10 year old patient. Neurocognitive dysfunction could result from alterations to the white matter microstructure with subsequent white matter loss. The white matter injury may be more severe in infants owing to the active myelination process. It is worth noting, however, that it is often impossible to assess whether the intellectual defect results from radiotherapy rather than from previous treatments (surgery or chemotherapy) or from the tumour itself. Some studies, indeed, have stressed the role of the disease and of the surgical treatment as the cause of the neurocognitive impairment (Carpentieri *et al*., 2003).

Endocrine dysfunction is a well documented complication of radiotherapy, occurring in children as well as in adults. It usually results from the irradiation of suprasellar (optic-hypothalamic gliomas, craniopharyngiomas, germ cell tumours), third ventricle (ependymomas, astrocytomas), or posterior cranial fossa tumours. This complication is reported in up to 75 to 85 per cent of the treated children. The most common defect is growth hormone reduction with consequent short stature, followed by precocious puberty and hypothyroidism.

Radiation-induced tumours are the most feared complication of radiotherapy. A recent meta-analysis (Pettorini *et al*., 2008) found 142 radiation-induced tumours reported so far in the paediatric population (mean age, 7.04 years), with a 9.6 years latency period. High grade gliomas were the most common type of second malignancy, followed by meningiomas, low grade gliomas, sarcomas, PNETs, and atypical meningiomas. As for neurocognitive impairment, the possible role of concurrent factors in inducing second malignancy – such as chemotherapy or the individual susceptibility – cannot be excluded. In fact, only one third of the presumed radiation-induced tumours occur within the irradiation field.

Prognostic factors and outcome

The treatment of CNS tumours requires reliable indicators of prognosis to adequately tailor the therapy regimens, especially in infants where the late effects of treatment may have severe consequences. Despite the large number of studies addressing the prognosis of brain tumours, reliable prognostic factors are still lacking. Very few parameters are of any current value: the classical oncological parameters – age, histotype, location and type of treatment – plus some 'new' factors resulting from immunohistochemical marker analysis.

The *age at diagnosis* is recognized as an important prognostic factor for brain tumours. Among children, infants show a worse prognosis than older children and adolescents, in contrast to extracerebral childhood malignancies. The survival rates of patients less than 2 years old are significantly lower than those of children more than 10 years old (Rickert & Paulus, 2001). These data in part depend on age *per se*, as, for the reasons given above, infants cannot always tolerate definitive treatment and are prone to develop significant complications. However, the greater part of the age-related prognosis depends on other concurrent prognostic factors, such as the histology and location of the tumour. Brain tumours in infancy are more likely to be malignant than at any other age (Table 1).

The *grade of malignancy* is probably the most significant predictor of overall survival, even within the same group of tumours. Tumour morphology (anaplasia, necrosis, and so on) and proliferation (MIB-1/Ki-67 index) contribute to the assessment of grading and thus of prognosis. For example, anaplastic and large cell medulloblastomas have a significantly worse overall survival than the other variants of this tumour. The same is true for teratoma and germinoma *vs.* other germ cell tumours, for anaplastic *vs.* classic ependymoma, for choroid plexus carcinoma *vs.* papilloma, for high grade *vs.* low grade astrocytomas, and even for fibrillary *vs.* pilocytic astrocytoma. Ependymomas with a proliferation index (Ki-67) > 20 per cent have a worse overall survival than those <20 per cent, as have pilocytic astrocytomas with Ki-67 > 2 per cent compared with those with Ki-67 < 2 per cent. Other immunohistochemical markers seem to correlate with a worse prognosis, such as p53 overexpression in high grade gliomas and germ cells tumours, a GFAP/vimentin ratio < 1 and p53 expression in ependymomas, or HER2 expression and tenascin immunoreactivity in medulloblastomas. It is interesting that some malignant tumours such as medulloblastoma do not show a different prognosis between infants and older children, and in some cases infants tend to do better (high grade gliomas), while some benign neoplasms (namely optic-hypothalamic gliomas) do significantly worse. The explanation for this behaviour probably lies in differences in genetic patterns revealed by differences in marker expression.

Tumour location and size are the other important factors. IBTs tend to reach huge dimensions and to be located in critical supratentorial regions or infratentorially, two factors preventing radical surgery and reducing the effectiveness of adjuvant treatment. Total tumour resection is possible in only 24 to 51 per cent of children less than 1 year old and in 35 to 58 per cent of those less than 2 years old. For malignant IBTs, the *degree of surgical resection* is the most important predictor of survival. In the series of 198 children in the Baby POG 1 study of malignant IBTs (Duffner *et al.*, 1999), there were no significant differences in survival with respect to age (0–23 months *vs.* 24–36 months), degree of malignancy (presence *vs.* absence of metastases at diagnosis), or delay in starting radiotherapy (2 *vs.* 1 year); however, the 57 children who had a gross total tumour resection had a 61.8 ± 7 per cent 5-year survival, compared with 31 ± 4.8 per cent in those with subtotal resection.

Current treatment options have significantly increased the chances of survival in children with brain tumours. The three most common IBTs have shown a dramatic improvement in 5-year survival in recent decades, increasing from 66 per cent during the 1980s to 72 per cent during late 1990s for astrocytomas, from 36 per cent to 52 per cent for medulloblastoma, and from 32 per cent to 64 per cent for ependymoma. Nevertheless, overall long-term survival of children with IBTs remains low at around 45 to 50 per cent, the poor prognosis depending on the factors mentioned above, as well as the risks of treatment. Surgical mortality can be up to 26-33 per cent (Rivera-Luna *et al.*, 2003), mainly from intraoperative haemorrhage, anaesthesiological problems (hypothermia, electrolytic imbalance), and postoperative complications (severe neurological/endocrinological deficits, postoperative haemorrhage, persistent hydrocephalus and its complications). In some series, up to 70 per cent of patients with malignant IBTs die within an average of 9 months after surgery (Sala *et al.*, 1999).

Analysis of outcome in long term survivors shows moderate to severe limitation in substantial numbers of children. Progress in the treatment of IBTs has allowed better survival rates but not always a parallel improvement in the quality of life. In an analysis of 20 long term survivors from IBT, Suc and coworkers (1990) found impaired cognitive functions in 85 per cent of the cases, neurological deficits in 65 per cent, and endocrinological problems in 70 per cent. In the report by Gjerris *et al.* (1998) analysing 353 long term survivors in Denmark (both infants and children), severe and moderate neurological deficits were present in 2 per cent and 37 per cent of the cases, respectively, and severe, moderate, and mild dementia in 1.6 per cent, 6 per cent, and 15 per cent, while 1.6 per cent required nursing at home and 21 per cent were dependent in their daily life. In our personal series of 57 long term survivors (14 year mean follow-up) treated when under 1 year of age at a single institution (Di Rocco *et al.*, 2007), 3 per cent have severe psychomotor retardation, being completely dependent in their daily life, 27 per cent need some kind of support; 38 per cent have mild psychomotor delay, and 32 per cent live a normal life.

Synopsis of the main infantile brain oncotypes

Teratoma

Epidemiology – Rare, 0.2 per 100,000/year, 0.4–0.5 per cent of all intracranial neoplasms, 2 per cent of all paediatric brain tumours, 10–30 per cent under the 2nd year of life, 30–50 per cent in the neonatal period, 50 per cent of the neoplasms diagnosed *in utero*. Observed within the second decade of life, virtually absent after the fourth decade. M/F ratio, 1.5:3.

Genetics – X, 1q, and 6q mutations (infants and children), isochromosome 12p or 12p amplification (mainly adults).

Origin – Abnormal proliferation of ectopically located multipotent germ cells migrating from the yolk sac to the primordial gonads along the dorsal surface of the embryo during the 4th to 6th week of fetal life.

Location – Midline (suprasellar region, hypothalamic area, third ventricle, pineal region) > cerebral hemispheres. The exact site of origin is often unidentifiable owing to huge size. Massive tumours replace the intracranial content ('holocranic teratoma') and erode the skull; extension into orbit or neck reported. Teratoma can also appear as a large cystic mass, with solid areas, or as a relatively small and homogeneous tumour causing hydrocephalus.

Clinical features – (i) Perinatal: sudden increase in uterine size during pregnancy because of tumour growth and the associated polyhydramnios (15–20 per cent of the cases); dystocia and difficult passage through the maternal birth canal because of fetal macrocephaly; stillbirth in about 35 per cent of the cases, breech presentation in 14 per cent. (ii) Neonatal: macrocrania (up to 75 per cent), hydrocephalus (35–40 per cent), eye signs (11 per cent). Focal neurological deficits are rare, occurring late in the clinical history. Generalized brain dysfunction at birth (seizures, hypotonia) indicates a worse prognosis.

Pathology – All three germinal layers are involved. (i) *Mature teratoma* (WHO grade I): well differentiated tissues with very low cell mitotic activity, wide calcified portions, large cysts, and areas with ectodermal (skin, nervous and ocular tissues), mesodermal (cartilage, bone, fat, muscle), and endodermal differentiation (tissues of hepatic, pancreatic, intestinal and bronchial derivation). Well shaped organs (bronchi, teeth, bones) can be found in the tumour. (ii) *Immature teratoma* (WHO grade II/III): poorly differentiated embryonal-derived tissues with a higher proliferation rate and rarer calcifications. The neuroectodermal areas are composed of aberrant neural elements, rosettes and rudimentary skin glands, the mesenchymal portions by numerous spindle cells, rabdomyoblasts and immature cartilage, and the endodermal parts by undifferentiated cells. Immature teratoma sporadically differentiates into mature teratoma, spontaneously or after chemotherapy or radiotherapy. (iii) *Malignant teratoma* (WHO grade III): malignant transformation of a mature/immature teratoma into teratocarcinoma or occurrence of a mixed tumour (teratoma plus germinoma and/or yolk sac tumour and/or choriocarcinoma and/or embryonal carcinoma). In case of mixed tumour, blood or CSF fetal markers (α-FP, β-HCG) may be positive.

Neuroimaging – *Ultrasound*: Non-homogeneous solid-cystic intracranial mass associated with gross calcifications, distortion of the brain, fetal macrocrania, and polyhydramnios. *MRI*: Solid areas are heterogeneous, hyperintense on T1 (fat tissue) or on T2 and FLAIR (other soft tissues), with variable contrast enhancement; cystic areas are hypointense on T1 and FLAIR, and hyperintense on T2, and not enhanced by contrast medium; calcifications are hypo-hyperintense on T1 and hypointense on T2 (strongly hyperdense on CT); haemorrhagic areas (not infrequent) are hyperintense in all the sequences. The cerebral architecture is often distorted and the cerebral vessels encased by the tumour. Spinal MRI may show secondary localizations (immature or malignant teratoma). *MRI spectroscopy*: ↑ lipids. *Differential diagnosis*: Dermoid tumours (mainly cystic, smaller and not contrast-enhanced); astrocytomas (more homogeneous and less calcified); other germ cell tumours (more circumscribed (pineal region) and poorly cystic); craniopharyngioma (prevalently cystic, mainly suprasellar, regular edges; sometimes hard to differentiate from teratoma).

Management and prognosis – Surgery is the treatment of choice. Mature teratoma can be considered as cured after complete surgical removal owing to the benign biological behaviour (5-year survival, 70 to 80 per cent). The same is true for immature teratomas although there is a 20 per cent recurrence risk even after gross total surgical excision (adjuvant chemotherapy/radiotherapy has been proposed). Malignant teratoma requires chemotherapy and radiotherapy after surgery and, in spite of these, the prognosis remains poor (5-year survival, 20–40 per cent). The worst prognosis is with huge teratomas of the newborn, where radical surgery is not possible. In these instances, surgery is limited to biopsy or palliative partial removal of the tumour mass to obtain a cerebral decompression, and treatment of associated hydrocephalus. The 5-year survival is 10–20 per cent regardless of histological features.

Desmoplastic infantile ganglioglioma

Epidemiology – Rare, about 1.2 per cent of all paediatric brain tumours (0.4 per cent in autopsy series), up to 16 per cent in infants. Typically diagnosed within the second year of life (especially < 18 months); older patients are sporadically affected. M/F ratio, 1.7.

Genetics – No specific alterations. The typical chromosomal abnormalities or mutations of astrocytomas are absent.

Origin – Neurons > glial cells.

Location – Supratentorial, usually arising from the cerebral hemispheres, without side prevalence. The frontal and parietal lobes are most commonly involved.

Clinical features – Abnormal head growth and/or macrocephaly (60 per cent of the cases), bulging fontanelle and sunset sign. Cranial bulge overlying the tumour or even asymmetrical expansion of the homolateral hemicranium are common. Longer clinical history (6–9 months *vs.* 3–6 months) and focal neurological deficits in children > 12 months old more than in children < 12 months old; seizures occur in about 20 per cent of the cases.

Pathology – Deposition of dense collagen (desmoplastic areas) combined with neuroepithelial and fibroblastic elements. The neuroepithelial elements consists of both pleomorphic and elongated astrocytes, intermixed with collagen and reticulin fibres, and small polygonal or atypical ganglioid-cell-like neurons. Some tumour portions can contain more primitive and less differentiated neural cells with high mitotic activity and necrosis. The proliferative index is usually low (0.5–2 per cent); higher rates are reported (up to 15 per cent). Anaplasia and tumour progression with malignant course are exceptional. WHO grade I.

Neuroimaging – Very large uni- or multicystic tumour mass or plaque attached to the dura mater, exerting mass effect (Fig. 2). The solid portion is hypointense on both T1 and T2 and hyperdense on CT; cystic part usually hypo-isointense on T1 and hyperintense on T2, with intracystic septations. Cyst wall, intracystic septa and solid component strongly enhanced after gadolinium administration. *Differential diagnosis*: Ganglioglioma (usually smaller, calcified, and hyperintense on T2); pilocytic astrocytoma (rarely occurring within the cerebral hemispheres); dysembryoplastic neuroepithelial tumour (DNET) (smaller and not contrast-enhanced); haemangioblastoma (uncommon above the tentorium); pleomorphic xanthoastrocytoma (frequently located within the temporal lobe). All these tumours occur later than in infancy.

Management – Total surgical excision is the gold standard. Complete tumour removal is obtained only in about 35 per cent of the cases, in spite of the superficial location and the benign biological behaviour. This low percentage depends on the frequent lack of a cleavage between tumour and the surrounding brain, the firm texture of the mass (often strictly adherent to the dural sinuses and/or to eloquent brain areas), and the huge tumour size. In case of tumour recurrence/regrowth, second-look surgery is the best option, followed by chemotherapy and radiotherapy.

Prognosis – DIG often stabilizes after surgery, even with only partial removal, so that its prognosis remains good. Recurrence-free interval ranging from 6 months to 14 years are reported and the median survival rate 15 years after the diagnosis is about 75 per cent.

Atypical teratoid/rhabdoid tumour (AT/RT)

Epidemiology – Once classified as medulloblastoma, PNET or choroid plexus carcinoma, 75 per cent of the cases are diagnosed in infants and 90 per cent in children less than 5 years old. AT/RT accounts for 10 to 15 per cent of all brain tumours in infants and for a quarter of primary embryonal tumours (ratio of medulloblastoma-PNETs to AT/RT, 3.8/1). Described also in older children (30 per cent of children older than 3 years) and adults. No sex prevalence.

Genetics – See 'Cytogenetics and molecular genetics' and Table 3.

Origin – Possibly mesenchymal, neuroectodermal or histiocytic; the cell of origin is unknown.

Location – Posterior cranial fossa in about 60 per cent of cases, with a predilection for the cerebello-pontine angle. Remaining localizations: cerebral hemispheres, 20 per cent; suprasellar region, 5 per cent; pineal region, 5 per cent; spinal cord, 1 per cent; multifocal, 5 per cent. The

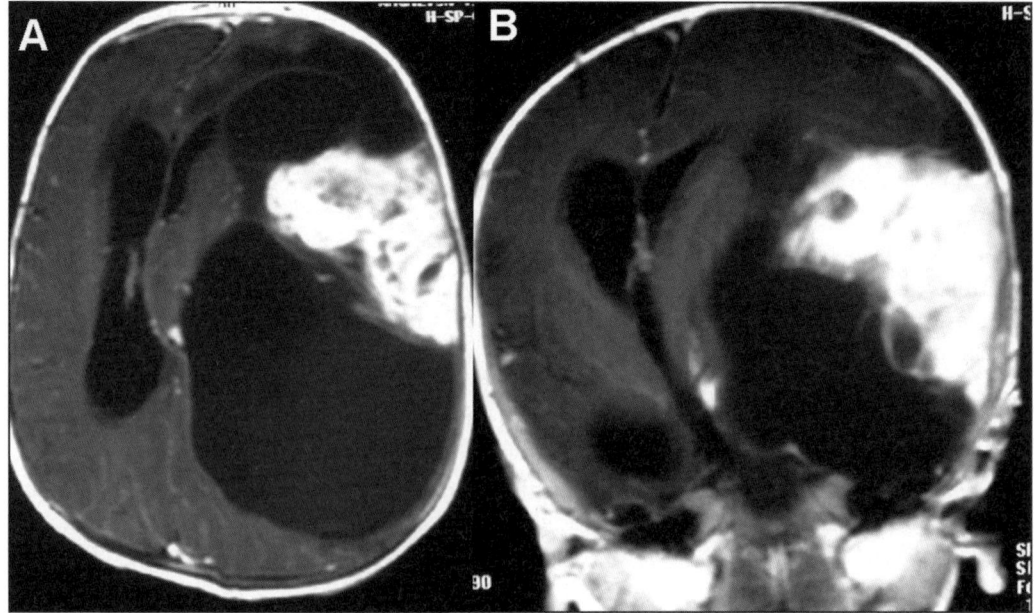

Fig. 2. Axial (A) and coronal (B) T1-MRI after contrast medium injection showing a huge tumour occupying an enlarged left hemicranium. The cystic portion is prevalent; the solid portion is adherent to the dura mater and strongly enhanced. The mass effect is impressive. Diagnosis: desmoplastic infantile ganglioglioma.

supratentorial location is prevalent in older children and adults compared with infants. Leptomeningeal dissemination and CSF tumour seeding in up to 30 to 35 per cent of cases. AT/RT may occur synchronously in the brain and in the kidney.

Clinical features – Often related to signs and symptoms of intracranial hypertension. Clinical history is significantly shorter than in other infantile neoplasms (length of symptoms measured in days or weeks) and focal neurological deficits are more likely to occur. *Infratentorial AT/RT*: cranial nerve palsies (VI and VII), ataxia and regression of motor skills. *Supratentorial AT/RT*: seizures, hemiparesis and visual field defects. Hydrocephalus is quite common.

Pathology – Sheets or nests of rhabdoid cells resembling a rhabdomyosarcoma in a mixed background consisting of primitive neuroectodermal cells (small size, little cytoplasm, large nucleus, positivity for neurofilament protein (NFP), glio-fibrillary acid protein (GFAP), actin and desmin) and/or mesenchymal elements (spindle-shaped and surrounded by pale ground substance). Rhabdoid cells are round or polygonal, with eccentric and round nuclei, prominent nucleoli, and abundant cytoplasm, and show immunohistochemical expression of vimentin, epithelial membrane antigen (EMA), and smooth muscle actin (SMA). Rhabdoid cells may be largely prevalent, being the only cells present in 10–15 per cent of cases, or alternating with areas resembling PNETs or medulloblastoma. Loss of immunohistochemical staining for INI1 is pathognomonic. The proliferative index is very high (50–70 per cent or more). WHO grade IV.

Neuroimaging – Not pathognomonic, appearances being similar to medulloblastoma and PNET. Usually a large and infiltrative mass (mean diameter at diagnosis, 2–4 cm), possibly showing necrotic components, cysts, haemorrhagic areas, and peritumoral oedema. *MRI*: Isointense in T1 (high cellularity), quite heterogeneous on T2 and FLAIR owing to the different components, heterogeneously contrast-enhanced (Fig. 3). *MRI spectroscopy*: ↑↑ choline (high cell turnover) and ↓↓ creatine and N-acetyl-aspartate (lack of neuronal differentiation). Calcifications may be detected. Leptomeningeal spread is evident in 20 per cent of the cases at diagnosis. *Differential diagnosis*: Medulloblastoma and PNET (often impossible to distinguish; AT/RT is more likely to have cysts and calcifications and to occur in the cerebello-pontine angle); ependymoma (same signal, especially with regard to calcifications, cysts and haemorrhages, but growing within the IV ventricle 'respecting' its limits and invading the cerebello-pontine angle through the lateral foramina); astrocytoma (more homogeneous solid portion and larger cysts, occurring in older children).

Management – Necessarily multimodal, consisting of surgical excision followed by chemotherapy and radiotherapy. *Surgery*: radical surgery is possible in 35–68 per cent of the patients owing to the large tumour size at diagnosis and the frequent infiltration of the nervous and vascular structures of the cerebello-pontine angle. Complete tumour resection correlates with a longer median survival. Second-look surgery can be considered after induction chemotherapy in cases of residual tumour. *Chemotherapy*: two main approaches based on rhabdomyosarcoma-like protocols and high dose chemotherapy with stem cell rescue, with or without intrathecal chemotherapy. Response to chemotherapy is quite good, up to half of the patients showing >50 per cent reduction in tumour volume, but generally short (less than 1 year). Chemotherapy in case of tumour progression is ineffective. *Radiotherapy*: AT/RT is radiosensitive, showing complete disappearance and even survival for > 3 years without chemotherapy. Because of its crucial role in survival, radiotherapy has recently begun to be used in children < 36 months old (irradiation of the tumour bed with or without craniospinal axis irradiation), with encouraging initial results.

Prognosis – Despite the sensitivity to chemotherapy and radiotherapy, prognosis of AT/RT remains very poor. The Paediatric Oncology Group 9923 reported a 193-day median survival, the tumour progressing in nearly 70 per cent of the children by 12–24 weeks on therapy, and in 83 per cent by 12 months. Mortality is 80–85 per cent.

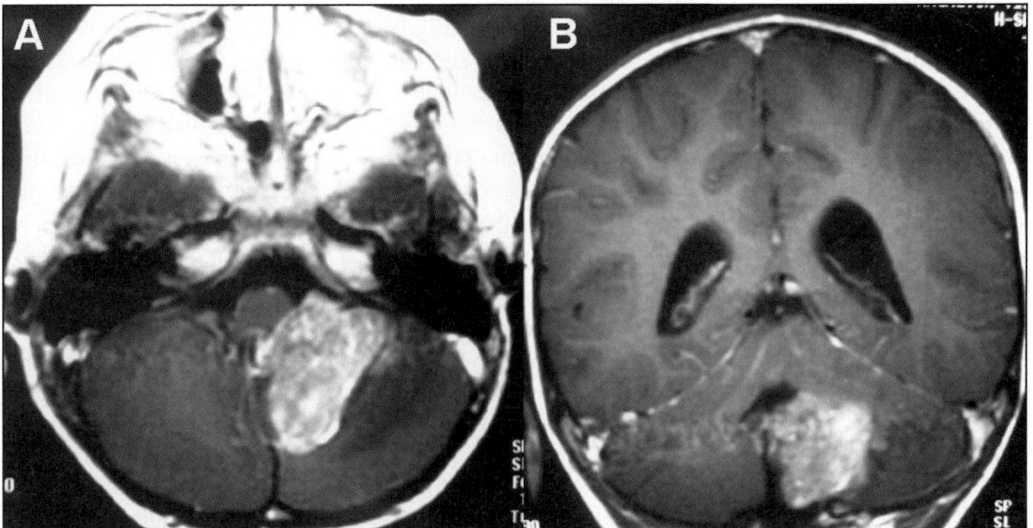

Fig. 3. Typical appearance of atypical teratoid/rhabdoid tumour (AT/RT) on axial (A) and coronal (B) contrast T1-MRI: large, heterogeneous enhanced, solid tumour extending into the left cerebello-pontine angle. The mass effect is moderate and the growth pattern is infiltrative.

Medulloblastoma

Epidemiology – The most frequent malignant IBT (13–15 per cent of all IBTs) and the most common paediatric brain tumour (15–20 per cent of all childhood neoplasms, peak incidence between 3 and 4 years), 40 per cent of all posterior cranial fossa tumours. M/F ratio, 1.5:4.

Genetics – See 'Cytogenetics and molecular genetics' and Table 3.

Origin – Primordial undifferentiated neuroectodermal elements from rests in the roof of the IV ventricle and/or the external granular layer of the cerebellum.

Location – Cerebellar vermis/superior medullary velum (site of origin) and IV ventricle; possible extension to cerebellar hemispheres and cerebello-pontine angle. Leptomeningeal seeding in 10–40 per cent (tumour cells possibly detected within the CSF); vascular infiltration and metastases outside the CNS are observed in 5–18 per cent of cases (lung, liver, bone marrow, lymph nodes).

Clinical features – Cleft palate, cerebellar agenesis. Medulloblastoma occurs in 3.5 per cent of patients with Gorlin syndrome and is possibly also associated with Li-Fraumeni, Turcot, Cowden and Gardner syndromes. Hydrocephalus and subsequently raised intracranial pressure are the main clinical findings, followed by signs of invasion of cerebellum and, later, the brain stem and lower cranial nerves. The clinical history is usually shorter than 3 months.

Pathology – Densely packed small cells with large hyperchromatic nuclei and scarce cytoplasm, high cell density, moderate to high mitotic index, Homer-Wright rosettes/neuroblastic differentiation in one third of the cases ('classic' medulloblastoma). Medulloblastoma is now divided into four subtypes according to the WHO 2007 classification: (i) *desmoplastic*: uniform cells with low mitotic index within reticulin-free nodules, surrounded by hyperchromatic cells showing active proliferation and positivity for reticulin; immunostaining for neuron-specific enolase (NSE), synaptophysin and neurofilaments; (ii) *extensive nodularity and neuronal differentiation*: rare variant characterized by nodules of uniform cells resembling neurocytes and immunostaining for NSE, synaptophysin and neurofilaments; (iii) *large cells*: sheets and lobules of large round cells with pleomorphic nuclei and prominent nucleoli, abundant cytoplasm, and high proliferative index, showing apoptosis and necrosis phenomena; immunostaining for vimentin and synaptophysin; (iv) *anaplastic*: cells with large nuclei with markedly atypical coarse chromatin and irregular shapes, anaplasia, high mitotic index, apoptosis, necrosis and immunostaining for vimentin and synaptophysin. The first two variants have a significantly better prognosis, the third and fourth variants show frequent CSF dissemination and metastases and low survival rates. WHO grade IV.

Neuroimaging – Grossly round 3–5 cm mass in the IV ventricle, displacing the IV ventricle anteriorly/superiorly and the surrounding brain in all directions; associated with hydrocephalus in 90–95 per cent of the cases. *CT*: Hyperdense (high cellularity), necrosis in 40–50 per cent of the cases, calcifications in 20 per cent. *MRI*: Hypointense on T1, isointense on T2, hyperintense on FLAIR, heterogeneously contrast-enhanced; frequent cranial and/or spinal leptomeningeal enhancement due to tumour spreading (Fig. 4). Cystic and haemorrhagic areas are rare. *MRI spectroscopy*: ↑ choline and ↓ N-acetyl-aspartate; lactate may be present (brain infiltration and damage). *Differential diagnosis*: AT/RT (often indistinguishable; see above); ependymoma (extension outside IV ventricle, more heterogeneous, calcification and haemorrhages more frequent, less vigorous contrast enhancement); pilocytic astrocytoma (more frequently hemispheric and cystic with mural nodule); choroid plexus tumour (stronger and more homogeneous enhancement, rarely within the IV ventricle).

Management – Multimodal (surgery + chemotherapy + possible radiotherapy). *Surgery*: gross total removal should be the goal; immediate second-look surgery is required by modern protocols for resectable tumour remnants. Gross total resection is achievable in 60–85 per cent of the cases. A typical complication of surgery is cerebellar mutism. *Chemotherapy*: medulloblastoma responds well to alkylating agents and platinum compounds. Many different regimens and protocols (mainly based on high dose chemotherapy) are currently available, all of them aimed at prolonging survival and delaying or avoiding radiation and/or reducing its dose. High risk infants benefit from specific protocols. *Radiotherapy*: currently feasible in most infants as it can be delayed by chemotherapy; it ensures the most stable results if associated with both surgery and chemotherapy. It is the best option in cases of chemotherapy failure. Achieved through 24-Gy irradiation to the cranio-spinal axis plus a 50–55 total boost on the tumour bed.

Prognosis – Classic unfavourable prognostic factors are age < 2 years (higher risk of metastases at diagnosis, lower rate of gross total resection, not always amenable to radiotherapy), presence of more than 1–1.5 cm^3 residual tumour (radical resection is one of the most important prognostic factors), metastases at neuroimaging or CSF sampling, M3–4 and/or T4 Chang's staging, and relapse during adjuvant treatment. Histomorphological and immunohistochemical negative predictors are large cell and anaplastic variants, apoptotic index > 1.5, MYCC and HER2 overexpression, and p53 expression. The 5-year survival in patients with 'standard' risk (no large cell/anaplastic variants, no gross residual tumour, no metastases, no HER2 expression) is 65–85 per cent; 'high' risk patients show a 20–25 per cent 5-year survival.

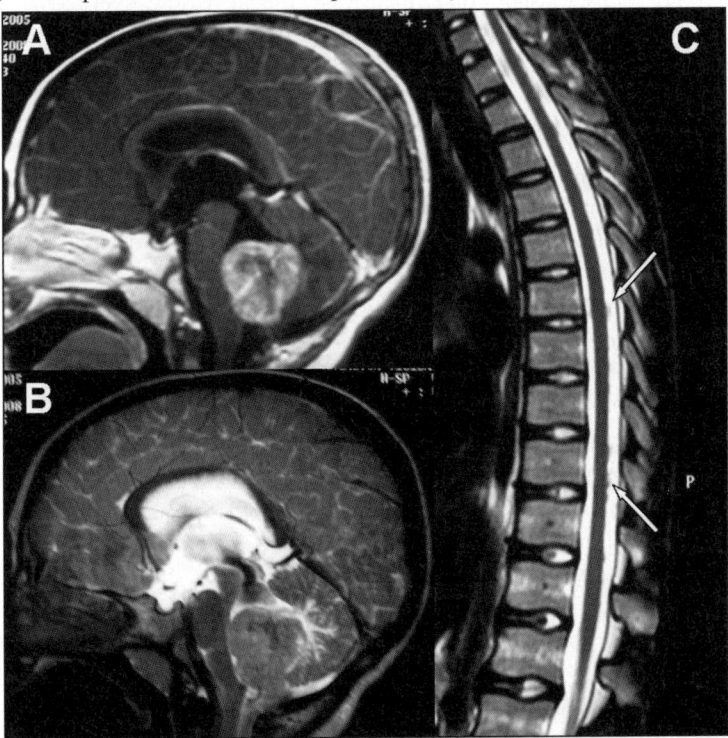

Fig. 4. Large midline tumour arising from the cerebellar vermis and filling almost the whole fourth ventricle, thus causing supratentorial triventricular hydrocephalus. The mass heterogeneously enhances after contrast medium administration (sagittal T1-MRI, A) and shows an isointense signal on sagittal T2-MRI (high cellularity, B). Diagnosis: medulloblastoma. Note the nodular leptomeningeal dissemination (arrows) on the sagittal T2-MRI of the spine (C).

Supratentorial primary neuroectodermal tumours

Epidemiology – Group of CNS malignant tumours with predilection for the paediatric population, morphologically indistinguishable from medulloblastoma but occurring elsewhere than the cerebellum. According to the recent WHO recommendations, the more general term CNS PNETs should be used to designate all the PNETs of the CNS (supratentorial tumours but also those located within the brain stem and the spinal cord) except for medulloblastoma. Supratentorial PNETs comprise 5–10 per cent of all CNS PNETs. They account for 1–2 per cent of all childhood tumours and 2–5 per cent of all IBTs. One quarter of them occur in infants. M/F ratio, 2.

Genetics – See 'Cytogenetics and molecular genetics' and Table 3.

Origin – Primordial undifferentiated neuroectodermal elements from the neural crest.

Location – Cerebral hemispheres (neuroblastoma and ganglioneuroblastoma), pineal region (pinealoblastoma), periventricular/intraventricular region (ependymoblastoma), olfactory nerve (esthesioneuroblastoma), and retina (retinoblastoma). The risk of CSF and vascular dissemination is similar to medulloblastoma.

Clinical features – *Neonates*: macrocephaly, bulging hemi-skull, seizures and, later, hemiparesis and disturbed consciousness. *Infants*: (i) cerebral hemisphere: seizures, hemiparesis, raised intracranial pressure, consciousness disturbance; (ii) pineal region: hydrocephalus, Parinaud's syndrome, other ocular signs; (iii) anterior skull base/suprasellar region: endocrine deficits, visual impairment, seizures. Possibly associated with Gorlin, Turcot and Rubinstein-Taybi syndromes. Median age at diagnosis, 35 months.

Pathology – Supratentorial PNETs can differentiate along neuronal, astrocytic, ependymal, muscular and melanotic cell lines. Histological features are quite similar to classic medulloblastoma: small undifferentiated or poorly differentiated, 'blue' cells, with pleomorphic and large nuclei, high cellular density, frequent mitoses, possible haemorrhagic areas, calcification, Homer-Wright and Flexner-Wintersteiner rosettes (Fig. 5). Additional findings depend on the possible differentiation (focal ganglion elements, peripheral astrocytic elements, mesenchymal components, ependymal, melanocytic or retinal elements). Immunostaining for synaptophysin and neurofilaments is present; immunostaining for GFAP indicates glial differentiation and a worse prognosis. WHO grade IV.

Neuroimaging – Large, moderately oedematous mass varying from solid and homogeneous to cystic and necrotic. CSF spread is common. *CT*: Calcifications, haemorrhages and necrosis more frequently than in medulloblastoma. *MRI*: Hypo-isointense on T1, iso-hyperintense on T2, hyperintense on FLAIR, heterogeneously contrast-enhanced. *MRI spectroscopy*: Suggestive of malignant tumour (↑↑ choline, ↓ creatine and N-acetyl-aspartate, lipids and lactate present). *Differential diagnosis*: AT/RT (often infratentorial, otherwise indistinguishable); malignant glioma (abundant oedema, ring enhancement, rare calcifications); ependymoma (in one third of the cases intraventricular, otherwise hard to differentiate); choroid plexus carcinoma (intraventricular with brain invasion, strong enhancement and extensive oedema).

Management – The treatment strategy is similar to that for medulloblastoma. Supratentorial PNETs are poorly responsive tumours, being prone to recur during chemotherapy and/or radiotherapy (median time of relapse, 5–6 months). Supratentorial PNETs of the pineal region seem to be more chemosensitive than others.

Prognosis – Unfavourable prognostic factors similar to medulloblastoma (surgical resection, age < 2 years, metastases at diagnosis, necrosis, staging) but poorer prognosis regardless of the different location (5-year survival, 15–35 per cent).

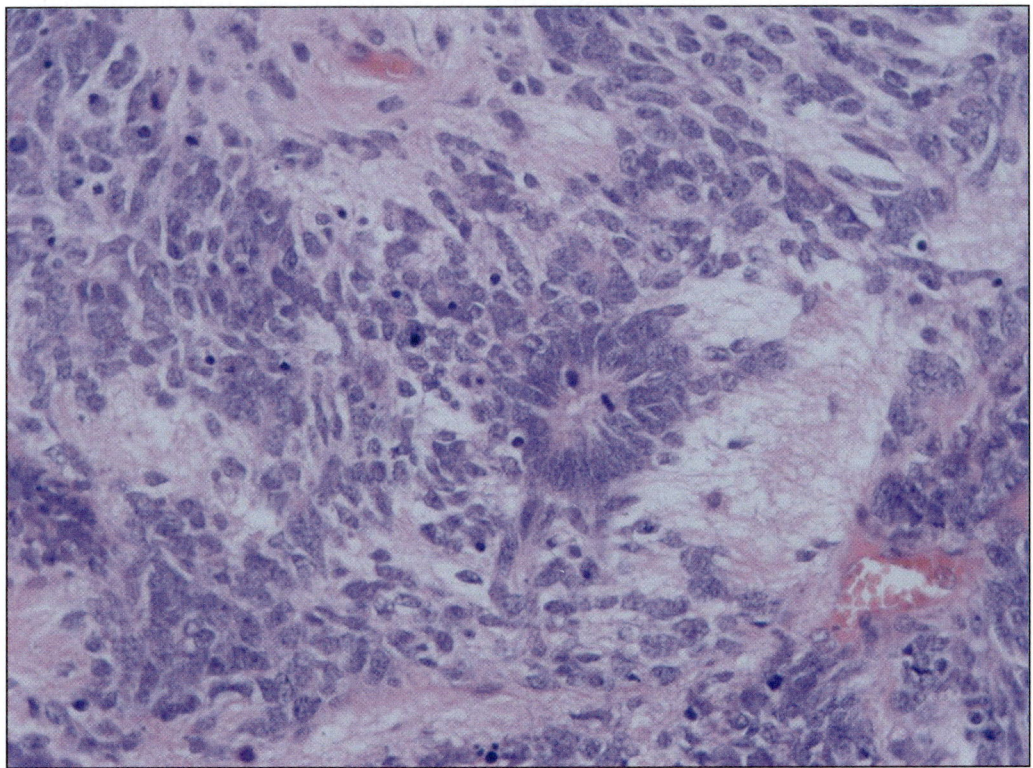

Fig. 5. Typical appearance of supratentorial primitive neuroectodermal tumour with standard haematoxylin & eosin stain. Note the very high density of poorly differentiated cells, the large and pleomorphic nuclei ('blue' cells), the Homer-Wright rosette (central area).

Ependymoma

Epidemiology – The third most common brain tumour in infants (16 per cent) after pilocytic astrocytoma and medulloblastoma; 15 per cent of all posterior fossa tumours and 5–10 per cent of all intracranial tumours. Peak of incidence between 1 and 5 years.

Genetics – See 'Cytogenetics and molecular genetics' and Table 4.

Origin – Ependymal cells or periventricular ependymal rests. Possible association with simian virus 40 (DNA of SV40 expressed in some ependymomas). SV40 has been found to induce ependymoma in experimental models.

Location – Infratentorial space in two thirds of cases: tumour of the IV ventricle often extending into the cisterna magna (foramen of Magendie), the cerebello-pontine angle cistern (foramina of Lushka), and even reaching the cisterns anterior to the brain stem; the brain stem is often compressed and/or infiltrated and the cranial nerves enveloped (Fig. 6). Supratentorial compartment is involved in the remaining one third of cases: intraventricular in 25–30 per cent of patients, mainly periventricular and intra-axial (70–75 per cent). CSF dissemination is not infrequent (5–7 per cent), especially in cases of IV ventricle ependymomas (drop metastases of the spinal cord).

Clinical features – Raised intracranial pressure is the main symptom (especially in infratentorial ependymomas because of the frequently associated hydrocephalus). Other signs in infratentorial ependymomas: ataxia, dizziness, torticollis, neck pain. Other signs in supratentorial ependymomas: seizures, irritability, psychomotor delay. Perinatally: stillbirth, dystocia and haemorrhages (frequent).

Pathology – (i) Ependymoma (WHO grade II): quite differentiated, uniform, darkly staining cells, low mitotic index, moderate cellular density, poor nuclear atypia, vascular pseudorosettes and true ependymal rosettes (more characteristic but rarer), immunostaining for vimentin, GFAP, S-100. (ii) Anaplastic ependymoma (WHO grade III): less differentiated cells with hyperchromatism and nuclear atypia, high cellular density and raised proliferative index, possible microvascular proliferation, pseudopalisading and necrosis (the last three features indicative of greater malignancy). The WHO 2007 classification distinguishes four ependymomas variants: *cellular* (common in the IV ventricle); *papillary* (showing extensive epithelial surface); *clear-cell* (small rounded oligodendroglioma-like cells with homogeneous nucleus and clear cytoplasm); and *tanycytic* (with elongated, pilocytic-like cells).

Neuroimaging – Large mass (2–5 cm), with 'plastic' growth within the ventricles, more irregular outside them. *CT*: Cysts, calcifications and haemorrhages are common (~50 per cent of cases). *MRI*: Very heterogeneous, usually hypo-isointense on T1, iso-hyperintense on T2 and FLAIR, moderate or slight enhancement with contrast medium. *MRI spectroscopy*: Non-specific (↑ choline, ↓ N-acetyl-aspartate). *Differential diagnosis*: Medulloblastoma/PNET (more homogeneous, less frequently haemorrhagic, arising from the cerebellar vermis if infratentorial, no plastic growth if intraventricular); choroid plexus tumour (stronger and more homogeneous enhancement, rare within the IV ventricle in infants); low grade astrocytoma (cerebellar hemisphere if infratentorial, often with strongly enhancing mural nodule); high grade astrocytoma (very similar features, more frequently necrotic, uncommon in posterior cranial fossa).

Management and prognosis – Ependymoma (WHO grade II) responds poorly to chemotherapy and moderately to radiotherapy, therefore surgery is the best treatment option. Second-look surgery is often considered in cases of tumour regrowth/recurrence. Once considered cured after radical surgical excision, supratentorial ependymoma is now treated with radiotherapy because of the high risk of relapse in infants. Infratentorial ependymoma is very hard to remove radically (brain stem and cranial nerve invasion) and, even if apparently totally resected, often tends to recur so radiotherapy is given according to the new protocols. Overall 5-year survival, 50–70 per cent. The younger the age, the poorer the survival (5-year survival in 0–24 month children, 25–30 per cent; in 24–36 months children, 65 per cent). Chemotherapy is used in several protocols to delay radiotherapy or to consolidate its results, especially in cases of anaplastic ependymoma. Anaplasia is an unfavourable prognostic factor (5-year survival in anaplastic ependymomas, 35 per cent).

Choroid plexus tumours: choroid plexus adenoma and carcinoma

Epidemiology – 0.5 to 6 per cent incidence in the overall population, 2–4 per cent of all paediatric tumours; 65–70 per cent diagnosed in infants, 10 per cent of all IBTs; median age at diagnosis, 26 months. Choroid plexus tumours are one of the most common tumours in the first year of life: 50 per cent of choroid plexus adenomas (CPA) and 30 per cent of choroid plexus carcinomas (CPC) are diagnosed in this period. M/F ratio, 1 (IV ventricle: M/F, 1.5).

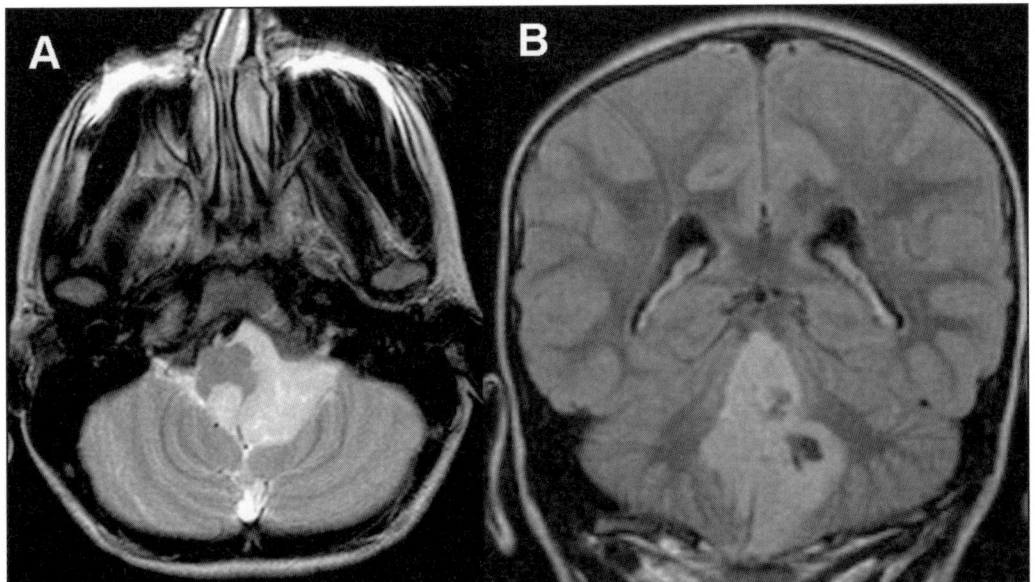

Fig. 6. Ependymoma usually presents as a heterogeneous mass, iso-hyperintense on both T2-MRI (axial, A) and FLAIR-MRI (coronal, B), plastically occupying the fourth ventricle (B). In this case, the tumour compresses the brain stem from behind, extends into the left cerebello-pontine angle cistern and crosses anterior to the medulla oblongata upwards to reach the prebulbar cistern (A).

Genetics – See 'Cytogenetics and molecular genetics' and Tables 3 and 4.

Origin – Choroid plexus epithelium. SV 40 DNA expressed in half the cases.

Location – 50 per cent lateral ventricles (mainly infants and children), 40 per cent IV ventricle (mainly adults), 10 per cent III ventricle, 5 per cent multiple sites. CSF seeding is reported (CPC > CPA).

Clinical features – Hydrocephalus frequently encountered (CSF hypersecretion and obstruction by the tumour + failure of resorption because of microhaemorrhages). Clinical signs and symptoms are thus related to raised intracranial pressure. Focal signs suggest brain invasion (CPC). Choroid plexus tumours may be associated with Li-Fraumeni and Aicardi syndromes.

Pathology – (i) CPA: often resemble normal choroid plexus (microvilli, cilia and zonula adherens junction at electron microscopy); connective finger-like papillary formations covered by mature epithelial cells disposed in columns, without mitotic activity and necrosis; immunostaining for S-100, cytokeratin, GFAP and vimentin. WHO grade I. (ii) CPC: grossly similar to CPA but with high density of pleomorphic cells with raised mitotic index, necrotic and haemorrhagic areas and microcalcifications, poorly formed papillary structures, microvascular proliferation and brain invasion. WHO grade III.

Neuroimaging – Large cauliflower-shaped mass (usually > 5 cm) located in the atrium of the lateral ventricle (the left side more affected) or close to the posterior medullary velum, exerting mass effect and filling the ventricle. Brain invasion in cases of CPC. (i) CPA: *CT*: Iso-hyperdense, calcifications in 25 per cent of cases, possible tumour haemorrhage. *MRI*: Iso-intense on T1, iso-hyperintense on T2, occasionally necrotic-cystic areas, strong and homogeneous contrast enhancement (Fig. 7). *MRI spectroscopy*: Non-specific (↑ choline, ↓ N-acetyl-aspartate). *Differential diagnosis*: CPC (hard to differentiate, see below);

ependymoma (heterogeneous, frequently in the IV ventricle, brain invasion if supratentorial); astrocytomas (less enhanced, usually III ventricle, cysts). (ii) CPC: Same CT and MRI characteristics and differential diagnosis as CPA. CPC shows more heterogeneous contrast enhancement, possible peritumoral oedema, more frequent CSF seeding and necrosis (? lactate on MRI spectroscopy).

Management and prognosis – CPA can be cured by surgery alone (complete removal), with 5-year survival near 90 to 100 per cent in many series. Surgery may be risky because of possible tumour haemorrhages. Preoperative chemotherapy to reduce mass size and/or preoperative embolization to reduce vascularity are two useful preoperative options. Surgery followed by careful monitoring is the best therapeutic choice for CPC. The chemo- and radiosensitivity of CPC have still to be assessed, although encouraging results have been obtained with multimodal treatment (5-year survival, 65 per cent). The overall 5-year and 10-year survival of CPC remains poor (40 per cent and 25 per cent, respectively), especially in cases of brain infiltration and CSF spread.

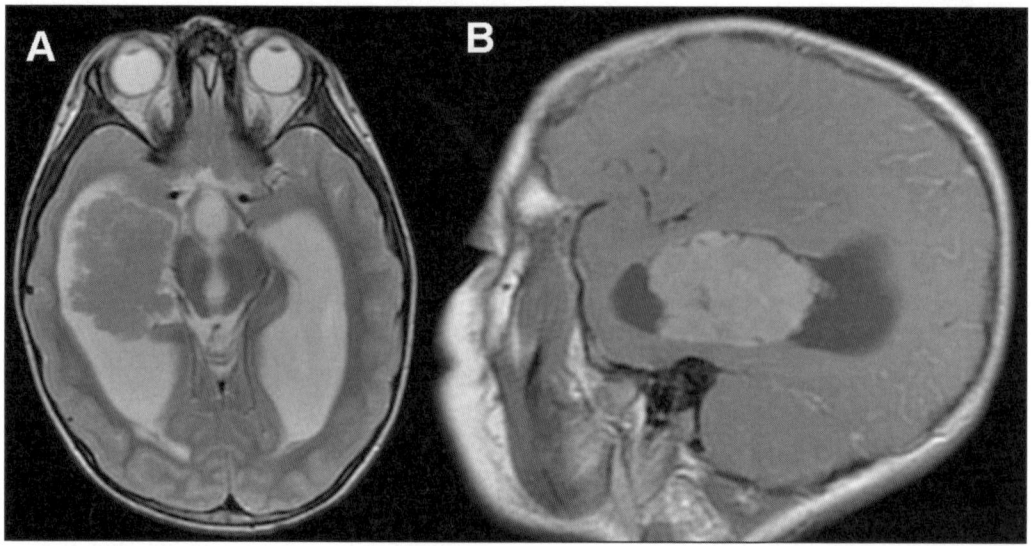

Fig. 7. Typical aspect of a choroid plexus papilloma located within the temporal horn of the right lateral ventricle. This large cauliflower tumour is isointense on axial T2-MRI (A) and homogeneously enhanced by gadolinium (B).

Low grade and high grade astrocytomas

Epidemiology – The most common primary brain tumour in all ages, > 50 per cent of all paediatric tumours, 30 per cent of all IBTs. Pilocytic astrocytoma is the most common histotype in infants (25–35 per cent). M/F ratio, 1. High grade astrocytomas comprise about 10–12 per cent of IBTs (M/F ratio, 1.5).

Genetics – See 'Cytogenetics and molecular genetics' and Tables 3 and 4.

Origin – Astroglia (differentiated astrocytes or precursor cells).

Location – Potentially anywhere within the neuraxis; *posterior cranial fossa*: children > infants >> adults, cerebellar hemisphere > vermis (pilocytic astrocytoma) and brain stem (both low grade and high grade, diffuse intrinsic or focal or exophitic tumours); *pineal region*: children > infants > adults, low grade ≥ high grade; cerebral hemispheres: adults > infants > children, high grade > low grade; *optic pathways-hypothalamus*: infants ≥ children > adults, low grade > high grade, 25–30 per cent associated with NF-1; *intraventricular*: children ≥ infants > adults, low grade > high grade.

Clinical features – (i) *Posterior cranial fossa*: raised intracranial pressure (hydrocephalus), cerebellar/brain stem dysfunction, lower cranial nerves impairment; (ii) *pineal region*: raised intracranial pressure (hydrocephalus), Parinaud's syndrome, brain stem dysfunction; (iii) *cerebral hemispheres*: raised intracranial pressure (large mass > hydrocephalus), seizures, motor deficits, psychomotor delay; (iv) *optic pathways-hypothalamus*: raised intracranial pressure (large mass, hydrocephalus) (Fig. 8), visual deficits, endocrine disturbances; (v) *intraventricular*: hydrocephalus, seizures. Low grade astrocytomas have a long clinical history (months or even years) while high grade astrocytomas have a short duration of symptoms (weeks to a few months).

Pathology – (i) Pilocytic astrocytoma (WHO grade I): *infants and children*, biphasic pattern with small bipolar and stellate-shaped cells with abundant cytoplasm, distributed either in loose or compact areas; microcystic areas, microcalcifications, Rosenthal fibres and eosinophilic granular bodies are typical but not always present; Ki-67 usually < 1 per cent but possibly > 5 per cent, immunostaining for GFAP. (ii) Pilomixoid astrocytoma (WHO grade II): *infants*, optic-hypothalamic region, aggressive behaviour, monophasic bipolar pattern with a myxoid background, proliferative index often > 3 per cent, high rate of brain infiltration and CSF seeding. (iii) Diffuse atrocytoma (WHO grade II): *adults* (infants only for the brain stem location), differentiated fibrillary or gemistocytic astrocytes within loose and microcystic matrix, occasional atypia, moderate cellularity, proliferative index usually < 5 per cent, immunostaining for GFAP. (iv) Anaplastic astrocytoma (WHO grade III): *adults > infants > children*, hypercellularity, cell and nuclear pleomorphism, coarse nuclear chromatin, high mitotic index (> 5–10 per cent), immunostaining for GFAP and vimentin. (v) Glioblastoma (WHO grade IV): *adults > infants > children*, high cellular density and marked pleomorphism, spindle-shaped cells forming palisades around central necrotic foci (palisading necrosis), haemorrhagic areas, microvascular proliferation, high mitotic index (> 15–20 per cent), immunostaining for GFAP, vimentin and p53 (variable).

Neuroimaging – (i) *Pilocytic astrocytoma*: Cerebellum (60 per cent, children), optic pathways (25–30 per cent, infants and children), third ventricle/hypothalamus (5–7 per cent, infants and children), brain stem (3–5 per cent, infants and children), usually large size, frequently (multi-)cystic, calcifications common, haemorrhages and oedema rare, heterogeneous, solid portions iso-hypointense on T1 and hyperintense on T2 and FLAIR, intense and heterogeneous contrast enhancement, spectroscopy suggesting malignant tumour (↑ choline and lactate, ↓ N-acetyl-aspartate), differential diagnosis with other tumours of the posterior cranial fossa. (ii) *Diffuse astrocytoma*: Cerebral hemispheres (65 per cent, adults), brain stem (30 per cent, infants and children), variable size, rare cysts, possible calcifications, homogeneous, circumscribed but also infiltrating, hypointense on T1 and hyperintense on T2, no contrast enhancement, ↑ choline, ↓ N-acetyl-aspartate, ↑ myoinositol/creatine ratio, differential diagnosis with other astrocytomas, ischaemia and infections. (iii) *Anaplastic astrocytoma*: Cerebral hemispheres (adults) > brain stem and thalamus (infants and children), sometimes circumscribed but usually ill-defined, rare calcifications and haemorrhages, heterogeneous, iso-hypointense on T1, hyperintense on T2 and FLAIR, usually no contrast enhancement, spectroscopy similar to diffuse astrocytoma but with lower myoinositol/creatine ratio, white matter and CSF spreading, differential diagnosis with other astrocytomas, ischaemia and infections. (iv) *Glioblastoma*: Cerebral hemispheres (adults > infants) >> brain stem > cerebellum (infants and children), diffused and ill-defined, highly infiltrating and oedema-forming, sometimes bilateral across the corpus callosum ('butterfly' tumour), multifocal in up to 20 per cent of cases, frequently necrotic, possibly haemorrhagic and cystic, rare calcifications, heterogeneously isointense on T1 and iso-hyperintense on T2, contrast-enhanced with variable patterns (ring pattern typical), nodular, patchy, solid), ↑↑ choline, lactate and lipids, ↓ myoinositol and N-acetyl-aspartate, frequent white matter and CSF spread, differential diagnosis with other astrocytomas, metastases, ischaemia, abscesses.

Management – (i) *Low grade astrocytomas*: Surgery ± chemotherapy ± radiotherapy. (ii) *Pilocytic astrocytoma*: Cerebellar: gross total surgical resection is curative; after subtotal or partial removal observation is recommended (the tumour may involute or regrow very slowly). Chemotherapy and/or radiotherapy are limited to recurrent or unresectable tumours. Optic pathways: observation + chemotherapy and/or surgery and/or radiotherapy in case of tumour progression. (iii) *Diffuse astrocytoma*: Gross total resection is the best option; chemotherapy and/or radiotherapy can improve survival in case of subtotal removal. (iv) *Pontine diffuse astrocytoma*: Radiotherapy and chemotherapy (poor response). (v) *High grade astrocytoma*: Surgery + chemotherapy + radiotherapy. (vi) *Anaplastic astrocytoma and glioblastoma*: Resection followed by radiotherapy ± chemotherapy (temozolamide). Several additional treatment have been introduced (mainly in adults), for example: intraoperative fluorescence with 5-aminolevulinic acid to improve surgical excision, interstitial brachytherapy, and radioimmunotherapy with monoclonal antibodies.

Prognosis – (i) Low grade astrocytoma: 5-year survival 80 to 100 per cent according to different series and location. Best prognosis is for cerebellar pilocytic astrocytoma (70 per cent median survival rate at 20 years). (ii) Optic-hypothalamic: 5-year survival > 70–80 per cent but poor quality of life. CSF dissemination and pilomixoid variant are unfavourable prognostic factors. (iii) Diffuse astrocytoma: high rate of recurrence (50–70 per cent), possible malignant differentiation (usually within 4–5 years), median survival 5–10 years. (iv) Brain stem diffuse astrocytoma: very poor prognosis; 90 per cent of deaths within 18 months of diagnosis. (v) High grade astrocytoma: 5-year survival, 45–50 per cent (much higher than in adults and higher than in older children), in some cases even without radiotherapy. Infant age, gross total resection, absence of contrast enhancement and low proliferative index are indicators of better survival.

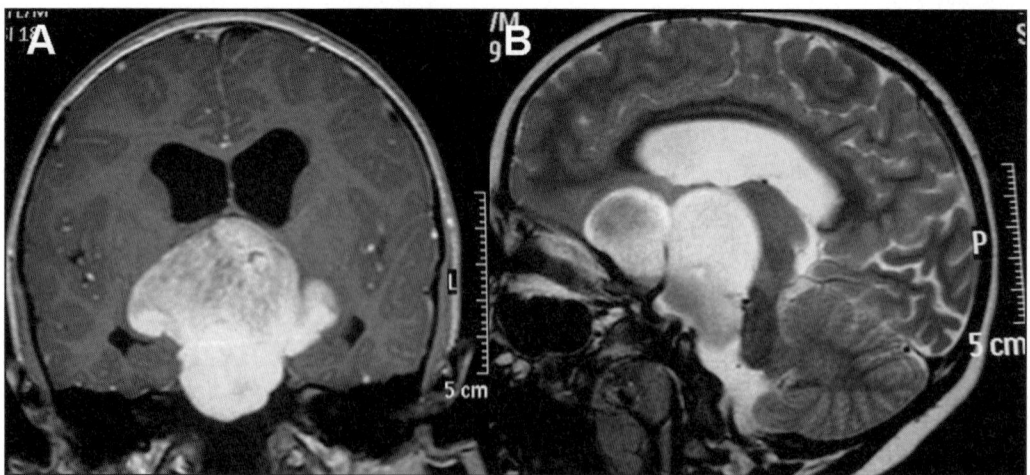

Fig. 8. *Very large, lobulated tumour arising from the optic chiasm/hypothalamus (no longer identifiable), invading the anterior skull base and completely obliterating the third ventricle, causing biventricular hydrocephalus. The demarcation with the surrounding brain is clear. The mass shows strong and homogeneous contrast enhancement (coronal T1-MRI, A) and presents hyperintense signal on T2-MRI (sagittal, B), revealing low cellularity. Imaging picture of an optic-hypothalamic low grade astrocytoma.*

Craniopharyngioma

Epidemiology – 0.5 to 2.5 per million/year, 1–5 per cent of all intracranial tumours; 5–10 per cent of all paediatric intracranial tumours (peak incidence, 5–15 years), 5 per cent of all IBTs; most common non-glial IBTs. Craniopharyngioma accounts for > 50 per cent of sellar/suprasellar tumours in children. M/F ratio, 1.

Genetics – Unknown (β-catenin mutation found in some adamantinomatous craniopharyngioma).

Origin – Rathke pouch epithelium (remnants of hypophyseal duct or squamous epithelial cells of the pars tuberalis of the adenohypophysis). If Rathke pouch fails to develop, the remnants can differentiate into primordial tooth tissue, giving rise to the adamantinomatous craniopharyngioma (most common, typical of infants and children), or into oral mucosal tissue, giving rise to the papillary craniopharyngioma (rare, typical of adults).

Location – Sellar (3–5 per cent), suprasellar prechiasmatic or retrochiasmatic (with or without III ventricle invasion/compression) (70–75 per cent), sellar + suprasellar (20 per cent), rarely ectopic (purely III ventricular, optic chiasm, nasopharynx, clivus, sphenoid sinus). Huge or giant craniopharyngioma often extends into the anterior (30 per cent), middle (25 per cent), or posterior cranial fossa (20 per cent). Optic chiasm and hypothalamus are often compressed.

Clinical features – Raised intracranial pressure is the most common clinical feature. Endocrine and visual disturbances also have an important place in the clinical profile, especially in infants: short stature (growth hormone deficiency) is the main sign, followed by hypothyroidism, adrenal failure and diabetes insipidus. Bitemporal hemianopia (or other visual field defects) and, less frequently, visual acuity deficits complete the picture.

Pathology – Macroscopic: solid portions contain squamous cells aggregates and gross calcifications; cyst are filled by cholesterol-rich, motor-oil-like, thick brownish-yellow fluid sometimes with crumbly debris. Microscopic: broad strands, cords and bridges of multistratified squamous epithelium with peripheral palisading of nuclei, nodules of compact 'wet' keratin and dystrophic calcifications, low proliferative index (usually < 1 per cent), immunostaining for cytokeratin and β-catenin. WHO grade I.

Neuroimaging – Multilobulated and multicystic large mass (> 5 cm at diagnosis) displacing or encasing the neighbouring structures (Fig. 9). Adamantinomatous craniopharyngioma is solid and cystic (90 per cent) or 'purely' cystic (10 per cent), and usually has a calcified capsule and/or gross tumour calcification. Papillary craniopharyngioma is mainly solid and poorly calcified. *CT*: Gross calcifications, solid-isodense, cystic-hypodense. *MRI*: Cysts are hyperintense on T1, FLAIR and T2 (high protein and cholesterol content), solid portion are heterogeneous on both T1 and T2, heterogeneous contrast enhancement of the solid part and strong enhancement of the cyst wall. *MRI spectroscopy*: Broad lipid spectrum of the cystic content. *Differential diagnosis*: Rathke cleft cyst (small size, usually sellar, no calcifications, no solid areas, no enhancement); optic-hypothalamic gliomas (mainly solid with multiple small cysts, more homogeneous enhancement, possible necrosis, only small calcifications).

Management – Craniopharyngioma is a benign, slowly growing tumour but its surgical and medical management is one of the most difficult among IBTs, the recurrence rate is high, and the outcome is often poor. This is due to the huge tumour size and the critical location that limits the extent of surgery and is associated with severe pre- and postoperative sequelae. For that reason, the standard approach to craniopharyngioma (attempt at radical surgery) is now changing in favour of more conservative strategies, such as subtotal/partial excision

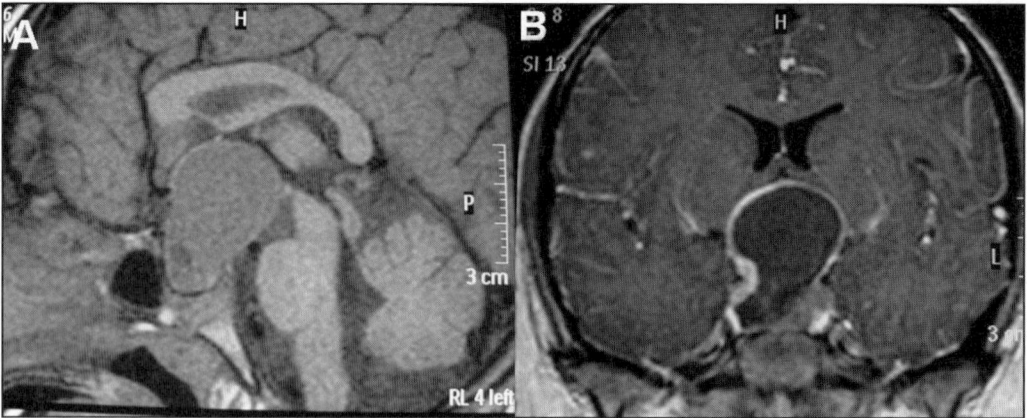

Fig. 9. Midline large cystic tumour, with well demarcated margins, occupying the sellar and suprasellar region and compressing and displacing the third ventricle. The fluid content is iso-hyperintense on sagittal T1-MRI (A), as for high protein levels, and the cyst wall enhances with gadolinium on coronal T1-MRI (B). Diagnosis: craniopharyngioma.

+ radiotherapy, biopsy/cyst fenestration + radiotherapy. Injection of sclerosing agents within the tumour cyst is an interesting alternative: thanks to new non-neurotoxic agents such as interferon-α, which can induce cyst shrinkage without the toxic effects of old drugs (bleomycin) or radioisotopes, it is now possible to postpone the direct surgical approach, making it also easier (smaller and less adherent tumour). To postpone the surgical approach is crucial in infants, as they are given the opportunity to grow and mature.

Prognosis – 10-year survival ranges from 64 to 96 per cent. The quality of life of treated patients is often poor, mainly because of obesity, permanent visual deficits, the need for chronic hormone replacement, and severe neurological postoperative sequelae (hemiparesis, seizures). The most important factors predicting craniopharyngioma recurrence are: size at diagnosis (> 5 cm, high risk of relapse; < 5 cm, low risk); completeness of surgical resection (gross total, low risk; subtotal/partial, high risk); and histological type (adamantinomatous craniopharyngiomas are more aggressive than papillary craniopharyngiomas).

References

Ater, J.L., Eys, J., Woo, S.Y., Moore, B., Copeland, D.R. & Bruner, J. (1997): MOPP chemotherapy without irradiation as primary postsurgical therapy for brain tumours in infants and young children. *J. Neurooncol.* **32**, 243–252.

Biegel, J.A. (1999): Cytogenetics and molecular genetics of childhood brain tumours. *Neuro-Oncology* **1**, 139–151.

Biernat, W. & Żawrocki, A. (2007): Molecular alterations in ependymomas. *Fol. Neuropathol.* **45**, 155–163.

Carpentieri, S.C., Weber, D.P., Pomeroy, S.L., Scott, R.M., Goumnerova, L.C., Kieran, M.W., Billet, A.L. & Tarbell, N.J. (2003): Neuropsychological functioning after surgery in children treated for brain tumour. *Neurosurgery* **52**, 1348–1357.

Carstensen, H., Juhler, M., Bøgeskov, L. & Laursen, H. (2006): A report of nine newborns with congenital brain tumours. *Childs Nerv. Syst.* **22**, 1427–1431.

CBTRUS (2008): *Statistical report: Primary brain tumours in the United States, 2000-2004*. Central Brain Tumours Registry of the United States (http://www.cbtrus.org).

Chen, W. (2007): Clinical applications of PET in brain tumours. *J. Nucl. Med.* **48**, 1468–1481.

Chi, S.N., Gardner, S., Levy, A.S., Knoop, E.A., Miller, D.C., Wisoff, J.H., Weiner, H.L. & Finlay, J.L. (2004): Feasibility and response to induction chemotherapy intensified with high dose methotrexate for young children with newly diagnosed high risk disseminated medulloblastoma. *J. Clin. Oncol.* **22**, 4881–4887.

Davis, F.S. (2007): Epidemiology of brain tumours. *Expert Rev. Anticancer Ther.* **7**, S3–S6.

Di Rocco, C., Iannelli, A. & Ceddia, A. (1991): Intracranial tumours of the first year of life. A cooperative survey of the 1986-1987 Education Committee of the ISPN. *Childs Nerv. Syst.* **7**, 150–153.

Di Rocco, C., Ceddia, A. & Iannelli, A. (1993): Intracranial tumours in the first year of life. A report of 51 cases. *Acta Neurochir.* **123**, 14–24.

Di Rocco, C., Iannelli, A. & Massimi, L. (2007): Characteristics and long term outcome of infants with intracranial tumours diagnosed in the first year of life. *Pan Arab J. Neurosurg.* **11**, 10–15.

Duffner, P.K., Horowitz, M.E., Krischer, J.P., Burger, P.C., Cohen, M.E., Sanford, R.A., Friedman, H.S. & Kun, L.E. (1999): The treatment of malignant brain tumours in infants and very young children: an update of The Pediatric Oncology Group. *Neuro-Oncology* **1**, 152–161.

Garré, M.L., Cama, A., Milanaccio, C., Gandola, L., Massimino, M. & Dallorso, S. (2006): New concepts in the treatment of brain tumours in very young children. *Expert Rev. Neurother.* **6**, 489–500.

Geyer, J.R., Zeltzer, P.M., Boyett, J.M., Rorke, L., Stanley, P., Albright, A.L., Wisoff, J.H., Milstein, J.M., Allen, J.C., Finlay, J.L., Ayers, G.D., Shurin, S.B., Stevens, K. & Bleyer, W.A. (1994): Survival of infants with primitive neuroectodermal tumours or malignant ependymomas of the CNS treated with eight drugs in 1 day: a report from the Childrens Cancer group. *J. Clin. Oncol.* **12**, 1607–1615.

Gjerris, F., Agerlin, N., Børgesen, S.E., Buhl, L., Haase, J., Klinken, L., Mortensen, A.C., Olsen, J.H., Ovensen, N., Reske-Nielsen, E. & Schmidt, K. (1998): Epidemiology and prognosis in children treated for intracranial tumours in Denmark 1960-1984. *Childs Nerv. Syst.* **14**, 302–311.

Hakin-Smith, V., Jellinek, D.A., Levy, D., Carrol, T., Teo, M., Timperley, W.R., McKay, M.J., Reddel, R.R. & Royds, J.A. (2003): Alternative lengthening of telomeres and survival in patients with glioblastoma multiforme. *Lancet* **361**, 836–838.

Inda, M.M., Perot, C., Guillaud Bataille, M., Danglot, G., Rey, J.A., Bello, M.J., Fan, X., Eberhart, C., Zazpe, I., Portillo, E., Tuñon, T., Martìnez-Peñuela, J.M., Bernheim, A. & Castresana, J.S. (2005): Genetic heterogeneity in supratentorial and infratentorial primitive neuroectodermal tumours of the central nervous system. *Histopathology* **47**, 631–637.

Isaacs, H.I. (2002): Perinatal brain tumours: a review of 250 cases. *Pediatr. Neurol.* **27**, 249–261.

Jellinher, K. & Sunder-Plassman, M. (1973): Congenital intracranial tumours. *Neuropaediatrie* **4**, 46–63.

Kalifa, C. & Grill, J. (2005): The therapy of infantile malignant tumours: current status? *J. Neuro-Oncol.* **75**, 279–285.

Kalifa, C., Hartmann, O., Demeocq, F., Vassal, G., Couanet, D., Terrier-Lacombe, M.J., Valteau, D., Brugieres, L. & Lemerle, J. (1992): High dose busulfan and thiotepa with autologous bone marrow transplantation in childhood malignant brain tumours: a phase II study. *Bone Marrow Transpl.* **9**, 227–233.

Kellie, S.J. (1999): Chemotherapy of central nervous system tumours in infants. *Child's Nerv. Syst.* **15**, 592–612.

Kleihues, P., Burger, P.C. & Scheitauer, B.W., editors (1993): *Histological typing of tumours of the central nervous system*. Heidelberg: Springer-Verlag.

Kleihues, P. & Cavenee, W.K. (2000): *World Heath Organization classification of tumours. Pathology and genetics of tumours of the nervous system*. Lyon: IARC Press.

Knab, B. & Connell, P.P. (2007): Radiotherapy for paediatric brain tumours: when and how. *Expert Rev. Anticancer Ther.* **7**, S69–S77.

Kurmasheva, R.T. & Houghton, P.J. (2007): Paediatric oncology. *Curr. Opin. Chem. Biol.* **11**, 424–432.

Louis, D.N., Ohgaki, H., Wiestler, O.D. & Cavenee, W.K. (2007): *WHO classification of tumours of the central nervous system*. Lyon: IARC Press.

MacDonald, T.J., Rood, B.R., Santi, M.R., Vezina, G., Bingaman, K., Cogen, P.H. & Packer, R.J. (2003): Advances in the diagnosis, molecular genetics, and treatment of pediatric embryonal CNS tumours. *Oncologist* **8**, 174–186.

Malinger, G., Ben-Sira, L., Lev, D., Ben-Aroya, Z., Kidron, D. & Lerman-Sagie, T. (2004): Fetal brain imaging: a comparison between magnetic resonance imaging and dedicated neurosonography. *Ultrasound Obstet. Gynecol.* **23**, 333–340.

Marsh, G.M., Youk, A.O., Buchanich, J.M., Kant, I.J. & Swaen, G. (2007): Mortality patterns among workers exposed to acrylamide: updated follow up. *J. Occup. Environ. Med.* **49**, 82–95

Massimi, L., Tufo, T. & Di Rocco, C. (2007): Management of optic-hypothalamic gliomas in children: still a challenging problem. *Expert Rev. Anticancer. Ther.* **7**, 1591–1610.

Massimino, M., Gandola, L., Cefalo, G., Lasio, G., Riva, D., Fossati-Bellani, F., Gianni, M.C., Luksch, R., Tesoro-Tess, J.D. & Lombardi, F. (2000): Management of medulloblastoma and ependymoma in infants: a single-institution long-term restrospective report. *Childs Nerv. Syst.* **16**, 15–20.

Merchant, T.E. & Fouladi, M. (2005): Ependymoma: new therapeutic approaches including radiation and chemotherapy. *J. Neuro-Oncol.* **75**, 287–299.

Merchant, T.E., Mulhern, R.K., Krasin, M.J., Kun, L.E., Williams, T., Li, C., Xiong, X., Khan, R.B., Lustig, R.H., Boop, F.A. & Sanford, S.A. (2004): Preliminary results from a phase II trial of conformal radiation therapy and evaluation of radiation-related CNS effects for paediatric patients with localized ependymoma. *J. Clin. Oncol.* **22**, 3156–3162.

Ohgaki, H. & Kleihues, P. (2007): Genetic pathways to primary and secondary glioblastoma. *Am. J. Pathol.* **170**, 1445–1453.

Pettorini, B., Park, Y.S., Caldarelli, M., Massimi, L., Tamburini, G. & Di Rocco, C. (2008): Radiation-induced brain tumours after central nervous system irradiation in childhood: a review. *Childs Nerv. Syst.* **24**, 793–805.

Pollack, J.F., Hamilton, R.L., Finkelstein, S.D., Campbell, J.W., Martinez, A.J., Shervin, R.N., Bozik, M.E. & Gollin, S.M. (1997): The relationship between TP53 mutation and overexpression of p53 and prognosis in malignant gliomas of childhood. *Cancer Res.* **57**, 304–309.

Reddy, A. & Packer, R. (1999): Chemotherapy for low grade gliomas. *Childs Nerv. Syst.* **15**, 506-513.

Rickert, C.H. (1998): Epidemiological features of brain tumours in the first 3 years of life. *Childs Nerv. Syst.* **14**, 547–550.

Rickert, C.H. & Paulus, W. (2001): Epidemiology of central nervous system tumours in childhood and adolescence based on the new WHO classification. *Childs Nerv. Syst.* **17**, 503–511.

Rickert, C.H., Probst-Cousin, S. & Gullotta, F. (1997): Primary intracranial neoplasms of infancy and early childhood. *Childs Nerv. Syst.* **13**, 507–513.

Rivera-Luna, R., Medina-Sanson, A., Leal-Leal, C., Pantoja-Guillen, F., Zapata-Tarrés, M., Cardenas-Cardos, R., Barrera-Gómez, R. & Rueda-Franco, F. (2003): Brain tumours in children under 1 year of age: emphasis on the relationship of prognostic factors. *Childs Nerv. Syst.* **19**, 311–314.

Rutkowski, S., Bode, U., Deinlein, F., Ottensmeier, H., Warmuth-Metz, M., Soerensen, N., Graf, N., Emser, A., Pietsch, Y., Wolff, J.E., Kortmann, R.D. & Kuehl, J. (2005): Treatment of early childhood medulloblastoma by postoperative chemotherapy alone. *N. Engl. J. Med.* **352**, 978–986.

Sala, F., Colarusso, E., Mazza, C., Talacchi, A. & Bricolo, A. (1999): Brain tumours in children under 3 years of age. *Pediatr. Neurosurg.* **31**, 16–26.

Saunders, D.E., Thompson, C., Gunny, R., Jones, R., Cox, T. & Chong, W.K. (2007): Magnetic resonance imaging protocols for pediatric neuroradiology. *Pediatr. Radiol.* **37**, 789–797.

Solitaire, G.B. & Krigman, M.R. (1964): Congenital intracranial neoplasm: a case report and review of the literature. *J. Neuropathol. Exp. Neurol.* **23**, 280–292.

Spiegler, B.J., Bouffet, E., Greenberg, M.L., Rutka, J.T. & Mabbott, D.J. (2004): Change in neurocognitive functioning after treatment with cranial radiation in childhood. *J. Clin. Oncol.* **22**, 706–713.

Suc, E., Kalifa, C., Brauner, R., Habrand, J.L., Terrier-Lacombe, M.J., Vassal, G. & Lemerle, J. (1990): Brain tumours under the age of three. The price of survival. A retrospective study of 20 long-term survivors. *Acta Neurochir.* **106**, 93–98.

Tamburrini, G., Massimi, L., Caldarelli, M. & Di Rocco, C. (2008): Antibiotic impregnated external ventricular drainage and third ventriculostomy in the management of hydrocephalus associated with posterior cranial fossa tumours. *Acta Neurochir.* **150**, 1049–1055.

Volpe, J.J. (1995): Brain tumours and vein malformations. In: *Neurology of the newborn*, 3rd ed., ed. J.J. Volpe, pp. 795–807. Philadelphia: WB Saunders.

Wakai, S., Arai, T. & Nagai, M. (1984): Congenital brain tumours. *Surg. Neurol.* **1**, 597–609.

Wigertz, A., Lönn, S., Schwartzbaum, J., Hall, P., Auvinen, A., Christensen, H.C., Johansen, C., Klaeboe, L., Salminen, T., Schoemaker, M.J., Swerdlow, A.J., Tynes, T. & Feychting, M. (2007): Allergic conditions and brain tumour risk. *Am. J. Epidemiol.* **166**, 941–950.

Zülch, K.J. (1979): *Histological typing of tumours of the central nervous system*. Geneva: World Health Organization.

Chapter 10

Epilepsy in infancy

Francesco Guzzetta and Domenica Battaglia

Catholic University, Largo Agostino Gemelli 8, 00168 Rome, Italy
fguzzetta@rm.unicatt.it

Epilepsy incidence is higher in the first months of life than at any other time (Hauser, 1994; Hauser, 1995; Cowan, 2002). Immaturity of the brain accounts for the enhanced development and propagation of seizures, with typical clinical and EEG features at an early age (Holmes, 1997). Knowledge of the particular characteristics of epileptogenesis in the developing brain is essential for understanding the propensity of young infants to seizures.

Epileptogenesis in infancy

There are several potential neurobiological factors affecting the development of epileptogenesis in the immature brain, where circuits supporting neuronal hypersynchrony may develop (Johnston, 1996) (Table 1). It is well known that the numbers of synapses and synaptic junctions are normally increased in young infants (Huttenlocher & Courten, 1987). Abnormal connections can also arise from early injury to certain cortical areas (for example, the hippocampus or limbic cortex). And there is evidence that early in development, receptors of excitatory and inhibitory neurotransmitters are distributed in a different way from those of the adult brain, with developmental changes in their expression that increase brain excitability (Holmes, 1997).

Table 1. Potential neurobiological substrates for epileptogenesis in the immature brain (after Johnston, 1996)

Hypersynchrony of groups of neurons
Increased density of synapses
Increased number of gap junctions
Establishment of abnormal connections after injury
Increased expression of excitatory receptors
Synaptic plasticity
Kindling
Long term potentiation (LTP)
Presynaptic and postsynaptic mechanisms
Neuronal loss of function (e.g., GABA neurons)

The presence of many excitatory synapses and a high density of excitatory neurotransmitter receptors, together with a shortage of inhibitory receptors, enhances synaptic excitation in the immature brain (Swann, 1995); by their inherent nature, some neurotransmitters that are inhibitory in adult life are excitatory in the immature brain (Cherubini et al., 1991; Khazipov et al., 2001; Ben-Ari, 2002; Ben-Ari & Holmes, 2005). Moreover, at this early age the substantia nigra plays a role in amplifying the epileptic activity (Moshé & Sperber, 1998).

The proneness to seizures may arise from an activity change in existing excitatory circuits (Witter, 1989), supported by a plastic modulation of the balance between the excitatory and inhibitory neurotransmitter systems (Gulyás et al., 1996). That is what happens in 'kindling', in which repeated small electrical stimuli to the brain eventually provoke major epileptic seizures, the expression of which is possibly enhanced at a very young age. Long term potentiation (LTP) – that is, the long lasting enhancement in communication between neurons strengthening synaptic functions, with consequent activation of pathways – is another mechanism increasing epileptogenicity (Bliss & Lomo, 1973). Finally, as in excitatory receptors, there are developmental changes in the regional configuration of the γ-aminobutyric acid (GABA) receptors in young infants, eventually producing brain hyperexcitability (Laurie et al., 1992). In Table 2, we present the points to stress concerning seizure susceptibility in the developing brain, supported by clinical observations. Although the immature brain is prone to seizure activity for the reasons given above, it is important to emphasize its lesser vulnerability to seizure-related brain damage, and the greater harmfulness of antiepileptic drugs.

The main questions concerning the effects of seizures on the immature brain are, first, whether seizures produce permanent injury and if so, what are the brain areas most damaged by seizures; second, whether such damage results in epilepsy; and third, what kind of seizures (status epilepticus? repeated, even brief, seizures?) can provoke these chronic epileptogenic effects.

There are controversial conclusions about the permanent brain damage caused by status epilepticus in humans (Berg & Shinnar, 1997; Sutula et al., 2003) – in particular, in children the presence of hippocampal oedema preceding atrophy after status epilepticus is not an agreed finding (Nohria et al., 1994; Scott et al., 2002). Also in animals, there is much evidence of resistance of the immature brain to the morphological damage induced by recurrent febrile seizures or status epilepticus, in contrast to what happens in the mature brain (Haut et al., 2004). On the other hand, the frequency of epilepsy as a consequence of status epilepticus in children (Maytal et al., 1989) would seem to be linked rather to pre-existing neurological abnormalities (Berg & Shinnar, 1996) and to reflect a common primary cause of brain injury and status epilepticus such as early prenatal or perinatal accidents (hypoxia, ischaemia, trauma, and so on) (De Lorenzo et al., 1995). With respect to repeated brief seizures, there is no definite

Table 2. Seizure susceptibility in infants

Features	Clinical observations
Higher susceptibility to seizures of the immature brain	Higher incidence of seizure occurrence, recurrence, and duration in infancy; lesser resistance to occasional causes (e.g., fever)
Unbalanced excitation/inhibition	Greater age-dependent electro-clinical abnormalities
Less vulnerable to seizure-related brain damage	Less severe clinical effects after status epilepticus
Antiepileptic drugs harmful to the developing brain	Teratogenic and neurotoxic effects

evidence that they produce brain damage in humans. In animals, the immature brain seems more resistant to brief seizures than the adult brain (Haut et al., 2004). However, early-life seizures, without causing evident cellular injury, predispose the immature brain to the damaging effects of seizures later on. This condition is the basis of the so-called 'two-hit hypothesis', indicating the major risk of injury with subsequent seizures in children who were affected by seizures early in life (Hoffman et al., 2004).

Yet, despite a greater proneness to seizures, infants seem to have resistance to seizure-induced brain damage (Ben-Ari & Holmes, 2006). This deserves further study as so far human studies have been mainly retrospective, so that the distinction between seizure-induced pathology and the causes of the seizures is hard to define. Furthermore, this apparent resistance should be examined in the context of the various known aetiopathogenic factors such as genetics, primary injuries, and predisposing functional brain disorders.

Experimental studies on rodents show that epileptogenesis caused by acquired factors – for example, hyperthermic seizures or status epilepticus – is based on functional changes in the immature brain, with permanent changes in the expression of molecules such as receptors and ion channels (Bender & Baram, 2007), eventually supported by microscopic morphological abnormalities. For example, in animal models of febrile seizures, a change in molecular expression is mediated by interleukin release which enhances enduring alterations in gene expression – that is, activity-dependent plasticity facilitating the conversion of 'normal' developing circuits to 'epileptic' circuits (Dube et al., 2005; Heida & Pittman, 2005; Vezzani & Baram, 2007).

The microscopic changes in the immature networks of the developing brain also need to be considered. There is evidence that seizures may activate genes producing dendrites and neo-synaptogenesis (Represa & Ben-Ari, 1997), with a consequent synaptic reorganization (sprouting axons of mossy fibres in different brain regions such as the hippocampal fascia dentata) (Tauck & Nadler, 1985). These sprouting of mossy fibres, the privileged site of the glutamate neurotransmitter, result in enhanced excitation (Esclapez et al., 1999).

Thus, despite the fact that in the immature brain there is a lesser degree of neuron vulnerability (neuronal damage and cell loss) than in adults, early in life seizures disrupt the fundamental development phenomena such as the sequential expression of receptors and the formation and stabilization of synapses, besides having more general effects on cellular proliferation and migration. These phenomena are essential for the adequate formation of circuits and are thus conditioning seizure susceptibility, explaining the eventual development of epilepsy later in life (Berg et al., 2001).

These developmental changes in brain excitability are the basis for the variability in the evolution of epilepsies in infancy. Seizures occurring early in development could be the first manifestations of an early-onset epilepsy or occasional epileptogenic episodes (for example, acute symptomatic seizures, febrile seizures) that evolve to epilepsy later. In the latter case, early seizures could be the effect of an epileptic predisposition that will manifest later in life as epilepsy or may be associated with or be caused by acute brain damage that produces epilepsy after a silent period. A developmental approach to seizure disorders and an understanding of the complex underlying mechanisms is thus relevant for any strategy of antiepileptic treatment (Dulac et al., 2007).

Antiepileptic drugs produce adverse effects on the developing brain, including interference with cell proliferation and migration, axonal arborization, synaptogenesis, synaptic plasticity and physiological apoptotic cell death. In particular, drugs may interfere with neurotransmitters that are conditioning neural cell proliferation, differentiation and migration (Retz et al., 1996;

Nguyen *et al.*, 2001) and thus can cause permanent brain defects. Similarly, neurotransmitters as well as growth factors and cytokines are involved in apoptosis and loss of synapses (pruning), a relevant phenomenon in the period of CNS organization which may be compromised by drug administration (Webb *et al.*, 2001). These data are consistent with the teratogenic or simply neurotoxic/apoptotic effects of antiepileptic drugs. For detailed treatment of this subject see the review by Kaindl *et al.* (2006). Consideration of these morphological and molecular collateral negative effects of antiepileptic drugs in infancy may contribute to a more balanced strategy in antiepileptic treatment.

Classification

The first and most important step in the management of paediatric epilepsy, in order to establish effective treatment and prognosis, is an accurate diagnosis of the epileptic disorder. In the last century the scientific community underlined the importance of precise diagnostic criteria for identifying seizure types and epileptic syndromes. Continuous work by the International Collaborative Group For Epilepsy has led to the definition of recognized systems for seizure and epilepsy classification (ILAE Commission on Classification and Terminology, 1981, 1985 and 1989; Engel, 2001).

Before the current syndromic International League Against Epilepsy (ILAE) classification of 1989, epilepsy in infants and young children was limited to categories defined according to the dominant seizure type and included West syndrome in the presence of infantile spasms and partial or generalized epilepsy (Cavazzuti *et al.*, 1984; Chevrie & Aicardi, 1971; Chevrie & Aicardi, 1975; Chevrie & Aicardi, 1977). Dalla Bernardina *et al.* (1982), in a study on children younger than 3 years, introduced new categories other than partial and generalized epilepsy, such as 'epileptic encephalopathies', including West syndrome, Lennox-Gastaut syndrome, and other subtypes. After the publication of the ILAE classification in 1989, the applicability of a syndromic approach in infancy was thoroughly evaluated (Aicardi, 1994). A study of Sarisjulis *et al.* (2000) shows that the *syndromic classification* is practicable in infants, even though a quarter of seizures and epilepsies remain unclassifiable. The difficulty is caused by many factors concerning either the definition of seizure type or the definition of the epilepsy syndrome.

The definition of seizure type is often not easy because of the complexity of the semiology, the difficulty in differentiating partial from generalized seizures and evaluating consciousness, and the frequently scanty semeiological details. Consequently, it is often impossible to draw an anatomo-electro-clinical correlation. These problems probably reflect the immaturity of the cortical functional circuitries and thus of the interhemispheric synchrony.

The definition of an epileptic syndrome, often mandatory for therapeutic strategies and prognostic evaluation, cannot be related only to the seizure type, but is the result of a combination of different aspects concerning electroclinical features, aetiology, age, and evolution. In infants, a key issue relates to the difficulty in defining the epileptic syndrome at its onset or soon after, because of the incomplete expression of the age-dependent electroclinical pattern (for example, in Dravet syndrome) and the complexity of the clinical presentation (polymorphism of seizures, EEG features, neuro-cognitive impairment, and so on).

In the last decade, electroclinical studies using video-EEG monitoring, new genetic findings, and developments in neuroradiological techniques have led to the definition of new epileptic syndromes in infancy. The ILAE has proposed a 'diagnostic scheme', useful for the analysis of different aspects in patients with epilepsy (Engel, 2001). This scheme has five axes: ictal semeiology, seizure type, epileptic syndrome, aetiology, and the degree of impairment. In this diagnostic scheme the dichotomous classification of epileptic syndrome into 'partial' and 'generalized' is abandoned. The approach is flexible and dynamic because the list of epileptic syndromes or the aetiology or the seizure type can be adjusted with the introduction of possible new elements. With regard to infant epilepsy, the introduction of key terms in the definition is particularly interesting, namely:

Epileptic encephalopathy – this indicates a condition in which the epileptiform abnormalities themselves are believed to contribute to the progressive deterioration of cerebral function. This definition is particularly useful in infancy, when the condition is relatively frequent. In the new diagnostic scheme several syndromes (early myoclonic encephalopathy; Ohtahara syndrome; West syndrome; Dravet syndrome; myoclonic status in non-progressive encephalopathies) are included among epileptic encephalopathies of infancy.

Benign epilepsy – this indicates a syndrome characterized by epileptic seizures which are easily treated or require no treatment, and remit without sequelae.

Focal seizures and focal syndromes – replace the terms 'partial seizures' and 'localization-related syndromes'.

The 'epileptic seizure type' has a unique underlying pathophysiological mechanism and anatomical substrate; thus, it represents a diagnostic entity with aetiological, therapeutic, and prognostic implications. As already stressed (Arziamnoglou et al., 2004; Korff & Nordli, 2006), the first step in the diagnostic process should be an accurate seizure classification and subsequently the definition of an epileptic syndrome. Continuous effort is necessary to define an electroclinical diagnosis of seizures in infancy in order to achieve appropriate diagnostic precision. A list of the currently acknowledged epileptic syndromes in infancy is given in Table 3.

Epilepsies and epileptic syndromes

Epileptic encephalopathy with suppression-burst

Epileptic encephalopathy with suppression-burst is a rare and severe neurological condition with very early onset (within the third month of life). It is characterized by polymorphic seizures and an EEG pattern of suppression-burst in both awake and sleep states. The suppression-burst pattern consists of paroxysmal activity (polyspikes) lasting several seconds and alternating with episodes of flat or low amplitude activity. The ILAE classification (1989) defines two types of epileptic encephalopathies with suppression-burst pattern: early infantile epileptic encephalopathy (EIEE) or Ohtahara syndrome, described by Ohtahara *et al.* (1976), and early myoclonic encephalopathy (EME) described by Aicardi & Goutières (1978).

Early infantile epileptic encephalopathy – EIEE is the earliest of the age-dependent epileptic encephalopathies. The more frequent seizures are tonic spasms, in clusters or isolated. Focal seizures such as erratic motor seizures and hemiconvulsions can be observed, while myoclonic seizures are very rare (Ohtahara *et al.*, 2006). The interictal EEG is characterized by suppression-bursts, with bursts of paroxysmal activity (slow waves and multifocal spikes) lasting 2 to 3 seconds, alternating with suppression phases (Fig. 1A). This pattern occurs during both awake and sleep states, so that the EEG differentiation between them is impossible. Ictal EEG of tonic spasms is characterized by a high amplitude slow wave followed by diffuse desynchronization or fast activity (Fig. 1B). A case with a negative myoclonic phenomenon was reported by Guzzetta *et al.* (2002a) (Fig. 2). Psychomotor development is very impaired from the onset, and neurological findings evolve towards severe abnormalities, particularly spastic cerebral palsy.

Table 3. Epilepsies and epileptic syndromes in infancy

Specific syndromes	Age at onset	Main characteristics	Prognosis
Early infantile epileptic encephalopathy	First months	Tonic seizures, spasms; suppression-burst	Severe outcome
Early myoclonic epilepsy	First months	Myoclonias, spasms; suppression-burst	Severe outcome
Malignant migrating partial seizures of infancy	First year	Continuous multifocal electrographic seizures	Severe outcome
Infantile spasms	First year	Spasms; hypsarrhythmia; developmental delay	Variable outcome
Dravet syndrome	First year	Partial and generalized seizures, myoclonias; normal EEG at onset; later: generalized spike-waves and multifocal spikes	Severe outcome
Generalized epilepsy with febrile seizures (+)	Infancy or later	Variable seizure and developmental phenotype in addition to febrile and afebrile generalized seizures	Variable outcome
Benign myoclonic epilepsy	3 months to 3 years	Myoclonic seizures; normal interictal EEG; normal development	Good/variable outcome
Myoclonic astatic epilepsy	First year to 4 years	Generalized myoclonic and astatic seizures; interictal parietal theta activity and bilateral spike-waves	Variable outcome
Myoclonic status in non-progressive encephalopathies	First year to 4 years	Atypical absence; epileptic and non epileptic myoclonus; long lasting epileptic status	Severe outcome
Benign familial/non-familial seizures	First year	Partial seizures; normal development	Good outcome
Non-idiopathic partial epilepsy	Infancy or later	Semeiology according to cortical area involved	Variable outcome
Febrile seizure (not diagnosed as being epileptic)	3 months to 5 years	Brief tonic-clonic or clonic seizures	Good outcome

Usually, EIEE is associated with structural brain damage (Ohtahara et al., 1992). The heterogeneous aetiology includes destructive brain lesions (for example, porencephaly) and brain malformations such as hemimegalencephaly, focal cortical dysplasia, schizencephaly, Aicardi syndrome, and olivary-dentate dysplasia. A few cryptogenic cases with apparently normal magnetic resonance imaging (MRI) are found. In some cases, diffuse microscopical abnormalities of migration have been detected at autopsy without evident abnormalities on MRI (Robain & Dulac, 1992; Miller et al., 1998). Metabolic disorders have been observed in a few cases (Aicardi & Ohtahara, 2005).

Kato et al. (2007) reported two non-familial cases with EIEE associated with polyalanine expansion in the ARX gene (Aristales-related homeobox). Recently, four unrelated children with EIEE were found to have heterozygous missense mutations in the gene encoding syntaxin binding protein 1 (STXBP1) (Saitsu et al., 2008). The STXBP1 protein is a neuronal sec1-Munc-18 protein essential for vesicle release in several species (Verhage et al., 1997). This mutation may thus have led to impairment of synaptic vesicle release and neural cell death in the brain stem, although MRI did not show brain stem abnormalities (Saitsu et al., 2008).

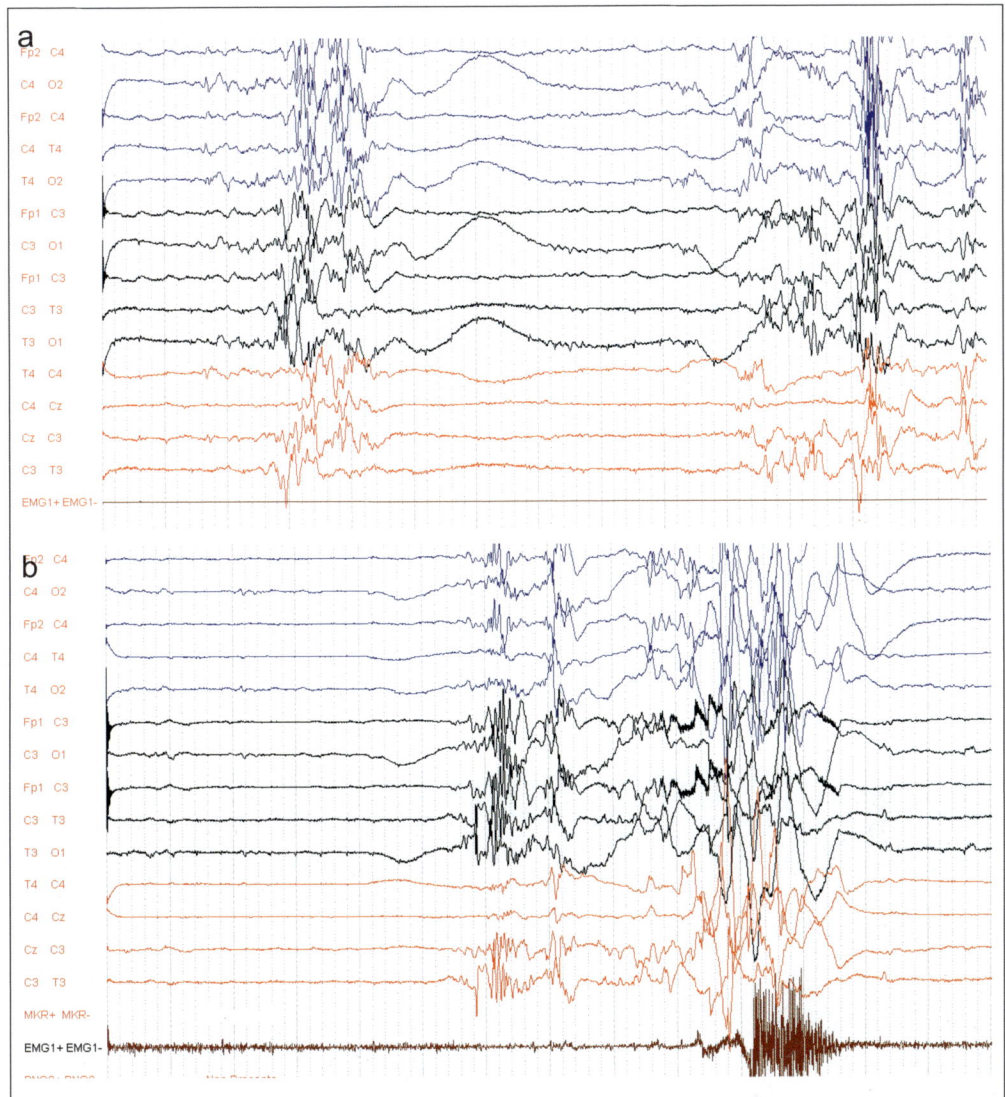

Fig. 1. Awake EEG of a 3-day-old infant affected by early infantile epileptic encephalopathy (Otahara's syndrome). (A) Brief bursts of diffuse spikes and polyspikes alternating with a suppression period lasting 6 seconds. (B) Tonic spasm correlated with polyspike discharges followed by slow waves.

Seizures are usually refractory to antiepileptic drugs. Surgical treatment has been undertaken in cases secondary to unilateral dysplasia such as hemimegalencephaly, sometimes with a good epilepsy outcome (Wyllie *et al.*, 1996; Battaglia *et al.*, 1999a; Devlin *et al.*, 2003; Jonas *et al.*, 2004; Lettori *et al.*, 2008).

Prognosis is very poor in almost all cases. Ohtahara reported a high early mortality (4 of 16 cases), and severe neurocognitive retardation in all cases. Among the cases with long follow-up, an evolution towards other epileptic encephalopathies – such as West syndrome and Lennox-Gastaut syndrome – is reported, though this remains controversial (Djukic *et al.*, 2006; Ohtahara & Yamatogi, 2006).

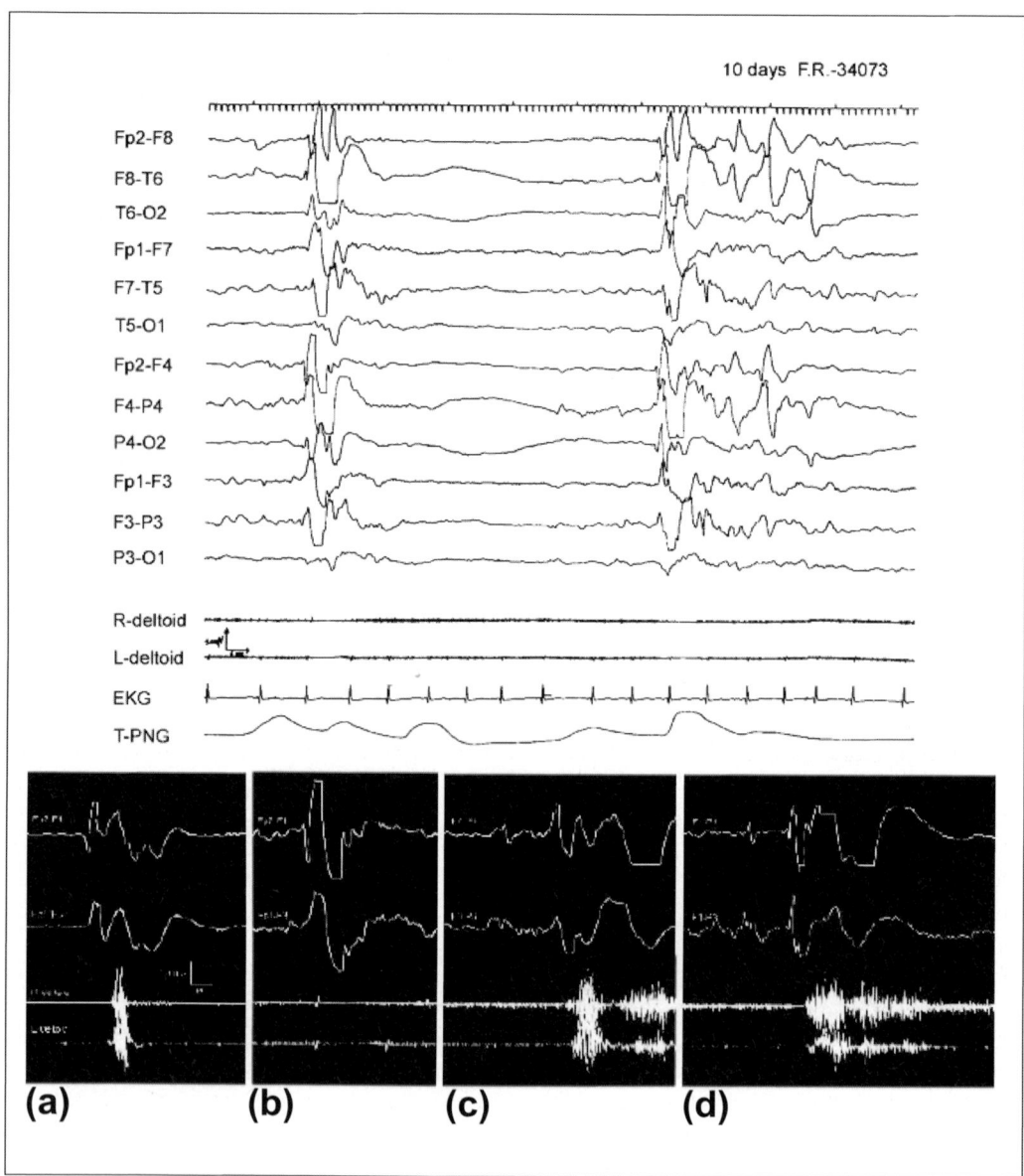

Fig. 2. Top: Suppression burst pattern with spikes more evident on the right hemisphere. Note the atonic events at the beginning of the bursts. Bottom: Paroxysmal events linked to EEG bursts: bilateral synchronous myoclonic jerks related to right high-voltage slow spike (a); deltoid electromyogram (EMG) silence associated with right spike-wave (b); typical spasm linked to a spike-wave; the spasm appears related to the wide high voltage slow wave (c); short EMG silence followed by a typical spasm (d). (From Guzzetta et al. Epilepsia 2002 Sep; 43(9): 1106-9)

Early myoclonic encephalopathy – EME has a very early onset, usually neonatal, and electro-clinical features similar to EIEE. The differential diagnosis is based on the predominance in EME of myoclonic seizures (segmental and erratic, rarely massive). Tonic spasms, absent at onset, may be observed after 3 to 4 months of life (Aicardi & Ohtahara, 2005). The electroclinical pattern consists of suppression-bursts in awake and sleep states. The aetiology is usually unknown or secondary to metabolic disorders, such as non-ketotic hyperglycinaemia, D-glyceric acidaemia, methylmalonic acidaemia, proprionic acidaemia, hyperammonaemia caused by carbamyl phosphate synthetase defect, Menkes disease, pyridoxine and pyridoxal phosphate dependencies, and glutamate transporter defect (Aicardi & Ohtahara, 2005). Familial cases are frequent. No abnormalities have been detected on MRI, except atrophy observed during follow-up. The epileptic and neurocognitive developmental prognosis is very poor; half the patients die during the first year of life.

The two epileptic encephalopathies are distinct entities according to the ILAE, presenting with different clinical and aetiological features. Nevertheless, the suppression-burst pattern is a common feature. The pathophysiology of the suppression-burst pattern is not clear. The presence of a suppression-burst pattern in both types of epileptic encephalopathy – as in other conditions (such as molybdenum cofactor deficit or Menkes disease) in which epileptic features are not compatible with a diagnosis of EIEE or EME – suggests possible underlying extensive brain damage causing a functional disruption of the neural network. According to some investigators, the responsiveness of cortical and thalamic neurons to orthodromic volleys is dramatically reduced, suggesting that the pattern is caused by disconnections in brain circuits involved in the genesis of the EEG (Steriade et al., 1994). Such dysfunction can be transitory or persistent, according to the aetiology and the maturation process.

Malignant migrant partial seizures of infancy

Malignant migrant partial seizures in infancy is an epileptic encephalopathy described in 1995 by Coppola et al. and characterized by partial seizures with onset in the first 6 months of life; these later become subcontinuous, involving multiple and independent cortical areas (Coppola et al., 1995; Gérard et al., 1999). Seizures are intractable. Infants present with normal psychomotor development before seizure onset, but then severe neurodevelopmental deterioration appears. After the first observations of Coppola et al. in 1995, other investigators reported small series in European, Asian and American countries (Okuda et al., 2000; Wilmurshurt et al., 2000; Veneselli et al., 2001; Gross-Tsur et al., 2004; Marsh et al., 2005). At onset, seizure semeiology is characterized by motor and autonomic signs, lasting several minutes; later on it becomes polymorphic and progressively tends to be generalized. After the first year of life, seizures occur in clusters and become continuous for weeks. During follow-up, progressive microcephaly and psychomotor deterioration are observed, especially when there are subcontinuous seizures.

The interictal EEG is normal or with slow background activity at onset; later on, multifocal spikes and sleep abnormalities appear. The ictal EEG is characterized by monomorphic rhythmic theta or alpha activity, involving a localized cortical area with progressive spread. Before the end or immediately after the end of the discharge, a new independent ictal event starts.

The aetiology remains unknown. Historical, biochemical, radiological, neuropathological and genetic investigations are negative. The outcome is very poor, with a high mortality. Conventional antiepileptic drugs are ineffective. Some investigators have reported a positive effect of bromide (Okuda et al., 2000) or stiripentol and clonazepam in combination (Perez et al., 1999). Carbamazepine and vigabatrin may exacerbate the seizures (Dulac, 2005). A few cases have been reported with a slightly better outcome (Marsh et al., 2005), suggesting a wider clinical spectrum of this syndrome.

Infantile spasms and West syndrome

Infantile spasms are a type of seizure disorder that generally occurs during the first year of life and is resistant to antiepileptic drugs. The triad of psychomotor retardation or deterioration, infantile spasms, and hypsarrhythmia is defined as *West syndrome*, which can be regarded as synonymous with infantile spasms (West, 1841; Gastaut *et al.*, 1964; Duncan, 2001). In a consensus conference of experts of the so-called West Delphi group, West syndrome is considered to be a subset of the syndrome of infantile spasms characterized by clinical spasms occurring in clusters with onset during the first year of life (Lux & Osborne, 2004). The term 'epileptic spasms' refers to the seizure type, regardless of age and the clinical context in which they occur. They can thus be observed during the whole of childhood or more rarely in adulthood (Dulac *et al.*, 1994; Bednarek *et al.*, 1998).

The first description of West syndrome was in 1841, when West reported the experiences of his son. The estimated incidence is 2.9–4.5/10,000 live births (Lúthvígsson *et al.*, 1994; Riikonen, 1995; Trevathan *et al.*, 1999), with a slight predominance of males (male/female ratio, 1.4:1) (Brna *et al.*, 2001).

The onset of the classical triad occurs during the first year of life. The peak is between 3 and 9 months (Lacy & Penry, 1976), though a few cases with onset after the first year have been reported (Bednarek *et al.*, 1998).

Hypsarrhythmia

Hypsarrhthmia, first described by Gibbs and Gibbs in 1952, represents the typical but not the only *interictal EEG* pattern associated with infantile spasms. Hypsarrhythmia, observed mainly during the awake state (Fig. 3A), consists of high amplitude slow waves, up to 500 µV, and spikes and sharp waves occurring asynchronously and randomly in all regions (Dalla Bernardina *et al.*, 2007). During slow sleep, discharges of diffuse and synchronous polyspikes and waves separated by low voltage and disorganized tracing are observed (Fig. 3B). This pattern is usually known as a pseudo-periodic pattern. Sometimes it is also detected in the awake state in patients who do not show typical hypsarrhythmia. Usually, during REM sleep the paroxysmal EEG activities almost disappear (Kellaway *et al.*, 1983; Lombroso, 1983a). Patterns defined as modified hypsarrhythmia have been reported, with atypical aspects such as a predominance of slow waves with few spikes, synchronous bursts of generalized spike-waves, significant asymmetry or suppression-burst patterns (Gastaut *et al.*, 1964; Jeavons & Bower, 1974; De Jong *et al.*, 1976; Lombroso, 1983a; Hrachovy *et al.*, 1984; Aicardi & Ohtahara, 2005). Hypsarrhythmia tends to disappear in older children, though spasms persist.

Spasms

Spasms consist of sudden, generally bilateral muscle contraction of the neck, trunk and extremities, more often in flexion (flexion of the upper limbs and extension of lower limbs) than in extension or mixed, lasting 0.2 to 2 seconds. Spasms occur usually in clusters of 20 to 40 up to 100, with 1 to 10 clusters/day, usually at the time of awakening or precipitated by drowsiness, feeding and handling (Plouin *et al.*, 1987).

The EEG findings in relation to spasms are variable. The ictal EEG pattern (Fig. 4) is usually characterized by a high voltage diffuse slow wave transient, with an inverse phase reversal over the vertex region (Fusco & Vigevano, 1993), followed by a voltage attenuation. Fast activity (beta or alpha) is observed coinciding with clinical spasms lasting 2 to 5 seconds.

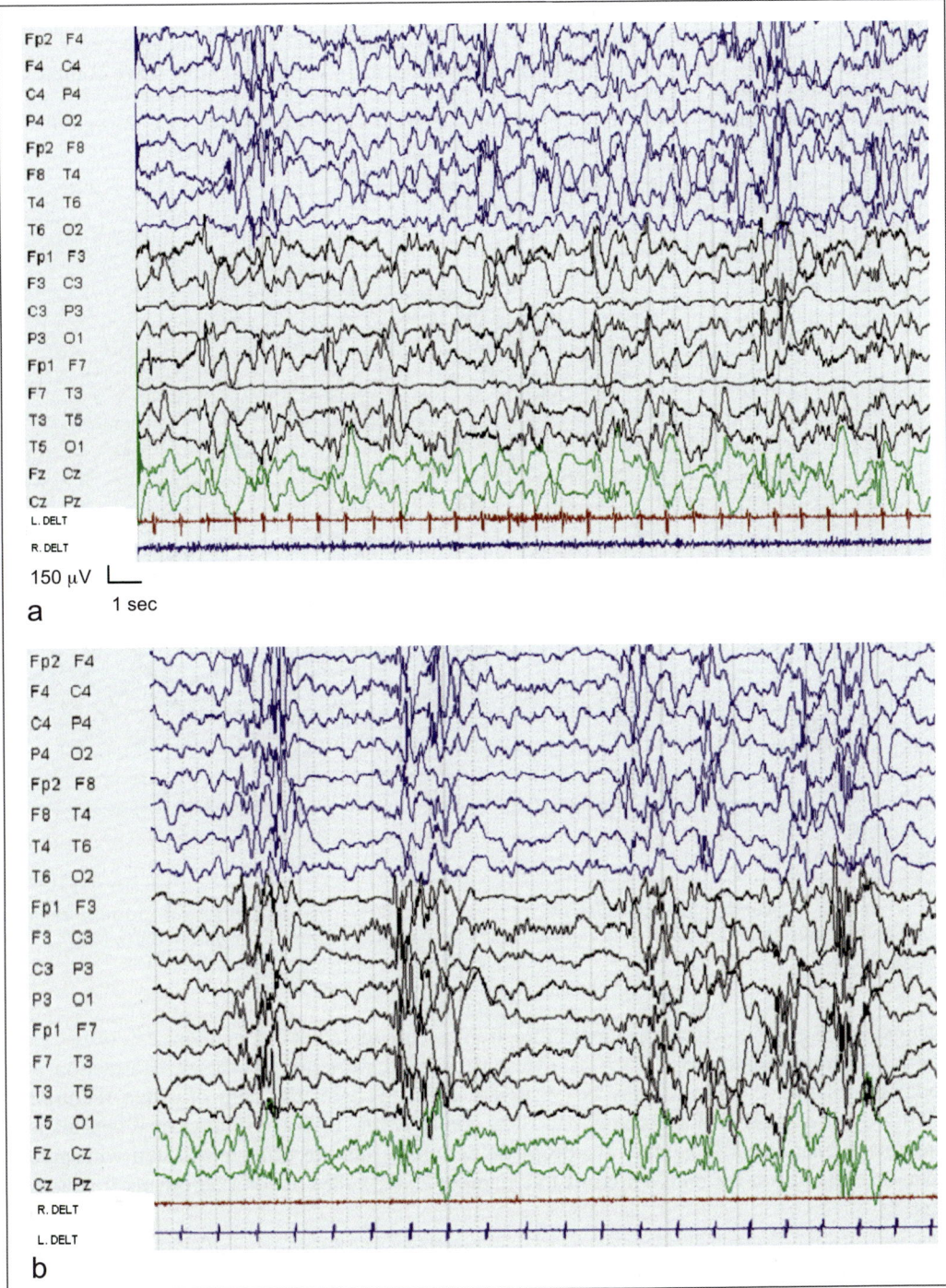

Fig. 3. EEG of a 5-month-old infant affected by cryptogenic West syndrome. (A) While awake: low background activity, repetitive multifocal spike-waves. (B) During sleep: pseudoperiodic, diffuse spike and spike-wave discharges. Spindles are evident on the left side.

A voltage attenuation (decremental discharge), with or without clinical signs, may also be detected (Gastaut *et al.*, 1964; Hrachovy *et al.*, 1984). Other ictal patterns include generalized slow wave transients, isolated fast rhythms, generalized sharp waves and slow wave complexes (Kellaway *et al.*, 1979).

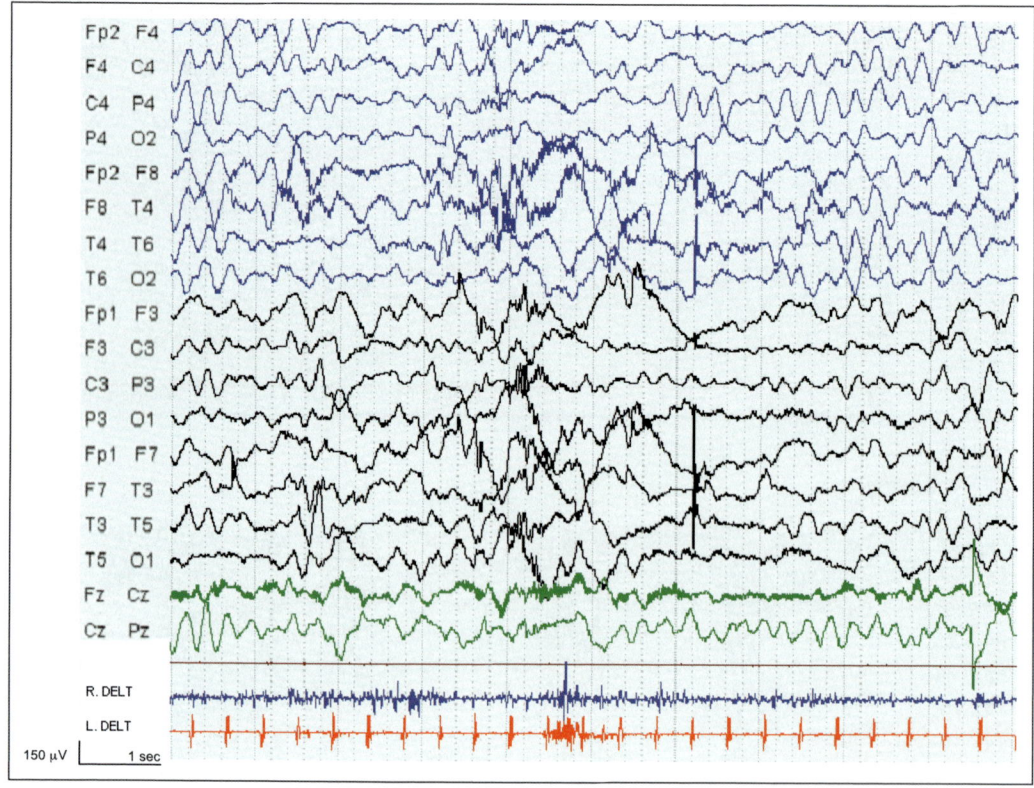

Fig. 4. EEG of a 5-month-old infant affected by cryptogenic West syndrome. Bilateral spasm is evident in the deltoid muscles, associated with diffuse slow waves with superimposed rapid activity.

Asymmetrical spasms with unilateral contraction or with an adversive element can occur. Lateralized motor phenomena – such as eye and or head deviation, eyebrow contraction and abduction of one shoulder – may be observed, generally with the help of video recordings (Kellaway *et al.*, 1979; Watanabe *et al.*, 1994; Gaily *et al.*, 1995). Asymmetrical spasms and lateralized phenomena indicate a symptomatic aetiology and are often associated with partial seizures occurring at the end of spasms (Yamamoto *et al.*, 1988) or soon before spasm clusters (Fig. 5).

Asymmetrical or unilateral spasms are associated with contralateral ictal paroxysms, usually homolateral to the side of the damage (Gaily *et al.*, 1995). The interpretation of spasm clusters, whether representing a single seizure or a series of individual seizures, remains controversial (Dalla Bernardina *et al.*, 2007). Dulac (2001) suggested that the disappearance of hypsarrhythmia during the cluster might indicate a symptomatic origin, whereas the resumption of hypsarrhythmia between single spasms suggests an idiopathic origin.

Chapter 10 Epilepsy in infancy

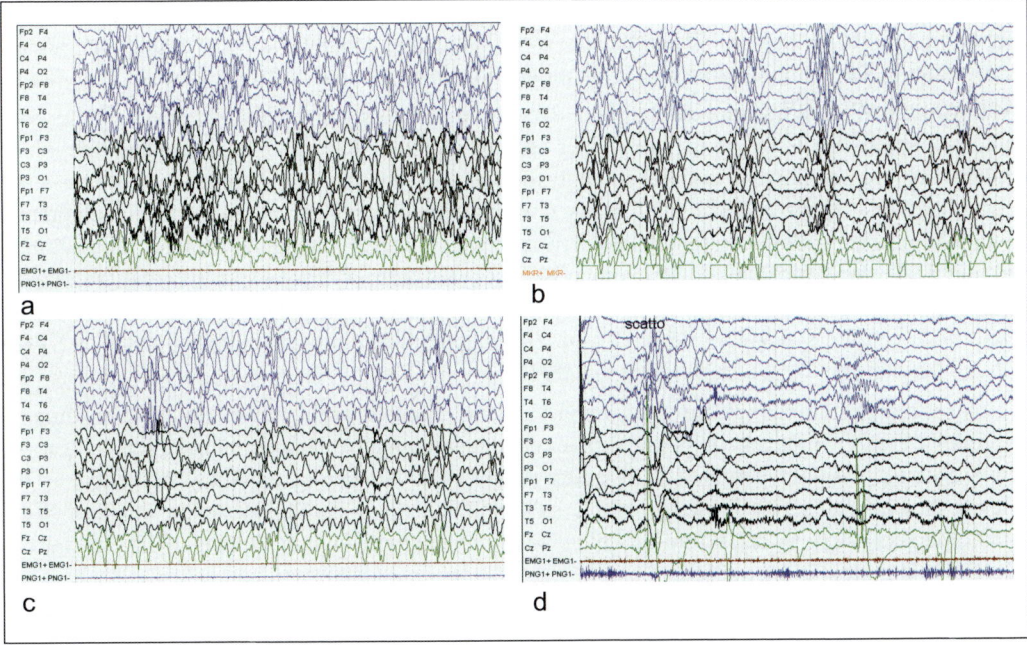

Fig. 5. EEG of a 5-month-old infant. (A) Awake hypsarrhythmic pattern with predominance of spikes on the posterior regions. (B) During sleep: pseudoperiodic diffuse bursts of spikes and waves, alternating with periods of lower theta-delta activity on the right. (C) Rhythmic spike-waves on the right posterior regions (electrical seizure). (D) Clusters of asymmetrical spasms, with eye deviation to the right, accompanied by focal rapid activity, localized on the temporal and posterior regions.

Developmental delay or deterioration

Psychomotor development before the spasm onset can be normal or delayed, possibly related to the aetiology. In the majority of patients (from 68 to 85 per cent) developmental retardation is present before the onset of infantile spasms, as reported by some investigators (Matsumoto, 1981; Kellaway et al., 1983). Although it is not easy to identify mild degrees of retardation retrospectively in apparently normal infants, a definite neurosensory and developmental regression seems to occur at the onset of spasms. Deterioration may also involve motor development, with loss of head control or reaching for and handling objects. Cognitive impairment and behavioural disorders, such as autistic withdrawals, may persist as long term sequelae (Chugani & Conti, 1996; Guzzetta et al., 2008).

Aetiology

The aetiology of West syndrome is heterogeneous. The ILAE classification (1989) recognizes the symptomatic and cryptogenic form, but there is no agreement about the definition of the two terms. Some authorities (Chevrie & Aicardi, 1971; Jeavons & Bower, 1974) consider West syndrome to be symptomatic when there is evidence of structural abnormalities in neuroimaging or of abnormal mental or neurological development before the onset of spasms. Others consider that infants with a definite predisposing aetiological factor are symptomatic (Matsumoto et al., 1981; Kellaway & Hrachovy, 1983). The distinction between the two aetiological groups,

255

however, may be important for its prognostic value. The prognosis in cryptogenic patients, including infants with possible idiopathic West syndrome and an excellent prognosis, seems better than in the symptomatic group (Plouin et al., 1987; Dulac, 2001).

Symptomatic West syndrome can be secondary to numerous causes. Neurocutaneous syndrome (tuberous sclerosis) is found in 7 to 27 per cent of patients. Aicardi syndrome, hemimegalencephaly, agyria-pachygyria, cortical focal dysplasia, and other brain malformations are possible causes of West syndrome detected using continuously improving neuroimaging techniques. Metabolic and neurodegenerative diseases (non-ketotic hyperglycinaemia, Menkes disease, pyridoxine deficiency, biotidinase deficiency, PEHO syndrome, X-linked spasms) may be associated with West syndrome (Guerrini et al., 2007). Possible genetic factors include chromosomal aberrations (Down syndrome, del 1p36) or single gene mutations (mutation of ARX or STK9 gene) (Scala et al., 2005; Guerrini et al., 2007).

Among the acquired causes, infectious and vascular diseases are common. West syndrome as a sequel of early injuries (hypoxic-ischaemic encephalopathy, haemorrhage, and so on) is observed in a variable percentage of cases (from 18 to 80 per cent) (Lacy & Penry, 1976; Aicardi & Chevrie, 1978; Battaglia et al., 1999b; Battaglia et al., 2005). A few cases of West syndrome secondary to brain tumours have been reported (Branch & Dyken, 1979; Mimaki et al., 1983; Ruggieri et al., 1989).

Treatment

West syndrome is usually refractory to common antiepileptic drugs. Early treatment seems to be correlated with a better prognosis (Gastaut et al., 1964; Lombroso et al., 1983b). The efficacy of therapy is often related to the underlying aetiology and neuropathological processes. Well controlled studies are very few, so many aspects of West syndrome treatment – such as the effective dosage, the duration of treatment, its effectiveness in the long term, especially concerning cognitive outcome – remain without an agreed solution.

ACTH is the most commonly used drug for West syndrome and is effective for short term treatment, but the optimum dosage and duration remain uncertain. Some studies have tried to compare the effectiveness of corticosteroid and ACTH therapy, but the schemes used are too variable to obtain uniform protocols or a definite cost/benefit evaluation in the two types of treatment (Hrachovy et al., 1979; Hrachovy et al., 1983; Glaze et al., 1988; Hrachovy et al., 1994; Baram et al., 1996).

In controlled studies vigabatrin seems effective for short term treatment, particularly in patients with tuberous sclerosis (Chiron et al., 1997; Vigevano & Cilio, 1997; Appleton et al., 1999; Lux et al., 2004). However, long term therapy is not recommended because of retinal toxicity and because of the difficulty in carrying out ophthalmological screening in infants.

According to published reports there is not enough evidence to recommend any other treatment for infantile spasms. Anecdotal use of most conventional drugs – such as benzodiazepines (Dreifuss et al., 1986; Silva et al., 2006), valproic acid (Pavone et al., 1981), lamotrigine (Veggiotti et al., 1994), topiramate (Glauser et al., 1998), levetiracetam (Lawlor & Devlin, 2005), zonisamide (Suzuki et al., 1997), or felbamate (Hosain et al., 1997) – does not give better results than steroids. Some investigators have proposed the use of pyridoxine before starting any other antiepileptic drugs (Blennow & Starck, 1986; Toribe, 2001), but without significant benefit. The results of ketogenic diet (Rubenstein et al., 2005) and palliative surgery (callosotomy, vagus nerve stimulation) (Wong et al., 2006) have been only anecdotal. Surgical treatment may be useful in resistant and selected cases secondary to localized cortical lesions (Chugani et al., 2007).

Prognosis

The prognosis is dependent on the aetiology and severity of the disease (Dulac & Tuxhorn, 2005). Idiopathic and cryptogenic West syndrome are considered to have a better prognosis than symptomatic West syndrome. In the group of idiopathic cases selected by strict criteria, there is a high percentage of children with an excellent outcome (Dulac *et al.*, 1986; Vigevano *et al.*, 1993; Guzzetta, 2007).

Irrespective of the aetiology, published reports suggest that about 60 per cent of children with West syndrome develop other types of epilepsy, such as Lennox-Gastaut syndrome or partial epilepsy (Dravet *et al.*, 1973; Riikonen, 1982). Half the patients have permanent motor disabilities and 60 to 70 per cent have severe cognitive deficits (Riikonen, 1996; Guzzetta, 2006). Psychiatric disorders and particularly autistic behaviour are reported in patients as sequelae of West syndrome (Riikonen, 1984; Chugani *et al.*, 1996). The risk of mortality has decreased in recent years to approximately 5 per cent. Death seems to be related to the aetiology and to the side effects of treatment, in particular steroid therapy.

Dravet syndrome

Severe myoclonic epilepsy, the first definition of Dravet syndrome, was described in 1978. In the ILAE classification (1989) it was included in the group of 'epilepsy undetermined if partial or generalized'. The newly proposed ILAE classification (Engel, 2001) included it in the group of 'epileptic encephalopathies'. After the finding of genetic mutation of SCN1A in several patients (Claes *et al.*, 2001, Dravet *et al.*, 2005), this severe epileptic syndrome now represents a model of epileptic channelopathy.

The prevalence of Dravet syndrome is not yet well established (Dravet & Bureau, 2005). In the few series of patients with seizure onset before the age of 3, from 7 to 8.2 per cent of cases had Dravet syndrome (Dravet & Bureau, 2005). A predominance in males has been reported, with a ratio of 2:1 (Hurst, 1990; Yakoub *et al.*, 1992).

The onset is generally during the first year of life, with febrile or non-febrile prolonged unilateral or generalized convulsive seizures occurring in otherwise normal infants.

Clinical features can be subdivided into three subsequent phases (Dravet *et al.*, 1992; Dravet & Bureau, 2005). During the first phase (in the first year of life) infants have prolonged clonic or tonic-clonic or clonic-tonic-clonic unilateral or generalized seizures, often precipitated by fever, with involvement of both sides simultaneously or alternately in some patients. In this period they may often be indistinguishable from febrile seizures, but the long seizure duration, the age of onset and the recurrence can suggest the diagnosis of Dravet syndrome. The second stage, the so-called catastrophic stage, encompasses the period from 1 to 5 years. During the second and third year of life, other seizure types appear including atypical absences, partial seizures, and epileptic and non-epileptic myoclonus (Fig. 6A and 6B). Seizures continue to be precipitated by fever and, in about 25 per cent of children, photosensitivity to intermittent light and to visual patterns appears (Fig. 6C). Status epilepticus can occur. During this phase, developmental delay, neurological signs and behavioural disorders can be observed progressively, particularly language deficit, ataxia, and hyperkinesia. The third phase (stabilization stage) usually starts at around 4–5 years. Clinical conditions generally improve: atypical absences, myoclonic seizures and partial seizures may decrease or sometimes disappear, though clonic or tonic-clonic seizures persist, usually occurring during sleep. Cognitive abilities may slowly improve.

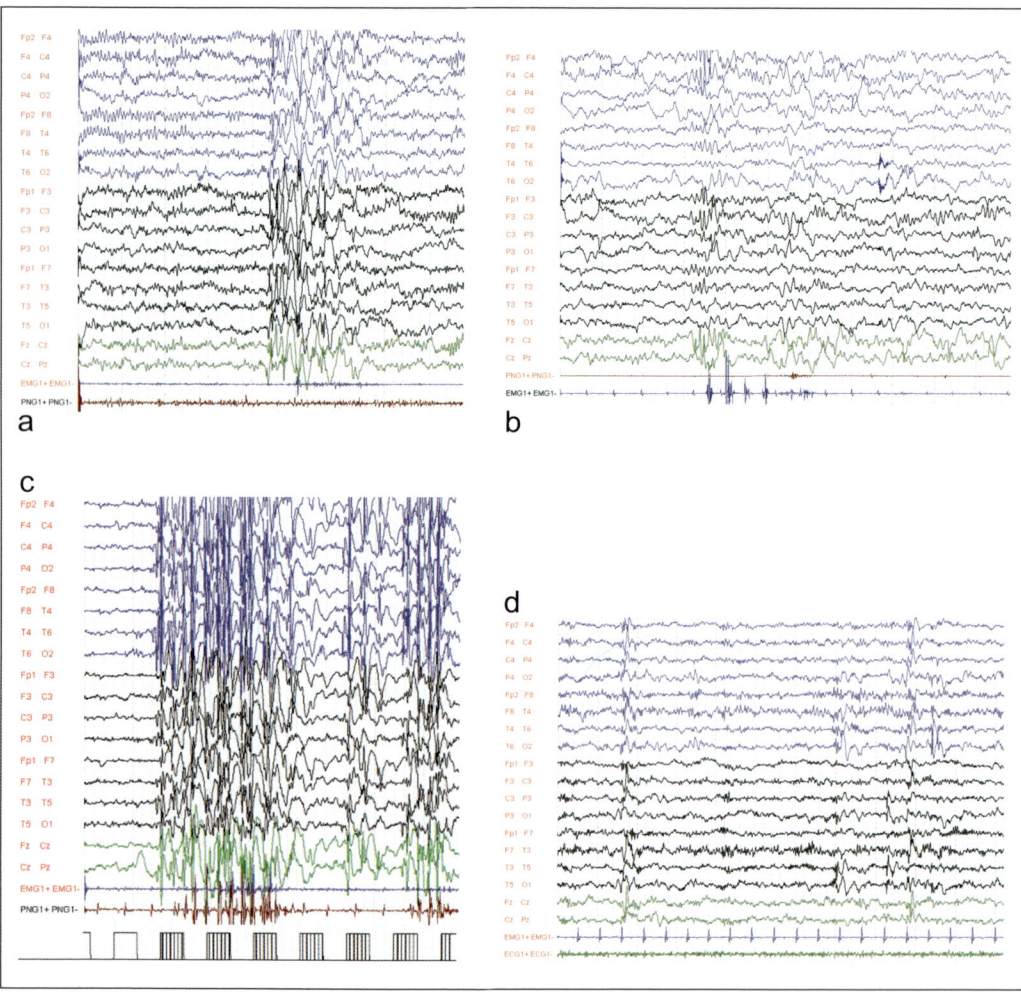

Fig. 6. Dravet syndrome. (A) Sleep EEG of a 2-year-old infant: diffuse discharge of irregular spike-waves, associated with an isolated myoclonia on the left deltoid. (B) same infant with non-epileptic rhythmic myoclonias of the left deltoid. (C) 20-month-old infant: diffuse discharges of irregular spike-waves and polyspikes during intermittent photo-stimulation at 20 Hz, associated with rhythmic myoclonias of the deltoid muscles. (D) 18-month-old infant: multifocal spikes and spike-waves during sleep.

The interictal EEG is normal at onset or during the first period; later on, paroxysmal activities such as focal or multifocal spikes or generalized irregular spike-waves appear (Fig. 6D).

The fever sensitivity suggests a mutation in the SCN1A gene (Claes et al., 2001). This mutation was previously described in families with febrile seizures + (FS+) (Scheffer & Berkovic, 1997). Thus, some investigators propose that Dravet syndrome is the most severe form of a broad spectrum of FS+ epilepsy (Singh et al., 2001). The SCN1A mutation was found in 60 to 70 per cent of patients with Dravet syndrome (Marini et al., 2007). Different types of SCN1A mutations and different involvements of the gene were reported (Marini et al., 2007). Recently, in almost 10 per cent of patients a complete deletion of the gene or rarely a duplication was found (Madia et al., 2006; Mulley et al., 2006). Parental mosaicism was identified in inherited cases (Depienne et al., 2006; Marini et al., 2006).

The *outcome* is generally poor. The seizures are resistant to antiepileptic drugs; developmental delay and behavioural disorders are present in almost all cases (Cassé-Perrot et al., 2001; Wolff et al., 2006; Caraballo & Fejerman, 2006). Neurological impairment is also observed, characterized by clumsiness and ataxia. Mortality is high (15.9 per cent in Dravet's series (Dravet & Bureau, 1992; Dravet & Bureau, 2005), mainly as a result of sudden death or accidents.

Some investigators describe a so-called borderline form of severe myoclonic epilepsy characterized by a lack of myoclonias and atypical absences and by a less severe outcome (Oguni et al., 2001a). Genetic studies show that the borderline severe myoclonic epilepsy is also largely due to SCN1A mutations (Fukuma et al., 2004; Kanai et al., 2004). As there are variable results of genetic studies and different clinical pictures, questions about phenotype-genotype correlations arise, such as: is Dravet syndrome a single disease with different forms reflecting different mutation types, or is it a part of a large spectrum of channelopathies including other myoclonic and non-myoclonic epilepsies? Further studies are needed to answer these questions.

Treatment

Usually, Dravet syndrome is refractory to antiepileptic drugs. Phenobarbital, valproate and benzodiazepines may be useful in reducing the frequency and duration of convulsive seizures (Dravet et al., 2005). A prospective randomized trial proved the efficacy of a combination of stiripentol, valproic acid and clobazam in reducing the episodes of status epilepticus (Chiron et al., 2000). Certain of the new antiepileptic drugs have shown relative efficacy, including topiramate, possibly levetiracetam, and recently zonisamide. Bromide (Oguni et al., 1994) and a ketogenic diet (Caraballo et al., 2005) seem also to be beneficial, but available data are scanty. In contrast, lamotrigine, carbamazepine and phenytoin usually cause seizure exacerbation (Guerrini et al., 1998; Dravet et al., 2005).

Generalized epilepsy with febrile seizures plus (GEFS+)

This entity was first described by Scheffer and Barkovich (Scheffer & Barkovich, 1997). It was characterized by the association of generalized febrile seizures beyond the age of 6 years and afebrile generalized convulsions, with a positive family history of epilepsy with variable phenotypes and a benign evolution in the majority of cases. The investigators reported a large multigenerational family with 25 affected members, presenting with febrile seizures and generalized epilepsy. The more frequent phenotype was an expansion of febrile seizures (FS+), usually with multiple recurrences consisting of febrile seizures persisting after 6 years of age and often associated with afebrile generalized seizures. In six family members, absences, myoclonic seizures or atonic seizures were also observed. The type of transmission suggested an autosomal dominant inheritance. A mutation in the SCN1B gene codifying for a β subunit of the sodium channel, located on chromosome 19q13.1 was identified in the first family described. To explain the phenotypic variability, the investigators suggested that there was a single major gene defect, with possible additive gene effects. Later on, in other families with GEFS+ different mutations were identified in SCN1A (Escayg et al., 2000), in GABRG2 (Baulac et al., 2001, Harkin et al., 2002) and in SCN1B genes (Bonanni et al., 2004). These genetic findings underline the complexity of the disorder and the difficulty in defining the relationship between genotype and phenotype.

Benign myoclonic epilepsy in infancy

The syndrome of benign myoclonic epilepsy in infancy (BMEI) was described in 1981 (Dravet & Bureau, 1981). It was defined as 'the occurrence of myoclonic seizures without other seizure types except rare simple febrile seizures', in normal infants of the first 3 years of life. The epileptic and cognitive prognosis was favourable. BMEI was classified among generalized idiopathic epilepsies in the 1989 International Classification (1989). Many other cases have now been published (Dravet & Bureau, 2005).

BMEI is a rare epileptic syndrome. The few *epidemiological data* suggest that it represents fewer than 1 per cent of all epilepsies (Dravet & Bureau, 2005), and 1.3 to 1.72 per cent of epilepsies with onset in the first year of life (Caraballo et al., 1997; Sarisjulis et al., 2000). It is predominant in males, with a male/female ratio of approximately 2:1 (Dravet & Bureau, 2005).

The genetics remain unknown. Although a family history of epilepsy or febrile convulsions is present in 50 per cent of cases, no family case of BMEI has been reported so far.

Clinical and EEG features

The age of onset is between 4 months and 3 years. Seizures consist of brief myoclonic jerks involving the axis of the body and upper limbs, rarely the lower limbs; they are facilitated by drowsiness, usually disappearing during sleep. In some cases activation by photic stimulation or sudden external stimuli such as sudden noise or sudden contact was reported (Dravet & Bureau, 2005). The duration is very brief (1–3 seconds), although there are cases with pseudo-rhythmically repeated jerks lasting no more than 5–10 seconds. Interictal EEG during awake and sleep states is normal. Rarely, generalized spike-wave discharges have been observed during REM sleep. The ictal EEG is characterized by fast generalized spike-wave or polyspike-wave discharges (Darra et al., 2006). Myoclonias are always associated with these discharges. Neuroradiological investigations show no abnormalities.

The *outcome* seems to depend on early diagnosis and treatment. Overall, 93.8 per cent of patients became seizure-free in the first 3 years of life (Dravet & Bureau, 2005). Seizure control is obtained with valproic acid. Other antiepileptic drugs used in a few patients are phenobarbital, ethosuximide and clonazepam, but valproic acid remains the drug of first choice. In rarely reported untreated patients, no other seizure types were observed during the follow-up: patients continue to experience myoclonic jerks and this may lead to a delay in psychomotor development and to behavioural disorders.

Long term outcome shows the disappearance of myoclonic seizures in all cases and 16 per cent of patients experience generalized tonic-clonic seizures during adolescence. Developmental and behavioural outcome is generally good (Dravet & Bureau, 2002; Auvin et al., 2006). Mild developmental delay was reported in 11.4 per cent of cases (Dravet & Bureau, 2005), partially interpreted as an effect of a delay in diagnosis and treatment. It is, however, possible that the abnormal biological process, the cause of the myoclonic attacks, also interferes with development when it occurs in a very immature brain.

Myoclonic astatic epilepsy

The first description of the syndrome was by Doose in 1970, using the term 'myoclonic astatic petit mal',which was changed to 'myoclonic astatic epilepsy' (MAE) later on (Doose et al., 1970). Doose considered MAE as a primary generalized epilepsy characterized by myoclonic attacks involving axial muscles or astatic seizures or both. From the first description the hypothesis of a genetic background was suggested by the absence of brain damage, peculiar EEG traits (a preponderance of generalized fast spike-waves or polyspike-waves) and a frequently positive family history.

Epidemiological data are difficult to collect owing to different classification systems adopted by various investigators. Males are more affected than females

Electroclinical features

The onset occurs in a wide range of ages (7 months up to 8 years), mostly between 2 and 6 years. Before the onset, the majority of patients have normal psychomotor development. Seizures consist of generalized jerks or astatic falls, with a high daily frequency. Polygraphic studies show an initial myoclonic component followed by an atonic phase (Oguni *et al.*, 2002), although purely atonic as well as myoclonic seizures are possible (Oguni *et al.*, 1993; Dravet *et al.*, 1997). In particular, the myoclonic-atonic seizures consist of brief axial symmetrical and massive myoclonias involving the neck, shoulders, arms, and legs, with head nodding or falling down. Myoclonias are generally followed by a loss of muscle tone (Guerrini *et al.*, 2005). The duration of each seizure is brief (2–3 seconds). The interictal EEG is characterized by bilateral, synchronous, irregular spike-wave discharges at 2–3 Hz and parietal rhythmic theta activity independent of the state of vigilance (Fig. 7A). The ictal EEG shows generalized and synchronous EEG discharges with jerks suggesting a primary generalized myoclonic attack (Fig. 7B); atonic seizures (Fig. 7C) may be associated with myoclonic jerks. This myoclonia is different from that seen in Lennox-Gastaut syndrome (Bonanni *et al.*, 2002; Guerrini *et al.*, 2002), in which an interhemispheric latency paralleling myoclonic jerks suggests a secondary generalization of focal myoclonic activity.

In MAE other types of seizure are often observed, including generalized tonic-clonic seizures, atypical absences (Fig. 7D) and non-convulsive status (Neubauer *et al.*, 2005). The non-convulsive status is very common, lasting for hours, days or weeks. It is characterized by a fluctuating blurring of consciousness and an erratic perioral and distal muscle twitching and brief head nods, caused by atonia or myoclonic jerks (Guerrini *et al.*, 2005). The EEG is characterized

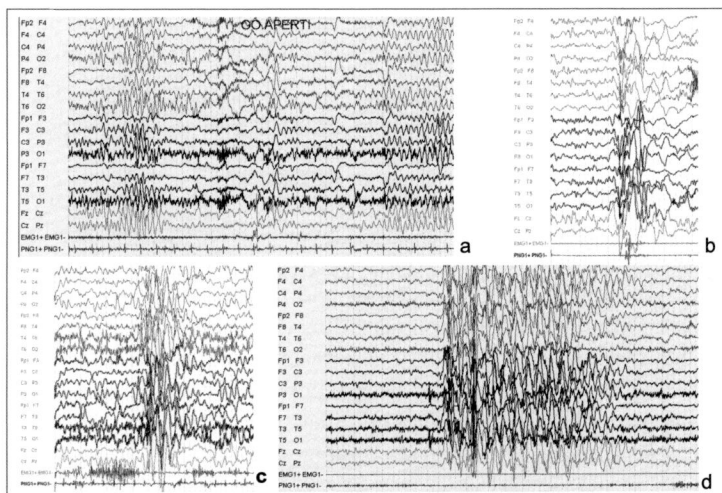

Fig. 7. Doose syndrome. (A) 2-year-old infant, while awake: theta activity at 5–6 Hz on the centroparietal regions and vertex. (B) 22-month-old infant: myoclonic jerks on the deltoids time-locked to diffuse polyspikes waves. (C) Axial atonic seizure associated with diffuse irregular spike-waves. (D) 2-year-old infant: atypical absence characterized by generalized irregular polyspikes and spike-waves followed by slow waves on the central regions.

by long runs of slow waves and spike-wave complexes, often associated with sequences of slow waves. Sometimes the EEG shows polymorphous paroxysmal activity simulating an hypsarrhythmic pattern (Guerrini et al., 2005). According to some investigators, such episodes can suggest a poor cognitive prognosis (Kaminska et al., 1999). Tonic seizures are generally absent in MAE (Oguni et al., 2002), even though some consider them very common and a sign of poor prognosis (Kaminska et al., 1999) as a sort of transition to Lennox-Gastaut syndrome.

A family history of seizures or EEG abnormalities was reported in up to 80 per cent of cases (Doose et al., 1970), suggesting a genetic origin. A genetic origin was shown in a particular family with GEFS+, in which MAE cases had missense mutations of SCN1A and GABRG2 genes (Meisler et al., 2001). However, very few cases of MAE have been reported in families with mutations for GEFS+, and in a study including 22 patients with MAE no mutation at all of the GEFS+ genes (SCN1A, SCN1B and GABRG2) was found (Nabbout et al., 2003). The genetics of MAE seem to be very complex and there is no evidence of a possible link between the genetic background and the type of outcome.

The outcome in MAE is variable. Most patients have a good outcome both for epilepsy and for development, with seizure control within 1 to 3 years, but a minority develops myoclonic status and severe cognitive deficit (Doose, 1992; Kaminska et al., 1999; Oguni et al., 2002). Highly effective antiepileptic drugs are valproate, ethosuximide, and benzodiazepines; in some cases with very frequent seizures, steroids are also indicated. The combination of valproate with lamotrigine appears also to be effective (Dulac & Kaminska, 1997). On the other hand, phenytoin, carbamazepine and vigabatrin cause seizure exacerbation (Guerrini et al., 2002). In patients resistant to antiepileptic drugs a trial with steroids is indicated (Oguni et al., 2005). Good results are obtained with the ketogenic diet, so that some authorities suggest starting such a diet as soon as possible and giving steroid treatment later, if the diet is ineffective or not tolerated (Oguni et al., 2001b; Caraballo et al., 2006).

Myoclonic status in non-progressive encephalopathies

Myoclonic status in non-progressive encephalopathies, considered a syndrome in the new ILAE diagnostic scheme, consists of recurrent episodes of prolonged and erratic atypical myoclonic absence status epilepticus. It was first described by Dalla Bernardina (Dalla Bernardina et al., 1992).

Range of onset age is from 3 months to 5 years, with a peak at 12 months. The prevalence and incidence are unknown. In selected populations of children with severe epilepsy, the incidence is 0.5–1 per cent, with a predominance of females.

Infants present with fixed encephalopathy (cerebral palsy), characterized by severe neurological deficits (axial hypotonia, ataxia, or dystonic-dyskinetic syndrome) and developmental impairment predating the onset of the epilepsy. Seizures consist of repetitive atypical absences and myoclonic jerks. Myoclonic jerks, asynchronous and erratic, involving the eyelids, face and limbs, are sometimes rhythmic and synchronous during absences. Sometimes they are very subtle or subclinical so that the infant appears only hyporeactive and ataxic. Negative myoclonus or mixed positive and negative myoclonus has been reported. Myoclonic status may be present at the onset of the epilepsy or may be preceded by other seizures such as focal motor, myoclonic absences or rarely generalized or unilateral clonic seizures. Tonic seizures are not reported.

The EEG is characterized by poorly reactive slow waves with mixed paroxysmal activity. The ictal EEG shows brief bursts of diffuse slow spike and waves associated with bilateral, more or less rhythmic myoclonias. During drowsiness and at the start of slow sleep, paroxysmal activity becomes continuous, followed during slow sleep by a decrease in myoclonia that reappears later on during REM sleep and arousal.

In the series by Dalla Bernardina *et al.* (2005), the aetiology included genetic causes in 47 per cent of patients (Angelman syndrome, Wolf syndrome, Rett syndrome and Prader Willi syndrome), fetal/neonatal anoxic injury in 15.6 per cent, and unknown causes in 37 per cent, among which there was a subgroup with cortical dysplasia on neuroimaging, probably genetic in origin.

In his series Dalla Bernardina (2005) described three electroclinical patterns with different diagnostic and prognostic implications. The first is characterized by a combination of absences, arrhythmic and rhythmic subcontinuous jerks, mainly positive, brief myoclonic absences and hypnagogic startles. This pattern is usually observed in Angelmann syndrome. The second consists of absence status and continuous rhythmic myoclonus, mainly negative, combined with continuous dyskinetic movements inducing a peculiar 'hyperkinetic motor inhibition'. This condition is usually associated with cortical malformations and is refractory to treatment. The third is characterized by a continuous spike activity over the rolandic regions persisting throughout life, associated with bilateral rhythmic myoclonia, and eventually by inhibitory phenomena with consequent motor deterioration. It corresponds to a form of progressive myoclonic epilepsy in the absence of a progressive disease. These cases are often produced by cortical dysplasia in the motor area. Treatment usually consists of benzodiazepines, valproic acid and ethosuximide. ACTH or steroids can be useful.

Diagnosis is important in order that adequate treatment can be started promptly, to limit developmental deterioration and to ensure that possible progressive diseases are excluded.

Syndromes with partial seizures of idiopathic origin

Benign familial/non-familial infantile seizures

This condition includes several electroclinical pictures reported in the last decades and not considered in the ILAE classification of 1989. The principal characteristics are the presence of partial seizures with onset in the first year of life in otherwise normal infants, and a genetic substrate. The most important forms are as follows: benign familial infantile convulsions (Vigevano *et al.*, 1992); benign partial epilepsy of infancy (Watanabe *et al.*, 1987; Watanabe *et al.*, 1990; Watanabe *et al.*, 1993); familial infantile convulsions and choreoathetosis (Szepetowski *et al.*, 1997); and benign infantile focal epilepsy with midline spikes and waves during sleep (Bureau & Maton, 1998; Bureau & Maton, 2002; Capovilla & Beccaria, 2000).

Clinical and EEG features

The various types of benign infantile convulsions have in common some clinical elements: partial seizures occurring in clusters, with onset during the first year of life, rarely in the second year, apparent absence of aetiological factors, normal psychomotor development, and a favourable outcome (Vigevano & Bureau, 2005).

In the *benign familial infantile convulsions* (BFIC) the onset of seizures occurs between 3 and 6 months. They are brief, organized in clusters of maximum 8 to 10 seizures which do not reach true status epilepticus. Infants have motor arrest with staring, impairment of consciousness and convulsive movements. The interictal EEG is normal. The ictal EEG, according to Vigevano *et al.*, (1992), is characterized by focal recruiting rhythms in the parieto-occipital area, spreading over the hemispheres and involving the entire brain (Fig. 8). It is possible to observe a hemispheric alternating pattern on both sides of the brain. The *benign partial epilepsy of infancy* described by Watanabe *et al.* (1987) shows similar clinical features except for the presence of limb or oral and facial automatisms in the cases reported as 'benign partial epilepsy of infancy with complex partial seizures' (Watanabe *et al.*, 1990). Prompt seizure generalization with tonic-clonic manifestations is described in 'benign partial epilepsy of infancy with secondary generalization' (Watanabe *et al.*, 1993).

Epileptic and developmental outcome in this type of epilepsy is good. In untreated cases, symptoms may be confined to isolated clusters before the end of the first year (Vigevano & Bureau, 2005). The antiepileptic drugs generally used are carbamazepine, phenobarbital and valproic acid. Because of the recurrence of seizures and the impossibility of confirming the diagnosis at the ontset, treatment is usually indicated, except in familial cases in which no continuative antiepileptic drug treatment may be advised.

In the form reported by Vigevano *et al.* (1992), the familial occurrence with first and second relatives affected by similar seizures suggests a transmission with autosomal dominant inheritance. A mutation of a locus on chromosome 19q12-q13.11 was identified in some patients (Guipponi *et al.*, 1997), but not in all (Gennaro *et al.*, 1999). Recently, a mutation at a different locus (2q24) codifying for the SCNA2 gene was reported (Striano *et al.*, 2006). Heron *et al.*, in 2002, had observed two families with seizure onset between 1 and 3 months of age and electroclinical manifestations similar to those in BIFC, associated with a mutation of the gene for subunit 2 of the sodium channel (SCN2A). A new entity called 'benign neonatal-infantile familial seizures' (BNIFC), considered an intermediate form between benign neonatal familial convulsions (BNFC) with only neonatal seizures (Rett & Teubel, 1964) and BIFC was thus proposed. Later on, Berkovic *et al.*, (2004) reported six families with the same mutation and with the seizure onset between 2 and 7 months. Therefore, it is difficult to define the new entity exclusively on the basis of the onset age of seizures.

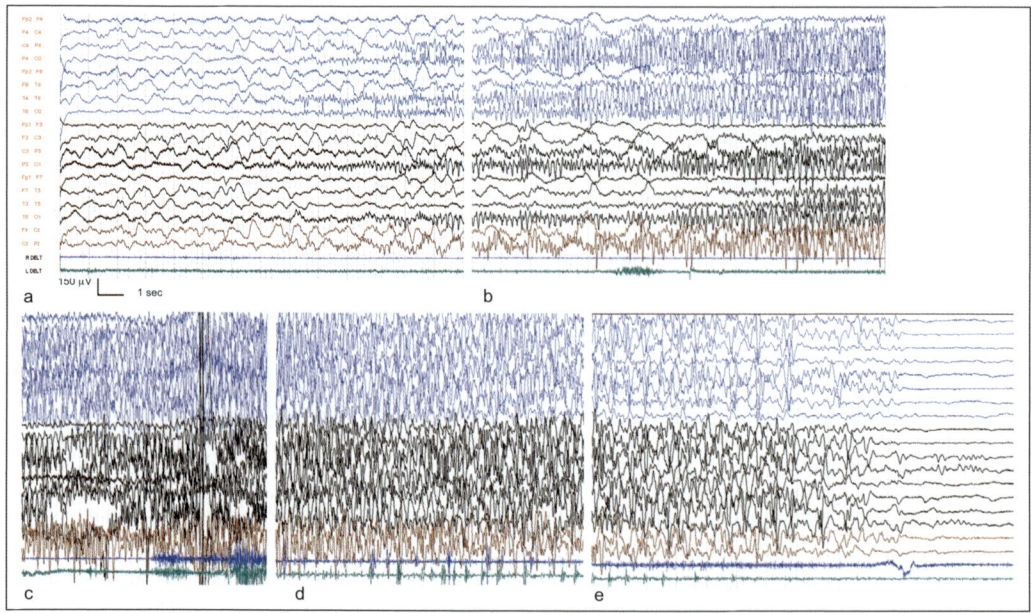

Fig. 8. *Four-month-old infant with benign familial infantile convulsions: ictal EEG of a seizure occurring during sleep, showing a recruiting rhythm with onset on the right occipital regions, spreading to the left occipital region (A, B) and then to the entire brain (C, D). The end of the discharge was asynchronous between the two sides (E). The seizure was characterized by staring, eye deviation to the left, left arm hypertonus and flexion followed by diffuse hypertonia, followed after 10 seconds by asynchronous limb jerks.*

In 1997, Szepetowski reported a family with electroclinical manifestation similar to BIFC followed by paroxysmal choreoathetosis. Movement disorders consisting of choreoathetosis or dystonia at rest or induced by anxiety or exertion may appear during infancy. In this form, there was a linkage in chromosome 16p12-q12 in four French families (Szepetowski et al., 1997) and in one Chinese family (Lee et al., 1998).

In 1998, 'benign infantile focal epilepsy with midline spikes and waves during sleep', described by Bureau & Maton (1998) and later confirmed by Capovilla & Beccaria (2000), was included in the context of the partial seizures of idiopathic origin in infancy. This condition presents characteristics similar to the other forms of the same group, so that there is some doubt as to whether it is really an entity distinct from the benign partial epilepsy of infancy reported by Watanabe (Arzimanoglou et al., 2004). However, clinical manifestations present some peculiarities: seizures are not in clusters but isolated, the mean age at onset is 9.9 months (range 1 to 20 months), secondary generalization is uncommon, and the interictal EEG during sleep shows low voltage spikes, followed or not by a slow wave localized over the fronto-central region or the vertex of one or both hemispheres. The outcome is good: seizures disappear with or without treatment at 3 to 4 years of age. These cases are sporadic; a positive history of febrile convulsions is reported, but no gene mutations have been identified so far.

All these findings suggest that several idiopathic syndromes of benign partial seizures exist in infancy. Some of them have been genetically identified, and they have a strong genetic heterogeneity.

Non-idiopathic focal (partial) epilepsy

Non-idiopathic focal epilepsy in infancy is rare according to some investigators (Oller-Dorella & Oller, 1989), probably because it is not easy to define seizures as focal at this early age. The identification of focal signs clinically using an interictal EEG is not easy. In the last decade, however, the widespread use of ictal video-EEG has resulted in an improved ability to define ictal semeiology in infancy.

The incidence reported in the few series examining early onset epilepsy varies between 12 and 28 per cent (Okumura et al., 1996; Caraballo et al., 1997; Kramer, 1999, Battaglia et al., 1999b). The symptomatic form is more frequent than the cryptogenic form.

Aetiology

The most frequent cause of non-idiopathic focal epilepsy with early onset is focal cortical dysplasia. The exact identification of the lesion on neuroimaging is very important, in order to evaluate surgical options in a form of epilepsy that is often resistant to antiepileptic drugs. Several other causes have been reported although less frequently, including different types of abnormal cortical development, low grade tumours, neurocutaneous syndrome, prenatal or perinatal hypoxic ischaemic injury, metabolic diseases, and so on.

Electroclinical semeiology

The seizure semeiology of early onset non-idiopathic focal epilepsy has only rarely been reported (Duchowny, 1987; Luna et al., 1989; Acharya et al., 1997; Rathgeb et al., 1998; Lortie et al., 2002). Seizures are usually characterized by behavioural arrest and are lateralized or bilateral motor phenomena (tonic posturing, sometimes clonic); rarely, facial or oral automatism

(Duchowny et al., 1987) and vegetative signs (flushing, mydriasis, pallor, apnoea, tachypnoea) are also observed. The seizure semeiology may depend on the localization of the ictal EEG or of the lesion on neuroimaging. Seizures arising from the temporo-parietal or parieto-occipital regions are hypomotor seizures, whereas those arising from frontal or fronto-central areas presents localized or generalized motor phenomena (clonic, atonic, or tonic) (Acharya et al., 1997; Battaglia et al., 2007). A posterior location may be associated with abnormal eye movements, whereas the localization to the central regions can produce partial clonic activity and in frontal regions, tonic posturing seizures (Rathgeb et al., 1998; Lortie et al., 2002).

During infancy, is not rare to observe epileptic spasms, usually asymmetrical, isolated or associated with partial seizures. The association of partial seizures with asymmetrical spasms is not uncommon, particularly in epilepsy secondary to cortical dysplasia (Watanabe et al., 1994). Usually, in several forms of epilepsy of early onset an age-dependent change in seizure semeiology occurs. However, Watanabe et al. (2005) reported no change of semeiology in 80 per cent of 183 children with focal symptomatic epilepsy with onset before the age of 6. In a few patients focal epilepsy is followed by West syndrome or undetermined epilepsy with focal and generalized seizures. These cases are considered affected by a focal epilepsy with transient generalized seizures. Some investigators suggest that epileptic spasms could be considered an unusual type of partial seizures. Although in the 1981 ILAE Seizure Classification, epileptic spasms belong to the group of generalized seizures, frequently in infants with focal lesions there are asymmetrical spasms or spasms with focal elements. However, infantile spasms, as the first manifestation or during the course of partial epilepsy, have been reported in the context of partial epilepsy by several investigators (Dravet et al., 1989; Ohtsuka et al., 2000; Fogarasi et al., 2001; Lortie et al., 2002; Pachatz et al., 2003; D'Agostino et al., 2004). Spasms may follow partial seizures and rarely precede them; the association with a hypsarrhythmic pattern is not constant.

These findings are relevant for surgical management in cases resistant to medical treatment. The recent surgical results suggest that the presence of epileptic spasms associated with partial seizures is not a contraindication to surgery (Asano et al., 2001; Jonas et al., 2005).

EEG features

The interictal EEG is not usually characterized by a specific pattern. Background activity with localized slow waves may possibly be coincident with the lesion. Paroxysmal activity, such as focal or multifocal spikes or spike-waves, is not always of diagnostic significance, in particular during early infancy. However, frequent paroxysmal discharges including high amplitude spikes and spike-waves may occur (Fig. 9), with changes with age towards a hypsarrhythmic pattern (Tagawa et al,. 1996). Dalla Bernardina et al. (1996) observed an unusual fast activity in patients with focal or bilateral dysplasia. Similar rapid activity, rarely appearing early in life and sometimes evident only during sleep, was also reported by Bureau et al. (1996).

The ictal EEG is not specific; in infancy it is sometimes associated with epileptic spasms, and often shows focal paroxysmal discharges such as semi-rhythmic theta/delta activity followed by slow sharp waves (Fig. 10).

Outcome

Published data suggest that the earlier the onset, the more severe the prognosis (Arzimanoglou et al,. 2004; Watanabe et al., 2005). Symptomatic aetiology, seizures with early onset, polymorphic seizure types or complex partial seizures, and high frequency seizures at onset are

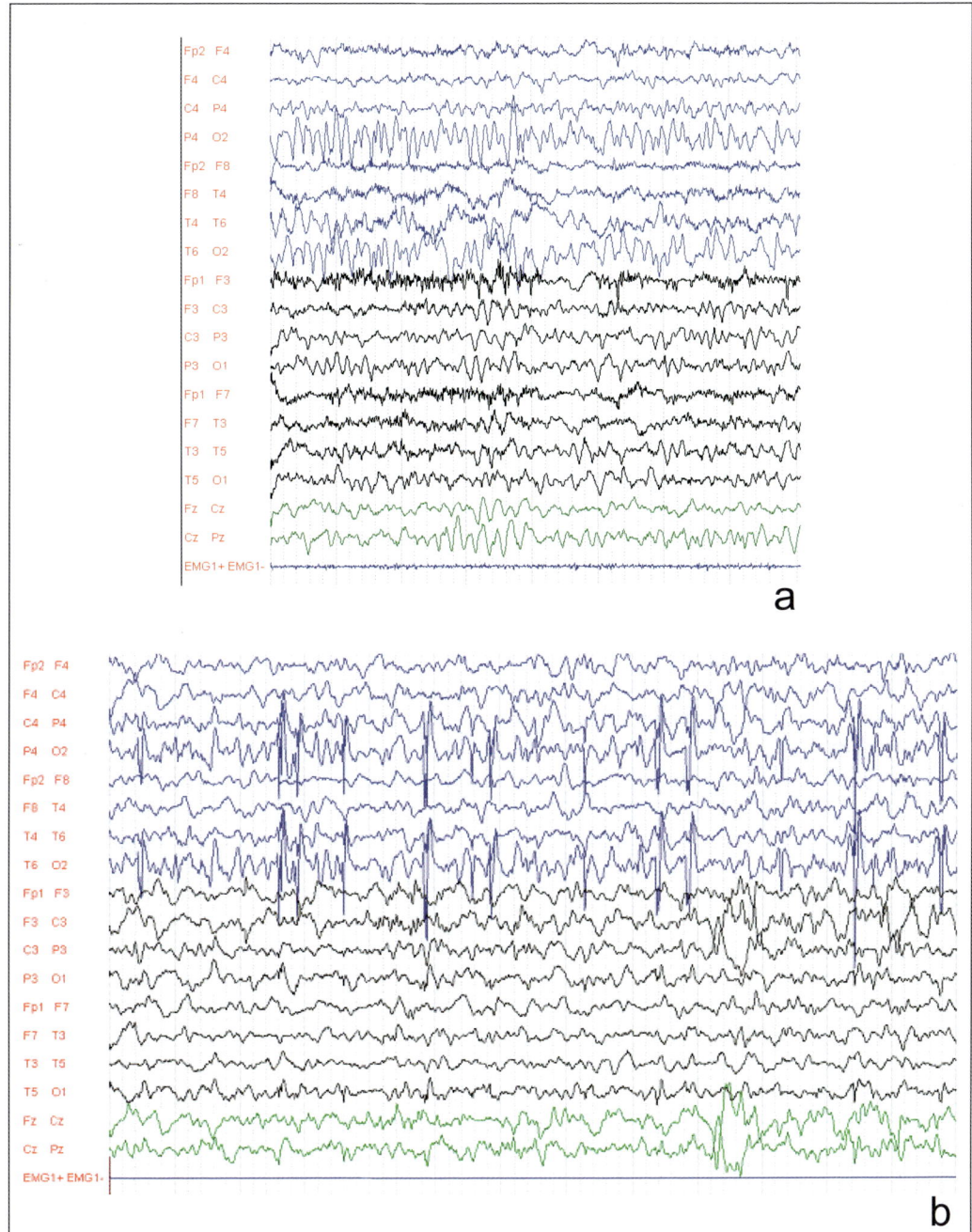

Fig. 9. (A) Awake EEG of a 16-month-old infant affected by right occipital dysplasia: continuous high voltage rhythmic activity localized to the right occipital region. (B) Sleep EEG: very high voltage spikes and spike-waves on the same region, sometimes spreading onto the homologous contralateral areas.

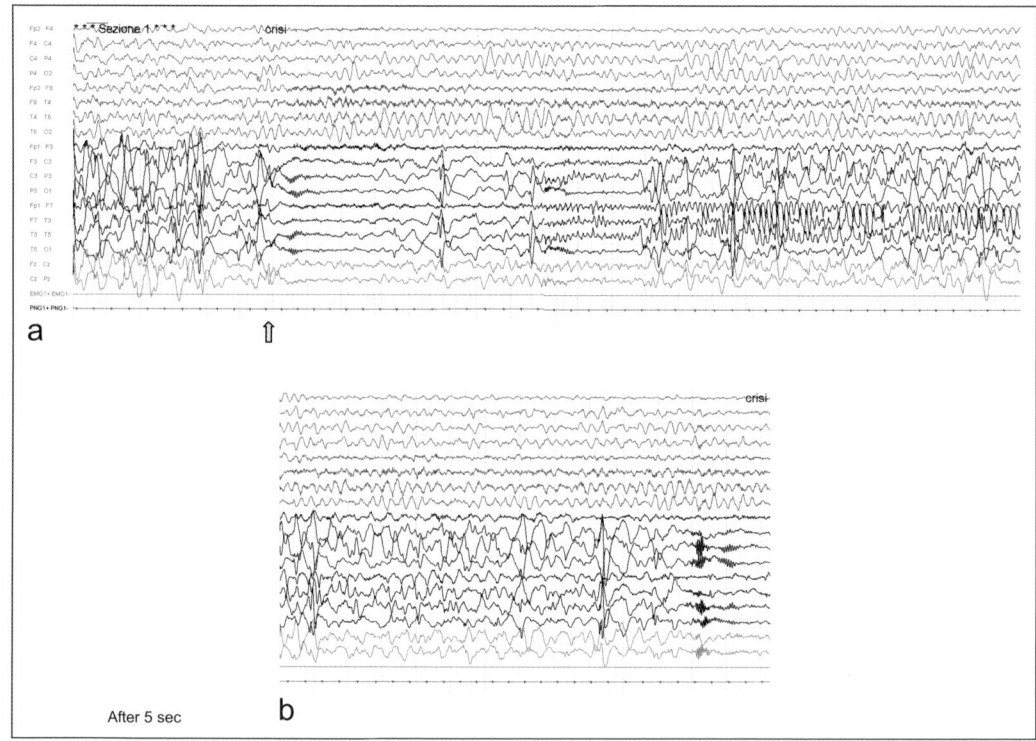

Fig. 10. Girl, 14 months old: focal seizures, characterized by brief eye and head deviation to the right associated with decremental activity with superimposed rapid activity on the left hemisphere (arrow); after 6 seconds, rhythmic theta activity on the temporal regions was correlated with staring and oral automatisms; at the end of the discharge the same initial ictal pattern reappeared.

considered signs of an unfavourable prognosis (Roger et al., 1981; Revol, 1992; Sillanpää, 1993; Berg et al., 1996; Battaglia et al.,1998; Watanabe et al., 2005). One of the greatest problems in the prognostic evaluation of non-idiopathic partial epilepsy is the fluctuating evolution of the epilepsy, with periods of transient seizure remission alternating with periods of seizure recurrence (Battaglia et al., 1998; Takenaka et al., 2000; Watanabe et al., 2005). Unfortunately, this may cause a delay in taking decisions about surgical treatment.

Treatment

The first choice pharmacological treatment recommended in newly diagnosed partial epilepsy in infancy is carbamazepine or valproate; new antiepileptic drugs are indicated in non-responding patients (French et al., 2004a, 2004b). The treatment of non-idiopathic partial epilepsy in infancy should take into consideration the high risk of resistance to antiepileptic drugs and the consequent negative effects produced by epileptic disorders on the cognitive development of infants. Thus it is important to evaluate whether surgical treatment is possible. To verify the response to many different antiepileptic drugs in the individual case would take a very long time, so surgery should be considered soon after the demonstration of resistance to two appropriate drugs (Kwan & Brodie, 2000; Berg et al., 2003; Cross et al., 2006; Harvey et al., 2008). In recent decades, investigators have reported that partial seizures in early life may be catastrophic and be associated with poor long term cognitive and epileptic outcome. These conditions are usually linked to extensive brain lesions, suggesting the need for early surgical treatment (Wyllie *et al.*, 1998; Di Rocco *et al.*, 2006). As reported in recent studies (Battaglia *et al.*, 2006; Harvey *et al.*, 2008), the most frequent types of surgical treatment in children under 4 are hemispherectomy and multilobar resections. The post-surgical results show a generally good epileptic outcome (Devlin *et al.*, 2003; Wyllie *et al.*, 1998; Battaglia *et al.*, 2006; Lettori *et al.*, 2008). Cognitive postsurgical outcome seems to be related to aetiological factors, with a better outcome in patients with acquired lesions (Devlin *et al.*, 2003; Pulsifier *et al.*, 2004; Delalande *et al.*, 2007; Battaglia *et al.*, 2006; Lettori *et al.*, 2008).

Febrile seizures

'Febrile seizures' is the preferred term for febrile convulsions according to the proposed Task Force Classification (Engel, 2001).

In 1980, the Consensus Development Panel in USA defined a febrile convulsion as 'an event in infancy or childhood, usually occurring between 3 months and 5 years of age, associated with fever but without evidence of intracranial infection or other definable cause. Seizures with fever in children who have suffered a previous non-febrile seizure are excluded.'

Febrile seizures are characterized by brief generalized tonic-clonic seizures; in 8 per cent of the cases seizures are partial and in 5 per cent they last longer than 20 minutes (Nelson & Ellenberg, 1976; Annegers *et al.*, 1987). The body temperature is usually higher than 38.5° C. Febrile seizures are the most frequent convulsive event in humans: 4–5 per cent of the general population will be affected at least once (Nelson & Ellenberg, 1978; Verity *et al.*, 1985). In some ethnic groups the prevalence is higher (7 per cent in Japan). Males are slightly more affected than females (60 per cent *vs.* 40 per cent). The annual incidence is 460 per 100,000 children in the age group 0–4 years (Forsgren *et al.*, 1990).

A significant risk of occurrence of febrile seizures in the 24 hours after receiving diphtheria-pertussis-tetanus vaccination and 8 to 14 hours after receiving mumps, measles, and rubella vaccination is reported (Barlow *et al.*, 2001). Brown *et al.* (2007) underlined the fact that no controlled study has been carried out comparing the risk of febrile seizures following vaccination with the risk of febrile seizures from other causes. There is also evidence that children experiencing their first febrile seizure after vaccination are no more likely to have recurrent seizures or to develop epilepsy or neurological disability than those with febrile seizures not temporally related to the vaccination (Barlow *et al.*, 2001; Vestergaard *et al.*, 2004). Furthermore, rates of febrile seizures are lower with newer vaccines. According to Brown *et al.* (2007), an established diagnosis of febrile seizures or epilepsy is not a contraindication to vaccination, although fever may precipitate a seizure.

Aetiology

Despite the high frequency in the general population, the biological mechanisms of febrile seizures are unknown. They appear to be linked to three conditions: an immature brain, fever, and a genetic predisposition.

The immaturity of the brain and its thermoregulatory mechanisms, as well as its capacity to implement cellular metabolism during fever, together with circulating toxins, immune reaction products and viral or bacterial invasion of the central nervous system, have been implicated in the seizure pathogenesis. Recently, the role of the activation of the cytokine network has been investigated, suggesting that specific interleukins may be involved in susceptibility to febrile seizures (Tsai *et al.*, 2002; Kanemoto *et al.*, 2003). A genetic predisposition seems to have a defined role in the occurrence of febrile seizures (Berkovic & Scheffer, 1998; Baulac *et al.*, 2004). The recurrence of febrile seizures is greater in the presence of positive family histories.

At the moment at least six susceptibility febrile seizure loci have been identified, on chromosomes 8q13-q21 (FEB1), 19p (FEB2), 2q23-q24 (FEB3), 5q14-q15 (FEB4), 6q22-q24 (FEB5), and 18p11 (FEB6) (Nakayama & Arinami, 2006). The identification of mutations of SCN1A and GABRG2 genes in families with GEFS+ suggests the involvement of sodium channel or GABA A receptors in the pathogenesis of febrile seizures as well as in FS+.

The mode of inheritance is unknown, but it is probably polygenic or autosomal dominant inheritance with reduced penetrance (Annegers et al., 1982).

Clinical features

Generalized tonic-clonic seizures are the most frequent seizure type (80 per cent). In the remaining 20 per cent seizures are tonic (13 per cent), atonic (3 per cent), unilateral or focal onset tonic (4 per cent). Rarely, seizures are characterized by staring associated with stiffness or floppiness or rhythmic jerking movements without stiffness. Myoclonic fits or absences are not considered to be febrile seizures.

Febrile seizures are classified as simple and complex, with a distinct prognostic significance. About 60 to 70 per cent of febrile seizures are simple and 30 to 40 per cent complex (Nelson & Ellenberg, 1976; Berg & Shinnar, 1996). Simple febrile seizures are generalized, lasting less than 15 minutes and not recurring within 24 hours. Complex febrile seizures are prolonged (more than 15 minutes), repetitive (occurring in clusters of two or more within 24 hours), and focal (with focal onset or with the Todd's postictal paresis).

Postictal symptoms are rare and Todd's paralysis is exceptional (0.4 per cent) (Nelson & Ellenburg, 1978).

Factors predisposing to recurrence of febrile seizures are as follows: a) occurrence of febrile seizures during the first year of life; b) occurrence during a low grade febrile temperature; c) short duration of the febrile illness before febrile seizures; d) a family history of febrile seizures. Neurological dysfunction and complex febrile seizures are not considered among the predisposing factors in all studies (Offringa, 1994). In a study by Berg et al. (1992) involving 428 infants with a first febrile seizure, the risk of recurrence in those without predisposing factors was 14 per cent, and increased progressively with an increase in the number of predisposing factors, up to 76 per cent when all the four factors were present.

Febrile seizures and subsequent epilepsy

Children without predisposing factors have a 2 per cent risk of developing epilepsy. Each of the risk factors increases the likelihood of developing epilepsy by 5 per cent.

Falconer in 1964 reported that among 100 children surgically treated for temporal lobe epilepsy, 41 had mesial temporal sclerosis (MTS) and in this group 30 per cent of temporal epilepsies were preceded by a history of prolonged febrile seizures during the first years of life, vs. 6 per cent in the group without MTS. The relationship between prolonged and unilateral febrile seizures and mesial temporal sclerosis, however, is nowadays controversial (Scott et al., 2003; Cendes, 2004; Lewis, 2005; Provenzale et al., 2008).

Management of febrile seizures

Usually, clinical assessment is sufficient, without any laboratory, EEG or neuro-imaging studies. Lumbar puncture is indicated if there are signs of meningism. The indication for lumbar puncture in all infants during the first year of life, when meningeal signs may be subclinical, is controversial (Camfield & Camfield, 2005).

Febrile seizures lasting longer than several minutes should be treated with rectal diazepam. Prophylactic treatment is only justified in children with prolonged febrile seizures. Intermittent prophylaxis at times of fever should be discouraged. Continuous antiepileptic drug treatment is not indicated to prevent recurrences, and antipyretic treatment is also ineffective (Rantala *et al.*, 1997).

Infantile epilepsy and development

Cognitive impairment is a frequent consequence of epilepsy, especially in infants, although it is not clear whether it is due to seizures or to the epilepsy, and in the latter case to the epileptic disorder or to a pre-existing brain injury (Niemann *et al.*, 1985; Ellenberg *et al.*, 1989; Hermann *et al.*, 2002); moreover, it is not easy to disentangle the possible role of medication (Mandelbaum & Burack, 1997) (Table 4).

Studies on the effects of epilepsy on cognitive development in infancy may follow different approaches. We will focus on the following: a) the role of seizures *per se* and electroencephalographic abnormalities ('related to paroxysmal electric activity'), and of a stable epileptic disease ('disease-related stable epileptic factors') (Aldenkamp & Arends, 2004a, 2004b); b) the study of functional or structural brain changes produced by seizures early in life and associated with cognitive impairment; c) the cognitive impairment of specific epileptic diseases, seizure-induced or linked to the disease itself; and d) analysis of the main developing functions that become impaired in epilepsies of infants.

It is well known that interictal epileptiform discharges (IED) can disrupt cortical functions and, possibly through local plastic changes associated with cognitive functions, produce transient cognitive impairment (Tassinari & Rubboli, 2006). That is what happens in benign childhood epilepsy with centrotemporal spikes (BCECTS); cognitive and behavioural disorders are reported in such epilepsies, correlated with IED (Nicolai *et al.*, 2006).

Some workers have suggested that the initial transitory impairment can, when chronic, lead to stable long term cognitive impairment (Stores, 1990; Aldenkamp *et al.*, 2001; Aldenkamp & Arends, 2004a; Jaseja, 2007a). Moreover, there is evidence of a strong correlation between IED and cognitive dysfunctioning, with a possible interference of IED with learning and memory in the waking state and with memory consolidation during sleep. Experimental support for such a notion is given by studies on the effects of seizures on the hippocampus, a region linked to learning and memory functions. A model of *in vitro* 'epilepsy', based on hippocampal neuronal culture, produces spontaneous recurrent epileptiform discharges provoking changes in intracellular calcium ions (prolonged elevation) after exposure to glutamate (Pal *et al.*, 2000), which leads to neuronal death (Limbrick *et al.*, 2003).

Table 4. Main factors involved in cognitive impairment due to epilepsy in infants

- Possible primary 'structural' brain injury
- Electroencephalographic abnormalities
- Seizures
- Epilepsy (characteristics of the type)
- Acquired brain damage due to epilepsy: structural or functional
- Abnormally developing functions (cognitive or pre-cognitive abilities)
- Negative collateral effects of antiepileptic drugs

Thus, even with subclinical interictal electrical discharges antiepileptic treatment is advised by some authorities (Ronen et al., 2000; Jaseja, 2007b) in order to prevent the deleterious effects of EEG abnormalities on cognitive abilities and psychosocial development (Binnie, 2003; Pressler et al., 2005).

The distinction proposed by Aldenkamp between a stable condition, linked to the epileptic disease (and possibly chronic IED), and a transitory condition, related to electrical paroxysmal discharge, refers to two different partly overlapping clinical situations: in the latter there is a transient reversible effect of seizures/EEG abnormalities in controlled forms of epilepsy or subclinical epilepsy; in the former there is a chronic disease, in which basal pathology, seizures and EEG abnormalities play a complex but stable role in development. In both, the mechanism underlying cognitive impairment is mediated by seizures/EEG abnormalities. In the transitory form, cognitive assessment during EEG monitoring shows an involvement of attention and speed processing; in the chronic form more complex and stable defects are observed, reflecting an uncontrolled repetition of seizures with brain damage caused by either a primary or a secondary effect of the repeated seizures.

Experimental seizure models and clinical studies show evidence that recurrent seizures early in life are associated with developmental and cognitive disorders (Sutula & Pitkänen, 2002; Motamedi & Meador, 2003; Haut et al., 2004; Ben-Ari & Holmes, 2006; Stafstrom, 2006). The forms with the worst developmental impairment of cognitive as well as sensory and motor functions – produced by frequent seizures and/or relevant interictal paroxysmal activity – are the so-called epileptic encephalopathies.

In animal models early life seizures induced by chemical convulsants or hyperthermia produce impairment of learning and memory (Lee et al., 2001; Chang et al., 2003), by altering the expression of NMDA receptors, particularly those located at synapses on dendritic spines, consequently causing cognitive deficits. These effects were obtained by Swann and colleagues (Swann et al., 2007a), who induced seizures in rodents in the first days of life by impairing GABAergic (inhibitory) synapses by the intrahippocampal injection of tetanus toxin or the inhalation of the volatile convulsant flutothyl. The study showed a downregulation of NMDA receptors. These findings are associated with a spectacular loss of dendritic spines, the main site of excitatory synapses – a possible basis for cognitive impairment (Jiang et al., 1998). Thus, there is evidence that early-life seizures may cause cognitive impairment through deep changes in glutamatergic receptors, especially those located at synapses on dendritic spines, possibly as an adaptive compensation employed by the nervous system to try to stabilize the network activity to prevent seizures (Wong, 2005; Swann et al., 2007b; Stafstrom & Benke, 2008).

If the affected regions are specific cortical areas with consequent changes in their projections, the development of superior functions may be altered later in life (Grigoris & Murphy, 1994). Also, behaviour abnormalities such as increased emotionality have been observed in adult animals which had suffered early seizures (Holmes et al., 1993).

In human infants, intractable epilepsy during the first 24 months leads to a significant risk of developmental arrest or deterioration, independently of aetiology (Vasconcellos et al., 2001). Studies on the long term effects of neonatal seizures report neurological sequelae, including psychomotor impairment, in 30 to 49 per cent of cases (Lombroso, 1983b; Ellenberg et al., 1984), the severity and quality of which are dependent on the distribution of the brain injuries (Legido, 1991; Bye et al., 1997; Mizrahj, 1999). This detrimental impact of seizures on development in the first months of life may be explained by the cortical damage caused by seizure activity (Hermann *et al.*, 2002) whatever the mechanism (see above) – as shown, for example, by studies on the impact of age at onset of epilepsy on development in children with temporal lobe epilepsy (Cormack *et al.*, 2007). This is the rationale for advising early intervention in cases of resistant epilepsy who are potential candidates for surgery (Freitag & Tuxhorn, 2005; Lettori *et al.*, 2008).

Another relevant issue concerning the effects of epileptic seizures at an early age is the known ability of the immature brain to reorganize its functions (plasticity). This is particularly evident in language development. A transfer of language functions to the right hemisphere is significantly related to earlier age at onset of left hemisphere epilepsy. However, after left hemispherectomy done at a very early age for right sided refractory epilepsy, difficulties in complex language tasks can persist.

Development in specific epileptic diseases

West syndrome

Infantile spasms, the most frequent age-dependent severe epileptic syndrome in infancy, consists of a heterogeneous group of epilepsies caused by a broad array of brain insults, including genetic mutations. A certain uniformity of clinical epileptic presentation suggests a possible unique mechanism, to which the cognitive involvement as well as other clinical aspects seem linked. An excellent review considers the main hypotheses about the mechanisms involved in the developmental impairment (Rho, 2004).

The aberrant neuronal excitotoxicity should first be evoked. Changes in NMDA receptors involved in cellular plasticity, migration and neurite outgrowth may occur, with excessive activation eventually leading to cell death. An imbalance between inhibitory and excitatory factors may thus explain the neuronal injury observed in infantile spasms (Riikonen *et al.*, 1997).

A second possible mechanism concerns corticotropin-releasing hormone (CRH) (Baram, 1993; Brunson *et al.*, 2002), which plays a central role in the pathogenesis of early epileptic encephalopathies. There is evidence in infantile spasms of activation of the brain's stress response with excessive release of CRH, enhancing seizure susceptibility (Baram & Hatalski, 1998). Desensitization of CHR receptors after chronic activation decreases ACTH release, and ACTH administration in turn suppresses excessive production of CRH. Thus, ACTH inhibits proconvulsant CRH release by the amygdala, hypothalamus and hippocampus, produced by various non-specific stressors (Rho, 2004).

A serotonin hypothesis is supported by several pieces of evidence. A decreased CSF level of 5-hydroxyindoleacetic (5-HIAA) was observed in infantile spasms (Yamamoto, 1991; Chugani *et al.*, 1998) by undertaking positron emission tomography using a novel radiotracer, an analogue of tryptophan (a precursor for serotonin synthesis): α-$[^{11}C]$ methyl-L-tryptophan, AMT. This technique was successful in differentiating epileptogenic tubers (with increased AMT) from non-epileptogenic tubers in children with tuberous sclerosis, a disease often associated with infantile spasms. Another possible hypothesis based on serotonin metabolism concerns the kynurenine pathway, which ultimately leads to the production of quinolinic acid, activating the NMDA receptor and causing excitotoxicity.

Focusing on the main developing functions impaired in West syndrome, one should distinguish symptomatic and cryptogenic forms, with various brain injuries or supposed brain injuries, from the generally benign idiopathic form. In the first, it is not always easy to disentangle the effects, both cognitive and behavioural, of underlying brain damage from any supervening further deterioration produced by the epileptic disorder. The normalization in idiopathic forms may be explained by the transitory nature of the epileptic activity or by a reorganization of neuronal circuitries, or both. Indeed, cognitive arrest or deterioration may be approached through the analysis of mechanisms impairing the early development of functions. The functioning of emerging abilities is involved in early onset epilepsies, especially in catastrophic forms. West syndrome is a paradigmatic syndrome that generally shows such kinds of impairment, beginning at the acute stage of the disease (at the onset of spasms and hypsarrhythmia) as an evident deterioration of responsiveness and of the sensory abilities of the infant, even of alertness itself. This deterioration, perceived by parents, can often be the cause of medical consultation. Associated with a lack of contact and impairment of social skills, it presents as a 'developmental arrest or regression', one of the three elements of the West triad. Sensory, especially visual, impairment is the predominant feature.

The mental deterioration at the onset of West syndrome – described many decades ago (Illingworth, 1955; Dongier et al., 1964) – has recently been confirmed by several studies on functional (visual and auditory) and cognitive skills (Jambaqué et al., 1993; Guzzetta et al., 2002b; Randò et al., 2005). Impairment of visual function in particular seems to be related to posterior brain areas (parieto-occipital), where injury has been demonstrated by electroclinical (Suzuki et al., 2003), neuroimaging (Jambaqué et al., 1993), and neuropathological findings (Chugani et al., 1993) in patients with West syndrome. Accordingly, the parieto-occipital regions could represent age-dependently sensitive areas involved in the mechanism of infantile spasms, especially when their onset is very early (Koo & Hwang, 1996). As well as high level disorders affecting the processing of visual stimuli (Guzzetta et al., 2002b), impairment of the arousal system is also possible, mediated by the reticular formation (Guzzetta et al., 1993), supported by the well known neuroradiological and neuropathological brain stem changes in West syndrome (Chugani et al., 1992; Miyazaki et al., 1993; Hayashi et al., 2000).

Similarly, there is evidence in West syndrome of high level and low level disorders of processing of auditory stimuli (Kaga et al., 1982; Baranello et al., 2006). Thus, multiple sensory functions appear to be impaired during the first stages of the disease, possibly preventing the laying of the first building blocks of cognition. This is why the finding of early impairment of sensory functions may predict developmental outcomes (Guzzetta et al., 2007). Also in early-brain-injured infants without epilepsy, visual impairment seems to be related to disorders of neurodevelopment, confirming that visual function is strongly related to cognitive outcome (Cioni et al., 1996, Lanzi et al., 1998, Mercuri et al.,1999). In fact, a model based on information processing theories considers visual maturation to be a kind of prerequisite of cognitive development. The pervasive epileptic disorder can thus prevent the normal maturation of neural connectivity and, if persistent, impairs cognitive development.

Results of developmental follow-up of patients with West syndrome (Guzzetta et al., 2008) may suggest that the specific epileptic disorder – eventually worsened by primary structural brain injuries involving eloquent cortical areas – can interfere with physiological functions in neural circuitries encompassing sensory domains, with consequent impairment of proper processing of sensory stimuli and of their higher integration. If the epileptic disorder subsides, sensory impairment is transient; otherwise, functional reorganization is prevented and cognitive development itself is compromised, resulting in progressive deterioration (Fig. 11), consistent with the notion of sensitive periods in normal brain development (Knudsen, 2004). Similar results, although less severe, seem to occur in other forms of early onset epilepsy (personal data).

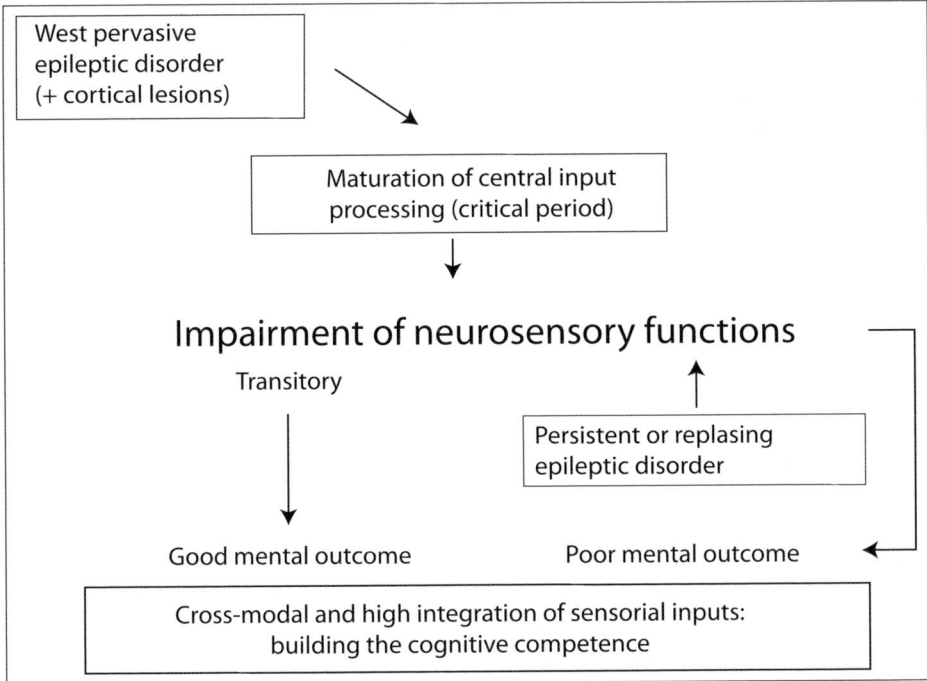

Fig. 11. A possible mechanism of cognitive impairment in West syndrome. (From Guzzetta F. In: Progress in Epileptic Spasms and West Syndrome. Paris: John Libbey Eurotext, 2007: 131-42).

One should anyway consider the greater functional plasticity in early-onset epilepsies, which makes recovery easier than in the later-onset forms. That is shown in focal lesion epilepsies, where successful drug or surgical treatment results in a good cognitive outcome in children; what does not happen in persisting forms of epilepsy where the epileptic disorder leads to progressive developmental deterioration, ultimately aggravated by additional impairment of compensating functional reorganization. Nevertheless, there are cases of chronic epilepsy in which processes of reorganization can be activated (Rasmussen & Milner, 1977; Janszky *et al.*, 2003).

Benign myoclonic epilepsy in infancy

In general, only sporadic cognitive and behavioural abnormalities have been found in such children, although there are reports of cases with more severe evolution (Mangano *et al.*, 2005); family anxiety together with a possible associated pathology would account for these disorders (Dravet & Bureau, 2002).

Severe myoclonic epilepsy in infancy (Dravet syndrome)

A few neuropsychological studies on the evolution of Dravet syndrome are available. A retrospective study (Cassé-Perrot *et al.*, 2001) showed, after an apparently normal first year, a marked psychomotor delay in the second and third year, followed by a persistent although slower deterioration. The psychomotor retardation associated with behavioural problems up to autistic traits seemed dependent on the severity of seizures in the first years of life. There were some cases with an apparently milder form.

In a more recent prospective study (unpublished data), an initially good sensorimotor and cognitive development was confirmed. Deterioration was abrupt during the second to third year and was followed by a progressive but mild decrease in developmental quotient except in sporadic cases. No apparent relationship was found between deterioration and seizure severity.

Idiopathic and/or benign focal epilepsies in infancy

There is no abnormal developmental evolution or outcome in these conditions. However, there are still no studies on an eventual influence of centrotemporal spikes on development.

References

Acharya, J.N., Wyllie, E., Lüders, H.O., Kotagal, P., Lancman, M. & Coelho, M. (1997): Seizure symptomatology in infants with localization-related epilepsy. *Neurology* **48**, 189–196.

Aicardi, J. (1994): Syndromic classification in the management of childhood epilepsy. *J. Child Neurol.* **9** (suppl. 2), 14–18.

Aicardi, J. & Chevrie, J.J. (1978): [Infantile spasms.] *Arch. Fr. Pediatr.* **35**, 1015–1023.

Aicardi, J. & Goutières, F. (1978): Encéphalopathie myoclonique néonatale. *Rev. Electroencephalogr. Neurophysiol. Clin.* **8**, 99–101.

Aicardi, J. & Ohathara, S. (2005): Several neonatal epilepsies with suppression-burst pattern. In: *Epileptic syndromes in infancy, childhood and adolescence*, eds. J. Roger, M. Bureau, Ch. Dravet, F.E. Dreifuss, A. Perret & P. Wolf. London: John Libbey.

Aldenkamp, A.P., Arends, J., Overweg-Plandsoen, T.C., et al. (2001): Acute cognitive effects of nonconvulsive difficult-to-detect epileptic seizures and epileptiform electroencephalographic discharges. *J. Child Neurol.* **16**, 119–123.

Aldenkamp, A.P. & Arends, J. (2004a): The relative influence of epileptic EEG discharges, short nonconvulsive seizures, and type of epilepsy on cognitive function. *Epilepsia* **45**, 54–63.

Aldenkamp, A.P. & Arends, J. (2004b): Effects of epileptiform EEG discharges on cognitive function: is the concept of 'transient cognitive impairment' still valid? *Epilepsy Behav.* **5** (Suppl. 1), S25–S34.

Annegers, J.F., Hauser, W.A., Anderson, V.E. & Kurland, L.T. (1982): The risks of seizure disorders among relatives of patients with childhood onset epilepsy. *Neurology* **32**, 174–179.

Annegers, J.F., Hauser, W.A., Shirts, S.B. & Kurland, L.T. (1987): Factors prognostic of unprovoked seizures after febrile convulsions. *N. Engl. J. Med.* **316**, 493–498.

Appleton, R.E., Peters, A.C., Mumford, J.P. & Shaw, D.E. (1999): Randomised, placebo-controlled study of vigabatrin as first-line treatment of infantile spasms. *Epilepsia* **40**, 1627–1633.

Arzimanoglou, A., Guerrini, R. & Aicardi, J. (2004): Partial epilepsy. In: *Aicardi's epilepsy in children*, 3rd ed., eds. A. Arzimanoglou, R. Guerrini & J. Aicardi, pp. 213–219. Philadelphia: Lippincott Williams & Wilkins.

Asano, E., Chugani, D.C., Juhász, C., Muzik, O. & Chugani, H.T. (2001): Surgical treatment of West syndrome. *Brain Dev.* **23**, 668–676.

Auvin, S., Pandit, F., De Bellecize, J., et al. (2006): Benign myoclonic epilepsy in infants: electroclinical features and long-term follow-up of 34 patients. *Epilepsia* **47**, 387–393.

Baram, T.Z. (1993): Pathophysiology of massive infantile spasms: perspective on the putative role of the brain adrenal axis. *Ann. Neurol.* **33**, 231–236.

Baram, T.Z., Mitchell, W.G., Tournay, A., Snead, O.C., Hanson, R.A. & Horton, E.J. (1996): High-dose corticotropin (ACTH) versus prednisone for infantile spasms: a prospective, randomized, blinded study. *Pediatrics* **97**, 375–379.

Baram, T.Z. & Hatalski, C.B. (1998): Neuropeptide-mediated excitability: a key triggering mechanism for seizure generation in the developing brain. *Trends Neurosci.* **21**, 471–476.

Baranello, G., Randò, T., Bancale, A., et al. (2006): Auditory attention at the onset of West syndrome; correlation with EEG patterns and visual function. *Brain Dev.* **28**, 293–299.

Barlow, W.E., Davis, R.L., Glasser, J.W., et al. (2001): The risk of seizures after receipt of whole-cell pertussis or measles, mumps, and rubella vaccine. *N. Engl. J. Med.* **345,** 656–661.

Battaglia, D., Dravet, C., Gelisse, Ph., Bureau, M., Pinto, P. & Genton, P. (1998): Pronostic des epilepsies partielles non idiopathiques chez l'enfant de moins de 6 ans. In: *Epilepsies partielles graves pharmacoresistentes de l'enfant*, eds. M. Bureau et al., pp. 55–66. Paris: John Libbey Eurotext.

Battaglia, D., Di Rocco, C., Iuvone, L., et al. (1999a): Neuro-cognitive development and epilepsy outcome in children with surgically treated hemimegalencephaly. *Neuropediatrics* **30,** 307–313.

Battaglia, D., Randò, T., Deodato, F., et al. (1999b): Epileptic disorders with onset in the first year of life: neurological and cognitive outcome. *Eur. J. Paediatr. Neurol.* **3,** 95–103.

Battaglia, D., Pasca, M.G., Cesarini, L., et al. (2005): Epilepsy in shunted posthemorrhagic infantile hydrocephalus owing to pre- or perinatal intra- or periventricular hemorrhage. *J. Child Neurol.* **20,** 219–225.

Battaglia, D., Chieffo, D., Lettori, D., Perrino, F., Di Rocco, C. & Guzzetta, F. (2006): Cognitive assessment in epilepsy surgery of children. *Childs Nerv. Syst.* **22,** 744–759.

Battaglia, D., Lettori, D., Contaldo, I., et al. (2007): Seizure semiology of lesional frontal lobe epilepsies in children. *Neuropediatrics* **38,** 287–291.

Baulac, S., Huberfeld, G., Gourfinkel-An, I., et al. (2001): First genetic evidence of GABA(A) receptor dysfunction in epilepsy: a mutation in the gamma2-subunit gene. *Nat. Genet.* **28,** 46–48.

Baulac, S., Gourfinkel-An, I., Nabbout, R., et al. (2004): *Lancet Neurol.* **3,** 421–430.

Bednarek, N., Motte, J., Soufflet, C., Plouin, P. & Dulac, O. (1998): Evidence of late-onset infantile spasms. *Epilepsia* **39,** 55–60

Ben-Ari, Y. (2002): Excitatory actions of GABA during development: the nature of the nurture. *Nat. Rev. Neurosci.* **3,** 728–739.

Ben-Ari, Y. & Holmes, G.L. (2005): The multiple facets of gammaaminobutyric acid dysfunction in epilepsy. *Curr. Opin. Neurol.* **18,** 141–145.

Ben-Ari, Y. & Holmes, G.L. (2006): Effects of seizures on developmental processes in the immature brain. *Lancet Neurol.* **5,** 1055–1063.

Bender, R.A. & Baram, T.Z. (2007): Effects of early seizures. Epileptogenesis in the developing brain: what can we learn from animal models? *Epilepsia* **48** (Suppl. 5), 2–6.

Berg, A.T. & Shinnar, S. (1996): Complex febrile seizures. *Epilepsia* **37,** 126–133.

Berg, A.T. & Shinnar, S. (1997): Do seizures beget seizures? An assessment of the clinical evidence in humans. *J. Clin. Neurophysiol.* **14,** 102–110.

Berg, A.T., Shinnar, S., Hauser, et al. (1992): A prospective study of recurrent febrile seizures. *N. Engl. J. Med.* **327,** 1122–1127.

Berg, A.T., Levy, S.R., Novotny, E.J. & Shinnar, S. (1996): Predictors of intractable epilepsy in childhood: a case-control study. *Epilepsia* **37,** 24–30.

Berg, A.T., Shinnar, S., Levy, S.R., et al. (2001): Two-year remission and subsequent relapse in children with newly diagnosed epilepsy. *Epilepsia* **42,** 1553–1562.

Berg, A.T., Langfitt, J., Shinnar, S., et al. (2003): How long does it take for partial epilepsy to become intractable? *Neurology* **60,** 186–190.

Berkovic, S.F., Heron, S.E., Giordano, L., et al. (2004): Benign familial neonatal-infantile seizures: characterization of a new sodium channelopathy. *Ann. Neurol.* **55,** 550–557.

Berkovic, S.F. & Scheffer, I.E. (1998): Febrile seizures: genetics and relationship to other epilepsy syndromes. *Curr. Opin. Neurol.* **11,** 129–134.

Binnie, C.D. (2003): Cognitive impairment during epileptiform discharges: is it ever justifiable to treat the EEG? *Lancet Neurol.* **2,** 725–730.

Blennow, G. & Starck, L. (1986): High dose B6 treatment in infantile spasms. *Neuropediatrics* **17,** 7–10.

Bliss, T.V.P. & Lomo, T. (1973): Long-lasting potentiation of synaptic transmission in the dentate area of the anaesthetized rabbit following stimulation of the perforant pathway. *J. Physiol. (Lond.)* **232,** 331–336.

Bonanni, P., Parmeggiani, L. & Guerrini, R.(2002): Different neurophysiologic patterns of myoclonus characterize Lennox-Gastaut syndrome and myoclonic astatic epilepsy. *Epilepsia* **43,** 609–615.

Bonanni, P., Malcarne, M., Moro, F., et al. (2004): Generalized epilepsy with febrile seizures plus (GEFS+): clinical spectrum in seven Italian families unrelated to SCN1A, SCN1B, and GABRG2 gene mutations. *Epilepsia* **45,** 149–158.

Branch, C.E. & Dyken, P.R. (1979): Choroid plexus papilloma and infantile spasms. *Ann. Neurol.* **5,** 302–304.

Brna, P.M., Gordon, K.E., Dooley, J.M. & Wood, E.P. (2001): The epidemiology of infantile spasms. *Can. J. Neurol. Sci.* **28**, 309–312.

Brown, N.J., Berkovic, S.F. & Scheffer, I.E. (2007): Vaccination, seizures and 'vaccine damage'. *Curr. Opin. Neurol.* **20**, 181–187.

Brunson, K.L., Avishai-Eliner, S. & Baram, T.Z. (2002): ACTH treatment of infantile spasms: mechanism of its effects in modulation of neuronal excitability. *Int. Rev. Neurobiol.* **49**, 185–197.

Bureau, M. & Maton, B. (1998): Valeur de l'EEG dan le pronostic précoce des épilepsies partielles non idiopathiques de l'enfant. In: *Epilepsies graves pharmaco-résistantes de l'enfant: stratégies diagnostiques et traitements chirurgicaux*, eds. M. Bureau, P. Kahane & C. Munari, pp. 67–78. Paris: John Libbey Eurotext.

Bureau, M., Genton, P., Guerrini, R. & Roger, J. (1996): Sleep EEG in cortical dysplasias. In: *Dysplasias of the cerebral cortex and epilepsy*, eds. R. Guerrini, F. Andermann, R. Canapicchi, J. Roger, B.G. Zifkin & P. Pfanner, pp. 247–254. Philadelphia: Lippincott-Raven.

Bye, A.M.E, Cunningham, C.A., Chee, K.Y. & Flanagan, D. (1997): Outcome of neonates with electrographically identified seizures, or at risk of seizures. *Pediatr. Neurol.* **16**, 225–231.

Camfield, C. & Camfield, P. (2005): Febrile seizures. In: *Epileptic syndromes in infancy, childhood and adolescence*, 4th ed, eds. J. Roger, M. Bureau, C. Dravet, P. Genton & P. Wolf, pp. 159–169. London: John Libbey.

Capovilla, G. & Beccaria, F. (2000): Benign partial epilepsy in infancy and early childhood with vertex spikes and waves during sleep: a new epileptic form. *Brain Dev.* **22**, 93–98.

Caraballo, R.H. & Fejerman, N. (2006): Dravet syndrome: a study of 53 patients. *Epilepsy Res.* **70** (Suppl. 1), S231–S238.

Caraballo, R., Cersósimo, R., Galicchio, S. & Fejerman, N. (1997): Epilepsies during the first year of life. *Rev. Neurol.* **25**, 1521–1524.

Caraballo, R.H., Cersósimo, R.O., Sakr, D., Cresta, A., Escobal, N. & Fejerman, N. (2005): Ketogenic diet in patients with Dravet syndrome. *Epilepsia* **46**, 1539–1544.

Caraballo, R.H., Cersosimo, R.O., Sakr, D., Cresta, A., Escobal, N. & Fejerman, N. (2006): Ketogenic diet in patients with myoclonic-astatic epilepsy. *Epileptic Disord.* **8**, 151–155.

Casse-Perrot, C., Wolf, M. & Dravet, C. (2001): Neuropsychological aspects of severe myoclonic epilepsy in infancy. In: *Neuropsychology of childhood epilepsy*, eds. I. Jambaue, M. Lassonde & O. Dulac, pp. 131–140. New York: Plenum.

Cavazzuti, G.B., Ferrari, P. & Laba, M. (1984): Follow-up study of 482 cases with convulsive disorder in the first year of life. *Dev. Med. Child Neurol.* **26**, 425–437.

Cendes, F. (2004): Febrile seizures and mesial temporal sclerosis. *Curr. Opin. Neurol.* **17**, 161–164.

Chang, Y.-C., Huang, A.-M., Kuo, Y., Wang, S.T., Chang, Y.Y. & Huang, C.C. (2003): Febrile seizures impair memory and cAMP response-element binding protein activation. *Ann. Neurol.* **54**, 706–718.

Cherubini, E., Galarsa, J.L. & Ben-Ari, Y. (1991): GABA: an excitatory transmitter in early postnatal life. *Trends Neurosci.* **14**, 515–519.

Chevrie, J.J. & Aicardi, J. (1971): Psychiatric prognosis of infantile spasms treated by ACTH or corticoids. Statistical analysis of 78 cases followed for more than one year. *J. Neurol. Sci.* **12**, 351–357.

Chevrie, J.J. & Aicardi, J. (1975): Duration and lateralization of febrile convulsions. Etiological factors. *Epilepsia* **16**, 781–789.

Chevrie, J.J. & Aicardi, J. (1977): Convulsive disorders in the first year of life: etiologic factors. *Epilepsia* **18**, 489–498.

Chiron, C., Dumas, C., Jambaqué, I., Mumford, J. & Dulac, O. (1997): Randomized trial comparing vigabatrin and hydrocortisone in infantile spasms due to tuberous sclerosis. *Epilepsy Res.* **26**, 389–395.

Chiron, C., Marchand, M.C., Tran, A., et al. (2000): Stiripentol in severe myoclonic epilepsy in infancy: a randomised placebo-controlled syndrome-dedicated trial. STICLO study group. *Lancet* **356**, 1638–1642.

Chugani, D.C., Chugani, H.T., Muzik, O., et al. (1998): Imaging epileptogenic tubers in children with tuberous sclerosis complex using alpha-[^{11}C] methyl-L-tryptophan positron emission tomography. *Ann. Neurol.* **44**, 858–866.

Chugani, H.T. & Conti, J.R. (1996): Etiologic classification of infantile spasms in 140 cases: role of positron emission tomography. *J. Child Neurol.* **11**, 44–48

Chugani, H.T., Shewmon, D.A., Sankar, R., Chen, B.C. & Phelps, M.E. (1992): Infantile spasms : lenticular nuclei and brain stem activation on positron emission tomography. *Ann. Neurol.* **31**, 212–219.

Chugani, H.T., Shewmon, D.A., Shields, W.D., et al. (1993): Surgery for intractable infantile spasms: neuroimaging perspective. *Epilepsia* **34**, 764–771.

Chugani, H.T., Da Silva, E. & Chugani, D.C. (1996): Infantile spasms. III. Prognostic implications of bitemporal hypometabolism on positron emission tomography. *Ann. Neurol.* **39**, 643–649.

Chugani, H.T., Asano, E. & Sood, S. (2007): Surgical treatment of West syndrome. In: *Progress in epileptic spasms and West syndrome*, eds. F. Guzzetta, B. Dalla Bernardina & R. Guerrini, pp. 143–152. London: John Libbey Eurotext.

Cioni, G., Fazzi, B., Ipata, A., Canapicchi, R. & van Hoof-van Duin, J. (1996): Correlation between cerebral visual impairment and magnetic resonance imaging in children with neonatal encephalopathy. *Dev. Med. Child Neurol.* **38**, 120–132.

Claes L, Del-Favero J, Ceulemans B, Lagae L, Van Broeckhoven C, De Jonghe P. (2001): De novo mutations in the sodium-channel gene SCN1A cause severe myoclonic epilepsy of infancy. *Am. J. Hum. Genet.* **68**, 1327–1332.

Consensus Development Panel (1980): Febrile seizures: long-term management of children with fever-associated seizures. *Pediatrics* **66**, 1009–1012.

Coppola, G., Plouin, P., Chiron, C., Robain, O. & Dulac, O. (1995): Migrating partial seizures in infancy: a malignant disorder with developmental arrest. *Epilepsia* **36**, 1017–1024.

Cormack, F., Cross, J.H., Isaacs, E., et al. (2007): The development of intellectual abilities in pediatric temporal lobe epilepsy. *Epilepsia* **48**, 201–204.

Cowan, L.D. (2002): The epidemiology of the epilepsies in children. *Ment. Retard. Dev. Disabil. Res. Rev.* **8**, 171–181.

Cross, J.H., Jayakar, P., Nordli, D., et al.; International League against Epilepsy, Subcommission for Paediatric Epilepsy Surgery; Commissions of Neurosurgery and Paediatrics (2006): Proposed criteria for referral and evaluation of children for epilepsy surgery: recommendations of the Subcommission for Pediatric Epilepsy Surgery. *Epilepsia* **47**, 952–959.

D'Agostino, M.D., Bastos, A., Piras, C., et al. (2004): Posterior quadrantic dysplasia or hemi-hemimegalencephaly: a characteristic brain malformation. *Neurology* **62**, 2214–2220.

Dalla Bernardina, B., Capovilla, G., Gattoni, M.B., Colamaria, V., Bondavalli, S. & Bureau, M. (1982): Epilépsie myoclonique grave de la première année. *Rev. Electroencephalogr. Neurophysiol. Clin.* **12**, 21–25.

Dalla Bernardina, B., Fontana, E., Sgrò, V., Colamaria, V. & Elia, M. (1992): Myoclonic epilepsy ('myoclonic status') in non-progressive encephalopathies. In: *Epileptic syndromes in infancy, childhood and adolescence*, 2nd ed., eds. J. Roger, C. Dravet, M. Bureau, F.E. Dreifuss, A. Perret & P. Wolf, pp. 89–96. London: John Libbey.

Dalla Bernardina, B., Pérez-Jiménez, A., Fontana, E., Colamaria, V., Piardi, F. & Avesani, E. (1996): Electroencephalographic findings associated with cortical dysplasia. In: *Dysplasias of the cerebral cortex and epilepsy*, eds. R. Guerrini, F. Andermann, R. Canapicchi, J. Roger, B.G. Zifkin & P. Pfanner, pp. 235–245. Philadelphia: Lippincott-Raven.

Dalla Bernardina, B., Fontana, E. & Darra, F. (2005): Myoclonic status in nonprogressive encephalopathies. *Adv. Neurol.* **95**, 59–70.

Dalla Berbardina, B., Fontana, E., Osanni, R., Opri, R. & Darra, F. (2007): Epileptic spasms: interictal patterns. In: *Progress in epileptic spasms and West syndrome*, eds. F. Guzzetta, B. Dalla Bernardina & R. Guerrini, pp. 43–60. London: John Libbey Eurotext.

Darra, F., Fiorini, E., Zoccante, L., et al. (2006): Benign myoclonic epilepsy in infancy (BMEI): a longitudinal electroclinical study of 22 cases. *Epilepsia* **47** (suppl 5), 31–35.

De Jong, J.G., Delleman, J.W., Houben, et al. (1976): Agenesis of the corpus callosum, infantile spasms, ocular anomalies (Aicardi's syndrome). Clinical and pathologic findings. *Neurology* **26**, 1152–1158.

Delalande, O., Bulteau, C., Dellatolas, G., et al. (2007): Vertical parasagittal hemispherotomy: surgical procedures and clinical long-term outcomes in a population of 83 children. *Neurosurgery* **60** (2 Suppl. 1), ONS19–32.

DeLorenzo, R.J., Pellock, J.M., Towne, A.R. & Boggs, J.G. (1995): Epidemiology of status epilepticus. *J. Clin. Neurophysiol.* **12**, 316–325.

Depienne, C., Arzimanoglou, A., Trouillard, et al. (2006): Parental mosaicism can cause recurrent transmission of SCN1A mutations associated with severe myoclonic epilepsy of infancy. *Hum. Mutat.* **27**, 389.

Devlin, A.M., Cross, J.H., Harkness, W., et al. (2003): Clinical outcomes of hemispherectomy for epilepsy in childhood and adolescence. *Brain* **126**, 556–566.

Di Rocco, C., Battaglia, D., Pietrini, D., Piastra, M. & Massimi, L. (2006): Hemimegalencephaly: clinical implications and surgical treatment. *Childs Nerv. Syst.* **22**, 852–866.

Djukic, A., Lado, F.A., Shinnar, S. & Moshé, S.L. (2006): Are early myoclonic encephalopathy (EME) and the Ohtahara syndrome (EIEE) independent of each other? *Epilepsy Res.* **70** (Suppl. 1), S68–S76.

Dongier, S., Charles, C. & Chabert, F. (1964): Sémiologie psychiatrique et psychometrique. In: *L'encéphalopathie myoclonique infantile avec hypsarrhythmie (Syndrome de West)*, eds. H. Gastaut, J. Roger, R. Soulager & N. Pinsard. Paris: Masson.

Doose, H., Gerken, H., Leonhardt, R., Völzke, E. & Völz, C. (1970): Centrencephalic myoclonic-astatic petit mal. Clinical and genetic investigation. *Neuropadiatrie* **2**, 59–78.

Doose, H. (1992): Myoclonic-astatic epilepsy. *Epilepsy Res.* **Suppl. 6**, 163–168.

Dravet, C. & Bureau, M. (1981): L'épilepsie myoclonique bénigne du nourisson. *Rev. Electroencephalogr. Neurophysiol. Clin.* **11,** 438–444.

Dravet, C. & Bureau, M. (1992): Benign myoclonic epilepsy in infants. In: *Epileptic syndromes in infancy, childhood and adolescence*, 2nd edition, ed. J. Roger, C. Dravet, M. Bureau, F.E. Dreifuss, A. Perret & P.Wolf, pp. 67–74. London: John Libbey.

Dravet, C. & Bureau, M. (2002): Benign myoclonic epilepsy in infancy. In: *Epileptic syndromes in infancy, childhood and adolescence*, eds. J. Roger, M. Bureau, C. Dravet, *et al.*, pp. 69–79. London: John Libbey.

Dravet, C. & Bureau, M. (2005): Benign myoclonic epilepsy in infancy. In: *Epileptic syndromes in infancy, childhood and adolescence*, 4th ed., eds. J. Roger, M. Bureau, C. Dravet, P. Genton & P. Wolf, pp. 77–88. London: John Libbey.

Dravet, C., Munari, C. & Roger, J. (1973): Evolution de 39 cas de syndrome de West en relation avec l'épilepsie ultérieure. In: *Evolution and prognosis of epilepsies*, eds. E. Lugaresi, P. Pazzaglia & C.A. Tassinari, pp. 119–131. Bologna: A. Gaggi.

Dravet, C., Catani, C., Bureau, M. & Roger, J. (1989): Partial epilepsies in infancy: a study of 40 cases. *Epilepsia* **30,** 807–812.

Dravet, C., Bureau, M., Guerrini, R., Giraud, N. & Roger, J. (1992): Severe myoclonic epilepsy in infancy (Dravet syndrome). In: *Epileptic syndromes in infancy, childhood and adolescence*, 2nd ed., eds. J. Roger, C. Dravet, M. Bureau, F.E. Dreifuss, A. Perret, P. Wolf, pp. 75–88. London: John Libbey.

Dravet, C., Guerrini, R. & Bureau, M. (1997): Epileptic syndromes with drop seizures in children. In: *Falls in epileptic and non-epileptic seizures during childhood*, eds. A. Beaumanoir, F. Andermann, G. Avanzini & L. Mira, pp. 95–111. London: John Libbey.

Dravet, C., Bureau, M., Guerrini, R., Oguni, H., Fuujama, Y. & Cokar, O. (2005): Severe myoclonic epilepsy in infancy (Dravet syndrome). In: *Epileptic syndromes in infancy, childhood and adolescence*, 4th ed., eds. J. Roger, M. Bureau, C. Dravet, P. Genton & P. Wolf, pp. 89–113. London: John Libbey.

Dreifuss, F., Farwell, J., Holmes, G., *et al.* (1986): Infantile spasms. Comparative trial of nitrazepam and corticotropin. *Arch. Neurol.* **43,** 1107–1110.

Dreifuss, F.E., Perret, A. & Wolf, P. (1992): *Epileptic syndromes in infancy, childhood and adolescence*, 2nd ed., pp. 67–74. London: John Libbey.

Dube, C., Vezzani, A., Behrens, M., Bartfai, T. & Baram, T.Z. (2005): Interleukin-1beta contributes to the generation of experimental febrile seizures. *Ann. Neurol.* **57,** 152–155.

Duchowny, M.S. (1987): Complex partial seizures of infancy. *Arch. Neurol.* **44,** 911–914.

Dulac, O. (2001): What is West syndrome? *Brain Dev.* **23,** 447–452.

Dulac, O. (2005): Malignant migrating partial seizures in infancy. In: *Epileptic syndromes in infancy, childhood and adolescence*, 4th ed., eds. J. Roger, M. Bureau, C. Dravet, P. Genton, C.A. Tassinari & P. Wolf, pp. 73–76. London: John Libbey.

Dulac, O. & Kaminska, A. (1997): Use of lamotrigine in Lennox-Gastaut and related epilepsy syndromes. *J. Child Neurol.* **12** (Suppl. 1), 23–28.

Dulac, O. & Tuxhorn, I. (2005): Infantile spasms. In: In: *Epileptic syndromes in infancy, childhood and adolescence*, 4th ed., eds. J. Roger, M. Bureau, C. Dravet, P. Genton, C.A. Tassinari & P. Wolf, pp. 53–72. London: John Libbey.

Dulac, O., Plouin, P., Jambaque, I. & Motte, J. (1986): Benign epileptic infantile spasms. *Rev. Electroencephalogr. Neurophysiol. Clin.* **16,** 371–382

Dulac, O., Chiron, C., Robain, O., Plouin, P., Jambaque, I. & Pinard, J.M. (1994): Infantile spasms: a pathophysiological hypothesis. *Semin. Pediatr. Neurol.* **1,** 83–89.

Dulac, O., Nabbout, R., Plouin, P., Chiron, C. & Scheffer, I.E. (2007): Early seizures: causal events or predisposition to adult epilepsy? *Lancet Neurol.* **6,** 643–651.

Duncan, R. (2001): Infantile spasms: the original description of Dr West, 1841. *Epileptic Disord.* **3,** 47–48.

Ellenberg, J.H., Hirtz, D.G. & Nelson, K.B. (1984): Age at onset of seizures in young children. *Ann. Neurol.* **15,** 127–134.

Ellenberg, J.H., Hirz, D.G. & Nelson, K.B. (1989): Do seizures in children cause intellectual deterioration? *N. Engl. J. Med.* **314,** 1085–1088.

Engel, J., for the International League Against Epilepsy (ILAE) (2001): A proposed diagnostic scheme for people with epileptic seizures and with epilepsy: report of the ILAE Task Force on Classification and Terminology. *Epilepsia* **42,** 796–803.

Escayg, A., MacDonald, B.T., Meisler, M.H., *et al.* (2000): Mutations of SCN1A, encoding a neuronal sodium channel, in two families with GEFS_2. *Nat. Genet.* **24,** 343–345.

Esclapez, M., Hirsch, J., Ben-Ari, Y. & Bernard, C. (1999): Newly formed excitatory pathways provide a substrate for hyperexcitability in experimental temporal lobe epilepsy. *J. Comp. Neurol.* **408**, 449–460.

Falconer, M.A., Serafetinides, E.A. & Corsellis, J.A. (1964): Etiology and pathogenesis of temporal lobe epilepsy. *Arch Neurol.* **10**, 233–248.

Fogarasi, A., Janszky, J., Faveret, E., Pieper, T. & Tuxhorn, I. (2001): A detailed analysis of frontal lobe seizure semiology in children younger than 7 years. *Epilepsia* **42**, 80–85.

Forsgren, L., Sidenvall, R. & Blomquist, H.K. (1990): A prospective incidence study of febrile convulsions. *Acta Neurol. Scand.* **79**, 550–557.

Freitag, H. & Tuxhorn, I. (2005): Cognitive function in pre-school children after epilepsy surgery: rationale for early intervention. *Epilepsia* **46**, 561–567.

French, J.A., Kanner, A.M., Bautista, J., et al. (2004a): Efficacy and tolerability of the new antiepileptic drugs I: Treatment of new onset epilepsy: report of the Therapeutics and Technology Assessment Subcommittee and Quality Standards Subcommittee of the American Academy of Neurology and the American Epilepsy Society. *Neurology* **62**, 1252–1260.

French, J.A., Kanner, A.M., Bautista, J., et al. (2004b): Efficacy and tolerability of the new antiepileptic drugs II: Treatment of refractory epilepsy: report of the Therapeutics and Technology Assessment Subcommittee and Quality Standards Subcommittee of the American Academy of Neurology and the American Epilepsy Society. *Neurology* **62**, 1261–1273.

Fukuma, G., Oguni, H., Shirasaka, Y., et al. (2004): Mutations of neuronal voltage-gated Na+ channel alpha 1 subunit gene SCN1A in core severe myoclonic epilepsy in infancy (SMEI) and in borderline SMEI (SMEB). *Epilepsia* **45**, 140–148.

Fusco, L. & Vigevano, F. (1993): Ictal clinical electroencephalographic findings of spasms in West syndrome. *Epilepsia* **34**, 671–678.

Gaily, E.K., Shewmon, D.A., Chugani, H.T. & Curran, J.G. (1995): Asymmetric and asynchronous infantile spasms. *Epilepsia* **36**, 873–382.

Gastaut, H., Roger, J., Soulayrol, R. & Pinsard, N. (1964): *L'encéphalopathie myoclonique précoce avec hypsarythmie (syndrome de West)*. Paris: Masson.

Gennaro, E., Malacarne, M., Carbone, I., et al. (1999): No evidence of a major locus for benign familial infantile convulsions on chromosome 19q12-q13.1. *Epilepsia* **40**, 1799–1803.

Gérard, F., Kaminska, A., Plouin, P., Echenne, B. & Dulac, O. (1999): Focal seizures versus focal epilepsy in infancy: a challenging distinction. *Epileptic Disord.* **1**, 135–139.

Glauser, T.A., Clark, P.O. & Strawsburg, R. (1998): A pilot study of topiramate in the treatment of infantile spasms. *Epilepsia* **39**, 1324–1328.

Glaze, D.G., Hrachovy, R.A., Frost, J.D., Kellaway, P. & Zion, T.E. (1988): Prospective study of outcome of infants with infantile spasms treated during controlled studies of ACTH and prednisone. *J. Pediatr.* **112**, 389–396.

Grigonis, A.M. & Murphy, E.H. (1994): The effects of epileptic cortical activity on the development of callosal projections. *Dev. Brain Res.* **77**, 251–255.

Gross-Tsur, V., Ben-Zeev, B. & Shalev, R.S. (2004): Malignant migrating partial seizures in infancy. *Pediatr. Neurol.* **31**, 287–290.

Guerrini, R & Pellicani, S. (2007): Infantile spasms and West syndrome: anatomo-electroclinical patterns and aetiology. In: *Progress in epileptic spasms and West syndrome*, eds. F. Guzzetta, B. Dalla Bernardina & R. Guerrini, pp. 23–42. London: John Libbey Eurotext.

Guerrini, R., Dravet, C., Genton, P., Belmonte, A., Kaminska, A. & Dulac, O. (1998): Lamotrigine and seizure aggravation in severe myoclonic epilepsy. *Epilepsia* **39**, 508–512.

Guerrini, R., Bonanni, P., Rothwell, J. & Hallett, M. (2002): Myoclonus and epilepsy. In: *Epilepsy and movement disorder*, eds. R. Guerrini, J. Aicardi, F. Andermann & M. Hallet, pp. 165–210. Cambridge: Cambridge University Press.

Guerrini, R., Parmeggiani, L., Bonanni, P., Kaminska, A. & Dulac, O. (2005): Myoclonic astatic epilepsy. In: *Epileptic syndromes in infancy, childhood and adolescence*, 4th ed., eds. J. Roger, M. Bureau, C. Dravet, P. Genton & P. Wolf, pp. 115–124. London: John Libbey.

Guerrini, R., Moro, F., Kato, M., et al. (2007): Expansion of the first PolyA tract of ARX causes infantile spasms and status dystonicus. *Neurology* **69**, 427–433.

Guipponi, M., Rivier, F., Vigevano, F., et al. (1997): Linkage mapping of benign familial infantile convulsions (BFIC) to chromosome 19q. *Hum. Mol. Genet.* **6**, 473–477.

Gulyás, A.I., Hájos, N. & Freund, T.F. (1996): Interneurons containing calretinin are specialized to control other interneurons in the rat hippocampus. *J. Neurosci.* **16**, 397–411.

Guzzetta, F. (2006): Cognitive and behavioral outcome in West syndrome. *Epilepsia* **47** (Suppl. 2), 49–52.

Guzzetta, F. (2007): West syndrome: epilepsy-induced neuro-sensory disorders and cognitive development. In: *Progress in epileptic spasms and West syndrome*, eds. F. Guzzetta, B. Dalla Bernardina & R. Guerrini R, pp. 131–142. Montrouge: John Libbey Eurotext.

Guzzetta, F., Crisafulli, A. & Isaya Crinò, M. (1993): Cognitive assessment of infants with West syndrome: how useful is it for diagnosis and prognosis? *Dev. Med. Child Neurol.* **35**, 379–387.

Guzzetta, F., Battaglia, D., Lettori, D., *et al.* (2002a): Epileptic negative myoclonus in a newborn with hemimegalencephaly. *Epilepsia* **43**, 1106–1109.

Guzzetta, F., Frisone, M.F., Ricci, D., Randò, T. & Guzzetta, A. (2002b): Development of visual attention in West syndrome. *Epilepsia* **43**, 757–763.

Guzzetta, F., Cioni, G., Mercuri, E., *et al.* (2008): Neurodevelopmental evolution of West syndrome: a 2-year prospective study. *Eur. J. Paediatr. Neurol.* **12**, 387–397.

Harkin, L.A., Bowser, D.N., Dibbens, L.M., *et al.* (2002): Truncation of the GABA(A)-receptor gamma2 subunit in a family with generalized epilepsy with febrile seizures plus. *Am. J. Hum. Genet.* **70**, 530–536.

Harvey, S., Cross, H., Shinnar, S., and the ILAE Pediatric Epilepsy Surgery Survey Taskforce (2008): Defining the spectrum of international practice in pediatric epilepsy surgery patients. *Epilepsia* 49, 146–155.

Hauser, W.A. (1994): The prevalence and incidence of convulsive disorders in children. *Epilepsia* **35** (suppl. 2): S1–S6.

Hauser, W.A. (1995): Epidemiology of epilepsy in children. *Neurosurg. Clin. North. Am.* **6**, 419–429.

Haut, S.R., Veliskova, J. & Moshe, S.L. (2004): Susceptibility of immature and adult brains to seizure effects. *Lancet Neurol.* **3**, 608–617.

Hayashi, M., Itoh, M., Araki, S., Kumada, S., Tanuma, N., Kohji, T., Kohyama, J., Iwakawa, Y., Satoh, J. & Morimatsu, Y. (2000): Immuno-histochemical analysis of brainstem lesions in infantile spasms. *Neuropathology* **20**, 297–303.

Heida, J.G. & Pittman, Q.J. (2005): Causal links between brain cytokines and experimental febrile convulsions in the rat. *Epilepsia* **46**, 1906–1913.

Hermann, B.P., Seidenberg, M. & Bell, B. (2002): The neurodevelopmental impact of childhood onset temporal lobe epilepsy on brain structure and function and the risk of progressive cognitive effects. *Prog. Brain Res.* **135**, 429–438.

Hoffmann, A.F., Zhao, Q. & Holmes, G.L. (2004): Cognitive impairment following status epilepticus and recurrent seizures during early development: support for the 'two-hit hypothesis'. *Epilepsy Behav.* **5**, 873–877.

Holmes, G.L. (1997): Epilepsy in the developing brain: lessons from the laboratory and clinic. *Epilepsia* **38**, 12–30.

Holmes, G.L., Thurber, S.J., Liu, Z., Stafstrom, C.E., Gatt, A. & Mikati, M.A. (1993): Effects of quisqualic acid and glutamate on subsequent learning, emotionality, and seizure susceptibility in the immature and mature animal. *Brain Res.* **623**, 325–328.

Hosain, S., Nagarajan, L., Carson, D., Solomon, G., Mast, J. & Labar, D. (1997): Felbamate for refractory infantile spasms. *J. Child Neurol.* **12**, 466–468.

Hrachovy, R.A., Frost, J.D., Kellaway, P. & Zion, T. (1979): A controlled study of prednisone therapy in infantile spasms. *Epilepsia* **20**, 403–407.

Hrachovy, R.A., Frost, J.D., Kellaway, P. & Zion, T.E. (1983): Double-blind study of ACTH vs prednisone therapy in infantile spasms. *J. Pediatr.* **103**, 641–645.

Hrachovy, R.A., Frost, J.D. & Kellaway, P. (1984): Hypsarrhythmia: variations on the theme. *Epilepsia* **25**, 317–325.

Hrachovy, R.A., Frost, J.D. & Glaze, D.G. (1994): High-dose, long-duration versus low-dose, short-duration corticotropin therapy for infantile spasms. *J. Pediatr.* **124**, 803–806.

Hurst, D.L. (1990): Epidemiology of severe myoclonic epilepsy of infancy. *Epilepsia* **31**, 397–400.

Huttenlocher, P.R. & Courten, C. (1987): The development of synapses in striate cortex of man. *Hum. Neurobiol.* **6**, 1–9.

ILAE Commission on Classification and Terminology of the International League against Epilepsy (1981): Proposal for revised clinical and electroencephalographic classification of epileptic seizures. *Epilepsia* **22**, 489–501.

ILAE Commission on Classification and Terminology of the International League Against Epilepsy (1985): Proposal for classification of epilepsies and epileptic syndromes. *Epilepsia* **26**, 268–278.

ILAE Commission on Classification and Terminology of the International League Against Epilepsy (1989): Proposal for revised classification of epilepsy and epileptic syndromes. *Epilepsia* **30**, 389–399.

Illingworth, R.S. (1955): Sudden mental deterioration with convulsions in infancy. *Arch. Dis. Child.* **30**, 529–537.

Jambaqué, I., Chiron, C., Dulac, O., Raynaud, C. & Syrota, P. (1993): Visual inattention in West syndrome: a neuropsychological and neurofunctional imaging study. *Epilepsia* 34, 692–700.

Janszky, J., Jokeit, H., Heinemann, D., Schulz, R., Woermann, F.G. & Ebner, A. (2003): Epileptic activity influences the speech organization in medial temporal lobe epilepsy. *Brain* **126**, 2043–2051.

Jaseja, H. (2007a): Cerebral palsy: interictal epileptiform discharges and cognitive impairment Clin. Neurol. Neurosurg. **109**, 549–552.

Jaseja, H. (2007b): Treatment of interictal epileptiform discharges in cerebral palsy patients without clinical epilepsy: hope for a better outcome in prognosis. *Clin. Neurol. Neurosurg.* **109**, 221–224.

Jeavons, P.M & Bower, B.D. (1974): Infantile spasms. In: *Handbook of clinical neurology*, eds. P.J. Vinken & G.W. Bruyn. The epilepsies: Amsterdam: Elsevier North Holland, pp. 219-34.

Jiang, M., Lee, C.L., Smith, K.L. & Swann, J.W. (1998): Spine loss and other persistent alterations of hippocampal pyramidal cell dendrites in a model of early-onset epilepsy. *J. Neurosci.* **18**, 8356–8368.

Johnston, M.V. (1996): Developmental aspects of epileptogenesis. *Epilepsia* **37** (Suppl. I), S2–S9.

Jonas, R., Nguyen, S., Hu, B., Asarnow, R.F., LoPresti, C., Curtiss, S., de Bode, S., Yudovin, S., Shields, W.D., Vinters, H.V. & Mathern, G.W. (2004): Cerebral hemispherectomy: hospital course, seizure, developmental, language, and motor outcomes. *Neurology* **62**, 1712–1721.

Jonas, R., Asarnow, R.F., LoPresti, C., *et al.* (2005): Surgery for symptomatic infant-onset epileptic encephalopathy with and without infantile spasms. *Neurology* **64**, 746–750.

Kaga, K., Marsh, R.R. & Fukuyama, Y. (1982): Auditory brain stem responses in infantile spasms. *Int. J. Pediatr. Otorhinolaryngol.* **4**, 57–67.

Kaindl, A.M., Asimiadoua, S., Mantheya, D., Hagen, M.V., Turski, L. & Ikonomidou, C. (2006): Antiepileptic drugs and the developing brain. *Cell. Mol. Life Sci.* **63**, 399–413.

Kaminska, A., Ickowicz, A., Plouin, P., Bru, M.F., Dellatolas, G. & Dulac, O. (1999): Delineation of cryptogenic Lennox-Gastaut syndrome and myoclonic astatic epilepsy using multiple correspondence analysis. *Epilepsy Res.* **36**, 15–29.

Kanai, K., Hirose, S., Oguni, H., *et al.* (2004): Effect of localization of missense mutations in SCN1A on epilepsy phenotype severity. *Neurology* **63**, 329–334.

Kanemoto, K., Kawasaki, J., Yuasa, S., *et al.* (2003): Increased frequency of interleukin-1beta-511T allele in patients with temporal lobe epilepsy, hippocampal sclerosis, and prolonged febrile convulsion. *Epilepsia* **44**, 796–799.

Kato, M., Saitoh, S., Kamei, A., *et al.* (2007): A longer polyalanine expansion mutation in the ARX gene causes early infantile epileptic encephalopathy with suppression-burst pattern (Ohtahara syndrome). *Am. J. Hum. Genet.* **81**, 361–366.

Kellaway, P. & Hrachovy, R.A. (1983): Status epilepticus in newborns: a perspective on neonatal seizures. *Adv. Neurol.* **34**, 93–99.

Kellaway, P., Hrachovy, R.A., Frost, J.D. & Zion, T. (1979): Precise characterization and quantification of infantile spasms. *Ann. Neurol.* **6**, 214–218.

Kellaway, P., Frost, J.D. & Hrachovi, R.A. (1983): Infantile spasms. In: *Antiepileptic drug therapy in paediatrics,* eds. P.L. Morselli *et al.* New York: Raven Press, pp. 115–136.

Khazipov, R., Esclapez, M., Caillard, O., *et al.* (2001): Early development of neuronal activity in the primate hippocampus in utero. *J. Neurosci.* **21**, 9770–9781.

Knudsen, E.I. (2004): Sensitive periods in the development of the brain and behavior. *J. Cogn. Neurosci.* **16**, 1412–1425.

Koo, B. & Hwang, P. (1996): Localization of focal cortical lesions influences age of onset of infantile spasms. *Epilepsia* **37**, 1068–1071.

Korff, C.M. & Nordli, D.R. (2006): Epilepsy syndrome in infancy. *Pediatr. Neurol.* **34**, 253–263.

Kramer, U. (1999): Epilepsy in the first year of life: a review. *J. Child Neurol.* **14**, 485–489.

Kwan, P. & Brodie, M.J. (2000): Early identification of refractory epilepsy. *N. Engl. J. Med.* **342**, 314–319.

Lanzi, G., Fazzi, E., Uggetti, C., Cavallini, A., Danova, S. & Egitto, M.G. (1998): Cerebral visual impairment in periventricular leukomalacia. *Neuropediatrics* **29**, 145–150.

Lacy, J.R. & Penry, J.K. (1976): *Infantile spasms*. New York: Raven Press.

Laurie, D.J., Wisden, W. & Seeburg, P.H. (1992): The distribution of the thirteen GABA, receptor subunit mRNAs in the rat brain. III. Embryonic and postnatal development. *J. Neurosci.* **12**, 4151–4172.

Lawlor, K.M. & Devlin, A.M. (2005): Levetiracetam in the treatment of infantile spasms. *Eur. J. Paediatr. Neurol.* **9**, 19–22.

Lee, C.L., Hannay, J., Hrachovy, R., Rashid, S., Antalffy, B. & Swann, J.W. (2001): Recurrent seizures in infant rats produced spatial learning deficits without a substantial loss of hippocampal pyramidal cells. *Neuroscience* **107**, 71–84.

Lee, W.L., Tay, A., Ong, H.T., Goh, L.M., Monaco, A.P. & Szepetowski, P. (1998): Association of infantile convulsions with paroxysmal dyskinesias (ICCA syndrome): confirmation of linkage to human chromosome 16p12-q12 in a Chinese family. *Hum. Genet.* **103**, 608–612.

Legido, A. (1991): Postnatal epilepsy after EEG-confirmed neonatal seizures. *Epilepsia* **32**, 69–76.

Lettori, D., Battaglia, D., Sacco, A., *et al.* (2008): Early hemispherectomy in catastrophic epilepsy: a neuro-cognitive and epileptic long-term follow-up. *Seizure* **17**, 49–63.

Lewis, D.V. (2005): Losing neurons: selective vulnerability and mesial temporal sclerosis. *Epilepsia* **46** (suppl. 7), 39–44.

Limbrick, D.D., Sombati, S. & DeLorenzo, R.J. (2003): Calcium influx constitutes the ionic basis for the maintenance of glutamate-induced extended neuronal depolarization associated with hippocampal neuronal death. *Cell Calcium* **33**, 69–81.

Lombroso, C.T. (1983a): A prospective study of infantile spasms: clinical and therapeutic correlations. *Epilepsia* **24**, 135–158

Lombroso, C.T. (1983b): Prognosis in neonatal seizures. *Adv. Neurol.* **34**, 101–103.

Lortie, A., Plouin, P., Chiron, C., Delalande, O. & Dulac, O. (2002): Characteristics of epilepsy in focal cortical dysplasia in infancy. *Epilepsy Res.* **51**, 133–145.

Luna, D., Dulac, O. & Plouin, P. (1989): Ictal characteristics of cryptogenic partial epilepsies in infancy. *Epilepsia* **30**, 827–832.

Lúthvígsson, P., Olafsson, E., Sigurthardóttir, S. & Hauser, W.A. (1994): Epidemiologic features of infantile spasms in Iceland. *Epilepsia* 35, 802–805.

Lux, A.L. & Osborne, J.P. (2004): A proposal for case definitions and outcome measures in studies of infantile spasms and West syndrome: consensus statement of the West Delphi group. *Epilepsia* **45**, 1416–1428.

Lux, A.L., Edwards, S.W., Hancock, E., *et al.* (2004): The United Kingdom Infantile Spasms Study comparing vigabatrin with prednisolone or tetracosactide at 14 days: a multicentre, randomised controlled trial. *Lancet* **364**, 1773–1778.

Madia, F., Striano, P., Gennaro, E., *et al.* (2006): Cryptic chromosome deletions involving SCN1A in severe myoclonic epilepsy of infancy. *Neurology* 67, 1230–1235.

Mandelbaum, D.E. & Burack, G.D. (1997): The effect of seizure type and medication on cognitive and behavioural functioning in children with idiopathic epilepsy. *Dev. Med. Child Neurol.* **39**, 731–735.

Mangano, S., Fontana, A. & Cusumano, L. (2005): Benign myoclonic epilepsy in infancy: neuropsychological and behavioural outcome. *Brain Dev.* **27**, 218–223.

Marini, C., Mei, D., Cross, H.J. & Guerrini, R. (2006): Mosaic SCN1A mutation in familial severe myoclonic epilepsy of infancy. *Epilepsia* **47**, 1737–1740.

Marini, C., Mei, D., Temudo, T., *et al.* (2007): Idiopathic epilepsies with seizures precipitated by fever and SCN1A abnormalities. *Epilepsia* **48**, 1678–1685.

Marsh, E., Melamed, S.E., Barron, T. & Clancy, R.R. (2005): Migrating partial seizures in infancy: expanding the phenotype of a rare seizure syndrome. *Epilepsia* **46**, 568–572.

Matsumoto, A., Watanabe, K., Negoro, T., *et al.* (1981): Long-term prognosis after infantile spasms: a statistical study of prognostic factors in 200 cases. *Dev. Med. Child Neurol.* **23**, 51–65.

Maytal, J., Shinnar, S., Moshe, S.L. & Alvarez, L.A. (1989): Low morbidity and mortality of status epilepticus in children. *Pediatrics* **83**, 323–31.

Meisler, M.H., Kearney, J., Ottman, R. & Escayg, A. (2001): Identification of epilepsy genes in human and mouse. *Annu. Rev. Genet.* **35**, 567–588.

Mercuri, E., Haataja, L., Guzzetta, A., Anker, S., Cowan, F. & Rutherford, M. (1999): Visual function in term infants with hypoxic-ischaemic insults: correlation with neurodevelopment at 2 years of age. *Arch. Dis. Child. Fetal Neonatal Ed.* **80**, F99–F104.

Miller, S.P., Dilenge, M.E., Meagher-Villemure, K., O'Gorman, A.M. & Shevell, M.I. (1998): Infantile epileptic encephalopathy (Ohtahara syndrome) and migrational disorder. *Pediatr. Neurol.* **19**, 50–54.

Mimaki, T., Ono, J. & Yabuuchi, H. (1983): Temporal lobe astrocytoma with infantile spasms. *Ann. Neurol.* **14**, 695–696.

Miyazaki, M., Hashimoto, T., Tayama, M. & Kuroda, Y. (1993): Brainstem involvement in infantile spasms: a study emplying brainstem evoked potentials and magnetic resonance imaging. *Neuropediatrics* **24**, 126–130.

Mizrahj, E.M. (1999): Acute and chronic effects of seizures in the developing brain: lessons from clinical experience. *Epilepsia* **40** (Suppl. 1), S42–S50.

Moshé, S.L. & Sperber, E.F. (1998): Substantia nigra-mediated control of generalized seizures. In: *Generalized epilepsy: cellular, molecular and pharmacological approaches*, eds. G. Gloor, R. Kostopoulos, M. Naquet & P. Avoli, pp. 355–367. Boston: Birkhauser.

Motamedi, G. & Meador, K. (2003): Epilepsy and cognition. *Epilepsy Behav.* **4** (Suppl. 2), S25–S38.

Mulley, J.C., Nelson, P., Guerrero, S., et al. (2006): A new molecular mechanism for severe myoclonic epilepsy of infancy: exonic deletions in SCN1A. *Neurology* **67**, 1094–1095.

Nabbout, R., Kozlovski, A., Gennaro, E., et al. (2003): Absence of mutations in major GEFS genes in myoclonic astatic epilepsy. *Epilepsy Res.* **56**, 127–133.

Nakayama, J. & Arinami, T. (2006): Molecular genetics of febrile seizures. *Epilepsy Res.* **70** (Suppl. 1), S190–S198.

Nelson, K.B. & Ellenberg, J.H. (1976): Predictors of epilepsy in children who have experienced febrile seizures. *N. Engl. J. Med.* **295**, 1029–1033.

Nelson, K.B. & Ellenberg, J.H. (1978): Prognosis in children with febrile seizures. *Pediatrics* 61, 720–727.

Neubauer, B.A., Hahn, A., Doose, H. & Tuxhorn, I. (2005): Myoclonic-astatic epilepsy of early childhood – definition, course, nosography, and genetics. *Adv. Neurol.* **95**, 147–155.

Nguyen, L., Rigo, J.M., Rocher, V., et al. (2001): Neurotransmitters as early signals for central nervous system development. *Cell Tissue Res.* **305**, 187–202.

Nicolai, J., Aldenkamp, A.P., Arands, J., Weber, J.W. & Vles, J.S. (2006): Cognitive and behavioral effects of nocturnal epileptiform discharges in children with benign childhood epilepsy with centrotemporal spikes. *Epilepsy Behav.* **8**, 56–70.

Niemann, H., Boenick, H.E., Schmidt, R.C. & Ettlinger, G. (1985): Cognitive development in epilepsy: the relative influence of epileptic activity and brain damage. *Eur. Arch. Psychiatry Neurol. Sci.* **234**, 399–403.

Nohria, V., Lee, N., Tien, R.D., et al. (1994): Magnetic resonance imaging evidence of hippocampal sclerosis in progression: a case report. *Epilepsia* **35**, 1332–1336.

Offringa, M. (1994): Seizures associated with fever: current management controversies. *Semin. Pediatr. Neurol.* **1**, 90–101.

Oguni, H., Imaizumi, Y., Uehara, T., Oguni, M. & Fukuyama, Y. (1993): Electroencephalographic features of epileptic drop attacks and absence seizures:a case study. *Brain Dev.* **15**, 226–230.

Oguni, H., Hayashi, K., Oguni, M., et al. (1994): Treatment of severe myoclonic epilepsy in infants with bromide and its borderline variant. *Epilepsia* **35**, 1140–1145.

Oguni, H., Fukuyama, Y., Tanaka, T., et al. (2001a): Myoclonic-astatic epilepsy of early childhood – clinical and EEG analysis of myoclonic-astatic seizures, and discussions on the nosology of the syndrome. *Brain Dev.* **23**, 757–764.

Oguni, H., Hayashi, K., Awaya, Y., Fukuyama, Y. & Osawa, M. (2001b): Severe myoclonic epilepsy in infants – a review based on the Tokyo Women's Medical University series of 84 cases. *Brain Dev.* **23**, 736–748.

Oguni, H., Tanaka, T., Hayashi, K., et al. (2002): Treatment and long-term prognosis of myoclonic-astatic epilepsy of early childhood. *Neuropediatrics* **33**, 122–132.

Oguni, H., Hayashi, K., Imai, K., et al. (2005): Idiopathic myoclonic-astatic epilepsy of early childhood – nosology based on electrophysiologic and long-term follow-up study of patients. *Adv. Neurol.* **95**, 157–174.

Ohtahara, S., Ohtsuka, Y. & Oka, E. (1976): On the specific age-dependent epileptic syndromes: the early-infantile epileptic encephalopathy with suppression-burst. *No Tu Hattatsu* **8**, 270–279.

Ohtahara, S., Ohtsuka, Y., Yamatogi, Y., Oka, E. & Inoue, H. (1992): Early epileptic encephalopathy with suppression-bursts. In: *Epileptic syndromes in infancy, childhood and adolescence*, eds. J. Roger, M. Bureau, Ch. Dravet, F.E. Dreifuss, A. Perret & P. Wolf. London: John Libbey, 25–34.

Ohtahara, S. & Yamatogi, Y. (2006): Ohtahara syndrome: with special reference to its developmental spects for differentiating from early myoclonic encephalopathy. *Epilepsy Res.* **70** (suppl. 1), S58–S67.

Ohtsuka, Y., Yoshinaga, H. & Kobayashi, K. (2000): Refractory childhood epilepsy and factors related to refractoriness. *Epilepsia* **41** (Suppl. 9), 14–17.

Okuda, K., Yasuhara, A., Kamei, A., Araki, A., Kitamura, N. & Kobayashi, Y. (2000): Successful control with bromide of two patients with malignant migrating partial seizures in infancy. *Brain Dev.* **22**, 56–59.

Okumura, A., Hayakawa, F., Kuno, K. & Watanabe, K. (1996): Benign partial epilepsy in infancy. *Arch. Dis. Child.* 74, 19–21.

Oller-Daurella, L. & Oller, L.F. (1989): Partial epilepsy with seizures appearing in the first three years of life. *Epilepsia* **30**, 820–826.

Pachatz, C., Fusco, L. & Vigevano, F. (2003): Epileptic spasms and partial seizures as a single ictal event. *Epilepsia* **44**, 693–700.

Pal, S., Limbrick, D.D., Rafique, A. & DeLorenzo, R.J. (2000): Induction of spontaneous recurrent epileptiform discharges causes long-term changes in intracellular calcium homeostatic mechanisms. *Cell Calcium* **28**, 181–193.

Pavone, L., Incorpora, G., La Rosa, M., Li Volti, S. & Mollica, F. (1981): Treatment of infantile spasms with sodium dipropylacetic acid. *Dev. Med. Child Neurol.* **23**, 454–461.

Perez, J., Chiron, C., Musial, C., et al. (1999): Stiripentol: efficacy and tolerability in children with epilepsy. *Epilepsia* **40**, 1618–1626.

Plouin, P., Jalin, C., Dulac, O. & Chiron, C. (1987): Ambulatory 24-hour EEG recording in epileptic infantile spasms. *Rev. Electroencephalogr. Neurophysiol. Clin.* **17**, 309–318.

Pressler, R.M., Robinson, R.O., Wilson, G.A. & Binnie, C.D. (2005): Treatment of interictal epileptiform discharges can improve behavior in children with behavioral problems and epilepsy. *J. Pediatr.* **146**, 112–117.

Provenzale, J.M., Barboriak, D.P., VanLandingham, K., MacFall, J., Delong, D. & Lewis, D.V. (2008): Hippocampal MRI signal hyperintensity after febrile status epilepticus is predictive of subsequent mesial temporal sclerosis. *Am. J. Roentgenol.* **190**, 976–978.

Pulsifer, M.B., Brandt, J., Salorio, C.F., Vining, E.P., Carson, B.S. & Freeman, J.M. (2004): The cognitive outcome of hemispherectomy in 71 children. *Epilepsia* **45**, 243–254.

Randò, T., Baranello, G., Ricci, D., et al. (2005): Cognitive competence at the onset of West syndrome: correlation with EEG-patterns and visual function. *Dev. Med. Child Neurol.* **47**, 760–765.

Rantala, H., Tarkka, R. & Uhari, M. (1997): A meta-analytic review of the preventive treatment of recurrences of febrile seizures. *J. Pediatr.* **131**, 922–925.

Rasmussen, T. & Milner, B. (1977): The role of early left-brain injury in determining lateralization of cerebral speech functions. *Ann. N. Y. Acad. Sci.* **299**, 355–369.

Rathgeb, J.P., Ploin, P., Soufflet, C., Cieuta, C., Chiron, C. & Dulac, O. (1998): Les cas particuliers des crises partielles du nourisson: sémiologie électroclinique. In: *Epilepsies graves pharmaco-résistantes de l'enfant: stratégies diagnostiques et traitements chirurgicaux,* eds. M. Bureau, P. Kahane & C. Munari. Paris: John Libbey Eurotext.

Represa, A. & Ben-Ari, Y. (1997): Molecular and cellular cascades in seizure-induced neosynapse formation. *Adv. Neurol.* **72**, 25–34.

Rett, A.R. & Teubel, R. (1964): Neugeborenenkrample in Rhamen einer epileptish belasten Familie. *Wien Klein. Wschr.* **76**, 609–613.

Retz, W., Kornhuber, J. & Riederer, P. (1996): Neurotransmission and the ontogeny of human brain. *J. Neural Transm.* **103**, 403–419.

Revol, M. (1992): Non idiopathic partial epilepsies and epileptic syndromes in childhood. In: *Epileptic syndromes in infancy, childhood and adolescence,* 2nd ed., eds. J. Roger, C. Dravet, M. Bureau, F.E. Dreifuss, A. Perret & P. Wolf, pp. 347–362. London: John Libbey.

Rho, J.M. (2004): Basic science behind catastrophic epilepsies. *Epilepsia* **45**, S5–S11.

Riikonen, R. (1982): A long-term follow-up study of 214 children with the syndrome of infantile spasms. *Neuropediatrics* 13, 14–23.

Riikonen, R. (1984): Infantile spasms: modern practical aspects. *Acta Paediatr. Scand.* **73**, 1–12.

Riikonen, R. (1995): Decreasing perinatal mortality: unchanged infantile spasm morbidity. *Dev. Med. Child Neurol.* **37**, 232–238.

Riikonen, R. (1996): Long-term otucome of West syndrome: a study of adults with a history of infantile spasms. *Epilepsia* 37, 367–372.

Riikonen, R., S?derstr?m, S., Vanhala, R., Ebendal, T. & Lindholm, D. (1997): West' syndrome: cerebrospinal fluid nerve growth factor and effect of ACTH. *Ped. Neurol.* **17**, 224–229.

Robain, O. & Dulac, O. (1992): Early epileptic encephalopathy with suppression bursts and olivary-dentate dysplasia. *Neuropediatrics* **23**, 162–164.

Roger, J., Dravet, C., Menendez, P. & Bureau, M. (1981): The partial epilepsies in childhood – evolution and prognosis factors. *Rev. Electroencephalogr. Neurophysiol. Clin.* **11**, 431–437.

Ronen, G.M., Richards, J.E., Cunningham, C., Secord, M. & Rosenbloom, D. (2000): Can sodium valproate improve learning in children with epileptiform bursts but without clinical seizures? *Dev. Med. Child Neurol.* **42**, 751–755.

Rubenstein, J.E., Kossoff, E.H., Pzyk, P.L., Vining, E.P., McGrogan, J.R. & Freeman, J.M. (2005): Experience in the use of ketogenic diet as early therapy. *J. Child Neurol.* **20**, 31–34

Ruggieri, V., Caraballo, R. & Fejerman, N. (1989): Intracranial tumors and West syndrome. *Pediatr. Neurol.* **5**, 327–329.

Saitsu, H., Kato, M., Mizuguchi, T., et al. (2008): De novo mutations in the gene encoding STXBP1 (MUNC18-1) cause early infantile epileptic encephalopathy. *Nat. Genet.* **40**, 782–788.

Sarisjulis, N., Gamboni, B., Plouin, P., Kaminska, A. & Dulac, O. (2000): Diagnosing idiopathic/cryptogenic epilepsy syndromes in infancy. *Arch. Dis. Child.* **82,** 226–230.

Scala, E., Ariani, F., Mari, F., *et al.* (2005): CDKL5/STK9 is mutated in Rett syndrome variant with infantile spasms. *J. Med. Genet.* **42,** 103–107.

Scheffer, I.E. & Berkovic, S.F. (1997): Generalized epilepsy with febrile seizures plus. A genetic disorder with heterogeneous clinical phenotypes. *Brain* **120,** 479–490.

Scott, R.C., Gadian, D.G., King, M.D., *et al.* (2002): Magnetic resonance imaging findings within 5 days of status epilepticus in childhood. *Brain* **125,** 1951–1959.

Scott, R.C., King, M.D., Gadian, D.G., Neville, B.G. & Connelly, A. (2003): Hippocampal abnormalities after prolonged febrile convulsion: a longitudinal MRI study. *Brain* **126,** 2551–2557.

Sillanpää, M. (1993): Remission of seizures and predictors of intractability in long-term follow-up. *Epilepsia* **34,** 930–936.

Silva, R.C., Montenegro, M.A., Guerreiro, C.A. & Guerreiro, M.M. (2006): Clobazam as add-on therapy in children with epileptic encephalopathy. *Can. J. Neurol. Sci.* **33,** 209–213.

Singh, R., Andermann, E., Whitehouse, W.P., *et al.* (2001): Severe myoclonic epilepsy of infancy: extended spectrum of GEFS+? *Epilepsia* **42,** 837–844.

Stafstrom, C.E. & Benke, T.A. (2008): Early-life seizures and cognitive impairment: a spiny problem? *Epilepsy Curr.* **8,** 27–28.

Stafstrom, C.E. (2006): Behavioral and cognitive testing procedures in animal models of epilepsy. In: *Models of seizures and epilepsy*, eds. A. Pitkanen, P.A. Schwartzkroin & S.L. Moshe, pp. 613–628. Amsterdam: Elsevier.

Steriade, M., Amzica, F. & Contreras, D. (1994): Cortical and thalamic cellular correlates of electroencephalographic burst-suppression. *Electroencephalogr. Clin. Neurophysiol.* **90,** 1–16.

Stores, G. (1990): Electroencephalographic parameters in assessing the cognitive function of children with epilepsy. *Epilepsia* **31** (Suppl. 4), 45–49.

Striano, P., Bordo, L., Lispi, M.L., *et al.* (2006): A novel SCN2A mutation in family with benign familial infantile seizures. *Epilepsia* **47,** 218–220.

Sutula, T. & Pitkänen, A. (2002): *Do seizures damage the brain?* Amsterdam: Elsevier.

Sutula, T.P., Hagen, J. & Pitkanen, A. (2003): Do epileptic seizures damage the brain? *Curr. Opin. Neurol.* **16,** 189–195.

Suzuki, Y., Nagai, T., Ono, *et al.* (1997): Zonisamide monotherapy in newly diagnosed infantile spasms. *Epilepsia* **38,** 1035–1038.

Suzuki, M., Okumura, A., Watanabe, K., *et al.* (2003): The predictive value of electroencephalogram during early infancy for later development of West syndrome in infants with cystic periventricular leukomalacia. *Epilepsia* **44,** 443–446.

Swann, J.W. (1995): Synaptogenesis and epileptogenesis in developing neural networks. In: *Brain development and epilepsy*, eds. P.A. Schwartzkroin, S.L. Moshe, J.L. Noebels & J.W. Swann, pp. 195-233. New York: Oxford University Press.

Swann, J.W., Le, J.T., Lam, T.T., Owens, J. & Meyer, A.T. (2007a): The impact of chronic network hyperexcitability on developing glutamatergic synapses. *Eur. J. Neurosci.* **26,** 975–991.

Swann, J.W., Le, J.T. & Lee, C.L. (2007b): Recurrent seizures and the molecular maturation of hippocampal and neocortical glutamatergic synapses. *Dev. Neurosci.* **29,** 168–178.

Szepetowski, P., Rochette, J., Berquin, P., Piussan, C., Lathrop, G.M. & Monaco, A.P. (1997): Familial infantile convulsions and paroxysmal choreoathetosis: a new neurological syndrome linked to the pericentromeric region of human chromosome 16. *Am. J. Hum. Genet.* **61,** 889–898.

Tagawa, T., Otani, K., Futagi, Y., Wakayama, A., Morimoto, K. & Morita, Y. (1996): Clinical and electroencephalographic studies in children with hemimegalencephaly. *No To Hattatsu* **28,** 53–59.

Takenaka, J., Aso, K., Watanabe, K., Okumura, A. & Negoro, T. (2000): Transient seizure remission in intractable localization-related epilepsy. *Pediatr. Neurol.* **23,** 328–331.

Tassinari, C.A. & Rubboli, G. (2006): Cognition and paroxysmal EEG activities: from a single spike to electrical status epilepticus during sleep. *Epilepsia* **47,** 40–43.

Tauck, D. & Nadler, J.V. (1985): Evidence of functional mossy fiber sprouting in the hippocampal formation of kainic acid-treated rats. *J. Neurosci.* **5,** 1016–1022.

Toribe, Y. (2001): High-dose vitamin B(6) treatment in West syndrome. *Brain Dev.* **23,** 654–657.

Trevathan, E., Murphy, C.C. & Yeargin-Allsopp, M. (1999): The descriptive epidemiology of infantile spasms among Atlanta children. *Epilepsia* 40, 748–751.

Tsai, F.J., Hsieh, Y.Y., Chang, C.C., Lin, C.C. & Tsai, C.H. (2002): Polymorphisms for interleukin 1 beta exon 5 and interleukin 1 receptor antagonist in Taiwanese children with febrile convulsions. *Arch. Pediatr. Adolesc. Med.* **156**, 545–548.

Vasconcellos, E., Wyllie, E., Sullivan, S., *et al.* (2001): Mental retardation in pediatric candidates for epilepsy surgery: the role of early seizure onset. *Epilepsia* **42**, 268–274.

Veggiotti, P., Cieuta, C., Rex, E. & Dulac, O. (1994): Lamotrigine in infantile spasms. *Lancet* **344**, 1375–1376.

Veneselli, E., Perrone, M.V., Di Rocco, M., Gaggero, R. & Biancheri, R. (2001): Malignant migrating partial seizures in infancy. *Epilepsy Res.* **46**, 27–32.

Verhage, M., de Vries, K.J., Røshol, H., Burbach, J.P., Gispen, W.H. & Südhof, T.C. (1997): DOC2 proteins in rat brain: complementary distribution and proposed function as vesicular adapter proteins in early stages of secretion. *Neuron* **18**, 453–461.

Verity, C.M., Butler, N.R. & Golding, J. (1985): Febrile convulsions in a national cohort followed fron the birth. Prevalence and recurrence in the first years of life. *BMJ* **290**, 1307–1310.

Vestergaard, M., Hviid, A., Madsen, K.M., *et al.* (2004): MMR vaccination and febrile seizures: evaluation of susceptible subgroups and long-term prognosis. *JAMA* **292**, 351–357.

Vezzani, A. & Baram, T.Z. (2007): New roles for interleukin-1 beta in the mechanisms of epilepsy. *Epilepsy Curr.* **7**, 45–50.

Vigevano, F. & Cilio, M.R. (1997): Vigabatrin versus ACTH as first-line treatment for infantile spasms: a randomized, prospective study. *Epilepsia* **38**, 1270–1274.

Vigevano, F. & Bureau, M. (2005): Idiopathic and/or benign localization-related epilepsies in infants. In: *Epileptic syndromes in infancy, childhood and adolescence*, 4th ed., eds. J. Roger, M. Bureau, C. Dravet, P. Genton, & P. Wolf, pp. 171–179. London: John Libbey.

Vigevano, F., Fusco, L., Di Capua, M., Ricci, S., Sebastianelli, R. & Lucchini, P. (1992): Benign infantile familial convulsions. *Eur. J. Pediatr.* **151**, 608–612.

Vigevano, F., Fusco, L., Cusmai, R., Claps, D., Ricci, S. & Milani, L. (1993): The idiopathic form of West syndrome. *Epilepsia* **34**, 743–746.

Watanabe, K., Yamamoto, N., Negoro, T., *et al.* (1987): Benign complex partial epilepsies in infancy. *Pediatr. Neurol.* **3**, 208–211.

Watanabe, K., Yamamoto, N., Negoro, T., Takahashi, I., Aso, K. & Maehara, M. (1990): Benign infantile epilepsy with complex partial seizures. *J. Clin. Neurophysiol.* **7**, 409–416.

Watanabe, K., Negoro, T. & Aso, K. (1993): Benign partial epilepsy with secondarily generalized seizures in infancy. *Epilepsia* **34**, 635–638.

Watanabe, K., Haga, T., Negoro, T., Aso, K. & Maeda, N. (1994): Focal spasms in clusters, focal delayed myelination, and hypsarrhythmia: unusual variant of West syndrome. *Pediatr. Neurol.* **11**, 47–49.

Watanabe, K., Okumura, A., Aso, K. & Duchowny, M. (2005): Non-idiopathic localization-related epilepsies in infants and young children. In: *Epileptic syndromes in infancy, childhood and adolescence*, 4th ed., eds. J. Roger, M. Bureau, C. Dravet, P. Genton & P. Wolf, pp. 181–202. London: John Libbey.

Webb, S.J., Monk, C.S. & Nelson, C.A. (2001): Mechanisms of postnatal neurobiological development: implications for human development. *Dev. Neuropsychol.* **19**, 147–171.

West, W.J. (1841): On particular form of infantile convulsions. *Lancet* I, 724–725.

Wilmshurst, J.M., Appleton, D.B. & Grattan-Smith, P.J. (2000): Migrating partial seizures in infancy: two new cases. *J. Child Neurol.* **15**, 717–722.

Witter, M.P. (1989): Connectivity of the rat hippocampus. In: *Neurology and neurobiology, vol. 52: The hippocampus – new vistas*, eds. V. Chan-Palay & C. Kohler, pp. 53–69. New York: Alan R. Liss.

Wolff, M., Cassé-Perrot, C. & Dravet, C. (2006): Severe myoclonic epilepsy of infants (Dravet syndrome): natural history and neuropsychological findings. *Epilepsia* **47** (Suppl. 2), 45–48.

Wong, M. (2005): Modulation of dendritic spines in epilepsy: cellular mechanisms and functional implications. *Epilepsy Behav.* **7**, 569–577.

Wong, T.T., Kwan, S.Y., Chang, K.P., Hsiu-Mei, W., Yang, T.F., Chen, Y.S. & Yi-Yen, L. (2006): Corpus callosotomy in children. *Childs Nerv. Syst.* **22**, 999–1011.

Wyllie, E. (1998): Surgical treatment of epilepsy in children. *Pediatr. Neurol.* **19**, 179–188.

Wyllie, E., Comair, Y.G., Kotagal, P., Raja, S. & Ruggieri, P. (1996): Epilepsy surgery in infants. *Epilepsia* **37**, 625–637.

Wyllie, E., Comair, Y.G., Kotagal, P., Bulacio, J., Bingaman, W. & Ruggieri, P. (1998): Seizure outcome after epilepsy surgery in children and adolescents. *Ann. Neurol.* **44**, 740–748.

Yakoub, M., Dulac, O., Jambaque, I. & Plouin, P. (1992): Early diagnosis of severe myoclonic epilepsy in infancy. *Brain Dev.* **14,** 299–303.

Yamamoto, H. (1991): Studies on CSF triptophan metabolism in infantile spasms. *Pediatr. Neurol.* **17**, 411–414.

Yamamoto, N., Watanabe, K., Negoro, T., *et al.* (1988): Partial seizures evolving to infantile spasms. *Epilepsia* 29, 34–40.

Chapter 11

Paroxysmal non-epileptic disorders

Federico Vigevano, Raffaella Cusmai and Nicola Specchio

*Division of Neurology, Bambino Gesù Children's Hospital, IRCCS,
Piazza S. Onofrio, 00165 Rome, Italy*
Vigevano@opbg.net

Paroxysmal non-epileptic disorders (PNED) are events characterized by clinical elements that need to be clearly differentiated from epileptic seizures. PNED may appear at any age, although the major incidence is in the paediatric age range, especially during the first years of life. In clinical practice, paediatricians are not infrequently asked to diagnose such events, which could be misdiagnosed as epileptic seizures. A correct diagnosis will avoid useless investigations and unnecessary medication.

The diagnosis of PNED requires a careful history of the episodes and the conditions of their occurrence. This is necessary to determine when the episodes occur, and inquiries should be made about the following: 1) Is the child asleep or awake when they occur? 2) What are the precipitating factors (emotion, anger, tiredness, happiness)? 3) Is there a specific posture when they occur (sitting, walking, high chair or car chair, vertical position)? 4) What is the duration and frequency of the episodes? 5) Are there any other accompanying features? 6) Is there anything that can terminate an episode?

It could also be useful to document the episode by a home video recording. A laboratory polygraphic video-electroencephalographic recording (video-EEG) may provide useful support to prove the absence of epileptiform discharges during the episodes.

Although some patients with epilepsy may also have PNED, interictal epileptiform abnormalities that may appear during an EEG are not proof of epileptic seizures in the absence of definitive ictal symptomatology.

Differential diagnosis can be difficult. PNED and epileptic seizures may have similar semeiology: syncope may appear with diffuse tonic and clonic manifestations mimicking generalized tonic-clonic epileptic seizures, and epileptic myoclonus is hardly distinguishable from non-epileptic myoclonus by clinical observation alone.

Epileptic seizures and PNED may coexist in the same patient: a patient affected by 'alternating hemiplegia of childhood' might have both non-epileptic paroxysmal manifestations and epileptic seizures, and many adolescents with epilepsy may experience pseudo-seizures.

Epileptic seizures and PNED may occur in close sequence, as one could be the consequence of the other. During breath-holding spells, the child has prolonged hypoxia that causes syncope with subsequent rapid recovery; in rare cases, this hypoxia may cause a prolonged clonic epileptic seizure. This condition is called 'anoxic-epileptic-seizures' (Horrocks *et al.*, 2005). In contrast, some epileptic seizures – especially in temporal lobe epilepsy – may cause severe bradycardia and therefore inducing syncope (Schuele *et al.*, 2008). In both cases, 'epileptic' and 'non-epileptic' events are not easily distinguishable.

Finally, epileptic seizures and PNED may have the same pathogenesis. Some children with 'benign familial infantile seizures', an autosomal dominant form of epilepsy, could have paroxysmal choreoathetosis during late childhood or even later (Szepetowski *et al.*, 1997). In these cases, the same genetic mutation is responsible for epileptic and non-epileptic seizures during two different stages of life.

Classification

PNED are episodes of a different nature, with variable aetiology and symptomatology; therefore it is difficult to classify them by univocal clinical criteria. In fact, some episodes are 'physiological', such as hypnic myoclonias, while some are only a temporary dysfunction related to maturation of the central nervous system, such as 'benign myoclonus of early infancy' or 'tonic reflex seizures'. Moreover, some have a benign prognosis with spontaneous age-related remission, while others are seen in severe neurological diseases, such as Niemann-Pick disease type C, in which some affected children may have cataplectic attacks.

We propose a classification for PNED according to symptomatology and aetiological criteria (Table 1).

Unusual movements, the most frequent type of PNED in the early years of life, will be described in detail. In *anoxic-ischaemic PNED* we include syncopes and pre-syncopes of cardiac or extracardiac origin. During the first 2 years of life syncope can be triggered by breath-holding spells. In the majority of cases, the characteristics of events such as crying, breath arrest, cyanosis, and loss of consciousness can allow a correct diagnosis.

Sleep-related PNED include myoclonia, jerks, 'sursaut', pavor nocturnus, nightmares, and sleep walking.

Periodic PNED include phenomena which are considered 'migraine equivalents', such as 'paroxysmal vertigo', 'abdominal pain', 'benign paroxysmal torticollis', and 'aura without migraine' (Al-Twaijri & Shevell, 2002).

Breathing disorders such as polypnoea or apnoea may be frequent in children with cognitive delay and pervasive disorders. In Rett syndrome, episodes of polypnoea and apnoea are both present in the same children. In these patients, because of severe mental retardation, apnoea may be misdiagnosed as epileptic absences. Moreover, in some cases prolonged apnoea may be self-induced, leading to syncope.

Table 1: Classification of paroxysmal non-epileptic disorders (PNED)

- Unusual movements
- Anoxic-ischaemic PNED
- Sleep-related PNED
- Periodic PNED
- Breathing disorders
- Drug induced PNED
- Pseudoseizures

Drug-induced: dystonic or athetotic paroxysmal phenomena may also occur as side effects in children treated with certain drugs, such as domperidone.

Pseudo-seizures are clinical manifestations that mimic epileptic seizures and occur in patients with behavioural disturbances.

PNED may occur at any time during the life, the incidence changing according to the age. Particularly frequent in adolescence are behavioural disorders, such as somatoform phenomena and psychotic seizures. Especially relevant during early childhood are PNED related to sleep, such as pavor nocturnus, somnambulism and confused awakening.

Unusual movements

Several types of unusual movements may be noticed during the first years of life. Table 2 gives the unusual movements in chronological order of appearance. About half of these clinical conditions have in common the presence of 'myoclonic jerks', with different types of myoclonus.

Unusual movements characterized by myoclonus

Myoclonus is a motor manifestation with different pathophysiological mechanisms and different aetiologies. There are pathological entities in which myoclonus is the major symptom, and others in which it is part of a wider clinical picture. Myoclonus may also be a physiological event. For these reasons it is not easy to classify the different types of myoclonus and so classifications are subject to continuous revision.

Myoclonus is defined as a sudden, brief, shock-like involuntary movement caused by muscular contractions or inhibitions. Muscular contractions produce a 'positive' myoclonus, whereas muscular inhibitions produce a 'negative' myoclonus. Depending on the distribution, myoclonus can be 'massive' or 'generalized' if it involves all four limbs, or 'segmental' when it involves only a segment of the body, or 'focal', when it is limited to one or more muscle districts. Myoclonus can be 'continuous' or 'intermittent'. When observing a myoclonus, it is important to determine whether it is 'spontaneous', elicited by motion, or by action ('action myoclonus'), or induced by tactile or sound stimuli ('reflex myoclonus').

Myoclonus can be classified into four major categories: physiological, essential, symptomatic and epileptic.

Table 2. Unusual movements of newborns and infants listed following age at onset

- Benign neonatal sleep myoclonus
- Hyperekplexia or startle disease
- Tonic reflex seizures of early infancy
- Benign myoclonus of early infancy
- Alternating hemiplegia of childhood
- Paroxysmal torticollis
- Cataplectic attacks
- Repetitive sleep starts
- Infantile masturbation or self-stimulation
- Tics and Tourette syndrome
- Opsoclonus-myoclonus syndrome

Physiological myoclonus may occur in healthy individuals in particular circumstances, without causing any discomfort. 'Sleep jerks' are a phenomenon occurring in almost the entire population, at all ages, during phases I and II of non-REM sleep. Physiological myoclonus may be present in two well known age-related types of PNED: 'benign neonatal sleep myoclonus' and 'benign myoclonus of early infancy'.

Essential myoclonus is a condition, in most cases inherited, involving the upper limbs in particular, with onset during adolescence.

Symptomatic myoclonus may be evident in different diseases. Myoclonia could be present in many types of both static or progressive encephalopathy including neurodegenerative and metabolic diseases, paraneoplastic syndromes, and infectious or autoimmune encephalitis. We will describe three types of symptomatic myoclonus that start in infancy or childhood: 'exaggerated startle syndrome' or 'hyperekpexia', 'tics and Tourette syndrome', and 'opsoclonus-myoclonus syndrome'.

Epileptic myoclonus is defined (Caviness & Brown, 2004) as 'the presence of myoclonus in the setting of epilepsy, that is a chronic disorder'.

On the basis of the pathophysiological mechanism, myoclonus it is classified as cortical, subcortical or spinal. Epileptic myoclonus originates from cortical or subcortical structures, whereas non-epileptic myoclonus may originate from cortical, subcortical or spinal structures.

Neurophysiological investigations – such as EEG, electromyography (EMG) and somatosensory evoked potentials – may help in understanding the pathophysiological mechanisms underlying the different types of myoclonus (Shibasaki & Hallett, 2005). In epileptic myoclonus an ictal EEG shows epileptiform discharges, while in non-epileptic myoclonus epileptiform discharges are absent. However, it should be born in mind that epileptic myoclonus may not always have a clear epileptiform EEG counterpart.

Benign neonatal sleep myoclonus

This syndrome is characterized by myoclonic jerks occurring solely during 'quiet sleep' in otherwise healthy newborn infants. It is a benign phenomenon spontaneously disappearing within the third to fourth month of life. Myoclonia may occur either in isolation or in clusters of four to five jerks, which can involve the entire body, or, more frequently, the upper limbs only. They occur daily, though not always during quiet sleep (Coulter & Allen, 1982; Di Capua *et al.*, 1993). The EEG is normal, even during the myoclonus. During awakening or active sleep the myoclonia disappear, this feature being of diagnostic value. Frequently, benign neonatal sleep myoclonus is misdiagnosed as epilepsy, and patients receive antiepileptic drugs without any effect (Egger *et al.*, 2003).

Exaggerated startle syndrome or hyperekplexia

Hyperekplexia is an inherited autosomal dominant disease with onset in the neonatal period, characterized by the presence of pathological startles (Gastaut & Villeneuve, 1967; Andermann *et al.*, 1980). Startle is a normal phenomenon, present at all ages. It consists of a massive myoclonus occurring as a response to violent and unexpected stimuli, disappearing when the stimulus is repeated. A startle response becomes pathological when even minor unexpected stimuli provoke an excessive response, which persists when the stimulus is repeated (Bakker *et al.*, 2006).

Chapter 11 Paroxysmal non-epileptic disorders

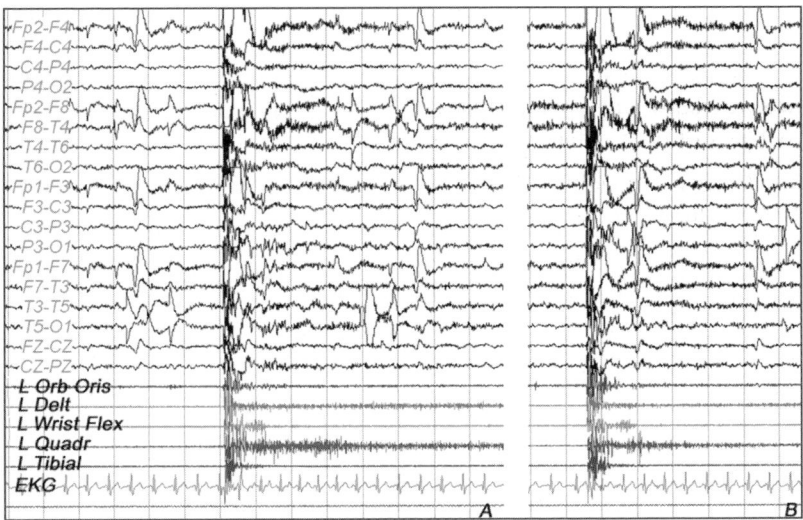

Fig. 1. Two massive myoclonias triggered by sudden and unexpected acoustic stimulus in a patient with symptomatic hyperekplexia.

Neonates with hyperekplexia present with diffuse hypertonia and poor spontaneous movements associated with massive myoclonia, both spontaneous and induced by tactile and acoustic stimuli. The most powerful trigger is tactile stimulation of the face, and, in particular of the nose: repetitive patting of the child's nose provokes a massive myoclonus at each stimulation. During the first months of life the response can be so intense as to provoke prolonged, sometimes life-threatening, stiffness seizures, with cyanosis and bradycardia.

One of us discovered – and this was subsequently confirmed by other investigators – that abrupt flexion of the trunk during the seizure may interrupt it, and this manœuvre should be used to stop the event (Vigevano et al., 1989). Cardiorespiratory monitoring in the first year would enable parents to react promptly when a seizure occurs. After the first year of life, manifestations are less frequent. Stiffness seizures disappear within the first 2 years.

The disease is caused by a genetic glycine receptor defect, with low levels of α-aminobutyric acid (GABA) being found in the liquor in some of the patients. Different mutations in the α1 subunit of inhibitory glycine receptor (GLRA1) gene have been identified in many affected families, usually inherited in an autosomal dominant manner, although there is also evidence of a recessive form. Mutations in the same gene, *GLRA1*, mapping on 5q33.2-q33.3 and encoding for the α1 subunit of the inhibitory glycine receptor chloride channel, determine an increased excitability in pontomedullary reticular neurons and abnormal spinal reciprocal inhibition (Ryan et al., 1992; Gomeza et al., 2003).

Encephalitis and anoxic-ischaemic cerebral injuries especially affecting cerebral trunk and basal nuclei may also cause the hyperekplexia phenomenon, with a poor prognosis (Fig. 1).

Tonic reflex seizures of early infancy

In 2001 Vigevano and Lispi described a new clinical entity – 'tonic reflex seizures of early infancy'(Vigevano & Lispi, 2001). It is a phenomenon observed in normal children usually at the age of 2 to 3 months, in most cases male, who experience tonic contractions, predominantly of the limbs, provoked by shaking or tactile stimulation. Upright rhythmic movements result in a diffuse tonic contraction, associated with breathing arrest and cyanosis which lasts between 3 and 10 seconds. Some mothers become aware of this phenomenon if they descend the stairs while holding the child in an upright position. All the children we observed were born after an uneventful pregnancy with a normal delivery. The phenomenon seems to have a familial occurrence, as we observed the same event in more than one brother. The onset is in most cases during the second month, more rarely during the third. The frequency of the episodes is variable because it is clearly related to the stimulus. The phenomenon could be triggered by tactile proprioceptive stimulation, or sudden postural changes, forward, upward or downward. Sensitivity to stimuli may vary at different times.

Following stimulation, the child has a sudden and sustained diffuse tonic contraction with extension and abduction of all four limbs, more evident in the arms, apnoea and cyanosis without impairment of consciousness (Fig. 2). At the end of the episode the child usually cries for a few seconds, with no other signs. The EEG is normal during both ictal and interictal periods. The phenomenon has a benign outcome and disappears by the age of 4 to 5 months. Psychomotor development is normal and no patients have presented with other paroxysmal events.

Tonic reflex seizures of early infancy need to be differentiated from both non-epileptic and epileptic phenomena. The Monroe reflex is a physiological reflex seen in neonates and characterized by rapid upper limb abduction induced by a stimulus such as 'shivering'. It disappears by the end of the first month. In our experience, the Monroe reflex vanishes before the onset of tonic reflex seizures.

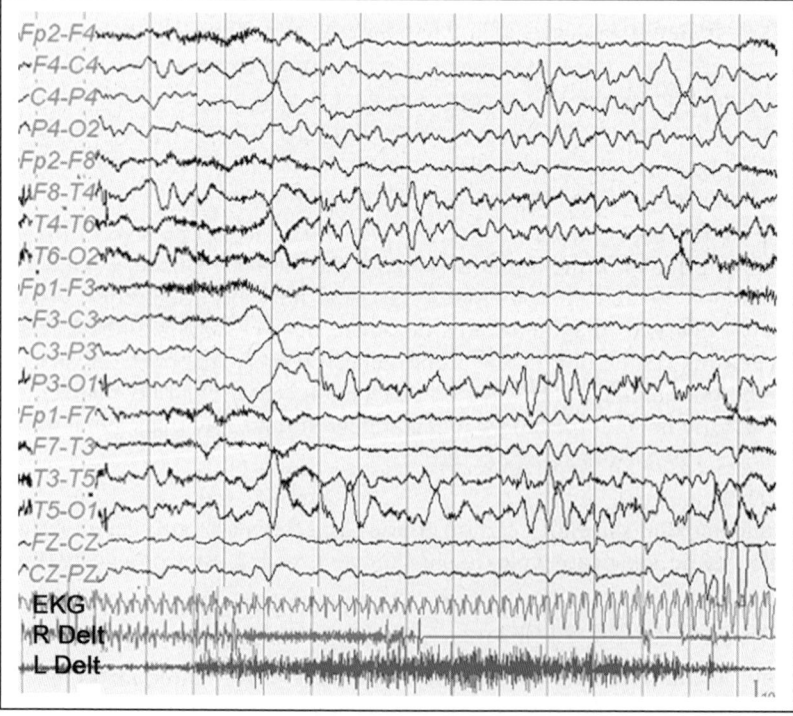

Fig. 2. A sustained tonic contraction induced by shaking in a 2 month old boy.

Children affected by 'paroxysmal extreme pain disorder' (Fertleman *et al.*, 2007) have more prolonged tonic contractions during pain attacks, which are associated with vegetative phenomena and severe bradycardia.

Though epileptic spasms are similar to tonic reflex seizures of early infancy, they usually appear later and are not triggered by sensory stimuli.

In our opinion, tonic reflex seizures of early infancy are the result of an age-dependent hyperexcitability of the labyrinthic system, and the maturation of the latter determines the disappearance of the phenomenon.

Benign myoclonus of early infancy

Benign myoclonus of early infancy (BMEI) was first described by Lombroso and Fejerman, who reported children with episodes resembling infantile spasms but with different clinical, EEG and outcome features, allowing a clear differential diagnosis from West syndrome (Lombroso & Fejerman, 1977). In the original report, the episodes were not recorded electrophysiologically and only a detailed clinical description was provided. Later, the syndrome was more fully delineated by Fejerman (2005).

This is a non-epileptic paroxysmal phenomenon which occurs in healthy children during the first year of life. It is self-limited, with variable duration. The phenomenon usually disappears within the second year of life. The episodes are characterized by repetitive jerks of the neck or upper limbs leading to abrupt flexion or rotation of the head and extension with abduction of limbs without changes in consciousness. Sometimes, a brief tonic flexion involving the upper limbs is associated with the movement. In other cases, head-dropping or a reduction in muscle tone in the trunk imitating epileptic atonia has been observed.

In some patients, the movements are described as a shuddering of the head, shoulders or upper limbs. The intensity and the duration of the motor phenomena can vary, ranging from a single episode to a series of contractions. In the most typical forms the main symptom is a shuddering motor manifestation predominantly involving the axial muscles. No focal signs are observed during the episodes. The EEG is unremarkable during the episodes.

The attacks are usually triggered by alert status, excitation or frustration, and in most cases the events appear in clusters, with intervals of 3–4 minutes between the events. The phenomenon typically occurs in the awake state. With respect to the EMG pattern, the episodes could be classified as myoclonus, spasms and brief tonic contractions, shuddering, atonia or negative myoclonus. The non-epileptic origin of the phenomenon has been demonstrated with polygraphic recordings obtained using video-EEG.

To define the movements the term 'non-epileptic infantile spasms' was proposed by Dravet *et al.* (1986). Pachatz *et al.* (1999), describing five cases, emphasized the 'shuddering' aspect of the event, and, analysing the EMG pattern which lasted more than 200 ms, defined the contractions as brief tonic and not truly myoclonic.

The differential diagnosis of BMEI includes all the non-epileptic conditions displaying abnormal movements with their onset in the first year of life, most of which are described in this chapter. The differential diagnosis must also include epileptic phenomena, as epileptic infantile spasms may resemble BMEI (Maydell *et al.*, 2001). The clinical aspects share common features: infantile spasms, like BMEI, may vary in intensity, ranging from brief movements of the head to typical spasms which consist in an abrupt axial contraction lasting from 1 to 2 seconds. Infantile spasms appear in clusters while in BMEI there is no periodic recurrence. An accurate diagnosis is possible by analysing the interictal and ictal EEG findings.

Alternating hemiplegia of childhood

Alternating hemiplegia is a very rare disease characterized by recurrent attacks of loss of muscular tone causing hypomobility of one side of the body (Andermann et al., 1995). The aetiology of the disease remains unknown. A few familial cases have been described (Kanavakis et al., 2003). Alternating hemiplegia has its onset in the first few months of life. Hemiplegic episodes are often accompanied by other paroxysmal manifestations, such as lateral eye and head deviation toward the hemiplegic side and a peculiar monocular nystagmus. As the attack progresses, hemiplegia can shift to the other side of the body. Sometimes the attack can provoke bilateral paralysis, and these patients may have severe clinical impairment, with difficulty in swallowing and breathing. A unilateral attack, in particular when accompanied by eye and head deviation, may be confused with partial motor seizures. Hemiplegic attacks may be triggered by various stimuli such as a warm bath, motor activity or emotion. The frequency of attacks is high, usually several in a month or in a week. The length is variable from a few minutes to several hours. Sleep can stop the attack. Movement disorders such as dystonia may be present in these patients. Cognitive delay of variable degree is a common feature. Epilepsy has been reported in 50 per cent of the cases, but seizure onset is usually during the 3rd or 4th year of life.

Benign paroxysmal torticollis

Benign paroxysmal torticollis consists of lateral head flexion, sometimes associated with trunk torsion. Its duration ranges from a few seconds to several hours. The deviation side can vary from attack to attack. Onset is generally in early infancy, with symptoms occurring around the first year of life, often associated with neurovegetative disturbances and occasional crying (Drigo et al., 2000). Attacks tend to recur more or less frequently, and generally disappear before the age of 2 years. The differential diagnosis is epileptic seizures. Careful examination is necessary to exclude a posterior cranial fossa tumour. Paroxysmal dizziness and episodes of transient ataxia have been observed in these patients on long term follow up. Benign paroxysmal torticollis may recur periodically and has been considered a migraine equivalent. A linkage to the *CACNA1A* gene has been reported in familial cases (Giffin et al., 2002).

Cataplectic attacks

A cataplectic attack is a sudden loss of muscular tone with preserved consciousness, commonly triggered by a sudden emotional reaction such as fear or laughter. Loss of muscle tone may cause the patient to fall, or experience head dropping. A video-EEG recording during the attack is necessary to exclude atonic epileptic seizures. Cataplexy may have a cryptogenic aetiology or appear during the course of neurodegenerative disorders, such as Niemann-Pick disease type C. It may be also symptomatic of a diencephalic lesion, and has been reported in Prader-Willi syndrome (Tobias et al., 2002). Cataplexy occurs either as an isolated phenomenon or in association with narcolepsy (Challamel et al., 1994).

Repetitive sleep starts

Sleep starts, also known as hypnic or hypnagogic jerks, are a physiological accompaniment of falling asleep. They are brief body jerks, mainly bilateral and sometimes asymmetrical. When excessive at the onset of sleep, they are considered to be parasomnias. Sleep starts are included in the category of sleep-wake transition parasomnias by the *International Classification of Sleep Disorders* (American Sleep Disorders Association, 2001). At times, sleep starts may be extremely numerous and represent a true sleep disorder, characterized by frequent awakenings and difficulty in getting to sleep.

This peculiar type of event consists of a massive myoclonic jerk in which the axial muscles are the main ones involved. Sleep starts may be accompanied by a dream, or by the impression of falling. They represent partial activation of the central nervous system, producing skeletal muscle activity. Their pathogenesis is unknown. A possible mechanism is a synchronous volley of pyramidal tract activity arising during the transition from wakefulness to sleep (Broughton, 1994). The involvement of the axial muscles, the possible reflex origin, and the absence of EEG abnormalities make a subcortical origin likely. Other studies have suggested a possible role of N-methyl-D-aspartic acid (NMDA) and serotoninergic system dysfunction in the pathogenesis (Lai & Siegel, 1997).

Sleep starts are very common, with a prevalence of about 60 to 70 per cent of the population. Rarely, intensified sleep starts produce a sleep-onset insomnia. Excessive sleep starts have been reported in normal subjects after caffeine intoxication, excessive physical exercise or non-specific stress, and in patients with parkinsonism, in post-polio syndrome (Bruno, 1998), or in children with migraine (Bruni *et al.*, 1999). A syndrome of excessive sleep starts occurring in clusters at the onset of sleep has been reported by one of us in neurologically impaired children (Fusco *et al.*, 1999). We observed and described the repetitive occurrence of sleep starts in epileptic children with spastic-dystonic diplegia, with pyramidal or extrapyramidal features and cognitive deficits. Patients previously experienced epileptic seizures during the first year, and sometimes they had a diagnosis of West syndrome or more often focal motor epilepsy. The onset of repetitive sleep starts was reported during the second year of life. Children begin to have 'multiple spasms' during the initial phase of sleep which appeared to the parents to be a new type of epileptic seizure. Video/EEG recordings of the episodes usually show the presence of clusters of massive myoclonic/tonic contractions, in the transition phase between wakefulness and sleep stage I, without any EEG changes. Each muscle contraction usually lasts from 500 ms to 5 s (Fig. 3), depending on the rapidity of the contraction, which can be more or less tonic. No epileptiform activity is seen during the episode and an arousal response often follows the jerks.

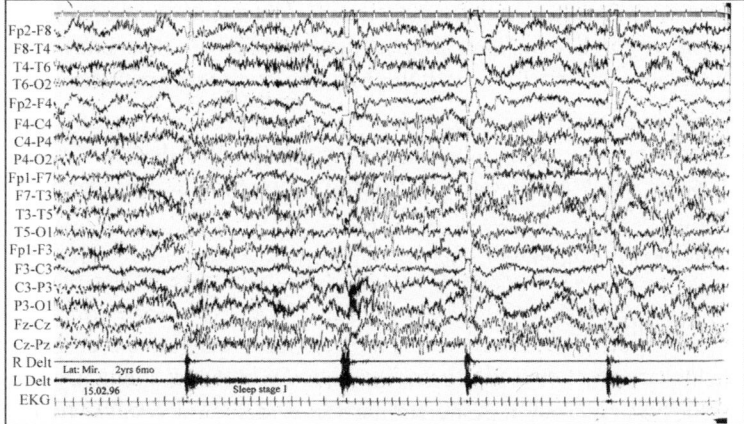

Fig. 3. Periodic brief tonic contraction, with an EMG counterpart resembling epileptic spasms, in a 2‰ year old boy during sleep stage I.

Sleep starts needs to be differentiated from other paroxysmal movements occurring during sleep, such as physiological hypnic myoclonus, which is a normal sleep phenomenon. Another condition to be excluded is benign neonatal sleep myoclonus, described above. Sleep starts may be similar to proprio-spinal myoclonus which occurs during the transition between wakefulness and sleep: affected individuals experience myoclonic jerks when they try to sleep or during awakening.

Clinical characteristics are similar to a startle, although the duration exceeds that usually accepted for physiological sleep starts. Even in normal subjects sleep starts can occur as a brief cluster, reflecting the physiological oscillation between sleep and wakefulness during the period of falling asleep. In neurologically impaired subjects, this oscillation can be enhanced by the lack of physiological inhibition of the pyramidal tract caused by pyramidal lesions.

Sleep starts usually remit spontaneously. Where they are associated with sleep-onset insomnia, the use of low doses of benzodiazepines should be considered. Parents have suggested that the phenomenon can be reduced if the child lies in the prone position, and this position is now recommended rather than drug therapy. The prone position can limit the extent of the movements, preventing arousal and improving the child's ability to fall asleep.

Infantile masturbation or self-stimulation

Infantile masturbation, known as self-stimulation, is frequent. Onset usually occurs after the age of 3 months and before 3 years. Episodes are stereotyped with variable duration. Common features in infants are stereotyped posturing of the legs with pressure on the perineum, irregular breathing, facial flushing and diaphoresis, and vocalizations (Mallants & Casteels, 2008; Omran *et al.*, 2008). At the plateau stage, contractions become rhythmic and the body can then momentarily stiffen. This is followed by the resolution phase in which muscular tension decreases. Consciousness is preserved but some children appear to have altered consciousness with a glassy-eyed fixed gaze and stare; distraction stops the episodes. Duration is from seconds or minutes up to several hours, the frequency ranging from once to several times a day. All children are responsive to their parents during the episodes which can occur in a car seat, in a walker or high chair, or when child is tired or annoyed. The diagnosis of infantile masturbation is more difficult when the infant seems unhappy during the rhythmic movements. Differential diagnosis includes paroxysmal dyskinesia, dystonic posturing, abdominal pain and epilepsy. Direct observation, parental interrogation and videotaping are very useful for diagnosis and to avoid excessive and unnecessary investigations. One of the most important features of childhood masturbation is cessation when child is distracted by parents or becomes engaged in another activity. Although the phenomenon is more frequent in girls, it may also be present in a boys.

The term 'masturbation' may be not accepted by parents and we prefer use the term 'self-stimulation' or gratification. It is useful to suggest to parents that they distract the child during masturbatory activity. These behaviours are normal in infantile development.

Little information is available on the long term follow-up of children with masturbatory behaviour. Most have normal development and the masturbation behaviours subside.

Tics and Tourette syndrome

Tics are movement disorders that are very common during childhood, although rarely occurring in late infancy. Some simple tics may be similar to segmental or focal myoclonus, involving the face and limbs in particular. More complex tics resemble choreiform movements or obsessive-compulsive behaviours (Dooley, 2006).

Their aetiology is unknown. Psychological factors are undoubtedly important but seem to affect only whether the course is favourable or unfavourable. Because of the similarity to choreiform movements, some investigators have suggested that streptococcal infections may be important as triggers for several types of movement and behaviour disorder named 'paediatric autoimmune neuropsychiatric disorders associated with streptococcus' (PANDAS) (Murphy et al., 2007). The course of the tics is variable. The majority of patients have complete spontaneous remission within a few months.

Tics are also the cardinal feature of Tourette syndrome, a childhood-onset neurobehavioural disorder characterized by a chronic inability to suppress, or by an urge to perform, patterned repetitive movements. In addition to tics, patients with Tourette syndrome most commonly have attention deficit hyperactivity and obsessive-compulsive behaviour (Goodman et al., 2006; Canitano & Vivanti, 2007).

Tourette syndrome often has an unfavourable outcome because of the chronicity of the symptoms. The aetiology is unknown, but basal ganglia and frontal cortical circuits are involved. Recent anatomical and neuroimaging studies have provided evidence for abnormal basal ganglia and dopaminergic dysfunction (Albin & Mink, 2006).

Tics do not always require medical treatment. Education and reassurance for the child and parents and psychological counselling can be important. Medical treatment in selected cases can reduce tics but most probably will not eliminate them. The most widely used drugs are dopamine antagonists, the most successful being haloperidol and pimozide and, most recently, risperidone (Gilbert, 2006). Patients with drug-resistant Tourette syndrome have been treated with functional neurosurgery (Albin & Mink, 2006), apparently with good results.

Opsoclonus-myoclonus syndrome

The opsoclonus-myoclonus syndrome (OMS) is a rare disorder characterized by multidirectional chaotic eyes movements, myoclonus and ataxia. This syndrome is considered to be an autoimmune disease caused by a cell-mediated immune response (Sottini et al., 2007). OMS occurs in children mainly in association with neuroblastoma, and in adults with breast cancer, lymphoma or melanoma. OMS may also appear following minor viral infections or vaccination. The clinical features and course are not very different between the forms that are associated with tumours and those that are not (Plantaz et al., 2000; Tate et al., 2005; Baets et al., 2006). However, the high incidence of spontaneous regression of neuroblastoma suggests that, even when a tumour is not found, the aetiology of this syndrome is in most cases paraneoplastic and it should be treated accordingly.

The syndrome has been described at all ages, but in the majority of cases the onset is during the second year of life. The earliest symptoms are generally staggering and falling, leading to a misdiagnosis of acute cerebellitis. Subsequently, myoclonias appear, which are mostly segmental and multifocal, occurring both at rest and exacerbated by movements. Irregular eye movements in all directions occur (opsoclonus), and irritability, rage attacks and sleep disturbances are common.

Chronicity is the rule. Complete resolution of neurological symptoms after surgery for neuroblastoma is extremely rare. Thus all cases, whether associated with tumours or not, need pharmacological treatment. ACTH, prednisone and intravenous immunoglobulin have all been used successfully; however, ACTH seems to give the best results (Pranzatelli et al., 2005a). Trazodone may be useful for treating sleep disturbances and rage attacks (Pranzatelli et al., 2005b).

More than half the children have relapses. Mild behavioural, language and cognitive problems are seen on long term follow-up.

Experimental studies suggest that a CSF B-cell expansion in OMS is characteristic and often persistent, revealing local antibody production (Pranzatelli *et al.*, 2004a, 2004b). Rituximab, an anti-CD 20 monoclonal antibody, causes a reduction in CSF B-cell expansion, with clinical improvement (Pranzatelli *et al.*, 2006).

References

Albin, R.L. & Mink, J.W. (2006): Recent advances in Tourette syndrome research. *Trends Neurosci.* **29**, 175–182.

Al-Twaijri, W.A. & Shevell, M.I. (2002): Pediatric migraine equivalents: occurrence and clinical features in practice. *Pediatr. Neurol.* **26**, 365–368.

American Sleep Disorders Association (2001): *International classification of sleep disorders: diagnostic and coding manual (revised).* Rochester (MN): American Sleep Disorders Association.

Andermann, F., Aicardi, J. & Vigevano, F. (1995): *Alternating hemiplegia of childhood.* New York: Raven Press.

Andermann, F., Keene, D.L., Andermann, E. & Quesney, L.F. (1980): Startle disease or hyperekplexia: further delineation of the syndrome. *Brain* **103**, 985–997.

Baets, J., Pals, P., Bergmans, B., Foncke, E., Smets, K., Hauman, H., Vanderwegen, L. & Cras, P. (2006): Opsoclonus-myoclonus syndrome: a clinicopathological confrontation. *Acta Neurol. Belg.* **106**, 142–146.

Bakker, M.J., van Dijk, J.G., van den Maagdenberg, A.M. & Tijssen, M.A. (2006): Startle syndrome. *Lancet Neurol.* **5**, 513–524.

Broughton, R.J. (1994): Parasomnias. In: *Sleep disorders medicine: basic sciences, technical considerations, and clinical aspects*, ed. S. Chokroverty, pp. 381–399. Boston: Butterworth-Heinemann.

Bruni, O., Galli, F. & Guidetti, V. (1999): Sleep hygiene and migraine in children and adolescence. *Cephalalgia* **19** (suppl. 25), 57–59.

Bruno, R.L. (1998): Abnormal movements in sleep as a post-polio sequelae. *Am. J. Phys. Med. Rehabil.* **77**, 339–343.

Canitano, R. & Vivanti, G. (2007): Tics and Tourette syndrome in autism spectrum disorders. *Autism* **11**, 19–28.

Caviness, J.N. & Brown, P. (2004): Myoclonus: current concepts and recent advances. *Lancet Neurol.* **3**, 598–607.

Challamel, M.J., Mazzola, M.E., Nevsimalova, S., Cannard, C., Louis, J. & Revol, M. (1994): Narcolepsy in children. *Sleep* **17** (Suppl. 8), 17–20.

Coulter, D.L. & Allen, R.J. (1982): Benign neonatal sleep myoclonus. *Arch. Neurol.* **39**, 191–192.

Di Capua, M., Fusco, L., Ricci, S. & Vigevano, F. (1993): Benign neonatal sleep myoclonus: clinical features and video-polygraphic recordings. *Mov. Disord.* **8**, 191–194.

Dooley, J.M. (2006): Tic disorders in childhood. *Semin. Pediatr. Neurol.* **13**, 231–242.

Dravet, C., Giraud, N., Bureau, M., Roger, J., Gobbi, G. & Dalla Bernardina, B. (1986): Benign myoclonus of early infancy or benign non-epileptic infantile spasms. *Neuropediatrics* **17**, 33–38.

Drigo, P., Carli, G. & Laverda, A.M. (2000): Benign paroxysmal torticollis of infancy. *Brain Dev.* **22**, 169–172.

Egger, J., Grossmann, G. & Auchterlonie, I.A. (2003): Benign sleep myoclonus in infancy mistaken for epilepsy. *BMJ* **326**, 975–976.

Fejerman, N. (2005): Nonepileptic disorders imitating generalized idiopathic epilepsies. *Epilepsia* **46** (Suppl. 9), 80–83.

Fertleman, C.R., Ferrie, C.D., Aicardi, J., Bednarek, N.A., Eeg-Olofsson, O., Elmslie, F.V., Griesemer, D.A., Goutières, F., Kirkpatrick, M., Malmros, I.N., Pollitzer, M., Rossiter, M., Roulet-Perez, E., Schubert, R., Smith, V.V., Testard, H., Wong, V. & Stephenson, J.B. (2007): Paroxysmal extreme pain disorder (previously familial rectal pain syndrome). *Neurology* **69**, 586–595.

Fusco, L., Pachatz, C., Cusmai, R. & Vigevano, F. (1999): Repetitive sleep starts in neurologically impaired children: an unusual non-epileptic manifestation in otherwise epileptic subjects. *Epileptic Disord.* **1**, 63–67.

Gastaut, H. & Villeneuve, A. (1967): The startle disease. Pathological surprise reaction. *J. Neurol. Sci.* **5**, 523–542.

Giffin, N.J., Benton, S. & Goadsby, P.J. (2002): Benign paroxysmal torticollis of infancy: four new cases and linkage to CACNA1A mutation. *Dev. Med. Child Neurol.* **44**, 490–493.

Gilbert, D. (2006): Treatment of children and adolescents with tics and Tourette syndrome. *J. Child Neurol.* **21**, 690–700.

Gomeza, J., Ohno, K., Hulsmann, S., Armsen, W., Eulenburg, V., Richter, D.W., Laube, B. & Betz, H. (2003): Deletion of the mouse glycine transporter 2 results in a hyperekplexia phenotype and postnatal lethality. *Neuron* **40**, 797–806.

Goodman, W.K., Storch, E.A., Geffken, G.R. & Murphy, T.K. (2006): Obsessive-compulsive disorder in Tourette syndrome. *J. Child Neurol.* **21**, 704–714.

Horrocks, I.A., Nechay, A., Stephenson, J.B. & Zuberi, S.M. (2005): Anoxic-epileptic seizures: observational study of epileptic seizures induced by syncopes. *Arch. Dis. Child.* **90**, 1283–1287.

Kanavakis, E., Xaidara, A., Papathanasiou-Klontza, D., Papadimitriou, A., Valentza, S. & Youroukos, S. (2003): Alternating hemiplegia of childhood: a syndrome inherited with an autosomal dominant trait. *Dev. Med. Child Neurol.* **45**, 833–836.

Lai, Y.Y. & Siegel, J.M. (1997): Brainstem-mediated locomotion and myoclonic jerks. II. Pharmacological effects. *Brain Res.* **745**, 265–270.

Lombroso, C.T. & Fejerman, N. (1977): Benign myoclonus of early infancy. *Ann. Neurol.* **1**, 138–143.

Mallants, C. & Casteels, K. (2008): Practical approach to childhood masturbation – a review. *Eur. J. Pediatr.* **167**, 1111–1117.

Maydell, B.V., Berenson, F., Rothner, A.D., Wyllie, E. & Kotagal, P. (2001): Benign myoclonus of early infancy: an imitator of West's syndrome. *J. Child Neurol.* **16**, 109–112.

Murphy, T.K., Snider, L.A., Mutch, P.J., Harden, E., Zaytoun, A., Edge, P.J., Storch, E.A., Yang, M.C., Mann, G., Goodman, W.K. & Swedo, S.E. (2007): Relationship of movements and behaviors to group a streptococcus infections in elementary school children. *Biol. Psychiatry* **61**, 279–284.

Omran, M.S., Ghofrani, M. & Juibary, A.G. (2008): Infantile masturbation and paroxysmal disorders. *Indian J. Pediatr.* **75**, 183–185.

Pachatz, C., Fusco, L. & Vigevano, F. (1999): Benign myoclonus of early infancy. *Epileptic Disord.* **1**, 57–61.

Plantaz, D., Michon, J., Valteau-Couanet, D., Coze, C., Chastagner, P., Bergeron, C., Nelken, B., Martelli, H., Peyroulet, M.C., Carpentier, A.F., Armari-Alla, C., Pagnier, A. & Rubie, H. (2000): Opsoclonus-myoclonus syndrome associated with non-metastatic neuroblastoma. Long-term survival. Study of the French Society of Pediatric Oncologists. *Arch. Pediatr.* **7**, 621–628.

Pranzatelli, M.R., Hyland, K., Tate, E.D., Arnold, L.A., Allison, T.J. & Soori, G.S. (2004a): Evidence of cellular immune activation in children with opsoclonus-myoclonus: cerebrospinal fluid neopterin. *J. Child Neurol.* **19**, 919–924.

Pranzatelli, M.R., Travelstead, A.L., Tate, E.D., Allison, T.J. & Verhulst, S.J. (2004b): CSF B-cell expansion in opsoclonus-myoclonus syndrome: a biomarker of disease activity. *Mov. Disord.* **19**, 770–777.

Pranzatelli, M.R., Chun, K.Y., Moxness, M., Tate, E.D. & Allison, T.J. (2005a): Cerebrospinal fluid ACTH and cortisol in opsoclonus-myoclonus: effect of therapy. *Pediatr. Neurol.* **33**, 121–126.

Pranzatelli, M.R., Tate, E.D., Dukart, W.S., Flint, M.J., Hoffman, M.T. & Oksa, A.E. (2005b): Sleep disturbance and rage attacks in opsoclonus-myoclonus syndrome: response to trazodone. *J. Pediatr.* **147**, 372–378.

Pranzatelli, M.R., Tate, E.D., Travelstead, A.L., Barbosa, J., Bergamini, R.A., Civitello, L., Franz, D.N., Greffe, B.S., Hanson, R.D., Hurwitz, C.A., Kalinyak, K.A., Kelfer, H., Khakoo, Y., Mantovani, J.F., Nicholson, S.H., Sanders, J.M. & Wegner, S. (2006): Rituximab (anti-CD20) adjunctive therapy for opsoclonus-myoclonus syndrome. *J. Pediatr. Hematol. Oncol.* **28**, 585–593.

Ryan, S.G., Sherman, S.L., Terry, J.C., Sparkes, R.S., Torres, M.C. & Mackey, R.W. (1992): Startle disease, or hyperekplexia: response to clonazepam and assignment of the gene (STHE) to chromosome 5q by linkage analysis. *Ann. Neurol.* **31**, 663–668.

Schuele, S.U., Bermeo, A.C., Locatelli, E., Burgess, R.C. & Lüders, H.O. (2008): Ictal asystole: a benign condition? *Epilepsia* **49**, 168–171.

Shibasaki, H. & Hallett, M. (2005): Electrophysiological studies of myoclonus. *Muscle Nerve* **31**, 157–174.

Sottini, A., Micheli, R., Ghidini, C., Valotti, M., Airo, P., Caimi, L. & Imberti, L. (2007): T-lymphocyte production, function, and death in children who recovered from opsoclonus-myoclonus syndrome. *Pediatr. Hematol. Oncol.* **24**, 23–27;

Szepetowski, P., Rochette, J., Berquin, P., Piussan, C., Lathrop, G.M. & Monaco, A.P. (1997): Familial infantile convulsions and paroxysmal choreoathetosis: a new neurological syndrome linked to the pericentromeric region of human chromosome 16. *Am. J. Hum. Genet.* **61**, 889–898.

Tate, E.D., Allison, T.J., Pranzatelli, M.R. & Verhulst, S.J. (2005): Neuroepidemiologic trends in 105 US cases of pediatric opsoclonus-myoclonus syndrome. *J. Pediatr. Oncol. Nurs.* **22**, 8–19.

Tobias, E.S., Tolmie, J.L. & Stephenson, J.B. (2002): Cataplexy in the Prader-Willi syndrome. *Arch. Dis. Child.* **87**, 170.

Vigevano, F., Di Capua, M. & Dalla Bernardina, B. (1989): Startle disease: an avoidable cause of sudden infant death. *Lancet* i, 216.

Vigevano, F. & Lispi, M.L. (2001): Tonic reflex seizures of early infancy: an age related non-epileptic paroxysmal disorder. *Epileptic Disord.* **3**, 133–136.

Chapter 12

The infant with neuromuscular disorders

Eugenio Mercuri, Paolo Alfieri and Marika Pane

*Child Neuropsychiatry Unit, Policlinico Gemelli, Catholic University,
Largo Agostino Gemelli 8, 00168 Rome, Italy*
eumercuri@gmail.com

The field of neuromuscular disorders has been growing rapidly in the past few years, mainly as a result of a rapid improvement in our understanding of the genetic basis of these disorders. In the last two decades more than 200 responsible loci have been identified, allowing a much better definition of the clinical phenotypes associated with the various forms.

Many of these disorders have their onset at birth or in the first years after birth, with delayed motor milestones as the presenting clinical sign. In this chapter we will review the current state of knowledge of the neuromuscular disorders with their clinical onset in the first years, focusing on their clinical presentation and giving an update on the rational approach to the diagnosis for each form.

Clinical presentation

A neuromuscular disorder should be suspected when the infant has a problem such as weakness, hypotonia, contractures, feeding difficulty or persistent ventilatory failure. Hypotonia is the most typical and common symptom of neuromuscular involvement in infancy but it can frequently also be found in infants with genetic or metabolic diseases and central nervous system involvement (Dubowitz, 1980; Vasta *et al.*, 2005). The differential diagnosis is not always easy but a detailed clinical examination and a good clinical and obstetric history can provide important diagnostic clues to distinguish infants with peripheral involvement from those with a non-neuromuscular aetiology.

In a recent study (Vasta *et al.*, 2005) we have retrospectively assessed the main clinical features that present in infancy in association with hypotonia, establishing their sensitivity and specificity for identifying neuromuscular disorders. The results of our study suggest that marked weakness, with absent or extremely reduced antigravity movements and contractures, are the signs that can most reliably identify infants with neuromuscular disorders.

Weakness

Weakness can be investigated by looking for the presence or absence of antigravity movements. It is essential that movements are judged not only at rest but also during possible peaks of activity, such as when the infant is crying or stimulated. Weak children, such as those with neuromuscular involvement, will show little movement, even in response to stimulation. Infants with CNS insults, in contrast, may move little but are likely to show occasional antigravity movements. The observation of even isolated good resistance and antigravity movements – for example, in response to painful stimuli or during a seizure – is a sign that the muscle is 'strong enough' to perform the movements and therefore that there is no weakness. This suggests that in these cases the paucity of movement is related to an abnormal control of movements because of CNS involvement rather than a peripheral problem. *Facial weakness* is often a sign of muscle diseases – such as myotonic dystrophy, congenital myopathies and congenital muscular dystrophy – but normal facial movements do not exclude a neuromuscular problem, as observed in infants with spinal muscular atrophy.

Fixed joint contractures

Fixed joint contractures are also frequent in infants with neuromuscular disorders. Contractures are often severe at birth because of immobility *in utero*, but may also present after the neonatal period and in some cases may become more obvious after the first year. Bilateral talipes equinovarus is common and is classically described in infants with congenital myotonic dystrophy, congenital myopathies and in some forms of congenital muscular dystrophy. Extended talipes is more rarely observed and is found in central core disease and Ullrich congenital muscular dystrophy.

Reflexes

Reflexes are usually absent or reduced in neuromuscular disorders. Normal reflexes in a floppy infant can almost exclude spinal muscular atrophy or severe peripheral neuropathy but their absence does not necessarily suggest a muscle disorder.

Swallowing and respiratory movements

The assessment of swallowing difficulties and of respiratory muscle movements is also important, though these signs, when present, are not as specific as the presence of weakness or contractures. Children with severe weakness might be totally unable to swallow their own secretions and often have feeding difficulties. The pattern of respiratory involvement can, in some circumstances, help suggest a specific neuromuscular disorder. Diaphragmatic weakness with abdominal paradox can be found in some conditions, such as diaphragmatic spinal muscular atrophy (SMA), congenital muscular dystrophy, some of the congenital myopathies such as myotubular, nemaline and minicore, and congenital myasthenia. In contrast, in spinal muscular atrophy the weakness is mainly intercostal, the breathing pattern is abdominal and the rib cage moves paradoxically with the abdomen.

Other signs

Other signs, such as brisk reflexes or visual and auditory attention and level of alertness are generally (but not always) preserved in infants with neuromuscular disorders. In an encephalopathic infant who is also weak and has contractures, CNS involvement is associated with a neuromuscular disorder.

Onset and timing

Some disorders may already have an antenatal onset, while others present in the immediate newborn period and some are delayed for hours or days after birth. For example, myotonic dystrophy is associated with an antenatal onset, while neonatal myasthenia usually presents a few hours after birth, and the mitochondrial myopathies or spinal muscular atrophy may present a few days after birth, or there may be a period of normality before the onset of weakness.

In the cases with antenatal onset, an obstetric history can help to identify cases in whom reduced fetal movements throughout the pregnancy, or normal movements initially followed by later reduction or polyhydramnios, suggest weakness with onset *in utero*.

Family history

As most neonatal neuromuscular disorders are genetic, it is important to inquire about any family history of possible neuromuscular diseases or of neonatal death and stillbirth. When a dominant or an X-linked disorder is suspected, it is important to assess possible subclinical manifestations in the family.

Investigations

The determination of serum creatine kinase (CK) levels can be an important marker of possible muscle involvement in some forms of muscular dystrophy, but the levels can be normal or only mildly elevated in congenital myopathies or other forms of congenital muscular dystrophy. Electromyography (EMG) is generally not as useful as in older children.

Ultrasound imaging of muscle can help to demonstrate the presence of muscle involvement, and, in some cases, the selective involvement or sparing of muscles, which can be of considerable practical importance when taking a biopsy.

Muscle biopsy is indicated every time the clinical examination suggests a peripheral involvement, but in a few conditions such as myotonic dystrophy and spinal muscular atrophy the diagnosis can be reached rapidly and reliably using molecular genetic techniques.

Brain imaging (cranial ultrasound or brain magnetic resonance imaging or both) can help to identify structural brain lesions, such as cerebellar hypoplasia or cortical dysplasia, which are features of some conditions, for example Walker-Warburg syndrome, muscle-eye-brain disease, and mitochondrial disorders or pontocerebellar hypoplasia type I, with both central and peripheral involvement.

The muscular dystrophies

Congenital muscular dystrophy

The term congenital muscular dystrophy has been widely used for a group of infants presenting with muscle weakness at birth or within the first few months of life in association with a dystrophic pattern on muscle biopsy. There is often an associated hypotonia on clinical presentation but other patients may present with arthrogryposis and associated contractures of various joints. In recent decades it has become obvious that the term congenital muscular dystrophy includes a heterogeneous group of genetically, clinically, and biochemically distinct entities. Their classification has become increasingly complicated owing to the ever growing number of genes and proteins identified.

We can now recognize nine forms of CMD for which the genetic defect is known. It is anticipated that several additional forms exist on the basis of clinical and immunohistopathological data.

A description of the individual forms is beyond the scope of this chapter (Muntoni et al., 2001) but we will highlight the clinical features of the forms most commonly seen in infancy, providing clinical, pathological and imaging details to help their identification and the differential diagnosis.

From a practical point of view, the clinician should be able to identify three main groups that include the most common forms of CMD: congenital muscular dystrophies with rigid spine; merosin-deficient CMD; and congenital muscular dystrophies with deficit of α dystroglycan.

Congenital muscular dystrophies with rigid spine

This group includes two genetically distinct forms of CMD, Ullrich CMD and RSMD1, with overlapping clinical features, such as rigidity of the spine and early respiratory involvement, and normal or only mildly raised CK.

Ullrich CMD

Ullrich CMD is one of the most common forms of CMD (Mercuri et al., 2002a) and is characterized by proximal contractures associated with distal laxity, rigidity of the spine and early respiratory failure. Contractures and hypotonia are often present at birth but some children may only show delayed milestones as the presenting sign. Torticollis, hip dysplasia and congenital kyphosis are also frequent at birth or in the first months. Other clinical signs are a tendency to develop follicular hyperkeratosis and hypertrophic scars and cheloids.

All patients develop rigidity of the spine, often associated with scoliosis, irrespective of whether they have achieved independent ambulation.

Muscle biopsy may show variable pathology ranging from myopathic to clearly dystrophic patterns with a reduction of collagen VI in muscle and skin. The diagnosis can be confirmed on genetic studies, looking for mutations in the collagen VI genes (Camacho-Vanegas et al., 2001).

Rigid spine muscular dystrophy (RSMD1)

This form has some overlapping clinical features with Ullrich CMD (Mercuri et al., 2002b) but the onset is generally related to delayed motor milestones and the evolution of motor signs is more benign. The consistent clinical features are early rigidity of the spine and restrictive respiratory syndrome. These children may have mild hypotonia and weakness or contractures in the first few months of life but generally achieve independent walking by 18 months of age. The diagnosis can be confirmed by looking for mutations in *SEPN1*, a gene on chromosome 1p35-36 encoding selenoprotein N, a protein of unknown function (Moghadaszadeh et al., 2001).

Merosin-deficient CMD

This group accounts for approximately 40 per cent of all the forms of CMD and has a relatively homogeneous phenotype and raised serum CK (Dubowitz & Fardeau, 1995). It includes the forms with total or partial deficit of laminin α2 (merosin) on muscle biopsy because of mutations in the *LAMA* gene. Patients with a total deficit of laminin α2 have a peculiar phenotype with onset at birth or in the first few months of life, with hypotonia, weakness (respiratory and feeding problems) and, in some cases, contractures (hip flexion contractures; talipes).

Motor development is delayed and the maximum motor ability achievable is sitting unsupported. Children may be able to stand with some form of support or, in rare instances, walk with support (Philpot *et al.*, 1995).

Respiratory function is often reduced. This is observed by the end of the first decade, and night time hypoventilation is common even in early childhood. Feeding problems are also frequent and failure to thrive occurs in more than 80 per cent of affected children.

Another constant feature in patients with merosin-deficient CMD is the presence of diffuse white matter changes affecting both hemispheres, but sparing the internal capsule, corpus callosum, basal ganglia, thalami, and cerebellum (Mercuri *et al.*, 1996; Philpot *et al.*, 1999).

The muscle biopsy shows a classical dystrophic picture with reduction in or absence of the laminin α2 chain on immunofluorescence.

The diagnosis of merosin-deficient CMD should be always genetically confirmed by looking for mutations in the laminin α2 chain *(LAMA 2)* gene, which has been mapped to chromosome 6q22-23 (Helbling-Leclerc *et al.*, 1995).

Congenital muscular dystrophies with deficit of α dystroglycan

This group includes a several forms of CMD, often but not always associated with structural brain and eye changes and with mental retardation, which share several clinical features such as relative hypertrophy of the legs and a more severe involvement of the upper limbs. Serum CK is generally grossly elevated and α dystroglycan is reduced on muscle biopsy. The most frequent phenotypes are those with severe structural brain changes (Jimenez-Mallebrera *et al.*, 2008).

Walker-Warburg syndrome

This is a relatively common form that occurs worldwide. This is the most severe of the conditions with CNS involvement. Severe neonatal hypotonia and weakness, poor visual attention and decreased alertness are invariably present (Dobyns *et al.*, 1989), and accompanied by ocular abnormalities including retinal dysgenesis, microphthalmia, buphthalmos or anterior chamber malformations.

Brain MRI shows type II lissencephaly with the typical micropolygyric cobblestone cortex. The white matter is also severely abnormal, showing dysmyelination or cystic changes (Dobyns *et al.*, 1989) and cerebellar and brain stem involvement. Progressive hydrocephalus often develops. These infants may be thought to have a CNS malformation as the sole abnormality until a markedly elevated serum CK suggests the presence of skeletal muscle involvement as well. The presence of muscular dystrophy is confirmed by pathological studies. In a few cases, normal CK in the neonatal period has been documented, followed by progressive and marked subsequent elevation with time.

Muscle-eye-brain disease

Muscle-eye-brain disease is a rare form of CMD, initially believed to be confined to Finland and Turkey, but more recently shown to occur worldwide (Taniguchi *et al.*, 2003). Clinical signs are usually present at birth or in the first months of life, with hypotonia and weakness.

Ocular abnormalities may become evident only after the first years of life. These children invariably develop severe mental retardation and often epilepsy (Santavuori *et al.*,1989); approximately a quarter of affected children eventually learn to walk.

Brain MRI shows extensive abnormalities of neuronal migration, such as pachygyria and polymicrogyria, and often brain stem and cerebellar hypoplasia and periventricular white matter changes.

Other forms associated with dystroglycan deficiency

There are many clinical phenotypes in patients with CMD and a dystroglycan deficiency, ranging from cases with normal brain MRI and normal cognitive development to cases with cerebellar hypoplasia or dysplasia, or other structural brain changes.

So far mutations in six known or putative glycosyltransferase genes have been identified in these disorders: protein-*O*-mannosyl transferase 1 *(POMT1)*, protein-*O*-mannosyl transferase 2 *(POMT2)*, protein-*O*-mannose 1,2-N-acetylglucosaminyltransferase 1 *(POMGnT1)*, *fukutin*, fukutin-related protein *(FKRP)*, and *LARGE* (Kobayashi *et al.*, 1998; Brockington *et al.*, 2001; Yoshida *et al.*, 2001; Beltran-Valero de Bernabe *et al.*, 2002; Longman *et al.*, 2003; Van Reeuwijk *et al.*, 2005). Although each of these genes was originally reported in patients with distinct phenotypes (for example, Walker-Warburg syndrome for *POMT1* and *POMT2*, muscle-eye-brain disease for *POMGnT1*, Fukuyama CMD for *fukutin*, and so on), two things have become increasingly obvious:

1) Mutations in each gene can be associated with different phenotypes. *FKRP* gene mutations, for example – originally found in a form of CMD with a severe clinical phenotype and normal cognitive development and brain MRI (Brockington *et al.*, 2001) – have subsequently been associated with various phenotypes of different severity, ranging from mild limb girdle muscular dystrophy to Walker-Warburg syndrome (Mercuri *et al.*, 2003; Beltran-Valero de Bernabe *et al.*, 2004). A broad spectrum of phenotypes has also been reported for *POMT1* and *POMT2*, and, to a lesser extent, for *POMGnT1*, *fukutin* (Mercuri *et al.*, 2003) and more recently *LARGE*.

2) Individual phenotypes, such as Walker-Warburg or muscle-eye-brain disease, until recently thought to be separate nosographical entities, can be associated with mutations in many if not all of the six genes. From a practical viewpoint this means that there is no clear phenotype-genotype correlation and that all the six genes should be screened in patients presenting with these phenotypes.

Congenital myotonic dystrophy

The onset of congenital myotonic dystrophy is generally at birth following a pregnancy complicated by reduced fetal movements and polyhydramnios. Affected infants typically have hypotonia, facial weakness, with a striking facial diplegia and a triangular-shaped open mouth, bilateral equinovarus talipes deformity and other contractures. Respiratory muscle weakness is frequent and the severity of the respiratory involvement is one important prognostic marker of long term survival. Previous studies have indicated that ventilation for more than 4 weeks in a term infant is a negative prognostic factor for long term survival (Rutherford *et al.*, 1989). Severe neonatal feeding difficulties are also almost invariably present and require nasogastric tube feeding for several months, even in the infants who breath spontaneously. These feeding difficulties tend, however, to improve over the first months of life in the survivors and gastrostomy feeding is very rarely needed. Children affected by the congenital variant of myotonic dystrophy who survive after the first months generally improve in the first 10 years of life.

Mental retardation is a very frequent feature of children with congenital myotonic dystrophy. Cardiac involvement is also invariably present in older individuals with myotonic dystrophy, but is rare in infancy.

Diagnosis involves recognizing the clinical signs and paying attention to the pedigree. Examination of the mother often reveals either subtle facial weakness – with mild ptosis, a stiff smile and inability to bury the eyelashes – or grip myotonia (better evaluated not by shaking hands but by asking the mother to tighten her fists for a few seconds and observing the delay in fist release). The EMG in the mother will invariably demonstrate myotonic discharges, further supporting the diagnosis. The diagnosis is confirmed by molecular genetic testing, looking at the expansion (increase in the number of CTG trinucleotide repeats) in the *DMPK* gene on chromosome 19. There is no need for a muscle biopsy.

Congenital myopathies

The term 'congenital myopathy' includes a heterogeneous group of clinically, biochemically and genetically distinct diseases. While until recently their classification was mainly based on histochemical and electron microscopy findings, revealing the structural changes – such as cores, rods, and myotubules – that enabled the various forms to be classified, more recently the genetic basis of these disorders has become increasingly clear, allowing several different genetically distinct entities to be identified.

Some of these conditions are already detectable in the neonatal period, while in others the clinical signs become more obvious in the first years after birth. The forms that most often have an early onset are nemaline myopathy, central core disease, myotubular myopathy, and minicore disease. The names of these conditions are derived from the typical histopathological changes in muscle. Both minicore and central core disease present more often in early infancy rather than in the neonatal period, although earlier presentation is possible.

Nemaline myopathy

The two most common forms with early presentation are the 'classical' congenital form and the 'severe' congenital form. The classical congenital form is characterized by hypotonia, general weakness predominantly affecting facial and axial muscles, and disproportionate bulbar and feeding difficulties, requiring frequent suctioning, tube feeding and gastrostomy. The severe form has a much more severe phenotype with complete immobility, arthrogryposis and respiratory failure, generally following fetal akinesia and polyhydramnios. The serum CK levels are usually normal and the EMG is myopathic. Muscle biopsy shows an abundance of rod-like structures in muscle.

The prognosis is invariably poor for children in the 'severe' category, with no significant improvement in their limb, axial, bulbar and respiratory function. However, it is much better for children with the classical form, and most affected children acquire independent ambulation.

As previously mentioned, nemaline myopathy is a genetically heterogeneous condition and at least five genes are known to be involved in the pathogenesis. The early onset forms appear to be related mainly to two of these genes. While most infants affected by the severe form have *de novo* dominant mutations in the *ACTA1* gene, most of those with the classical milder congenital forms have recessive mutations in the *NEB* gene (Sewry et al., 2001).

Central core disease

Central core disease (CCD) is characterized by a variable degree of hypotonia and axial and proximal muscle weakness predominantly affecting the hip girdle. Presentation with weakness is usually in infancy or early childhood, although contractures at birth (equinovarus feet deformity; hip dislocation) are common. Severe facial and respiratory muscle weakness and bulbar dysfunction are not features. Serum CK activity is usually normal or only moderately increased. The natural course is static or only slowly progressive, with most affected individuals achieving the ability to walk. One important feature is that these children may have susceptibility to malignant hyperthermia and all cases should be considered to be at risk.

The biopsy typically shows predominantly central, core-like areas on oxidative stains; however, these striking abnormalities may only develop later on in life (Quinlivan et al., 2003).

CCD is commonly transmitted as an autosomal dominant trait with variable penetrance, though many sporadic cases have also been reported. Dominant missense mutations in the skeletal muscle ryanodine receptor (*RYR1*) gene are found in most affected cases.

Myotubular (centronuclear) myopathy

This form is characterized by the presence of numerous centrally placed nuclei with a surrounding central zone devoid of oxidative enzyme activity on muscle biopsy. There are two main early clinical phenotypes associated with different modes of inheritance. The X-linked form is more common and is more severe in male infants who are born with marked hypotonia, a variable degree of external ophthalmoplegia and respiratory failure, generally after a pregnancy complicated by polyhydramnios and reduced fetal movements. There is often a fatal course and although some infants who are ventilator-dependent in the neonatal period may survive if given continuous invasive ventilation they generally do not show any motor developmental progress. The autosomal recessive forms can range from early presentation with marked proximal weakness and inability to walk to milder variants characterized by generalized weakness and a variable degree of external ophthalmoplegia.

The gene for the X-linked variant is the myotubularin gene (*MTM1*) on chromosome Xq28.

Motor neuron disorders: spinal muscular atrophy

Spinal muscular atrophy is the most common motor neuron disorder in infancy. The form affecting the newborn is the most severe of the subtypes of SMA and is classified as SMA type 1 or Werdnig-Hoffmann disease. Infants affected by this form are very weak, never acquire the ability to sit. They have severe respiratory muscle weakness and usually die of intercurrent respiratory infection (Dubowitz, 1980).

SMA type 1

In infants with SMA type 1 the onset is early, either *in utero* or within the first 2–3 months of life. The clinical features are unique. The face is spared, and the posture reveals profound hypotonia with internally rotated arms, in a 'jug-handle' position by the side of the body. The lower limbs are more severely affected than the upper, and the proximal muscles more than the distal. These infants cannot raise their legs against gravity and are never able to roll over. There is generally poor head control in both the prone and the supine position, but some infants with SMA 1 will achieve head control and may be able to maintain it for several months. The intercostal muscles are severely affected, with a bell-shaped appearance of the chest, and breathing is almost entirely diaphragmatic. The tendon reflexes are always absent. The combination of these findings usually allows a spot diagnosis.

In the past few years there has been increasing evidence that infants with SMA type 1 should be treated with non-invasive ventilation as early as possible as this not only provides help for infants who already have breathing problems but also aids the expansion of the chest in infants who are still able to breath spontaneously (Bush *et al.*, 2005). Other measures such as performing gastrostomy at the onset of swallowing problems or even before their onset, at the time when there is a plateau in weight gain, have become part of the routine in many centres and this has produced an increase in mean survival.

The diagnosis can be suspected on the basis of clinical and EMG findings, showing fibrillation potentials at rest, but should be confirmed by genetic analysis looking for homozygous deletion of *SMN1* (motor neuron survival factor) exon 7, which is found in more than 98 per cent of SMA patients.

SMA type 2

Very often children with SMA type 2 progress quite normally in the first months of life and achieve the ability to sit unaided but never to stand independently or walk. In a proportion of cases the onset may appear acute and the infant may suddenly lose some of the abilities previously achieved.

The pattern of clinical signs is similar to that observed in the severe form but less pronounced. The proximal muscles are more affected than the distal, and the lower limbs more than the upper. The power in the arms may be relatively good with the ability to lift the arms against gravity. The intercostal muscles are affected, but usually not severely, and the diaphragm tends to be spared, so that breathing is predominantly diaphragmatic. Fasciculation and atrophy of the tongue and tremors of the hands are common features (Wang *et al.*, 2007).

These cases usually have a benign course and patients easily survive into adolescence or adulthood providing care is taken to monitor their respiratory function, which is the most important factor in determining prognosis.

Conclusions

Hopefully the description of all these diseases will alert the clinician to the wide range of neuromuscular and non-neuromuscular disorders that may present in infancy. We strongly believe that even where genetic tests, muscle MRI and several other tools are now available, a good clinical assessment of the infant and the mother remains the key to providing guidance about the most appropriate investigations to establish a definitive diagnosis.

References

Beltran-Valero de Bernabe, D., Currier, S., Steinbrecher, A., Celli, J., van Beusekom, E., van der Zwaag, B., Kayserili, H., Merlini, L., Chitayat, D., Dobyns, W.B., Cormand, B., Lehesjoki, A.E., Cruces, J., Voit, T., Walsh, C.A., van Bokhoven, H. & Brunner, H.G. (2002): Mutations in the O-mannosyltransferase gene POMT1 give rise to the severe neuronal migration disorder Walker-Warburg syndrome. *Am. J. Hum. Genet.* **71**, 1033–1043.

Beltran-Valero de Bernabe, D., Voit, T., Longman, C., Steinbrecher, A., Straub, V., Yuva, Y., Herrmann, R., Sperner, J., Korenke, C., Diesen, C., Dobyns, W.B., Brunner, H.G., van Bokhoven, H., Brockington, M. & Muntoni, F. (2004): Mutations in the FKRP gene can cause muscle-eye-brain disease and Walker-Warburg syndrome. *J. Med. Genet.* **41**, e61.

Brockington, M., Blake, D.J., Prandini, P., Brown, S.C., Torelli, S., Benson, M.A., Ponting, C.P., Estournet, B., Romero, N.B., Mercuri, E., Voit, T., Sewry, C.A., Guicheney, P. & Muntoni, F. (2001): Mutations in the fukutin-related protein gene (FKRP) cause a form of congenital muscular dystrophy with secondary laminin alpha2 deficiency and abnormal glycosylation of alpha-dystroglycan. *Am. J. Hum. Genet.* **69**, 1198–1209.

Bush, A., Fraser, J., Jardine, E., Paton, J., Simonds, A. & Wallis, C. (2005): Respiratory management of the infant with type 1 spinal muscular atrophy. *Arch. Dis. Child.* **90**, 709–711.

Camacho-Vanegas, O., Bertini, E., Zhang, R.Z., Petrini, S., Minosse, C., Sabatelli, P., Giusti, B., Chu, M.L. & Pepe, G. (2001): Ullrich scleroatonic muscular dystrophy is caused by recessive mutations in collagen type VI. *Proc. Natl. Acad. Sci. USA* **98**, 7516–7521.

Dobyns, W.B., Pagon, R.A., Armstrong, D., Curry, C.J., Greenberg, F., Grix, A., Holmes, L.B., Laxova, R., Michels, V.V., Robinow, M., et al. (1989): Diagnostic criteria for Walker-Warburg syndrome. *Am. J. Med. Genet.* **32**, 195–210.

Dubowitz, V. (1980): *The floppy infant*, 2nd ed. London: Heinemann.

Dubowitz, V. & Fardeau, M. (1995): Workshop report on 27th ENMC-sponsored meeting on congenital muscular dystrophy held in Baarn, The Netherlands. *Neuromuscul. Disord.* **4**, 253–258.

Helbling-Leclerc, A., Zhang, X., Topaloglu, H., Cruaud, C., Tesson, F., Weissenbach, J., Tomé, F.M., Schwartz, K., Fardeau, M., Tryggvason, K., et al. (1995): Mutations in the laminin alpha 2-chain gene (LAMA2) cause merosin-deficient congenital muscular dystrophy. *Nat. Genet.* **11**, 216–218.

Jimenez-Mallebrera, C., Torelli, S., Feng, L., Kim, J., Godfrey, C., Clement, E., Mein, R., Abbs, S., Brown, S.C., Campbell, K.P., Kröger, S., Talim, B., Topaloglu, H., Quinlivan, R., Roper, H., Childs, A.M., Kinali, M., Sewry, C.A. & Muntoni, F. (2008): Comparative study of alpha-dystroglycan glycosylation in dystroglycanopathies suggests that the hypoglycosylation of alpha-dystroglycan does not consistently correlate with clinical severity. *Brain Pathol.* Aug 7 [Epub ahead of print].

Kobayashi, K., Nakahori, Y., Miyake, M., Matsumura, K., Kondo-Iida, E., Nomura, Y., Segawa, M., Yoshioka, M., Saito, K., Osawa, M., Hamano, K., Sakakihara, Y., Nonaka, I., Nakagome, Y., Kanazawa, I., Nakamura, Y., Tokunaga, K. & Toda, T. (1998): An ancient retrotransposal insertion causes Fukuyama-type congenital muscular dystrophy. *Nature* **394**, 388–392.

Longman, C., Brockington, M., Torelli, S., Jimenez-Mallebrera, C., Kennedy, C., Khalil, N., Feng, L., Saran, R.K., Voit, T., Merlini, L., Sewry, C.A., Brown, S.C. & Muntoni, F. (2003): Mutations in the human LARGE gene cause MDC1D, a novel form of congenital muscular dystrophy with severe mental retardation and abnormal glycosylation of alpha-dystroglycan. *Hum. Mol. Genet.* **12**, 2853–2861.

Mercuri, E., Pennock, J., Goodwin, F., Sewry, C., Cowan, F., Dubowitz, L., Dubowitz, V. & Muntoni, F. (1996): Sequential study of central and peripheral nervous system involvement in an infant with merosin-deficient CMD. *Neuromuscul. Disord.* **6**, 425–429.

Mercuri, E., Yuva, Y., Brown, S.C., Brockington, M., Kinali, M., Jungbluth, H., Feng, L., Sewry, C.A. & Muntoni, F. (2002a): Collagen VI involvement in Ullrich syndrome: a clinical, genetic and immunohistochemical study. *Neurology* **58**, 1354–1359.

Mercuri, E., Talim, B., Moghadaszadeh, B., Petit, N., Brockington, M., Counsell, S., Guicheney, P., Muntoni, F. & Merlini, L. (2002b): Clinical and imaging findings in six cases of congenital muscular dystrophy with rigid spine syndrome linked to chromosome 1p (RSMD1). *Neuromuscul. Disord.* **12**, 631–638.

Mercuri, E., Brockington, M., Straub, V., Quijano-Roy, S., Yuva, Y., Herrmann, R., Brown, S.C., Torelli, S., Dubowitz, V., Blake, D.J., Romero, N.B., Estournet, B., Sewry, C.A., Guicheney, P., Voit, T. & Muntoni, F. (2003): Phenotypic spectrum associated with mutations in the fukutin-related protein gene. *Ann. Neurol.* **53**, 537–542.

Moghadaszadeh, B., Petit, N., Jaillard, C., Brockington, M., Roy, S.Q., Merlini, L., Romero, N., Estournet, B., Desguerre, I., Chaigne, D., Muntoni, F., Topaloglu, H. & Guicheney, P. (2001): Mutations in SEPN1 cause congenital muscular dystrophy with spinal rigidity and restrictive respiratory syndrome. *Nat. Genet.* **29**, 17–18.

Muntoni, F., Bertini, E., Bönnemann, C., Brockington, M., Brown, S., Bushby, K., Fiszman, M., Körner, C., Mercuri, E., Merlini, L., Hewitt, J., Quijano-Roy, S., Romero, N., Squarzoni, S., Sewry, C.A., Straub, V., Topaloglu, H.,

Haliloglu, G., Voit, T., Wewer, U. & Guicheney, P. (2001): 98th ENMC International Workshop on Congenital Muscular Dystrophy (CMD), 7th Workshop of the International Consortium on CMD, 2nd Workshop of the MYO CLUSTER project GENRE, 26–28th October, Naarden, The Netherlands. *Neuromuscul. Disord.* **12,** 889–896.

Philpot, J., Sewry, C., Pennock, J. & Dubowitz, V. (1995): Clinical phenotype in congenital muscular dystrophy: correlation with expression of merosin in skeletal muscle. *Neuromuscul. Disord.* **5,** 301–305.

Philpot, J., Cowan, F., Pennock, J., Sewry, C., Dubowitz, V., Bydder, G. & Muntoni, F. (1999): Merosin deficient congenital muscular dystrophy: the spectrum of brain lesions on magnetic resonance imaging. *Neuromuscul. Disord.* **9,** 81–85.

Quinlivan, R.M., Muller, C.R., Davis, M., Laing, N.G., Evans, G.A., Dwyer, J., Dove, J., Roberts, A.P. & Sewry, C.A. (2003)œ: Central core disease: clinical, pathological, and genetic features. *Arch. Dis. Child.* **88,** 1051–1055.

Rutherford, M.A., Heckmatt, J.Z. & Dubowitz, V. (1989): Congenital myotonic dystrophy: respiratory function at birth determines survival. *Arch. Dis. Child.* **64,** 191–195.

Santavuori, P., Somer, H., Sainio, K., Rapola, J., Kruus, S., Nikitin, T., Ketonen, L. & Leisti, J. (1989): Muscle-eye-brain disease (MEB). *Brain Dev.* **11,** 147–153.

Sewry, C.A., Brown, S.C., Pelin, K., Jungbluth, H., Wallgren-Pettersson, C., Labeit, S., Manzur, A. & Muntoni, F. (2001): Abnormalities in the expression of nebulin in chromosome-2 linked nemaline myopathy. *Neuromuscul. Disord.* **11,** 146–153.

Taniguchi, K., Kobayashi, K., Saito, K., Yamanouchi, H., Ohnuma, A., Hayashi, Y.K., Manya, H., Jin, D.K., Lee, M., Parano, E., Falsaperla, R., Pavone, P., Van Coster, R., Talim, B., Steinbrecher, A., Straub, V., Nishino, I., Topaloglu, H., Voit, T., Endo, T. & Toda, T. (2003): Worldwide distribution and broader clinical spectrum of muscle-eye-brain disease. *Hum. Mol. Genet.* **12,** 527–534.

Van Reeuwijk, J., Brunner, H. & van Bokhoven, H. (2005): Glyc-O-genetics of Walker-Warburg syndrome. *Clin. Genet.* **67,** 281–289.

Vasta, I., Kinali, M., Messina, S., Guzzetta, A., Kapellou, O., Manzur, A., Cowan, F., Muntoni, F. & Mercuri, E. (2005): Can clinical signs identify newborns with neuromuscular disorders? *J. Pediatr.* **146,** 73–79.

Wang, C.H., Finkel, R.S., Bertini, E.S., Schroth, M., Simonds, A., Wong, B., Aloysius, A., Morrison, L., Main, M., Crawford, T.O. & Trela, A., for the Participants of the International Conference on SMA Standard of Care (2007): Consensus statement for standard of care in spinal muscular atrophy. *J. Child Neurol.* **22,** 1027–1049.

Yoshida, A., Kobayashi, K., Manya, H., Taniguchi, K., Kano, H., Mizuno, M., Inazu, T., Mitsuhashi, H., Takahashi, S., Takeuchi, M., Herrmann, R., Straub, V., Talim, B., Voit, T., Topaloglu, H., Toda, T. & Endo, T. (2001): Muscular dystrophy and neuronal migration disorder caused by mutations in a glycosyltransferase, POMGnT1. *Dev. Cell* **1,** 717–724.

Chapter 13

Peripheral neuropathies

Francesco Guzzetta

Catholic University, Largo Agostino Gemelli 8, 00168 Rome, Italy
fguzzetta@rm.unicatt.it

Notes on developmental anatomy and physiology

The peripheral nerves are formed by myelinated and unmyelinated fibres supported by connective tissue. The structure of nerves changes with age, especially in the first months of life, when development is most active, and consequently neurophysiological features are age-dependent.

In the foetal period the fascicles of the sural nerve (the most studied of the human nerves) consist only of bundles of unmyelinated fibres surrounded by Schwann cell cytoplasm (several fibres per cell). The number of fibres per Schwann cell progressively decreases, and by the middle of fetal life the process of myelination begins in individual fibres, surrounded by the cytoplasm of a single cell covering a segment of the fibre. At birth, most fibres with a diameter over 3 µm are myelinated. The total transverse fascicular area is reduced, but the density of myelinated fibres seems much greater than in older children. In the first months of life, the histogram of fibres (distribution of fibres according to size) is unimodal with a reduced mean of fibre diameter (about 4 µm) in comparison with adult values (about 8 µm) (Ferrière *et al.*, 1985; Ouvrier *et al.*, 1999). Consistently, the mean internodal length is shorter. The density of unmyelinated fibres seems to decrease during the first years of life (Ferrière *et al.*, 1985).

As the conduction velocity is directly proportional to the largest myelinated fibres with the longest internodal distance, lower values of nerve conduction velocity (NCV) and of muscle action potential (MAP) amplitude should thus be observed in infancy. A table of normal motor and sensory values in various peripheral nerves of developing infants, to which patient results should be compared, is given in a paper by Miller & Kunz (1986).

General pathology

Fibre axons or myelin may be affected by pathology. Mechanical injury such as trauma, as well as inflammatory infiltration, may dissect the fibres, producing degeneration distal to the site of injury (wallerian degeneration). The degenerated axon may subsequently regenerate, be remyelinated by Schwann cells, and once again reach its distal target.

Pathological degeneration of the axon from metabolic or toxic causes is more common. Disorders of metabolism of the cell body impair axonal transport, primarily damaging the distal part of the fibre, causing a functional (motor, sensory, or autonomic) defect in the distal parts of the limbs. This is what normally happens in many acquired or hereditary neuropathies. Myelin may be secondarily affected by a process of degeneration, but in some disorders there may be primary degeneration that specifically targets the Schwann cells, characteristically producing segmental demyelination (degeneration of an internodal segment referring to a single Schwann cell). This process is specific to some hereditary polyneuropathies. A genetic lack of myelin protein may be the cause, or other factors may affect the process of forming or maintaining myelin.

Diagnosis

Peripheral neuropathies include a wide range of disorders in which the nerves outside the brain and spinal cord become damaged. Clinical manifestations consist of a combination of muscle weakness, sensory disorders including pain, and autonomic symptoms. In early infancy, when sensory disturbances and weakness are difficult to detect, hypotonia may be the major sign.

Diagnosis may be supported by the symptomatic context, but especially by electrodiagnostic studies of nerve function. NCV, late response (H reflex and F wave), and needle electromyography (Wein & Alpers, 2002; Van den Bergh & Pieret, 2004) can identify and characterize the neuropathy by the following features:

- the anatomical pattern, whether focally involving a single peripheral nerve (mononeuropathy), multiple separate non-contiguous peripheral nerves either simultaneously or serially (mononeuropathy multiplex), or affecting nerves systematically and symmetrically in a length-dependent way (polyneuropathy);
- the part of neuron involved, whether proximal or distal;
- the severity, based on the reduction of motor and sensory NCV and of the amplitude of the MAP;
- the quality, whether predominantly causing axonal degeneration, segmental demyelination, or showing conduction block.

As neurophysiological examinations measure the fastest fibres (the largest myelinated fibres), neuropathies with small fibre involvement are barely detectable by these techniques (Said, 2003). Delta fibres (small myelinated fibres) and C fibres (0.5 to 2 µm unmyelinated fibres) with various kinds of sensory and autonomic function may be damaged in some neuropathies (for example, hereditary sensory and autonomic neuropathies). Unfortunately, quantitative sensory testing is difficult in non-collaborating infants. However, autonomic testing (heart and respiratory rate, blood pressure, sympathetic skin responses following the intradermal injection of histamine) may be helpful in identifying and characterizing autonomic dysfunction (Lacomis, 2002).

In addition to the ancillary investigations aimed at exploring the specific functions involved in various neuropathic diseases, an important role is now played by genetic tests aimed at detecting specific gene mutations in the hereditary neuropathies. These tests have rendered invasive nerve biopsy obsolete in most cases, so that it is now only indicated in patients with otherwise ambiguous results.

Classification

There are few studies specifically reporting peripheral neuropathies in infancy. In fact, the wide array of human neuropathies is markedly reduced if one considers only those occurring or beginning in infancy. A seminal European multicentre study identified only 20 cases under 1 year of age from among 287 children with peripheral neuropathies (Hagberg & Lyon, 1981). Since then, other series have been published (Hagberg & Westerberg, 1983; Rossi et al., 1983) including patients showing symptoms in infancy. More recently in another series, 50 of 260 infants presented with symptoms or signs of neuropathy at under 1 year of age (Wilmhurst et al., 2003). We propose a simple classification of the main forms observed in infancy (Table 1).

Table 1. Peripheral neuropathies in infancy

Mononeuropathies	Brachial plexus palsy; other mechanical palsies	
Polyneuropathies • Acquired		
(a) Acute	Demyelinating	Common form of Guillain-Barré syndrome; diphtheria
	Axonal	Axonal form of Guillain-Barré syndrome
(b) Chronic	Demyelinating	Chronic inflammatory demyelinating polyradiculoneuropathy (CIDP)
	Axonal	B vitamin deficiencies; leprosy; Lyme disease; drugs; toxins
• Hereditary	Hereditary motor and sensory neuropathy (HMSN) Hereditary sensory and autonomic neuropathy (HSAN) Neuropathies in hereditary metabolic and neurodegenerative diseases	

Mononeuropathies

Mononeuropathies in infancy are represented almost exclusively by neonatal peripheral palsies.

Obstetric peripheral palsy

The most common of obstetric palsy is brachial plexus palsy, a possible complication of a dystocic delivery as a sequela of overstretching of the plexus. Further studies motivated by medico-legal requirements have been carried out exploring the possibility that such palsies may arise from intrauterine injuries (Gherman et al., 1999).

In most cases brachial plexus palsy is transient; only a few patients have persistent sequelae leading to long term motor disability. In these cases physiotherapy is mandatory and surgical intervention may be required to improve the innervation of the affected muscles.

The nerve network of the brachial plexus may be involved in different ways, causing various subgroups of brachial plexus palsy: i) Duchenne-Erb palsy, which affects nerves arising from C5 and C6 (arm supinated with the elbow bent and wrist extended); ii) Klumpke palsy with deficit involving C8 and T1 (arm adducted and internally rotated with the elbow extended, forearm pronated, wrist flexed, and clutched hand); iii) complete brachial plexus palsy affecting nerves at all levels (C5–T1) (limp arm with areflexia, asymmetrical Moro reflex); iv) bilateral brachial plexus palsy, with bilateral involvement.

Possible associated injuries are bone fractures (clavicular and humeral), torticollis, cephalhaematoma, and other traumatic palsies (for example, facial nerve palsy).

Neuroimaging, in particular high resolution magnetic resonance imaging (MRI), and electrodiagnostic studies are the best tools to evaluate brachial plexus palsy and its evolution. Electromyography (EMG) is useful for detecting the first signs of denervation 2 to 3 weeks after injury and thus the timing of the injury. It may also be useful to monitor the re-innervation process, to inform possible surgical interventions (Pitt & Vredeveld, 2005). Latencies of the musculocutaneous and axillary nerves and motor and sensory NCV of the medial, ulnar and radial nerves are other informative studies.

Among the tools aimed at the clinical follow-up of patients with neonatal brachial plexus palsy (the Mallet Classification, the Toronto Test Score, and the Hospital for Sick Children Active Movement Scale), the Active Movement Scale benefits from good controlled studies that include inter-rater reliability (Curtis *et al.*, 2002; Bae *et al.*, 2003).

Polyneuropathies

Acquired polyneuropathies

Acquired polyneuropathies caused by toxic and vascular factors are very uncommon in infants (Ouvrier *et al.*, 1999; Craig & Richardson, 2003). Among the rare non-hereditary forms of acute neuropathy (poliomyelitis, diphtheria, tick paralysis, and so on), Guillain-Barré syndrome seems the most common (Table 1).

Guillain-Barré syndrome

Guillain-Barré syndrome (GBS) is an autoimmune disorder that affects the peripheral nerves producing an acute or subacute inflammatory demyelinating polyneuropathy. Among different variants of the disease, acute inflammatory demyelinating polyradiculoneuropathy (AIDP) is the most common Western form. Another form observed more often in other parts of the world (for example, China) is acute motor axonal neuropathy (AMAN).

GBS occurs at all ages including infancy. Even neonatal or prenatal cases have been reported (al-Qudah *et al.*, 1988; Bamford *et al.*, 2002). There may be a history of respiratory or gastrointestinal infection a few days before the onset of the neuropathy. The classical evolution of the disease consists of a progressive proximal spread from the distal parts of the limbs of paraesthesiae, weakness and loss of stretch reflexes, eventually involving the cranial nerves (especially the facial and bulbar muscles) and the respiratory musculature, maximal after 3 to 4 weeks. In infancy, hypotonia – possibly misinterpreted as ataxia – may be a prominent sign. Hypotonia is symmetrical, generalized or sometimes predominantly proximal with loss of tendon reflexes, associated with paucity of lower limb movements. Though severe forms occur, a benign course is often observed in infancy.

Laboratory and electrophysiological investigations are useful in diagnosing the disease and particularly in differentiating it from botulism, a possibility in infancy. GBS should also be differentiated from rarely occurring toxic neuropathies and poliomyelitis or other paralyses caused by enteroviruses. However, the major criterion of a high level of CSF protein together with an absence of pleocytosis is far from being absolute. Consistent with the patchy though extensively distributed nature of the demyelination, neurophysiological studies may show conduction blocks and various degrees of involvement of nerve conduction, including normal values in paralysed muscles (Ouvrier et al., 1999). Fibrillation on EMG, caused by the loss of motor units, may be observed some weeks after the disease onset.

Therapy in the acute stage is mainly supportive. Respiratory function should be monitored, especially in infants, in whom respiratory assessment may be particularly difficult. Respiratory physiotherapy is indicated to improve ventilation. As regards medical treatment, steroids are not recommended in infants. Rather, intravenous immunoglobulin infusions at a dose of 0.4 g/kg body weight on 5 successive days have been shown to be effective (Hughes et al., 2001), and at least equal to plasmapheresis, which is not advised in very young children because of complications and technical difficulties.

Chronic acquired polyneuropathy

A chronic form of relapsing or gradually progressive acquired polyneuropathy is chronic inflammatory demyelinating polyradiculoneuropathy (CIDP). Generally, this primarily affects both distal and proximal motor fibres. In a few cases reported in infancy (Sladky et al., 1986), generalized and severe hypotonia was observed with marked delay of motor development. Pathology shows inflammatory infiltration of nerve roots, with segmental demyelination possibly secondary to distal axonal degeneration produced by the proximal inflammatory reaction (Dyck et al., 1975). Electrophysiologically, there is a slow mNCV, with possible conduction blocks and dispersion of compound MAPs. Noteworthy, CIDP is responsive to steroid treatment. Treatment may be effective at a dose of 1 mg/kg/d, increasing to 2 mg/kg/d if there is no response (Ouvrier et al., 1999). Higher dosages have, however, been used, in particular in infancy (Sladky et al., 1986).

Hereditary polyneuropathies

The classification by Dyck & Lambert (1968) – based on clinical, genetic, electrophysiological and nerve biopsy findings – considers two broad categories: hereditary motor and sensory neuropathies (HMSN) and hereditary sensory and autonomic neuropathies (HSAN). The first category was subsequently refined (Dyck et al., 1993a) and includes various types of HMSN, among which types I and II correspond to types 1 and 2 of Charcot-Marie-Tooth disease, and type III to Dejerine-Sottas disease. Demyelinating forms with a major reduction of NCV include HMSN I (Charcot-Marie-Tooth disease type 1), usually with autosomal dominant inheritance, and the most severe autosomal recessive HMSN III (Dejerine-Sottas disease), while neuronal types include axonal forms (HMSN II or Charcot-Marie-Tooth disease type 2) with a lesser reduction in the motor nerve conduction velocities (mNCV > 38 m/s). HSAN (Dyck et al., 1993b) consist of five subgroups of hereditary neuropathies with sensory and autonomic involvement (Table 2). The availability of molecular genetic analysis has allowed an improved classification of the hereditary neuropathies (Tyson et al., 1997; Wilmshurst et al., 2003).

Hereditary motor and sensory neuropathy

HMSNs stem from the original category of the Charcot-Marie-Tooth (CMT) syndrome. A clinical classification of these forms (Table 3), based on a simple distinction between pathological features (axonal vs. demyelinating) and neurophysiological features (nerve conduction velocities < 38 m/s vs. > 38 m/s), has been proposed more recently and is now largely used (Reilly, 2000).

Table 2. HMSN and HSAN classification (Dyck & Lambert, 1993b)

Acronyms	Equivalent names
HNMS	
HMSN I	CMT 1
HMSN II	CMT 2
HMSN III	DSS
HMSN IV	Refsum's (phytanic acid storage) disease (polyneuropathy, cerebellar ataxia and retinitis pigmentosa)
HMSN V	HMSN with spastic paraparesis
HMSN VI	HMSN with optic atrophy
HMSN VII	HMSN with retinitis pigmentosa
HSAN	
HSAN I	
HSAN II	
HSAN III	Familial dysautonomia (Riley-Day syndrome)
HSAN IV	CIPA (congenital insensitivity to pain with anhidrosis)
HSAN V	

CMT, Charcot-Marie-Tooth neuropathy; DSS, Dejerine-Sottas syndrome; HMSN, hereditary motor and sensory neuropathy; HSAN: hereditary sensory and autonomic neuropathy.

Table 3. Charcot-Marie-Tooth (CMT) classification (Reilly, 2000)

CMT1	Hypertrophic-demyelinating CMT (mNCV < 38 m/s)
CMT2	Autosomal dominant axonal CMT (mNCV > 38 m/s)
CMT4	Recessive hypertrophic-demyelinating CMT (mNCV < 38 m/s)
DI-CMT	Dominant intermediate forms (intermediate mNCV)

MNCV, motor nerve conduction velocity.

CMT neuropathies form more than 90 per cent of the hereditary diseases of the peripheral nervous system. In the past few years, many genetic defects underlying hereditary peripheral neuropathies have been identified in CMT phenotypes, several of which have their onset in infancy (Table 4), so that new and at times confusing classifications have been proposed, based on gene mutations (Auer-Grumbach et al., 1999; Nelis et al., 1999). Different types of mutation generally correspond to different phenotypes – for example, *PMP22* deletion is typical of HNPP (hereditary neuropathy with liability to pressure palsies, usually present in older children) whereas duplication is frequently observed in HMSN 1A, and point mutation is associated with more severe forms of both HMSN IA and HMSN III. On the other hand, a broad array of phenotypes is observed in point mutations of *MPZ*. The phenotype variability seems linked to the exact location of the mutation (Warner et al., 1996). As in other phenotype-genotype correlations, the same gene mutation is often associated with different clinical entities, whereas some particular clinical forms are based on different gene mutations. Thus clinically oriented classifications still continue to be fruitfully used (Kuhlenbäumer et al., 2002).

Table 4. Genetics of the hereditary motor and sensory neuropathies possibly occurring in infancy

Acronyms	Pathology	Gene	Locus	Inheritance	Gene product	Onset	Early symptoms	mNCVs (m/s)
HMSN IB, CMT 1B	Hypertrophic-demyelinating	MPZ	1q22-q23	AD	Myelin protein zero	1st decade	Distal motor	< 38
HMSN ID, CMT 1D	Hypertrophic-demyelinating	EGR2	10q21.1-q22.1	AD	Early growth response 2 transcription factor	Cong./1st decade	Distal motor	25-38
HMSN IIC, CMT2C	Axonal form	Unknown	12q23-q24	AD		1st decade	Distal motor	> 38
HMSN-IX, CMT1X	Alterations of paranodal myelin; axonal damage	GJB1 (CX32)	Xq13.1	XD	Gap junction protein, β-1 (Connexin 32)	1st decade	Distal motor	> 38
MSN3, DSS	Hypertrophic-demyelinating	MPZ	1q22-q23	AR	Myelin protein zero	Infancy	Severe motor	< 10
"	"	PMP22	17p11.2	AR	Peripheral myelin protein 22	Infancy	Severe motor	< 10
"	"	EGR2	10q21.1-q22.1	AD	Early growth response 2 transcription factor	Infancy	Severe motor	< 10
" (CMT4F)	Severe neuropathy	PRX	19q13.1-q13.3	AR	Periaxin	1st–2nd year	Hypotonia	< 10
CHN	Hypomyelinating	MPZ	8q13	AD	Myelin protein zero	Congenital	Severe hypotonia	< 10
"	Hypomyelinating	PMP22	17p11.2	Sporadic	Peripheral myelin protein 22	Infancy	Severe hypotonia	< 10
" (CMT4E)	Hypomyelinating	EGR2	10q21.1-q22.1	AR	Early growth response 2 transcription factor	Congenital	Severe hypotonia	< 10
HMSN IVA, CMT4A	Hypertrophic-demyelinating	GDAP1	8q13-q21	AR	Ganglioside-induced differentiation associated protein-1	2nd–4th year	Distal motor	< 38
HMSN IVB1, CMT4B1	Focally folded myelin	MTMR2	11q23	AR	Myotubularin-related protein 2	1st decade	Distal motor	< 38
HMSN IVB2, CMT4B2	Focally folded myelin	MTMR13	11p15	AR	Myotubularin-related protein 13	1st–2nd decade	Distal motor + sensory	< 38
HMSN IVD, CMT4D	Hypertrophic-demyelinating + progressive deafness	NDRG1	8q24	AR	N-myc downstream regulated gene-1 factor	1st decade	Walk delay	< 38

AD, autosomal dominant; AR, autosomal recessive; mNCV, motor nerve conduction velocity; Cong., congenital; XD, X-linked dominant.

With regard to the gene function, *PMP22* and *MPZ* are relevant components of the compacted myelin of peripheral nervous system myelinated fibres produced by Schwann cells. Many of the *EGR2* target genes are needed to synthesize normal myelin lipids, while *PRX* encodes proteins required to maintain peripheral nerve myelin. Both *GDAP1* and *NDRG1* genes may be involved in signal transduction pathways, playing a role in Schwann cell development. Neural membrane trafficking is supported by MTMR. Finally, *connexin 32* provides – through the intracellular gap junctions – the connection to the folds of the Schwann cell cytoplasm (fast transport of low-molecular-weight substances from the adaxonal to the outer myelin lamellae).

HMSN is very rare in infancy. Clinical clues are predominantly distal weakness and frequent absence of deep tendon reflexes; later on, distal atrophy with sensory signs and hand and foot deformities may appear. Nerve conduction studies will confirm the diagnosis and nerve biopsy may give useful information, though this can now be replaced by molecular genetic diagnosis. In the congenital forms – congenital hypomyelinating neuropathy (CHN) and Dejerine-Sottas disease (DSS/HMSN III) – hypotonia and delay in motor development can be the major symptoms, affected children presenting as floppy infants. In these forms NCVs are very low (<10 m/s), while nerve biopsy shows typical features: severe demyelination, associated with diffuse onion bulb formation (Fig. 1), possibly an expression of a recurrent demyelination and remyelination process causing deficient maintenance of myelin (Guzzetta *et al.*, 1982). In CHN, the very early onset with a major defect of myelination is often associated with arthrogryposis, severe respiratory disorders, and swallowing problems that may lead to death in the first months of life. A form of CHN has been described where there is an absolute lack of myelin (Palix & Coignet, 1978; Charnas *et al.*, 1988), possibly an extreme expression of mutations in the myelin proteins. An infantile form of CHN presenting at an older age and generally associated with longer survival has been reported (Philips *et al.*, 1999), as well as a sporadic form with predominant primary axonal changes (Guzzetta & Ferrière, 1985).

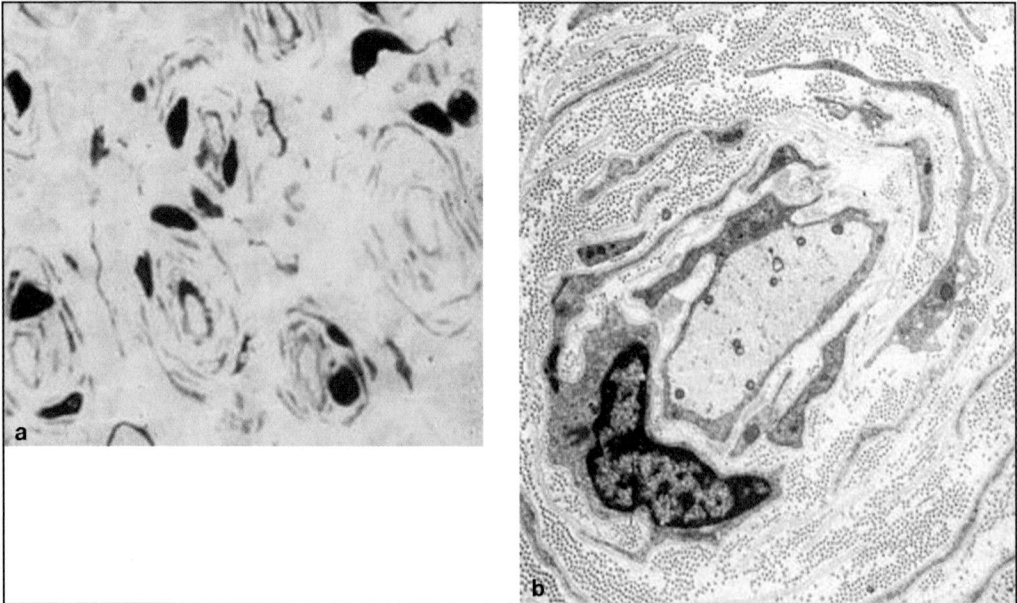

Fig. 1. (A) Electron micrograph from the sural nerve of a patient with congenital hypomyelinating neuropathy (CHN): only nude axons are seen, surrounded by typical 'onion bulb' formations. (B) Typical 'onion bulb': nude axon surrounded by multiple lamellae consisting of double basement membrane often filled with cytoplasm.

Later onset infantile forms (Deyerine-Sottas disease) present with a peroneal muscular atrophy syndrome, slowly progressive distal muscle weakness and atrophy with areflexia, and usually symmetrical sensory deficits that are hard to detect at this young age. Nerve biopsy findings are similar to those observed in CHN, but less severe (Fig. 2). The same genetic background (mutations of *PMP22*, *MPZ*, and *EGR2*) suggests a broad array of unique phenotypes with different degrees of severity, ranging from CHN to Dejerine-Sottas disease, down to some milder forms of HMSN-I (Warner *et al.*, 1996).

The autosomal dominant HMSN type I is possibly present in infancy (IB and ID). The peroneal atrophy syndrome, with a generally slower evolution, appears later on. The specific marker of the syndrome – nerve hypertrophy – is not evident during infancy. Nerve biopsy shows myelin degeneration with decreased numbers of fibres, which may appear to be surrounded by a reduced number of myelin sheaths (regenerating fibres), and some onion bulbs (Fig. 3). NCVs are slightly slower than normal (< 38 m/s).

An autosomal recessive form of HMSN, extremely rare, has been described as CMT4. Among these cases, CMT4B1 is the best characterized. Typical of this form is the focally folded myelin (Fig. 4) (Sabatelli *et al.*, 1994; Quattrone *et al.*, 1996). mNCVs are moderately slowed. The peroneal atrophy syndrome is more markedly progressive than the dominant forms (HMSN I), but is generally compatible with survival to the fourth or fifth decade of life.

There have been a few cases of HMSN II (type C) described in infancy, characterized by autosomal dominant inheritance and a relatively late onset. These present with a milder peroneal atrophy syndrome with normal or borderline mNCV (>38 m/s) and very slow progression. Pathological features in the peripheral nerves consist of various signs of axonal damage.

A few cases of severe forms of HMSN II have been reported in infancy, with early onset and rapid progression (Ouvrier *et al.*, 1981; Gabreels- Festen *et al.*, 1991). Axons of motor and especially sensory fibres are involved, and electrophysiology shows signs of severe denervation.

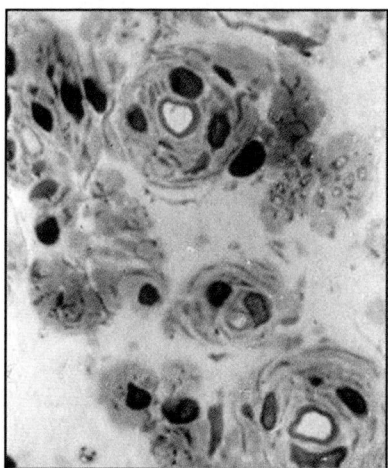

Fig. 2. Hereditary motor and sensory neuropathy (HMSN) type III: thinly myelinated fibres are observed, surrounded by multi-lamelled 'onion bulbs'.

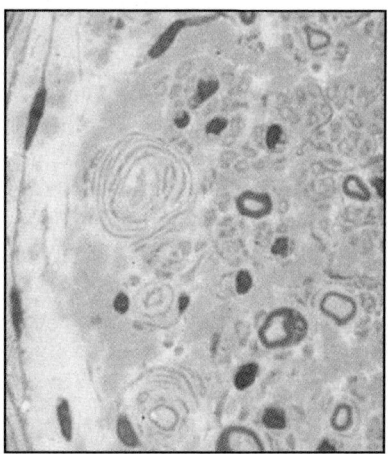

Fig. 3. Hereditary motor and sensory neuropathy (HMSN) type I: transverse section of sural nerve showing a decreased number of myelinated fibres, often surrounded by a reduced number of myelin sheaths (regenerating fibres), and some 'onion bulbs'.

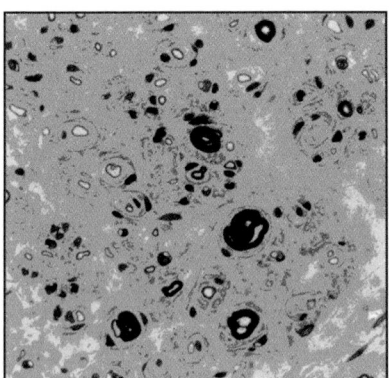

Fig. 4. Hereditary motor and sensory neuropathy (HMSN) with focally folded myelin sheaths: transverse section of sural nerve showing a moderate decrease in density of myelinated fibres. Several fibres are thinly myelinated or surrounded by hypertrophic and deformed myelin sheaths; also frequent faint 'onion bulb' formations.

CMTX is a dominant X-linked form and may present with an electrophysiological phenotype similar to CMT1 or CMT2 (mNCV between 25 and 40 m/s), but affected females have a less severe form. Nerve biopsy shows paranodal myelin changes and axonal damage. Nerve damage seems to be produced by a mutation of the *CX32* gene, expressed in Schwann cells corresponding to paranodal regions, but also in the CNS, which explains the associated minor CNS involvement.

Infantile distal spinal muscular atrophy with respiratory distress type 1 (SMARD1) largely overlapping the infantile proximal spinal muscular atrophy type 1 (SMA1) – a hereditary motor neuropathy described in chapter 12 – could be considered among the hereditary peripheral neuropathies. The phenotype of this form is characterized by an early onset of respiratory distress, in some cases even before the involvement of the distal muscles of the lower limbs, so that the respiratory symptoms may be mistaken for acute respiratory infection or near-miss sudden infant death syndrome (Grohmann *et al.*, 2003). This phenotype contrasts with that of SMA1, in which the symptoms present in the reverse order, proximal weakness preceding respiratory distress. Axonal and myelin pathology in the motor and sensory nerves is different from that found in SMA1, with irregular myelin thickening together with occasional basal lamina onion bulbs surrounding non-myelinated fibres (typical of some cases of CHN), reflecting severe impairment of maintenance and regeneration of axons, Schwann cells, and muscles (Diers *et al.*, 2005). Specific mutations of the gene encoding immunoglobulin μ-binding protein 2 (*IGHMBP2*) have been reported in SMARD1 (Grohmann *et al.*, 2001).

Hereditary sensory and autonomic neuropathies

Hereditary sensory and autonomic neuropathies (HSAN) are predominantly characterized by autonomic and peripheral sensory disturbances. The HSANs have been divided into five subgroups by Dyck *et al.* (1993b), four of which may occur in infancy (Table 5). They are extremely rare. In an important European series of affected children, they represented only 3 per cent of all neuropathies (Hagberg & Lyon, 1981).

Table 5. Hereditary sensory and autonomic neuropathies (HSAN) occurring in infancy

Acronym	Pathology	Gene	Locus	Inheritance	Gene product	Onset	Early symptoms	NCVs
HSAN II	Absence of myelinated fibres	HSN2	12p13.33	AR	HSN2 protein	Congenital-infancy	Sensory deficit (pain and temperature sensation), painless distal ulcerations, normal blood pressure	Reduced
HSAN III	Damage to motor, sensory and autonomic small fibres	IKBKAP	9q31-q33	AR	Inhibitor of kappa light-polypeptide	Infancy	Feeding problems and autonomic symptoms (body temperature control, high blood pressure, excessive sweating, disturbances of tear secretion)	Slowed
HSAN IV	Lack of unmyelinated fibres, decrease of small myelinated fibres	NTRK1	1q21-q22	AR	Neurotrophic, tyrosine kinase receptor, type 1	Infancy	Recurrent unexplained fever, anhidrosis, absence of reaction to noxious stimuli, self-mutilating-behaviour and developmental delay	Normal
HMSN V		NFGB	1p13.2-p11.2	AR	βNGF	Infancy	Less severe sensory and autonomic signs, no mental involvement	Normal

AR, autosomal recessive; NGF, nerve growth factor.

The onset of HSAN II is very early. Characteristically, infants are affected by loss of all types of sensation, especially pain, predominantly in the distal parts of the limbs. These signs are followed by ulceration and infections that lead to spontaneous amputations of digits. There is no major involvement of motor and autonomic functions. Consistently, nerve biopsy of the sural nerve shows severe loss of myelinated fibres with some loss of non-myelinated fibres (Fig. 5). The disease is generally slowly progressive, though non-progressive forms are described (Ferrière et al., 1992). Specifically, major autonomic disorders are typical of HSAN III (familial dysautonomia or Riley-Day syndrome). Even in the neonatal period, it is possible not only to observe feeding problems but also lack of control of body temperature, excessive sweating, absence of fungiform papillae on the tongue, miosis of the pupil after conjunctival instillation of 2.5 per cent methacholine chloride, absent deep tendon reflexes, diminished tear flow, and high blood pressure. Clinical symptoms occur later when sensory and motor problems appear. There is a slowing of mNCVs and a decrease in MAP amplitude. Neuropathological findings in the peripheral nerves show a reduced transverse fascicular area with diminished numbers of myelinated axons, especially those of small diameter, and very few non-myelinated axons. In addition, the neurons in the dorsal root ganglia appear to be reduced in number with increasing age. Techniques to detect autonomic signs (intradermal histamine, intraocular pilocarpine tests, urine excretion of homovanilic and vanilmandelic acid) may be useful.

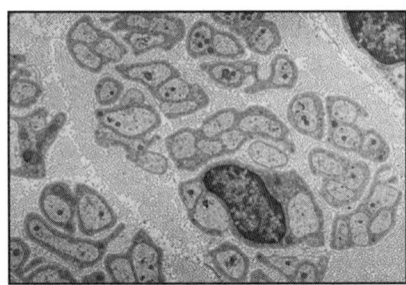

Fig. 5. Hereditary sensory and autonomic neuropathy (HSAN) type II: absence of myelinated fibres with apparently normal unmyelinated fibres.

Almost all HSAN III patients have a mutation of the *IKBKAP* gene coding for the IKAP protein, which is supposed to play a role in transcription control (Krappman et al., 2000). The disease occurs typically in Jewish families, although some sporadic non-Jewish cases have been described (Guzzetta et al., 1986).

HSAN IV, or CIPA (congenital insensitivity to pain with anhidrosis), is distinguished from previous forms by the presence of anhidrosis. As with the other forms, HSAN is recessively transmitted. The lack of sweating makes infants unable to cope with hot temperatures. Occasional deaths may occur in infancy from severe hyperthermia. Congenital insensitivity to pain is the other major sign. Developmental delay evolving towards mental retardation may be observed. The absence of nerve fibres in blood vessel walls as well as around the sweat glands and hair follicles, without degenerative changes, supports the hypothesis of a developmental defect of nerve outgrowth. The disease seems to be caused by mutations in the *NTRK1* gene, which encodes neurotrophic tyrosine kinase receptor type 1 and plays a crucial role in the function of the nociceptive reception system whereby thermoregulation is achieved in humans through sweating.

A similar phenotype is that of HSAN V, in which, however, symptoms are generally milder and mental abilities remain intact. There is always a severe loss of unmyelinated fibres, while the small myelinated fibres are relatively spared. A possible candidate gene of the disease is *NGFB*.

Polyneuropathies in systemic metabolic and neurodegenerative diseases

Several metabolic or neurodegenerative diseases are associated with an involvement of the peripheral nerves (Table 6).

Table 6. Neuropathies in hereditary metabolic and neurodegenerative diseases

Lysosomal diseases	• Sphingolipidosis (Krabbe and metachromatic leukodystrophies, Cockaine leukodystrophy, Chediak-Higashi syndrome, Farber, Niemann-Pick type A, Pelizaeus-Merzbacher) • Glycogenosis types III and IV
Mitochondrial disorders	• MNGIE, MELAS, MERRF, Kearns-Sayre, Leigh
Peroxisomal disorders	• Adrenoleukodystrophy, Zellweger syndrome, infantile Refsum
Other metabolic disorders	• Hereditary tyrosinaemia, infantile neuroaxonal dystrophy, Lowe syndrome, giant axonal neuropathy, Canavan disease
Other genetic diseases	• Merosin-deficient CMD • Andermann syndrome

CMD, congenital muscular dystrophy; MELAS, mitochondrial myopathy, encephalopathy, lactic acidosis and stroke; MERRF, myoclonic epilepsy associated with ragged red fibres; MNGIE, mitochondrial neurogastrointestinal encephalomyopathy.

Krabbe disease

The most common form of infantile Krabbe disease occurs in the first months of life. A deficiency of galactocerebroside β-galactosidase produced by mutations of the *GALC* gene mapped on locus 14q31 results in a disorder of white matter including the peripheral nerves. Symptoms caused by the latter represent a major marker, especially in the infantile form (Siddiqi *et al.*, 2006a). The association of a persistent hypertonia with areflexia is typical. A form with a floppy areflexic infant has also been described (Hagberg, 1984). Motor and sensory NCV are uniformly slow, consistent with diffuse demyelination. Infants genetically diagnosed *in utero* may have unequivocal and severe conduction abnormalities (Siddiqi *et al.*, 2006b). Nerve pathology shows evidence of active and diffuse demyelination and the characteristic features of intracellular inclusions, consisting of elongated profiles in Schwann cells or macrophages, representing deposits of galactocerebroside (Fig. 6). The effectiveness of treatment by haematopoietic stem cell transplantation is proven by an improvement in NCV, particularly when the transplantation is done in very early life (Siddiqi *et al.*, 2006b).

Metachromatic leucodystrophy

Similar changes of peripheral nerves (demyelination and intracellular inclusions) are observed in another leucodystrophy, metachromatic leucodystrophy (MLD), caused by an inborn error of metabolism resulting from a mutation in the *arylsulfatase A* gene. Storage of galactosphingosulphatides is found in the central and peripheral white matter (Fig. 7) – metachromatic material is seen in the perinuclear regions of Schwann cells, while electron microscopy shows tuff-stone bodies as well as prismatic lysosomal inclusions in macrophages and Schwann cells. The distinctive aspects of Krabbe and MLD, compared with other demyelinating polyneuropathies, have been underlined (Guzzetta *et al.*, 1995). Sensory and motor NCVs in MLD are markedly slow; in particular, motor responses may show multifocal slowing of nerve conduction velocities and conduction blocks, expression of a focal demyelination, mimicking an acquired neuropathy (Cameron *et al.*, 2004). The onset of the late infantile form occurs in the second year of life with hypotonia, muscle weakness and unsteady gait. This form generally leads to death by the age of 5.

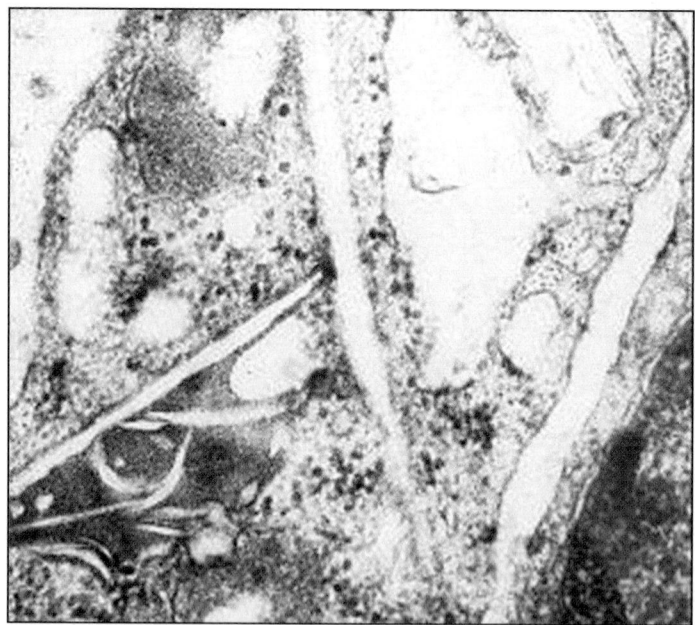

Fig. 6. Electron micrography from the sural nerve of a patient with globoid cell leucodystrophy (Krabbe disease): typical elongated inclusions observed in the cytoplasm of Schwann cells or macrophages.

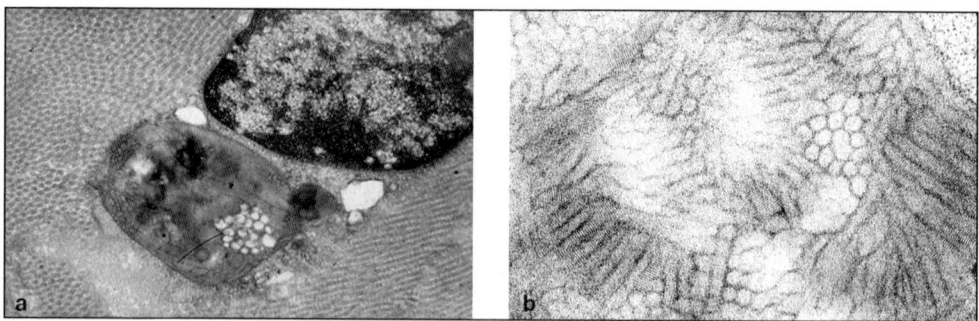

Fig. 7. (A) Tuff-stone body in a patient with metachromatic leucodystrophy. (B) At greater magnification, a pattern type 'pile of dishes' is observable.

Other sphingolipidoses

Other sphingolipidosis may be associated with disorders of the peripheral nerves. A demyelinating neuropathy has been described in cases of Cockaine leucodystrophy (Sasaki *et al.*, 1992). A motor-sensory axonal neuropathy was observed in the Chediak-Higashi syndrome (Tardieu *et al.*, 2005) and in Farber disease (lipogranulomatosis) (Pellissier *et al.*, 1986). Neuropathies have also been described rarely in type A Niemann-Pick disease (McGovern *et al.*, 2006), presenting as hypotonia, hyporeflexia and slowing of NCV, and in Pelizaeus-Merzbacher disease (Kaye *et al.*, 1994; Hodes *et al.*, 1995).

In glycogenosis type III, IV and VI, axonal, demyelinating or mixed polyneuropathies have been reported (Kotb *et al.*, 2004).

Genetic mitochondrial disorders

Peripheral neuropathy has a common though often unrecognized occurrence in genetic mitochondrial disorders. The neuropathy is always predominantly axonal with secondary demyelination (Mizusawa *et al.*, 1991; Colomer *et al.*, 2000; Sciacco *et al.*, 2001). Stickler *et al.* (2006) found a generalized reduction in motor NCV in a series of patients with congenital lactic acidosis, independent of age, sex, or congenital mitochondrial disorder. Cellular energy failure is supposed to be the common cause of peripheral neuropathy in patients with genetic mitochondrial diseases.

Peroxisomal disorders

Peroxisomal disorders (neonatal adrenoleucodystrophy, Zellweger syndrome, and infantile Refsum disease), particularly early in infancy – the so-called 'infantile Refsum disease' – are reported to show a mild non-specific loss of myelin and myelinated fibres. Classical Refsum disease (HMSN type IV) is not symptomatic in infancy.

Other genetic disorders

Other genetic disorders may be associated with peripheral neuropathies. Hereditary tyrosinaemia is caused by an inborn error of the final step of tyrosine metabolism, which leads to an accumulation of succinylacetone in the tissues. Recurrent neurological crises (pain, vomiting and constipation, autonomic signs) occur, with their onset in the first year of life, and even in newborn infants, with a predominantly motor neuropathy (limb weakness, reduction of NCV and histopathological features of axonal degeneration). Axonal neuropathy has also been observed in infantile neuro-axonal dystrophy, Lowe syndrome (oculo-cerebro-renal syndrome), giant axonal neuropathy (Wilmshurst *et al.*, 2003), and Canavan disease (spongy degeneration of the cerebral white matter) (Suzuki, 1968). However, it seems to be clinically silent in infancy (Lyon *et al.*, 1996).

Merosin, the α-2 subunit of laminin2, is defective in some congenital muscular dystrophies and this may be expressed in the Schwann cell. Studies on motor NCV in patients with merosin-deficient congenital muscular dystrophy (CMD) showed a definite reduction in conduction velocity (Shorer *et al.*, 1995), suggesting an associated neuropathy. A loss of myelinated fibres with a 'globular' hypermyelination characteristically located at the paranodal regions, with the laminin α-2 chain virtually absent in peripheral nerves (Fig. 8), was found in a girl affected by a form of merosin-deficient CMD (Deodato *et al.*, 2002), possibly showing the phenotypical heterogeneity of *LAMA2* gene mutations and their relation to myelination of the peripheral nerves.

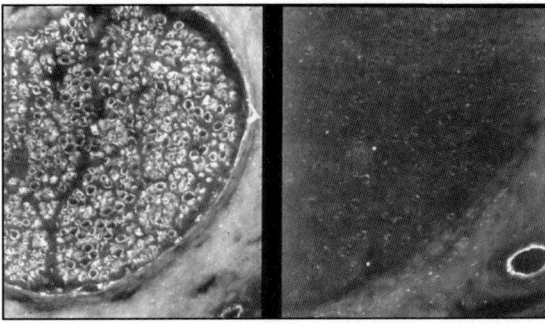

Fig. 8. Lack of the expression of laminin α-2 chain in peripheral (sural) nerve (right); on the left, normal nerve.

Finally, Andermann (1981) described children who, early in infancy, developed hypotonia with areflexia, caused by mutations in the *SLC12A6* gene. After an apparent improvement at preschool age, they had motor deterioration leading to wheel-chair dependency. On nerve biopsy, there was a significant loss of large myelinated fibres. Associated symptoms were mental retardation, epilepsy and psychotic features. Characteristically, there was complete agenesis of the corpus callosum.

References

al-Qudah, A.A., Shahar, E., Logan, W.J. & Murphy, E.G. (1988): Neonatal Guillain-Barré syndrome. *Pediatr. Neurol.* **4**, 255–256.

Andermann, E. (1981): Familial agenesis of the corpus callosum with sensorimotor neuropathy. In: *Handbook of clinical neurology*, vol. 42: *Neurogenetic directory, part I*, ed. N.C. Myrianthopoulos, pp. 100–103. Amsterdam: Elsevier.

Auer-Grumbach, M., Wagner, K., Fazekas, F., Loscher, W.N., Strasser-Fuchs, S. & Hartung, H.P. (1999): Hereditary motor-sensory neuropathies (Charcot-Marie-Tooth syndrome) and related neuropathies. Current classification and genotype-phenotype correlation. *Nervenarzt* **70**, 1052–1061.

Bae, D.S., Waters, P.M. & Zurakowski, D. (2008): Correlation of pediatric outcomes data collection instrument with measures of active movement in children with brachial plexus birth palsy. *J. Pediatr. Orthoped.* **28**, 584–592.

Bamford, N.S., Trojaborg, W., Sherbany, A.A. & De Vivo, D.C. (2002): Congenital Guillain-Barré syndrome associated with maternal inflammatory bowel disease is responsive to intravenous immunoglobulin. *Eur. J. Paediatr. Neurol.* **6**, 115–119.

Cameron, C.L., Kang, P.B., Burns, T.M., Darras, B.T. & Jones, H.R. (2004): Multifocal slowing of nerve conduction in metachromatic leukodystrophy. *Muscle Nerve* **29**, 531–536.

Charnas, L., Trapp, B. & Griffin, J. (1988): Congenital absence of peripheral myelin: abnormal Schwann cell development causes lethal arthrogryposis multiplex congenital. *Neurology* **38**, 966–974.

Colomer, J., Iturriaga, C., Bestué, M., Artuch, R., Briones, P., Montoya, J., Vilaseca, M.A. & Pineda, M. (2000): [Aspects of neuropathy in mitochondrial diseases.] *Rev. Neurol.* **30**, 1117–1121.

Craig, A.S. & Richardson, J.K. (2003): Acquired peripheral neuropathy. *Phys. Med. Rehabil. Clin. North Am.* **14**, 365–386.

Curtis, C., Stephens, D., Clarke, H.M. & Andrews, D. (2002): The active movement scale: an evaluative tool for infants with obstetrical brachial plexus palsy. *J. Hand Surg. (Am.)* **27**, 470–478.

Deodato, F., Sabatelli, M., Ricci, E., Mercuri, E., Muntoni, F., Sewry, C., Naom, I., Tonali, P. & Guzzetta, F. (2002): Hypermyelinating neuropathy, mental retardation and epilepsy in a case of merosin deficiency. *Neuromuscul. Disord.* **12**, 392–398.

Diers, A., Kaczinski, M., Grohmann, K., Hübner, C. & Stoltenburg-Didinger, G. (2005): The ultrastructure of peripheral nerve, motor end-plate and skeletal muscle in patients suffering from spinal muscular atrophy with respiratory distress type 1 (SMARD1). *Acta Neuropathol.* **110**, 289–297.

Dyck, P.J. & Lambert, E.H. (1968): Lower motor and primary sensory neuron diseases with peroneal muscular atrophy. I. Neurologic, genetic and electrophysiological findings in hereditary polyneuropathy. *Arch. Neurol.* **18**, 603-618.

Dyck, P.J., Lais, A.C., Ohta, M., Bastron, J.A., Okazaki, H. & Groover, R.V. (1975): Chronic inflammatory polyradiculoneuropathy. *Mayo Clin. Proc.* **50**, 621–637.

Dyck, P.J., Chance, P., Lebo, R. & Carney, J.A. (1993a): Hereditary motor and sensory neuropathy. In: *Peripheral neuropathy*, 3rd ed., vol. 2, eds. P.J. Dyck & P.K. Thomas, pp. 1094–1136. Philadelphia: W.B. Saunders.

Dyck, P.J., Chance, P., Lebo, R. & Carney, J.A. (1993b): Neuronal atrophy and degeneration predominantly affecting peripheral sensory and autonomic neurons. In: *Peripheral neuropathy*, 3rd edition, vol. 2, eds. P.J. Dyck & P.K. Thomas, pp. 1065–1193. Philadelphia: W.B. Saunders.

Ferrière, G., Denef, J.F., Rodriguez, J. & Guzzetta, F. (1985): Morphometric studies of normal sural nerves in children. *Muscle Nerve* **8**, 697–704.

Ferrière, G., Guzzetta, F., Kulakowski, S. & Evrard, P. (1992): Nonprogressive type II hereditary sensory autonomic neuropathy: a homogeneous clinicopathologic entity. *J. Child Neurol.* **7**, 364–370.

Gabreels-Festen, A.A.W.M., Jonsten, E.M.G., Gabreels, F.J., Jennekens, F.G., Gookens, R.H. & Stegeman, D.F. (1991): Hereditary motor and sensory neuropathy of neuronal type with onset in early childhood. *Brain* **114**, 1855–1850.

Gherman, R.B., Ouzounian, J.G. & Goodwin, T.M. (1999): Brachial plexus palsy: an in utero injury? *Am. J. Obstet. Gynecol.* **180**, 1303–1307.

Grohmann, K., Schuelke, M., Diers, A., Hoffmann, K., Lucke, B., Adams, C., Bertini, E., Leonhardt-Horti, H., Muntoni, F., Ouvrier, R., Pfeufer, A., Rossi, R., Van Maldergem, L., Wilmshurst, J.M., Wienker, T.F., Sendtner, M., Rudnik-Schöneborn, S., Zerres, K. & Hübner, C. (2001): Mutations in the gene encoding immunoglobulin mu-binding protein 2 cause spinal muscular atrophy with respiratory distress type 1. *Nat. Genet.* **29**, 75–77.

Grohmann, K., Varon, R., Stolz, P., Schuelke, M., Janetzki, C., Bertini, E., Bushby, K., Muntoni, F., Ouvrier, R., Van Maldergem, L., Goemans, N.M., Lochmüller, H., Eichholz, S., Adams, C., Bosch, F., Grattan-Smith, P., Navarro, C., Neitzel, H., Polster, T., Topalo?lu, H., Steglich, C., Guenther, U.P., Zerres, K., Rudnik-Schöneborn, S. & Hübner, C. (2003): Infantile spinal muscular atrophy with respiratory distress type 1 (SMARD1). *Ann. Neurol.* **54**, 719–724.

Guzzetta, F. & Ferrière, G. (1985): Congenital neuropathy with prevailing axonal changes. A clinical and histological report. *Acta Neuropathol.* **68**, 185–190.

Guzzetta, F., Ferrière, G. & Lyon, G. (1982): Congenital hypomyelination polyneuropathy. Pathological findings compared with polyneuropathies starting later in life. *Brain* **105**, 395–416.

Guzzetta, F., Tortorella, G., Cardia, E. & Ferrière, G. (1986): Familial dysautonomia in a non-Jewish girl, with histological evidence of progression in the sural nerve. *Dev. Med. Child Neurol.* **28**, 62–68.

Guzzetta, F., Rodriguez, J., Deodato, M., Guzzetta, A. & Ferrière, G. (1995): Demyelinating hereditary neuropathies in children: a morphometric and ultrastructural study. *Histol. Histopathol.* **10**, 91–104.

Hagberg, B. (1984): Krabbe's disease: clinical presentation of neurological variants. *Neuropediatrics* **15**, 11–15.

Hagberg, B. & Lyon, G. (1981): Pooled European series of hereditary peripheral neuropathies in infancy and childhood. A 'correspondence workshop' report of the European federation of child neurology societies (EFCNS). *Neuropediatrics* **12**, 9–17.

Hagberg, B. & Westerberg, B. (1983): The nosology of genetic peripheral neuropathies in Swedish children. *Dev. Med. Child Neurol.* **25**, 3–18.

Hodes, M.E., DeMyer, W.E., Pratt, V.M., Edwards, M.K. & Dlouhy, S.R. (1995): Girl with signs of Pelizaeus-Merzbacher disease heterozygous for a mutation in exon 2 of the proteolipid protein gene. *Am. J. Med. Genet.* **55**, 397–401.

Hughes, R.A.C., Raphael, J.-C., Swan, A.V. & van Doorn, P.A. (2001): Intravenous immunoglobulin for Guillain-Barré syndrome (Cochrane review). Cochrane Database of Systematic Reviews 3. Oxford: Update Software.

Kaye, E.M., Doll, R.F., Natowicz, M.R. & Smith, F.I. (1994): Pelizaeus-Merzbacher disease presenting as spinal muscular atrophy: clinical and molecular studies. *Ann. Neurol.* **36**, 916–919.

Kotb, M.A., Abdallah, H.K. & Kotb, A. (2004): Liver glycogenoses: are they a possible cause of polyneuropathy? A cross-sectional study. *J. Trop. Pediatr.* **50**, 196–202.

Krappmann, D., Hatada, E.N., Tegethoff, S., Li, J., Klippel, A., Giese, K., Baeuerle, P.A. & Scheidereit, C. (2000): The I kappa B kinase (IKK) complex is tripartite and contains IKK gamma but not IKAP as a regular component. *J. Biol. Chem.* **275**, 29779–29787.

Kuhlenbäumer, G., Young, P., Hünermund, G., Ringelstein, B. & Stögbauer, F. (2002): Clinical features and molecular genetics of hereditary peripheral neuropathies. *J. Neurol.* **249**, 1629–1650.

Lacomis, D. (2002): Small-fiber neuropathy. *Muscle Nerve* **26**, 173–188.

Lyon, G., Adams, R.D. & Kolodny, E.H. (1996): *Neurology of hereditary metabolic diseases of children*, 2nd ed. New York: McGraw Hill.

McGovern, M.M., Aron, A., Brodie, S.E., Desnick, R.J. & Wasserstein, M.P. (2006): Natural history of Type A Niemann-Pick disease: possible endpoints for therapeutic trials. *Neurology* **66**, 228–232.

Miller, R.G. & Kunz N.L. (1986): Nerve conduction studies in infants and children. *J. Child Neurol.* **1**, 19–26.

Mizusawa, H., Ohkoshi, N., Watanabe, M. & Kanazawa, I. (1991): Peripheral neuropathy of mitochondrial myopathies. *Rev. Neurol.* **147**, 501–507.

Nelis, E., Timmerman, V., De Jonghe, P., Van Broeckhoven, C. & Rautenstrauss, B. (1999): Molecular genetics and biology of inherited peripheral neuropathies: a fast-moving field. *Neurogenetics* **2**, 137–148.

Ouvrier, R.A., McLeod, J.G., Morgan, G.J., Wise, G.A. & Crouchin, T.E. (1981): Hereditary motor and sensory neuropathy of neuronal type with onset in early childhood. *J. Neurol. Sci.* **51**, 181–197.

Ouvrier, R.A., McLeod, J.G. & Polard, J.D. (1999): Toxic neuropathies. In: *Peripheral neuropathy in childhood*, 2nd ed., eds. R.A. Ouvrier, J.G. McLeod & J.D. Polard, pp. 201–210. London: Mac Keith Press.

Palix, C. & Coignet, J. (1978): Un cas de polyneuropathie périphérique néo-natale par amyélinisation. *Pédiatrie* **33**, 20–27.

Pellissier, J.F., Berard-Badier, M. & Pinsard, N. (1986): Farber's disease in two siblings: sural nerve and subcutaneous biopsies studied by light and electron microscopy. *Acta Neuropathol.* **72**, 178–188.

Phillips, J.P., Warner, L.E., Lupski, J.R. & Garg, B.P. (1999): Congenital hypomyelinating neuropathy: Two patients with long-term follow-up. *Pediatr. Neurol.* **20**, 228–234.

Pippa, P., Alto. S., Colminelli, E., Doni, L., Robassini, M., Marimelli, C. & Micozzi, S. (1992): Brachial plexus block using transcoracobrachial approach. *Eur. J. Anaesthesiol.* **9**, 235–239.

Pitt, M. & Vredeveld, J.W. (2005): The role of electromyography in the management of the brachial plexus palsy of the newborn. *Clin. Neurophysiol.* **116**, 1756–1761.

Quattrone, A., Gambardella, A., Bono, F., Aguglia, U., Bolino, A., Bruni, A.C., Montesi, M.P., Oliveri, R.L., Sabatelli, M., Tamburrini, O., Valentino, P., Van Broeckhoven, C. & Zappia, M. (1996): Autosomal recessive hereditary motor and sensory neuropathy with focally folded myelin sheaths. Clinical, electrophysiologic, and genetic aspects of a large family. *Neurology* **46**, 1318–1324.

Reilly, M.M. (2000): Classification of the hereditary motor and sensory neuropathies. *Curr. Opin. Neurol.* **13**, 561–564.

Rossi, L.N., Lütschg, J., Meier, C. & Vassella, F. (1983): Hereditary motor sensory neuropathies in childhood. *Dev. Med. Child Neurol.* **25**, 19–31.

Sabatelli, M., Mignogna, T., Lippi, G., Servidei, S., Manfredi, G., Ricci, E., Bertini, E., Lo Monaco, M. & Tonali, P. (1994): Autosomal recessive hypermyelinating neuropathy. *Acta Neuropathol.* **87**, 337–342.

Said, G. (2003): Small fiber involvement in peripheral neuropathies. *Curr. Opin. Neurol.* **16**, 601–602.

Sasaki, K., Tachi, N., Shinoda, M., Satoh, N., Minami, R. & Ohnishi, A. (1992): Demyelinating peripheral neuropathy in Cockaine syndrome: a histopathologic and morphometric study. *Brain Dev.* **14**, 114–117.

Sciacco, M., Prelle, A., Comi, G.P., Napoli, L., Battistel, A., Bresolin, N., Tancredi, L., Lamperti, C., Bordoni, A., Fagiolari, G., Ciscato, P., Chiveri, L., Perini, M.P., Fortunato, F., Adobbati, L., Messina, S., Toscano, A., Martinelli-Boneschi, F., Papadimitriou, A., Scarlato, G. & Moggio, M. (2001): Retrospective study of a large population of patients affected with mitochondrial disorders: clinical, morphological and molecular genetic evaluation. *J. Neurol.* **248**, 778–788.

Shorer, Z., Philpot, J., Muntoni, F., Sewry, C. & Dubowitz, V. (1995): Demyelinating peripheral neuropathy in merosin-deficient congenital muscular dystrophy. *J. Child Neurol.* **10**, 472–475.

Siddiqi, Z.A., Sanders, D.B. & Massey, J.M. (2006a): Peripheral neuropathy in Krabbe disease: effect of hematopoietic stem cell transplantation. *Neurology* **67**, 268–272.

Siddiqi, Z.A., Sanders, D.B. & Massey, J.M. (2006b): Peripheral neuropathy in Krabbe disease: electrodiagnostic findings. *Neurology* **67**, 263–267.

Sladky, J.T., Brown, M.J. & Berman, P.K. (1986): Chronic inflammatory demyelinating polyneuropathy of infant: a corticosteroid responsive disorder. *Ann. Neurol.* **20**, 76–81.

Stickler, D.E., Valenstein, E., Neiberger, R.E., Perkins, L.A., Carney, P.R., Shuster, J.J., Theriaque, D.W. & Stacpoole, P.W. (2006): Peripheral neuropathy in genetic mitochondrial diseases. *Pediatr. Neurol.* **34**, 127–131.

Suzuki, K. (1968): Peripheral nerve lesion in spongy degeneration of the central nervous system. *Acta Neuropathol.* **10**, 95–98.

Tardieu, M., Lacroix, C., Neven, B., Bordigoni, P., de Saint Basile, G., Blanche, S. & Fischer, A. (2005): Progressive neurologic dysfunctions 20 years after allogeneic bone marrow transplantation for Chediak-Higashi syndrome. *Blood* **106**, 40–42.

Tyson, J., Ellis, D., Fairbrother, U., King, R.H.M., Muntoni, F., Jacobs, J., Malcolm, S., Harding, A.E. & Thomas, P.K. (1997): Hereditary demyelinating neuropathy of infancy. A genetically complex syndrome. *Brain* **120**, 47–63.

Van den Bergh, P.Y. & Pieret, F. (2004): Electrodiagnostic criteria for acute and chronic inflammatory demyelinating polyradiculoneuropathy. *Muscle Nerve* **29**, 565–574.

Warner, L.E., Hilz, M.J., Appel, S.H., Killian, J.M., Kolodry, E.H., Karpati, G., Carpenter, S., Watters, G.V., Wheeler, C., Witt, D., Bodell, A., Nelis, E., Van Broeckhoven, C. & Lupski, J.R. (1996): Clinical phenotypes of different MPZ (P0) mutation may include Charcot-Marie-Tooth type 1B, Dejerine-Sotas, and congenital hypomyelination. *Neuron* **17**, 451–460.

Wein, T.H. & Albers, J.W. (2002): Electrodiagnostic approach to the patient with suspected peripheral polyneuropathy. *Neurol. Clin.* **20**, 503–526.

Wilmshurst, J.M., Pollard, J.D., Nicholson, G., Antony, J. & Ouvrier, R. (2003): Peripheral neuropathies of infancy. *Dev. Med. Child Neurol.* **45**, 408–414.

Mariani Foundation
Paediatric Neurology Series

1: Occipital Seizures and Epilepsies in Children
Edited by: *F. Andermann, A. Beaumanoir, L. Mira, J. Roger and C.A. Tassinari*
2: Motor Development in Children
Edited by: *E. Fedrizzi, G. Avanzini and P. Crenna*
3: Continuous Spikes and Waves during Slow Sleep – Electrical Status Epilepticus during Slow Sleep
Edited by: *A. Beaumanoir, M. Bureau, T. Deonna, L. Mira and C.A. Tassinari*
4: Metabolic Encephalopathies: Therapy and Prognosis
Edited by: *S. Di Donato, R. Parini and G. Uziel*
5: Neuromuscular Diseases during Development
Edited by: *F. Cornelio, G. Lanzi and E. Fedrizzi*
6: Falls in Epileptic and Non-Epileptic Seizures during Childhood
Edited by: *A. Beaumanoir, F. Andermann, G. Avanzini and L. Mira*
7: Abnormal Cortical Development and Epilepsy – From Basic to Clinical Science
Edited by: *R. Spreafico, G. Avanzini and F. Andermann*
8: Limbic Seizures in Children
Edited by: *G. Avanzini, A. Beaumanoir and L. Mira*
9: Localization of Brain Lesions and Developmental Functions
Edited by: *D. Riva and A. Benton*
10: Immune-Mediated Disorders of the Central Nervous System in Children
Edited by: *L. Angelini, M. Bardare and A. Martini*
11: Frontal Lobe Seizures and Epilepsies in Children
Edited by: *A. Beaumanoir, F. Andermann, P. Chauvel, L. Mira and B. Zifkin*
12: Hereditary Leukoencephalopathies and Demyelinating Neuropathies in Children
Edited by: *G. Uziel, F. Taroni*
13: Neurodevelopmental Disorders: Cognitive/Behavioural Phenotypes
Edited by: *D. Riva, U. Bellugi and M.B. Denckla*
14: Autistic Spectrum Disorders
Edited by: *D. Riva and I. Rapin*

15: Neurocutaneous Syndromes in Children
Edited by: *P. Curatolo and D. Riva*
16: Language: Normal and Pathological Development
Edited by: *D. Riva, I. Rapin and G. Zardini*
17: Movement Disorders in Children: a Clinical Update, with video recordings
Edited by: *N. Nardocci and E. Fernandez-Alvarez*
18: Mental Retardation
Edited by: *D. Riva, S. Bulgheroni and C. Pantaleoni*
19: Perinatal Brain Damage: From Pathogenesis to Neuroprotection
Edited by: L.A. Ramenghi, P. Evrard and E. Mercuri
20: Genetics of Epilepsy and Genetic Epilepsies
Edited by: G. Avanzini and J. Noebels

NJINGA OF NDONGO AND MATAMBA STICKERS

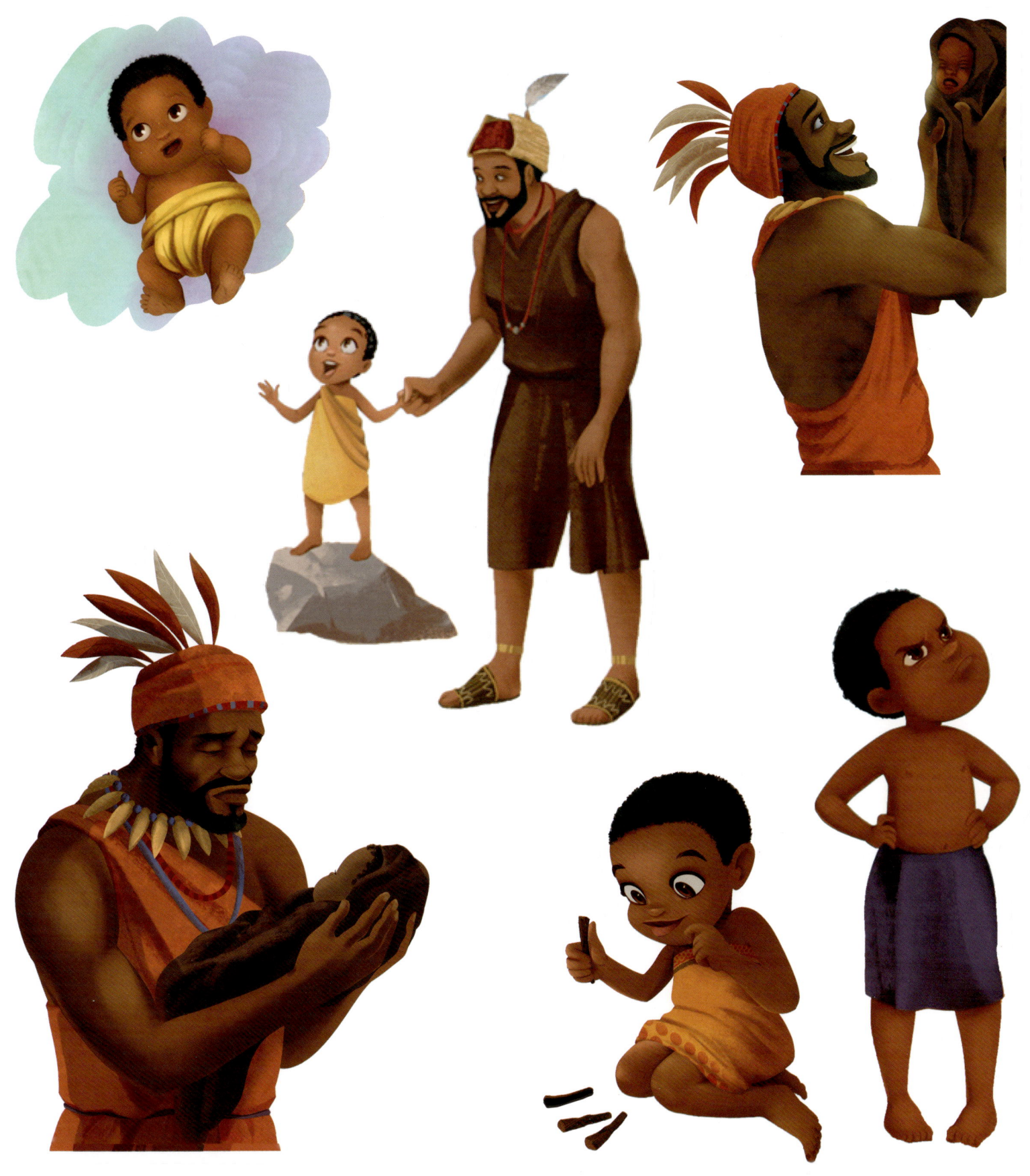

NJINGA OF NDONGO AND MATAMBA STICKERS

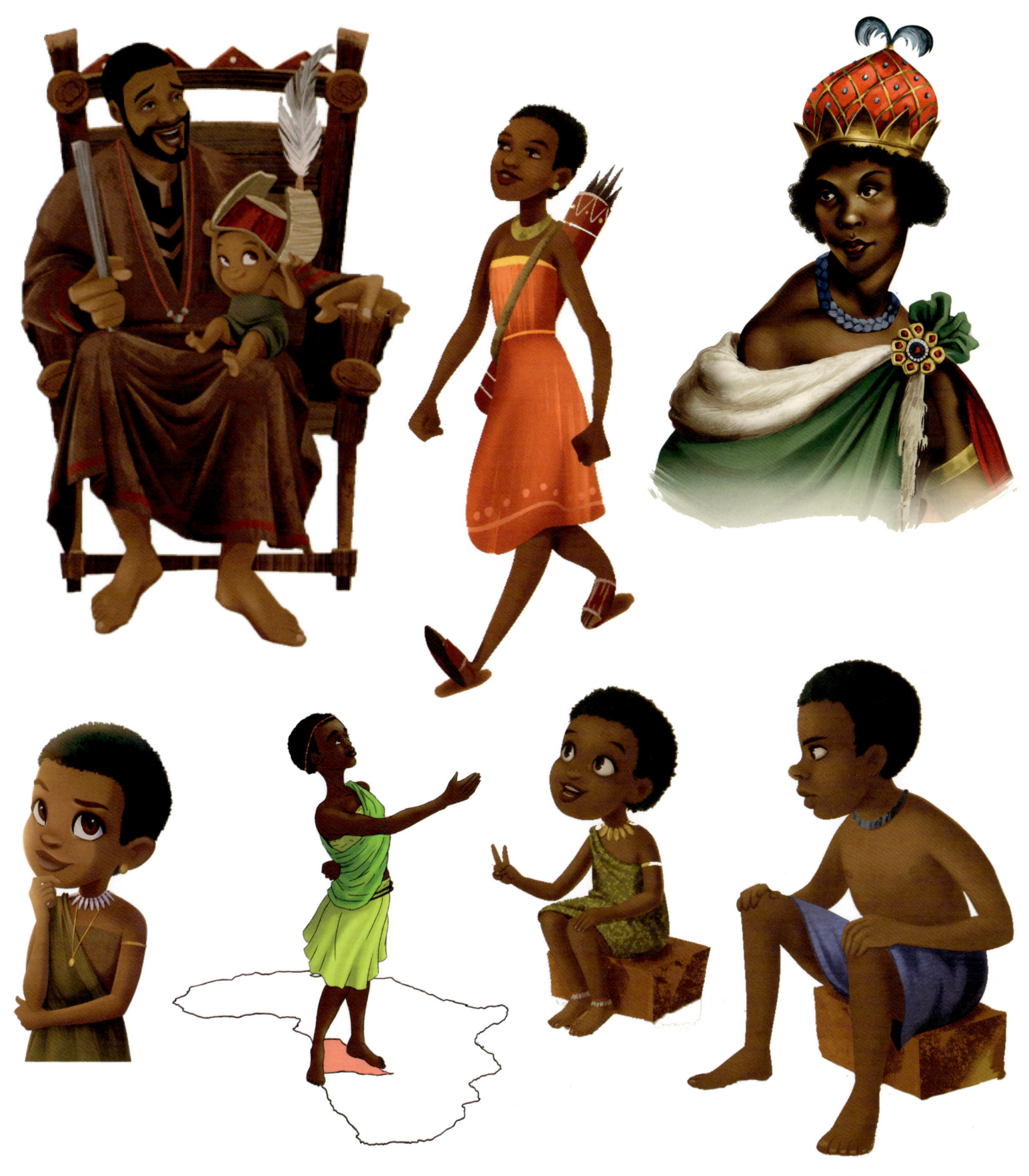